Posterior Hip Disorders

Hal D. Martin • Juan Gómez-Hoyos
Editors

Posterior Hip Disorders

Clinical Evaluation and Management

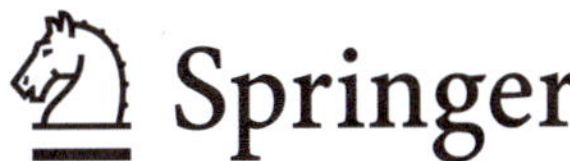 Springer

Editors
Hal D. Martin, DO
Medical and Research Director
Hip Preservation Center
Baylor University Medical Center
Dallas, TX
USA

Juan Gómez-Hoyos, MD
International Consultant
Hip Preservation Center / Baylor Scott
and White Research Institute
Baylor University Medical Center
Dallas, TX
USA

Department of Orthopaedic Surgery -
Health Provider
Clínica Las Américas / Clínica del
Campestre
Medellín, Antioquia
Colombia

Professor - School of Medicine - Sports
Medicine Program
Universidad de Antioquia
Medellín, Antioquia
Colombia

ISBN 978-3-030-08605-3   ISBN 978-3-319-78040-5   (eBook)
https://doi.org/10.1007/978-3-319-78040-5

This Springer imprint is published by the registered company Springer Nature Switzerland AG.
The registered company address is: Gewerbestrasse 11, 6330 Cham, Switzerland

To those who suffer posterior hip pain, and to those striving or supporting in the efforts to help in their care.

Hal D. Martin

For those who have not found an answer, I hope that this book will give light to their doctors to guide them out of the woods.
To my beautiful wife and my beloved family for their love and unconditional support.
To my mentors Dr. Johnny Marquez, Dr. Jaime Gallo and
Dr. Hal Martin for guiding me with patience and wisdom.

Juan Gómez-Hoyos

Foreword

The definition of genius is taking the complex and making it simple.
—Albert Einstein.

It is what it is.
—Bill Belichick, winning coach of five Super Bowls

The above two famous quotes describe a whole lot about this book and its editors. Hal Martin and Juan Gomez-Hoyos have brought together some brilliant minds and simplified *the* most poorly understood part of our musculoskeletal anatomy. They use colored diagrams, striking dissections of fresh cadavers, and photographs of actual pathology to make this anatomy simple. They unveil answers to anatomic and pathological mysteries within our deep derriere. Don't get me wrong. We readers cannot just sit back with a glass of sherry and read this book casually. Understanding this anatomy is not *all* that easy. There is a lot to it and a lot of it. New England Patriot Coach Belichick might say, "The anatomy is what it is." There are a lot of twists and turns. This anatomy remains treacherous. Many diagnoses dwell here that possibly explain the various types of suffering that we see.

The book's title, *Posterior Hip Disorders*, is brilliant. Among surgeons, there are currently two definitions of the hip. It is either *just* the ball and socket or, more inclusively, the entire side of our body between the top of the lower extremity and waist (https://www.collinsdictionary.com/us/dictionary/english/hip). The two editors deftly dodge this semantic issue. The definition of the hip remains however one wants to define it. The exact definition does not matter. The many anatomic sources of pain in this region apply no matter the definition. No doubt, we need to understand more. By creating this book, Martin and Gomez-Hoyos have now laid the anatomic foundation from which we can build our new understandings about this region.

As I see it, the entire unit of the body from mid-chest to mid-thigh remains largely unstudied. That is why I am coming out soon with a book called *Introducing the Core*. With their book, Martin and Gomez-Hoyos now make me look good. They have now tackled the part of the core anatomy that I struggled with the most. Thank you, Hal and Juan. You have done me, and everyone who wants to know a lot more about the core, a great service. And you are helping so many patients.

PA, USA   William C. Meyers

Preface

Posterior Hip Disorders: Clinical Evaluation and Management is a novel text intended for all health providers caring for patients with pain coming from anatomic structures around the posterior part of the hip.

Interest in posterior hip disorders has increased in recent years as new studies and theories have emerged regarding the disease process. Although most of the differential diagnoses mentioned in this text have traditionally been considered uncommon, recent reports suggest that these problems have instead been commonly overlooked. Understanding of the etiology and evolving research on intra- and extra-articular hip problems is essential to diagnose and treat the spectrum of posterior hip diseases.

Patients presenting with posterior hip pain require a methodical history and physical examination with specific diagnostic tests to assess all structures around the hip. These structures are categorized into five levels as osseous, capsulolabral, musculotendinous, neurovascular, and kinematic chain. The influence of the biomechanics in producing hip pathology has been marginalized for a long time; however recent scientific advances have proven that our human body works as a unit and any change in the normal range of motion of a joint could lead to compensatory changes both caudal and cephalic to that given joint. The complex biomechanics require a balanced interaction between anatomic structures, neuromuscular activity, and range of motion.

Apart from structural explanations for specific diseases, we truly believe in the mind-body-spirit connection as an essential part of the treatment of diseases generating chronic pain. Failure to identify the organic cause of posterior hip pain in a timely manner as well as an unnoticed mind-body-spirit connection problem can increase pain perception, deteriorate patient's hope, and consequently affect quality of life.

This book presents advances in physical examination, diagnostic tools, therapy, and surgical techniques from different parts of the world as valuable information to doctors to help ensure that the final result will give our patients a new hope. We are confident that this book on posterior hip disorders will be a valuable source of theoretical and applied knowledge enabling human-centered care.

Dallas, TX, USA   Hal D. Martin, DO
Dallas, TX, USA / Medellín, Colombia   Juan Gómez-Hoyos, MD

Contents

Contributors

Bernardo Aguilera-Bohórquez, MD Orthopaedics and Traumatology, Centro Médico Imbanaco de Cali, Young Adult Hip Arthroscopy and Preservation Unit, Cali, Colombia

Lorena Bejarano-Pineda, MD Duke University Health System, Department of Orthopaedic Surgery, Durham, NC, USA

Srino Bharam, MD Orthopaedic Surgery, Mount Sinai School of Medicine, Lenox Hill Hospital, New York, NY, USA

Valerie L. Bobb, PT, DPT, WCS, ATC Women's and Men's Health Pelvic Therapy, University of Washington Medical Center, Seattle, WA, USA

Joshua S. Bowler, MD Baylor University Medical Center, Department of Orthopedic Surgery, Dallas, TX, USA

Karen K. Briggs, MPH Center for Outcomes-Based Orthopaedic Research (COOR), Steadman Philippon Research Institute, Vail, CO, USA

Alexander Ortiz Castillo, MD Hip Arthroscopy and Sports Medicine, Hospital Clínica Mompía, Orthopedic Surgery Department, Santander, Cantabria, Spain

Luis Cerezal, MD, PhD Diagnóstico Médico Cantabria (DMC), Department of Radiology, Santander, Cantabria, Spain

Timothy S. Clark, PhD Comprehensive Interdisciplinary Program, Baylor University Medical Center, Center for Pain Management, Dallas, TX, USA

Hermelinda Fernandez Escajadillo, RN Clínica Mompia, Orthopedic Department, Santa Cruz de Bezana, Cantabria, Spain

Frank Feigenbaum, MD, FAANS, FACS Feigenbaum Neurosurgery, Dallas, TX, USA

Ana Alfonso Fernández, MD, PhD Hospital Sierrallana, Orthopedic Surgery, Torrelavega, Cantabria, Spain

Elan Jack Golan, MD Maimonides Medical Center, Department of Orthopaedic Surgery, Brooklyn, NY, USA

Juan Gómez-Hoyos, MD International Consultant, Hip Preservation Center / Baylor Scott and White Research Institute, Baylor University Medical Center, Dallas, TX, USA

Department of Orthopaedic Surgery - Health Provider, Clínica Las Américas / Clínica del Campestre, Medellín, Antioquia, Colombia

Professor - School of Medicine - Sports Medicine Program, Universidad de Antioquia, Medellín, Antioquia, Colombia

Carlos A. Guanche, MD Southern California Orthopedic Institute, Los Angeles, CA, USA

Manu Gupta, MD Division of Neuroradiology, Baylor University Medical Center—Dallas, Department of Radiology, Dallas, TX, USA

Lorien Hathaway, PT, DPT, WCS, BCB-PMD Baylor Scott & White Institute for Rehabilitation (a Division of Select Medical), Outpatient Services – Plano Alliance, Plano, TX, USA

Moisés Fernández Hernando, MD Diagnóstico Médico Cantabria (DMC), Musculoskeletal Radiology, Santander, Cantabria, Spain

Cyndi Hill, PT, DPT Kinetic Physical Therapy, Chester Springs, PA, USA

Anthony Nicholas Khoury, PhD Hip Preservation Center, Baylor University Medical Center, Baylor Scott and White Health, Dallas, TX, USA

Bioengineering Department, University of Texas at Arlington, Arlington, TX, USA

Benjamin R. Kivlan, PhD, PT, OCS, SCS Department of Physical Therapy, Rangos School of Health Sciences, Duquesne University, Pittsburgh, PA, USA

Nucelio L. B. M. Lemos, MD, PhD University of Toronto, Women's College Hospital and Mount Sinais Hospital, Department of Obstetrics and Gynecology, Toronto, ON, Canada

Jennifer Marland, DPT Intermountain Healthcare, Department of Orthopedics, Murray, UT, USA

William Henry Márquez-Arabia, MD Clínica Las Americas, Orthopaedic Surgery, Medellin, Antioquia, Colombia

Sports Medicine Program, School of Medicine, Medellin, Antioquia, Colombia

Hal D. Martin, DO Medical and Research Director, Hip Preservation Center, Baylor University Medical Center, Dallas, TX, USA

RobRoy L. Martin, PhD, PT, CSCS Department of Physical Therapy, Rangos School of Health Sciences, Duquesne University, Pittsburgh, PA, USA

Centers for Sports Medicine, University of Pittsburgh, Pittsburgh, PA, USA

Ryan P. McGovern, MS, ATC Rangos School of Health Sciences, Rehabilitation Sciences, Duquesne University, Pittsburgh, PA, USA

Justin J. Mitchell, MD The Steadman Clinic/Steadman Philippon Research Institute, Vail, CO, USA

Francisco Javier Monsalve, MD Orthopedic Department, Medellin, Antioquia, Colombia

Ivan Saenz Navarro, MD University of Barcelona, Funacio Hospitalaria de Mollet, Department of Anatomy and Human Embriology/Trauma and Orthopaedic Surgery, Mollet Del Valles, Spain

Miguel Eduardo Sánchez Otamendi, MD Orthopaedics and Traumatology, Centro Médico Imbanaco de Cali, Young Adult Hip Arthroscopy and Preservation Unit, Cali, Colombia

Andrew E. Park, MD Orthopaedic Surgery, Texas A&M Health Science Center, Bryan, TX, USA

Baylor University Medical Center, Dallas, TX, USA

Department of Orthopaedic Surgery, Methodist Hospital for Surgery, Addison, TX, USA

Luis Pérez-Carro, MD, PhD Clínica Mompia, Orthopedic Surgery Department, Santa Cruz de Bezana, Cantabria, Spain

Marc J. Philippon, MD The Steadman Clinic/Steadman Philippon Research Institute, Vail, CO, USA

Jeremy A. Ross, MD UMass Memorial Health Care, Orthopaedics and Physical Rehabilitation, Worcester, MA, USA

Ricardo Gonçalves Schröder, PT Hip Preservation Center, Baylor University Medical Center, Dallas, TX, USA

Luke Spencer-Gardner, MD Baylor University Medical Center, Hip Preservation Center, Dallas, TX, USA

Leon R. Toye, MD Radsource, Brentwood, TN, USA

David Vier, MD Baylor University Medical Center, Department of Orthopedic Surgery, Dallas, TX, USA

Hugh S. West Jr., MD Intermountain Healthcare, Department of Orthopedics, Murray, UT, USA

Sung-Jung Yoon, MD, PhD Chonbuk National University Hospital, Department of Orthopedic Surgery, Jeonju, South Korea

Gross and Endoscopic Posterior Hip Anatomy

1

Luis Pérez-Carro, Moisés Fernández Hernando,
Hermelinda Fernandez Escajadillo, Luis Cerezal,
Ivan Saenz Navarro, Ana Alfonso Fernández,
Alexander Ortiz Castillo,
and William Henry Márquez-Arabia

Introduction

The deep gluteal space is the cellular and fatty tissue located between the middle and deep gluteal aponeurosis layers [1, 2]. This space is anterior and beneath the gluteus maximus and posterior to the posterior border of the femoral neck, with the linea aspera (lateral), the sacrotuberous and falciform fascia (medial), the inferior margin of the sciatic notch (superior), and the hamstring origin (inferior) (Fig. 1.1). At its inferior margin, it continues into and with the posterior thigh. Laterally it is demarcated by the linea aspera and the lateral fusion of the middle and deep gluteal aponeurosis layers extending up to the tensor fasciae latae muscle via the iliotibial tract. The anterior limit is formed by the posterior border of the femoral neck and the greater and lesser trochanters (Table 1.1). Within the space, superior to inferior, the piriformis, superior gemellus, obturator internus, inferior gemellus, and quadratus femoris are included. The medial margin is comprised of the greater and minor sciatic foramina (Fig. 1.2). The greater sciatic foramen is bounded by the outer edge of the sacrum, greater sciatic notch (superior) and sacrospinous ligament (inferior). The limits of the lesser sciatic foramen are the lesser sciatic notch (external), sacrospinous lower border (superior), and the upper edge of the sacrotuberous ligament (inferior) [1–3]. Our aim is to describe gross and endoscopy anatomy of the structures within this space.

L. Pérez-Carro, MD, PhD
Clínica Mompia, Orthopedic Surgery Department,
Santa Cruz de Bezana, Cantabria, Spain

M. F. Hernando, MD (✉)
Diagnóstico Médico Cantabria (DMC), Musculoskeletal
Radiology, Santander, Cantabria, Spain

H. F. Escajadillo, RN
Clínica Mompia, Orthopedic Department,
Santa Cruz de Bezana, Cantabria, Spain

L. Cerezal, MD, PhD
Diagnóstico Médico Cantabria (DMC), Department
of Radiology, Santander, Cantabria, Spain

I. S. Navarro, MD
University of Barcelona, Funacio Hospitalaria de
Mollet, Department of Anatomy and Human
Embriology/Trauma and Orthopaedic Surgery,
Mollet Del Valles, Spain

A. A. Fernández, MD, PhD
Hospital Sierrallana, Orthopedic Surgery,
Torrelavega, Cantabria, Spain

A. O. Castillo, MD
Hip Arthroscopy and Sports Medicine, Hospital
Clínica Mompía, Orthopedic Surgery Department,
Santander, Cantabria, Spain

W. H. Márquez-Arabia, MD
Clínica Las Americas, Orthopedic Surgery, Medellin,
Antioquia, Colombia

Sports Medicine Program, School of Medicine,
Medellin, Antioquia, Colombia

© Springer International Publishing AG, part of Springer Nature 2019
H. D. Martin, J. Gómez-Hoyos (eds.), *Posterior Hip Disorders*,
https://doi.org/10.1007/978-3-319-78040-5_1

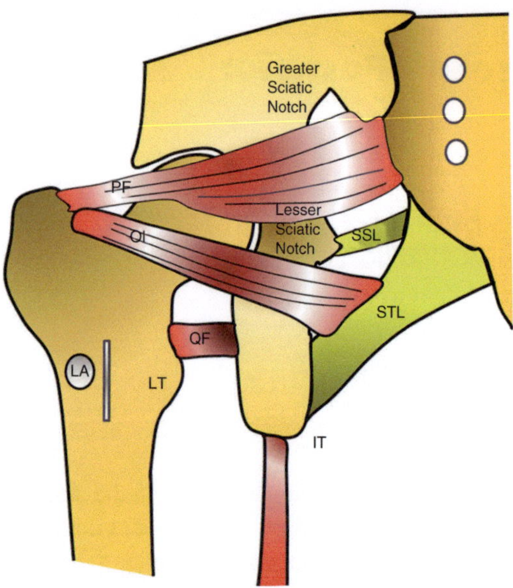

Fig. 1.1 Schematic of the deep gluteal space (Modified from Hal Martin et al. [2]) *IT* isquial tuberosity and hamstring origin, *LA* linea aspera, *LT* lesser trochanter, *OI* obturator internus, *PF* piriformis, *QF* quadratus femoris, *SSL* sacrospinous ligament *STL* sacrotuberous ligament

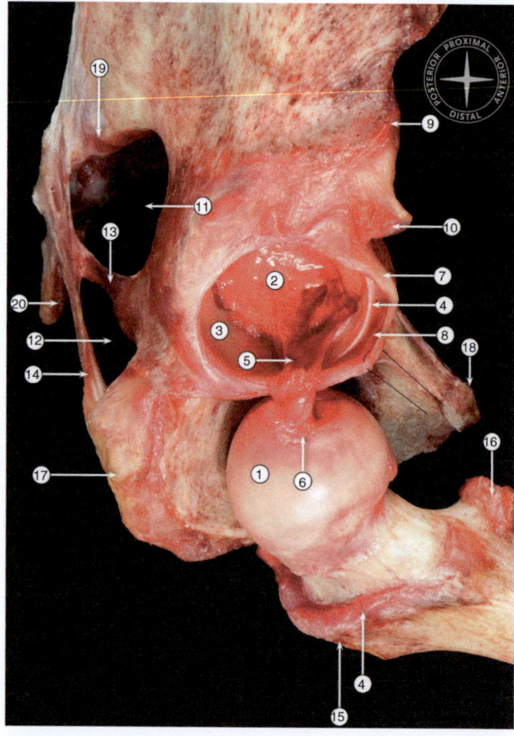

Fig. 1.2 Osteoarticular dissection of the hip joint (lateral view). (1) Head of femur. (2) Acetabular fossa or cotyloid fossa, with the pulvinar. (3) Lunate articular surface. (4) Acetabular labrum. (5) Ligamentum teres. (6) Fovea capitis. (7) Capsule of the hip joint (resected). (8) Paralabral sulcus, labrum-capsular sulcus, or perilabral recess. (9) Anterior inferior iliac spine. (10) Rectus femoris tendon cut (reflected and straight heads of the rectus femurs tendon). (11) Greater sciatic foramen. (12) Lesser sciatic foramen. (13) Sacrospinous ligament. (14) Sacrotuberous ligament. (15) Greater trochanter. (16) Lesser trochanter. (17) Ischial tuberosity. (18) Pubic tubercle. (19) Sacroiliac joint. (20) Coccyx

Table 1.1 Limits and contents of the deep gluteal space

Limits
- Posterior limit is the gluteus maximus muscle
- Anterior limit is formed by the posterior border of the femoral neck
- Laterally is limited by the linea aspera and the lateral fusion of middle and deep gluteal aponeurosis layers reaching the tensor fasciae latae muscle (iliotibial tract, ITT)
- Medial: sacrotuberous and falciform fascia
- Superior: inferior margin of the sciatic notch
- Inferior: hamstring origin

Content
- Sup/inf gluteal nerves
- Vessels, ACFM
- Ischium
- Sacrotuberous/sacrospinous ligaments
- Sciatic nerve
- Piriformis
- Obturator int/ext
- Gemelli
- Quadratus femoris
- Hamstrings

The Ligaments

Within the deep gluteal space of great importance are the sacrotuberous and sacrospinous ligaments and the ischiofemoral ligament and the femoral arcuate ligament (orbicularis ligament).

The *ischiofemoral ligament* arises from the ischiatic rim of the acetabulum, and attaches to the posterior aspect of the femoral neck (Fig. 1.3). Due to its posterior position, the main function is to restrict the internal rotation but also

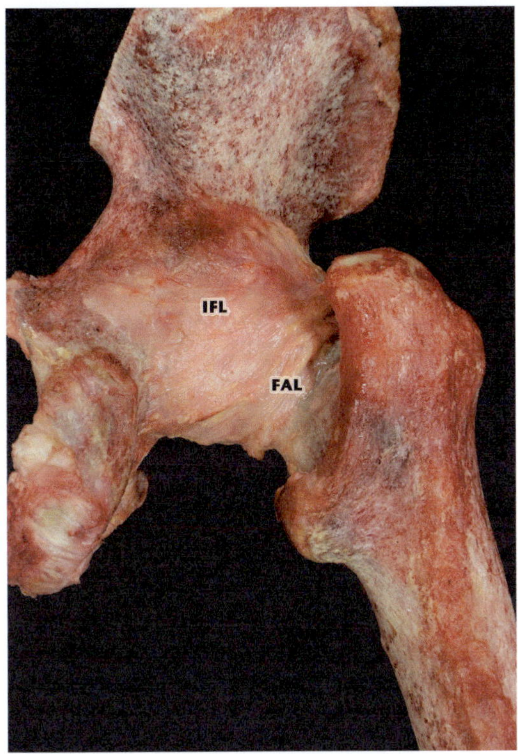

Fig. 1.3 Posterior view of the right hip joint. Observe the presence of the ischiofemoral ligament (IFL) and femoral arcuate ligament (orbicularis ligament) (FAL) that passes below the first one

the adduction when the hip is flexed. The femoral arcuate ligament (orbicularis ligament) originates at the greater trochanter; passes deep to the ischiofemoral ligament, around the posterior aspect of the femoral neck; and attaches to the lesser trochanter. This ligament acts tensioning the capsule in extreme flexion and extension of the hip. Previously this ligament was described as orbicularis zone because of the direction of its fibers [4, 5].

The *sacrotuberous and sacrospinous* ligaments create the greater and lesser sciatic foramen, which communicate the deep gluteal space with the true pelvis and ischioanal fossa (Fig. 1.4).

The *sacrospinous ligament (SSL)* consists of dense connective tissue and contributes to the stability of the bony pelvis. It attaches to the ischial spine laterally and lower part of the sacrum and coccyx medially. The internal pudendal and inferior gluteal vessels, sciatic nerve, and other branches of the sacral nerve plexus pass through the greater sciatic foramen in close proximity to the ischial spines and SSL.

The sacrotuberous ligament. From its broad superomedial attachments (posterior portion of

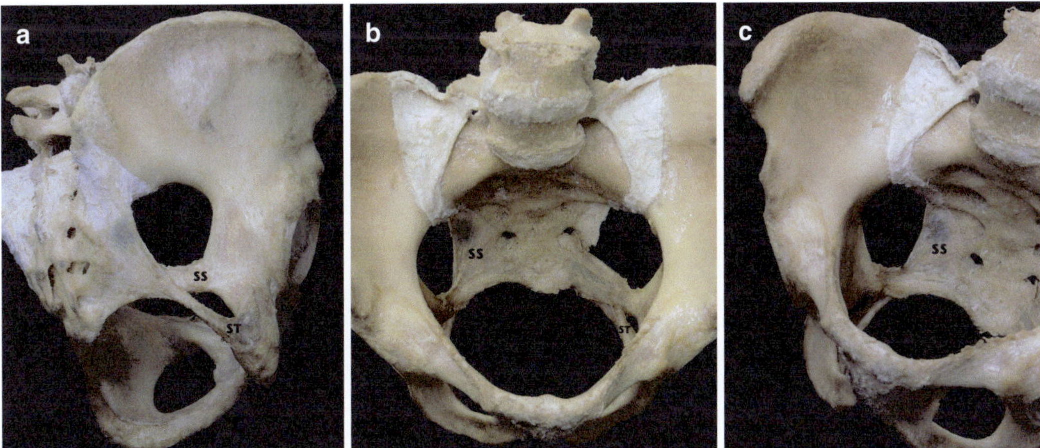

Fig. 1.4 (**a–c**) Sacrotuberous and sacrospinous ligaments. Sacrospinous ligament (SS): It attaches to the ischial spine laterally and lower part of the sacrum and coccyx medially. Sacrotuberous ligament (ST): From its broad superomedial attachments (posterior portion of the iliac crest, the lower three sacral vertebrae, and the coccyx), the fibers of the sacrotuberous ligament converge as they pass downward, laterally and slightly anteriorly toward the ischial tuberosity

the iliac crest, the lower three sacral vertebrae, and the coccyx), the fibers of the sacrotuberous ligament converge as they pass downward, laterally and slightly anteriorly toward the ischial tuberosity. A number of ligamentous and muscular structures are intimately associated with the sacrotuberous ligament. The sacrotuberous ligament is normally composed of two parts: a ligamentous band and a membranous falciform process [6]. Both sacrospinous and sacrotuberous ligaments are anatomically close to the pudendal nerve and may be involved in the entrapment of this nerve.

The Muscles

The muscles covering the posterior aspect of the hip joint form two layers. The outer layer consists of the gluteus maximus, which together with the fascia lata and the tensor fasciae latae form a continuous fibromuscular sheath that can be viewed as the "pelvic deltoid" as Henry noted, because it covers the hip much as the deltoid covers the shoulder [7] (Fig. 1.5). The inner layer consists of the short external rotators of the hip, the piriformis, the superior gemellus, the obturator internus, obturator externus muscle, the inferior gemellus, and the quadratus femoris. The gluteus medius and minimus cover the lateral pelvis, and

by their insertion to the greater trochanter, they act as hip abductors (Fig. 1.6).

The *gluteus medius muscle* has three different groups of fibers [8] that act over the hip joint in a different way: anterior fibers produce an abduction and internal rotation of the hip, posterior fibers produce also abduction but external rotation of the hip, and finally the middle fibers only produce abduction. The gluteus medius attachment can also be divided into three parts [9].

- The main tendon arose from the central posterior portion of the muscle, and it is attached to the superoposterior facet of the greater trochanter. The thickness of this main tendon is not homogeneous, so the medial part is thicker than the lateral one.
- The lateral part of the tendon takes its origin from the undersurface of the gluteus medius muscle, and it is usually thin. It is attached into the lateral facet of the greater trochanter and continues anteriorly covering the insertion of the gluteus minimus tendon.
- The anterior part of the tendon is surrounded and attached by the gluteus minimus muscle.

The *gluteus minimus muscle*, which is covered by the gluteus medius muscle, attaches to the greater trochanter through two different

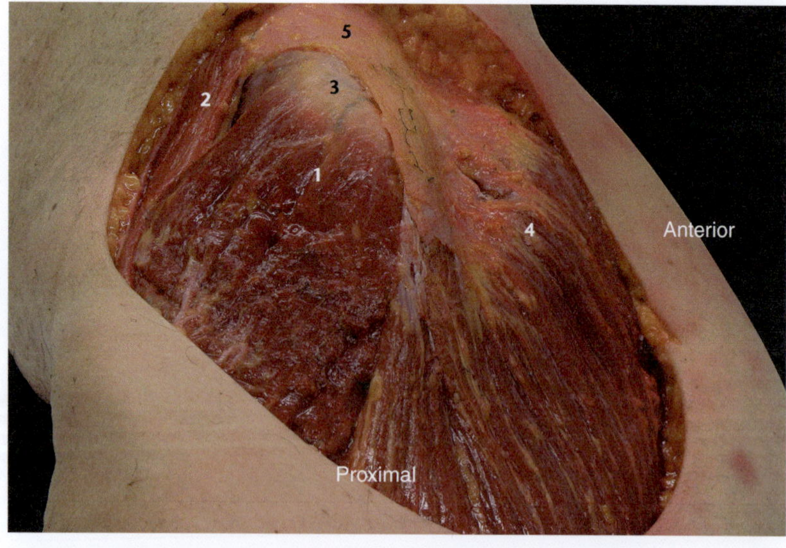

Fig. 1.5 Posterior view of the right gluteus region. The gluteus maximus has been partially resected to show the gluteus medius main attachment into the superoposterior facet of the greater trochanter. (1) Gluteus medius m. (2) Gluteus maximus m. (3) Greater trochanter. (4) Tensor fascia latae m. (5) Iliotibial band

components [9] (Figs. 1.7 and 1.8). The main tendon is attached mainly in the anterior (lateral and inferior aspect) facet of the greater trochanter. The fibers that compose this main tendon are the anterior muscle fibers. The secondary part of the gluteus minimus is attached through a muscular insertion into the anterior and superior aspect of the hip capsule.

The quadratus femoris muscle (QFM) is a flat and quadrilateral muscle, situated within the deep gluteal space of the hip [10]. It has a somewhat striated appearance, the fibers running along the axial plane. They are more closely opposed along the femoral end of the muscle. Along the ischial aspect, they are more loosely arranged and have more interspersed fat. Quadratus femoris nerve arose from the ventral surface of L4, L5, and S1 in 79.4% of population. It exits the pelvis through the greater sciatic notch, travels inferiorly along the anterior surface of the gemellus and obturator internus muscles, and enters the quadratus muscle along its anterior surface [8–10]. The QFM is bordered anteriorly by obturator externus muscle, iliacus-psoas distal tendon, the lesser trochanter, and the posteromedial intertrochanteric area of the femur; posteriorly by deep gluteal space fat, hamstring tendons, and the anterior surface of the gluteus maximus muscle; superiorly by obturator internus-gemelli complex; and inferiorly by the adductor magnus (Fig. 1.9). QFM is an adductor and external rotator of the thigh.

The obturator internus muscle originates from the pelvic surface of the obturator membrane and surrounding bones. It inserts on to the greater trochanter medial surface in union with the gemelli tendons. Its actions are the same as superior gemellus. It is innervated by the nerve to obturator internus from the sacral plexus containing fibers from the L5–S2 spinal nerves. The obturator internus muscle belly is located intrapelvically.

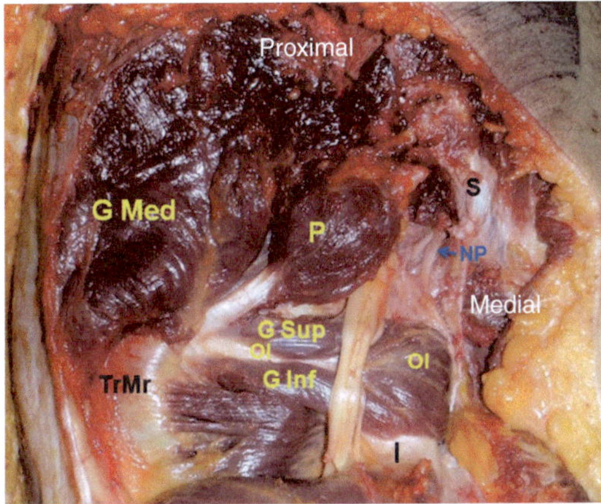

Fig. 1.6 View of the short external rotators of the hip. *P* piriformis, *G Sup* superior gemellus, *OI* obturator internus, *G Inf* inferior gemellus, *I* ischion, *TrMr* lesser trochanter, *G Med* gluteus medius, *NP* pudendal nerve, *S* sacrum

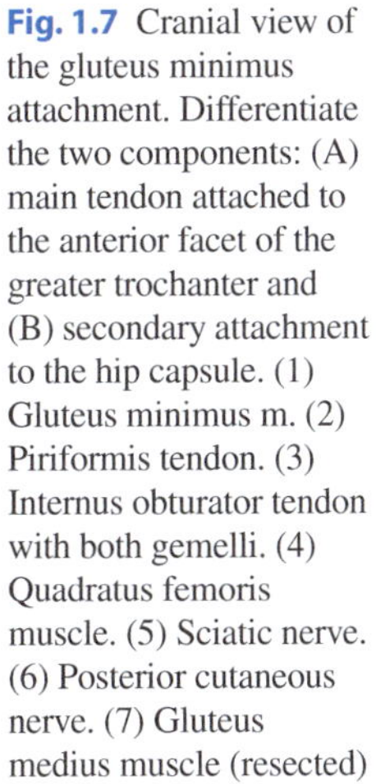

Fig. 1.7 Cranial view of the gluteus minimus attachment. Differentiate the two components: (A) main tendon attached to the anterior facet of the greater trochanter and (B) secondary attachment to the hip capsule. (1) Gluteus minimus m. (2) Piriformis tendon. (3) Internus obturator tendon with both gemelli. (4) Quadratus femoris muscle. (5) Sciatic nerve. (6) Posterior cutaneous nerve. (7) Gluteus medius muscle (resected)

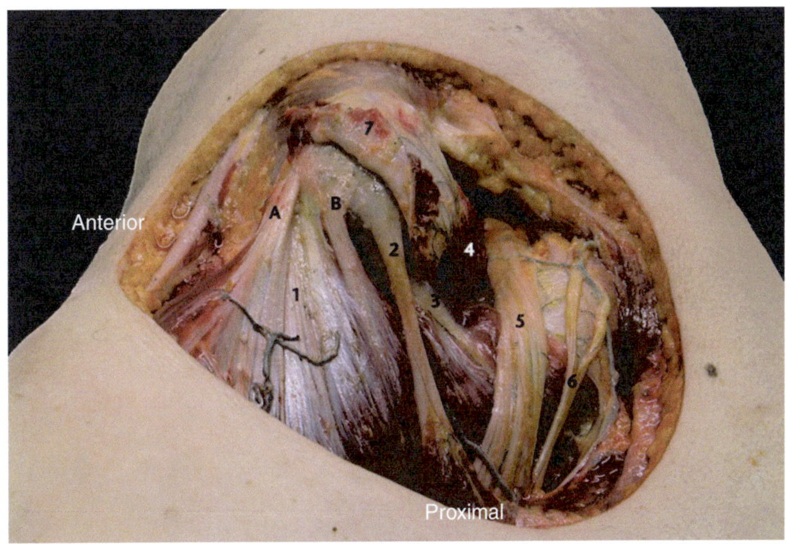

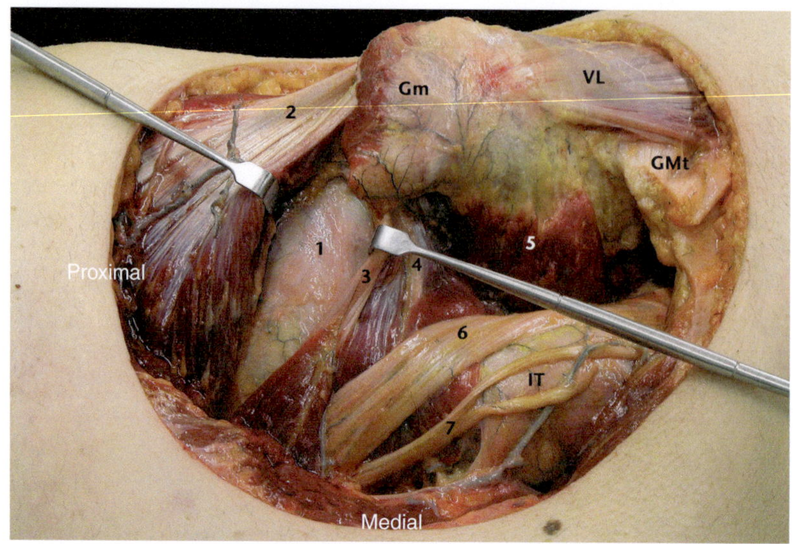

Fig. 1.8 View of the relationship of the hip capsule with the piriformis. (1) Posterior hip capsule. (2) Gluteus minimus. (3) Piriformis. (4) Internus obturator with both gemelli. (5) Quadratus femoris. (6) Sciatic nerve. (7) Posterior cutaneous nerve. *Gm* gluteus medius (resected), *GMt* gluteus max tendon, *IT* ischial tuberosity, *VL* vastus lateralis

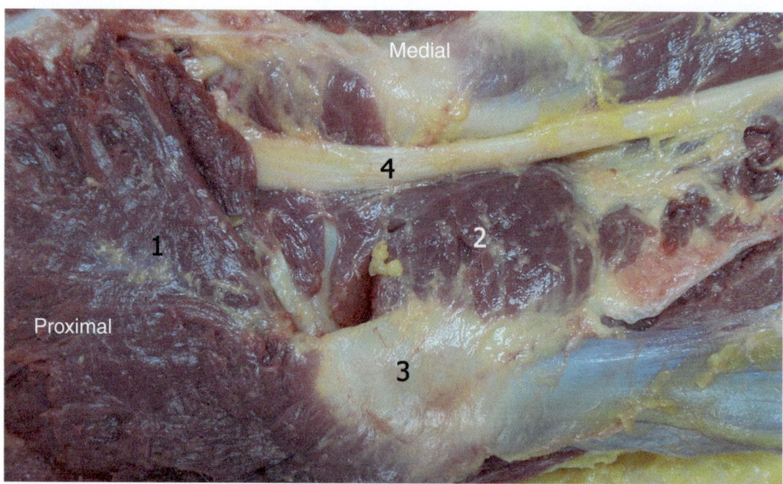

Fig. 1.9 Quadratus femoris muscle view. (1) Gluteus medius. (2) Quadratus femoris. (3) Greater trochanter. (4) Sciatic nerve

It usually turns tendinous as it exits the pelvis through the lesser sciatic foramen. Although the gemelli superior and inferior and obturator internus muscles are usually described separately, because they have a common insertion, they can be considered three heads of a single muscle, similar to the triceps brachii muscle [11] (Fig. 1.10).

The obturator externus has a proximal attachment to the obturator foramen and courses laterally, inferior to the femoral neck, to insert into the trochanteric fossa [12]. The tendon of the obtura-tor externus has been observed to connect to the hip joint capsule. The obturator externus muscle is technically considered a muscle of the medial thigh and receives innervation from the posterior division of the obturator nerve but is considered with the short rotators of the gluteal region given its shared function with these muscles.

The superior gemellus originates from the ischial spine and inserts on to the medial aspect of the greater trochanter in union with the tendon of obturator internus. The superior gemellus action is external rotation of the thigh; when the

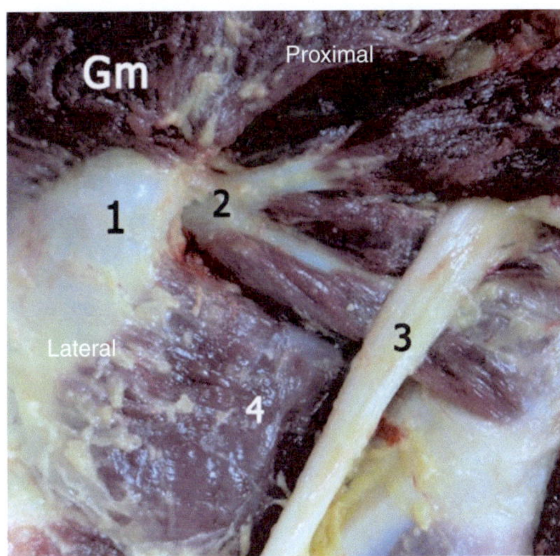

Fig. 1.10 Gemelli superior and inferior and obturator internus view. Because they have a common insertion, they can be considered three heads of a single muscle, similar to the triceps brachii muscle. (1) Greater trochanter. (2) Obturator internus. (3) Sciatic nerve. *Gm* gluteus medius

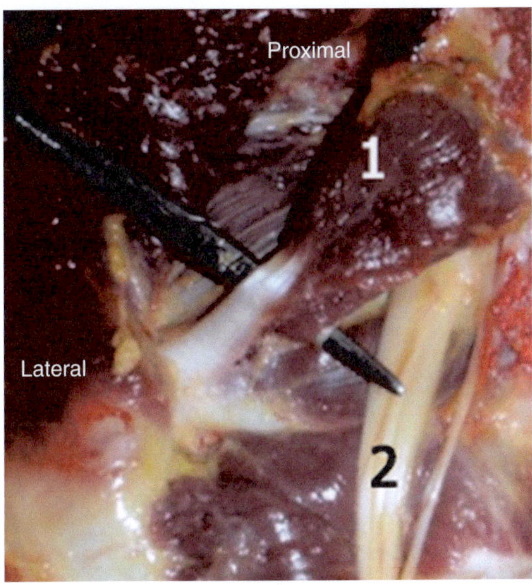

Fig. 1.11 Piriformis muscle. Tendon inserts to the piriformis fossa at the medial aspect of the greater trochanter of the femur often partially blended with the common tendon of obturator/gemelli complex. (1) Piriformis muscle. (2) Sciatic nerve

hip is flexed, it aids in thigh abduction. A branch from the nerve to the obturator internus from the sacral plexus containing fibers from the L5–S2 spinal nerves provides innervation to the superior gemellus. The superior gemellus may be absent or small or may be doubled and inserted into the hip joint capsule. It may fuse with the piriformis or gluteus minimus muscle [11].

The inferior gemellus muscle originates from the ischial tuberosity and also inserts on to the medial aspect of the greater trochanter in union with tendon of obturator internus. Its actions are the same as the superior gemellus. A branch of the nerve to the quadratus femoris from the sacral plexus and lumbosacral trunk containing fibers from the L4–S1 spinal nerves innervates the inferior gemellus. The inferior gemellus may be doubled and rarely absent. It may fuse with the quadratus femoris [11].

The piriformis muscle occupies a central position in the buttock and is an important reference for identifying the neurovascular structures emerging above and below it (Fig. 1.11). This muscle arises from the ventrolateral surface of the S2–S4 sacral vertebrae, gluteal surface of the ileum, and sacroiliac joint capsule. It runs later-ally through the greater sciatic foramen, becomes tendinous, and inserts to the piriformis fossa at the medial aspect of the greater trochanter of the femur often partially blended with the common tendon of obturator/gemelli complex. Distal to the piriformis muscle is the cluster of short external rotators: the gemellus superior, obturator internus, gemellus inferior, and quadratus femoris muscle [13, 14]. The branches of the L5, S1, and S2 spinal nerves innervate the piriformis muscle.

There are six possible anatomical relationships between the sciatic nerve and the piriformis muscle [15, 16] (Fig. 1.12): (1) Sciatic nerve passes below the piriformis muscle; (2) divided nerve passes through and below the muscle; (3) divided nerve passes through and above the muscle; (4) a divided nerve passes above and below the muscle; (5) undivided nerve passes through the piriformis; or (6) undivided nerve passes above the muscle. In 120 cadaver dissections, Beason and Anson [15] found that the most common arrangement was the undivided nerve passing below the piriformis muscle (84%) followed by the divisions of the sciatic nerve between and below the muscle (12%). In 130 anatomic dissections, Pecina [16]

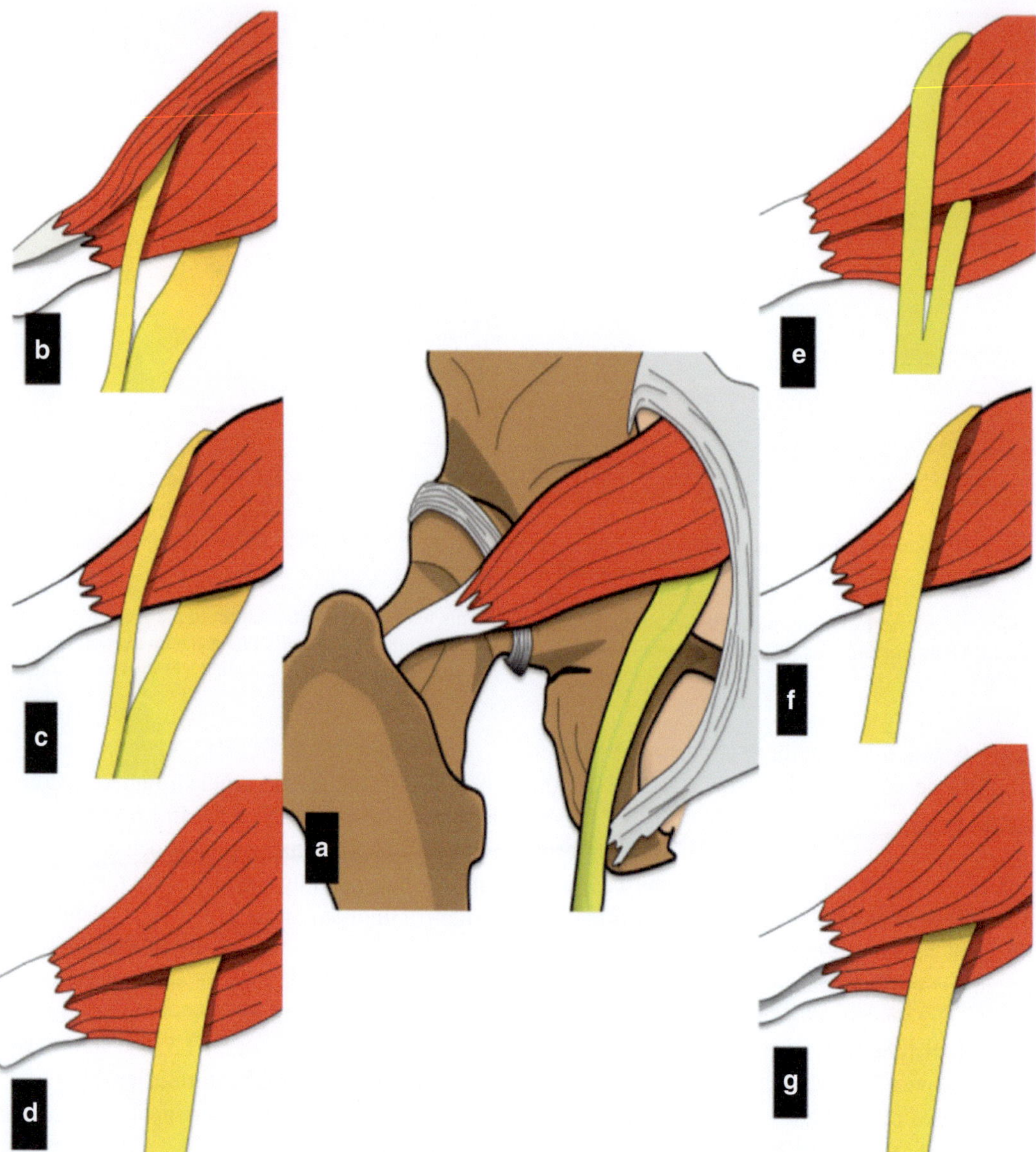

Fig. 1.12 Anatomic variations of the relationship between the piriformis muscle and sciatic nerve. Diagrams illustrate the six variants, originally described by Beaton and Anson. (**a**) An undivided nerve comes out below the piriformis muscle (normal course). (**b**) A divided sciatic nerve passing through and below the piriformis muscle. (**c**) A divided nerve passing above and below an undivided muscle. (**d**) An undivided sciatic nerve passing through the piriformis muscle. (**e**) A divided nerve passing through and above the muscle heads. (**f**) An undivided sciatic nerve passing above an undivided muscle. (**g**) Diagram showing an unreported additional B-type variation consisting of a smaller accessory piriformis (AP) with its own separate tendon

found that the undivided nerve passed below the muscle in 78% of his dissections and the divided nerve passed through and below the muscle in 21%. He noted the relation between high-level divisions of the sciatic nerve (i.e., in the pelvis) and the common peroneal nerve passing through the piriformis muscle.

Function: The piriformis muscle potentially plays a role not only in external rotation of the hip but also in restricting posterior translation of the femoral head when the joint is flexed due to the shift toward a more posterior position of this muscle with respect to the hip joint in hip flexion [17]. Hip flexion, adduction, and internal rotation stretch the piriformis muscle and cause narrowing of the space between the inferior border of the piriformis, superior gemellus, and sacrotuberous ligament.

Hamstrings

The long head of biceps femoris (BFlh) and the semitendinosus (ST) have a common origin and a common tendon originating from the ischial tuberosity which ultimately divides into two separate tendons at a mean distance of 9.1 ± 2.3 cm from the ischial tuberosity [18] (Fig. 1.13). These findings correspond well with those of Miller et al. and Garrett et al. who found this division at a mean distance of 9.9 ± 1.5 and approximately 10 cm from the ischial tuberosity. The semimebranosus origin is located lateral on the ischium, while the conjoined tendon is located distal and posterior. The most proximal part of the semimembranosus tendon is conjoint with the BFlh/ST common tendon and gets separated at a mean distance of 2.7 ± 1.0 cm from the ischial tuberosity. Garrett et al. described this division more distally, at approximately 5 cm from the ischial tuberosity [19, 20].

Bones Peritrochanteric Anatomy

Proximal Femur

The typical morphology of the greater trochanter is produced by the architecture of the abductor mechanism [21, 22]. Pfirrmann et al. [9] described the presence of four different facets in the greater trochanter.

- The anterior facet can be identified on the anterolateral surface of the trochanter and corresponds to the attachment of the gluteus minimus tendon and is oval in shape and shares a medial border with the intertrochanteric line. The anterior border is formed by the intertrochanteric line just posterior to the capsular insertion of the hip.
- The superoposterior facet is located in the top of the greater trochanter and has an oblique transverse orientation. It gives attachment to the gluteus medius tendon.
- The lateral facet has an inverted triangular shape. It is in contact with the superoposterior facet through its posterior-superior border. In the same way, that superoposterior facet is completely covered by the gluteus medius tendon.
- The posterior facet is placed in the posterior aspect of the greater trochanter. It is in close

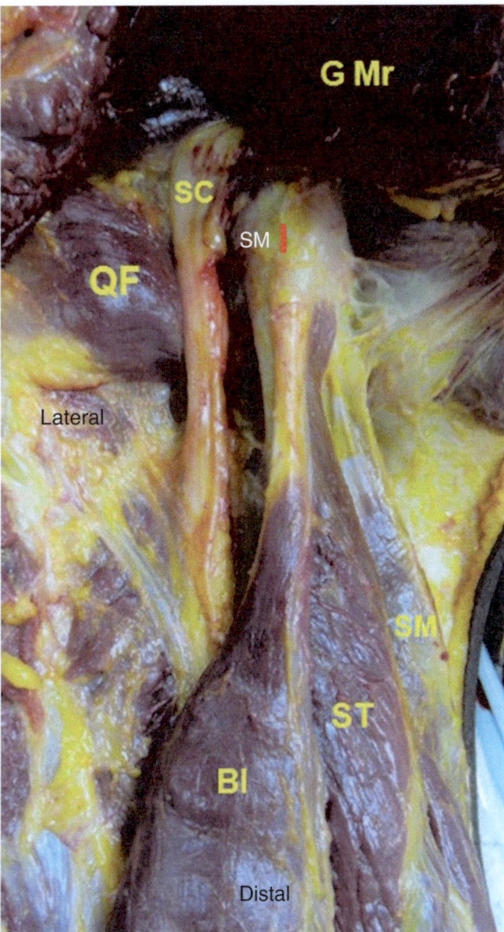

Fig. 1.13 Hamstring tendons. The long head of biceps femoris (BI) and the semitendinosus (ST) have a common origin and a common tendon originating from the ischial tuberosity which ultimately divides into two separate tendons. *G Mr* gluteus maximus, *QF* quadratus femoris, *SM* semimembranosus, *SC* sciatic nerve

contact with the lateral and superoposterior facets through its superior border. This facet does not receive any tendon attachment, but it is covered by the trochanteric bursa.

Hip Bursae Complex

A number of trochanteric bursae have been described. Three of the most important ones are: trochanteric bursa, subgluteus medius bursa, and subgluteus minimus bursa [21, 23, 24]. The description of the "bursae complex" was performed by Pfirrmann et al. [9]:

- The trochanteric bursa is the largest hip bursa. It is located beneath the gluteus maximus muscle and iliotibial tract. Its function is to cover the posterior facet of the greater trochanter, the gluteus medius tendon, and the proximal part of the vastus lateralis origin.
- The subgluteus medius bursa is placed deep to the lateral part of the gluteus medius tendon.
- The subgluteus minimus bursa lies beneath the gluteus minimus tendon, in a medial and superior position. It covers partially the anterior area of the hip capsule.

The Nerves

Seven neural structures exit the pelvis through the greater sciatic notch: posterior femoral cutaneous nerve (sensory innervation of the gluteal region, perineum, and posterior thigh and popliteal fossa), superior gluteal nerve (motor innervation: gluteus medius, gluteus minimus, and tensor fascia lata), inferior gluteal nerve (motor innervation of gluteus maximus), nerve to obturator internus (motor innervation of superior gemellus and obturator internus), nerve to quadratus femoris muscle (motor innervation of inferior gemellus and quadratus femoris and sensory innervation of hip capsule), pudendal nerve (motor innervation of perineal muscles, external urethral sphincter, and external anal sphincter and sensory innervation perineum, external genitalia), and sciatic nerve (motor innervation of semitendinosus, biceps femoris, semimembranosus, extensor portion

of the adductor magnus, and leg and foot musculature and sensory innervation of the leg and foot, except for the saphenous nerve dermatome) [25]. Accompanying the respective nerves are the superior gluteal vessels, inferior gluteal vessels, and internal pudendal vessels. It is important to differentiate normal neurovascular bundles and isolated nerves that normally run along the deep gluteal space and not to confuse them with fibrovascular bands.

The *superior gluteal nerve* is formed by the posterior roots of L4, L5, and S1and exits the pelvis through the greater sciatic foramen (sciatic notch), just superior to the piriformis muscle (sometimes the superior gluteal nerve can perforate the piriformis muscle) [26]. It courses with the superior gluteal artery between the gluteus medius and minimus muscles (Fig. 1.14). At a variable distance from the greater sciatic notch, it divides into a superior and an inferior branch

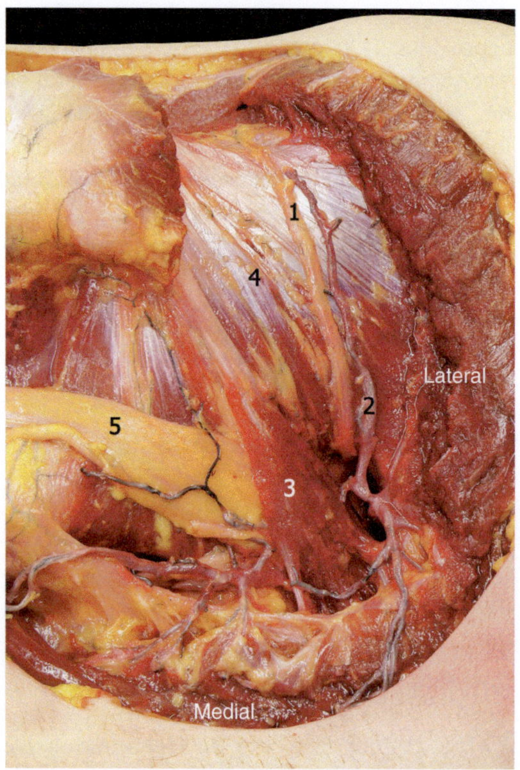

Fig. 1.14 Posterior view of a left hip showing the superior gluteal nerve and artery path (the gluteus maximus and medius muscles have been resected). (1) Superior gluteal nerve. (2) Superior gluteal artery. (3) Piriformis muscle. (4) Gluteus minimus muscle. (5) Sciatic nerve

[27]. Some authors described three branches [28, 29]. The superior branch accompanies the upper branch of the deep division of the superior gluteal artery and innervated the gluteus minimus muscle, gluteus medius muscle, and tensor fascia latae muscle. The inferior branch runs with the lower branch of the division of the superior gluteal artery across the gluteus minimus muscle and also innervates the gluteus medius muscle as well as the tensor fascia latae muscle. The inferior branch is thicker than superior one.

The inferior gluteal nerve, the main motor nerve of the gluteus maximus, originates from the dorsal L5, S1, and S2 rami and leaves the pelvis through the greater sciatic notch, just inferior to the piriformis muscle and medial regarding the sciatic nerve. After its pass inferior to the piriform muscle, it divides into different branches which pass posteriorly into the deep surface of the gluteus maximus muscle (the number of branches can vary from 3 to 7) [30]. Apaydin et al. measured the mean distance between the closest branch to the greater trochanter and the greater trochanter, and the result was 0.8 cm (0–2.2 cm) [30]. Ling and Kumar reported that the inferior gluteal nerve entered into the deep surface of the gluteus maximus muscles approximately at 5 cm from the tip of the greater trochanter of the femur, over the inferior one-third of the belly of the gluteus maximus muscle [31]. The nerve may also send a branch to the posterior femoral cutaneous nerve.

The Sciatic Nerve

The sciatic nerve, the terminal branch of the sacral plexus, exits the pelvis through the greater sciatic notch and courses anterior to the piriformis muscle in the pelvis. Descriptions of variations concerning the relationship between the piriformis muscle and sciatic nerve have been limited [15, 32–34]. It originates from the ventral rami of L4–L5 and S1–S3 spinal nerves. Part of the ventral ramus of L4 joins the ventral ramus of L5 to originate the lumbosacral trunk, which joins the first three sacral ventral rami to form the sciatic nerve. This nerve has two components, the tibial nerve (on the medial side), which is derived from the anterior divisions of L4–L5 and S1–S3, and the common peroneal nerve (on the lateral side), which is derived from the posterior divisions of L4–L5 and S1–S2. In the gluteal area and proximal thigh, a third component can be described. That corresponds to the most medial part of the nerve, and it is formed by the fibers providing the motor innervation to the hamstring muscles. The sciatic nerve may divide into its common fibular and tibial nerve components within the pelvis [33]. Prevalence was 16.9% in a meta-analysis of cadaveric studies and 16.2% in published surgical case series [32]. The nerve exits the greater sciatic foramen as distinct tibial and peroneal divisions, enclosed in a common nerve sheath. It is not infrequent (10–15% of cases) [35] that the two components of the sciatic nerve can be easily distinguished as separate nerves, during their entire course, from the pelvis to the popliteal fossa. In those cases, usually the common peroneal nerve pierces the piriformis instead of passing caudal to it. This variation is usually interpreted as an "early division" of the sciatic nerve and understood as a premature separation of both components. Anatomy dissections demonstrate instead that, regardless of their apparent single or obvious double macroscopic appearance, both components run invariably together, inside a common sheath, from the inferior border of the piriformis muscle to the popliteal fossa.

Six categories of anatomic variations of the relationship between the piriformis muscle and sciatic nerve were originally reported in 1938 by Beaton and Anson [15]. Smoll presented the overall reported incidence of these six variations in over 6,000 dissected limbs. Relationships A, B, C, D, E, and F occurred in 83.1, 13.7, 1.3, 0.5, 0.08, and 0.08% of limbs, respectively [32]. Therefore, with the exception of relationship A (normal course), the B-type piriformis-sciatic variation is the most commonly found. An additional and unreported B-type variation consisting of a smaller accessory piriformis with its own separate tendon is often seen. Nerve fibers of the fibular and tibial components maintain a pattern of fiber separation in these branches and in the sciatic nerve. The sciatic nerve physically splits in tibial and fibular divisions at highly variable locations from the pelvis to the popliteal fossa, although this split is more frequent at the distal thigh [36]. Often, the split is oblique and may not be seen in a uniplanar MRI view [37]. The nerve fibers of the sciatic nerve do not course between the tibial and fibular divisions [25]. Neural tissue and nonneural tissue compose the sciatic nerve. The ratio neural/nonneural tissue changes from 2/1 at the level of piriformis muscle to 1/1 at the midfemur, and there is an increase in the nonneural tissue contribution as the sciatic nerve courses distally [38].

After leaving the piriformis muscle, the sciatic nerve runs posteriorly to the obturator/gemelli complex and quadratus femoris muscle. It passes between the ischial tuberosity and the greater trochanter lying close to the posterior capsule of the hip (Fig. 1.15a, b). Miller et al. performed a cadaveric study and concluded that the sciatic nerve is located at a mean distance of 1.2 ± 0.2 cm from the most lateral aspect of the ischial tuberosity, and it has an intimate relation with proximal origin of the

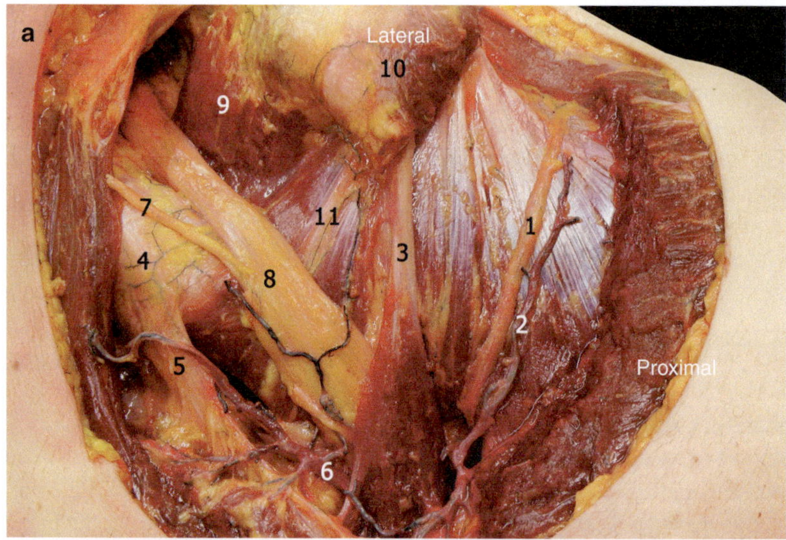

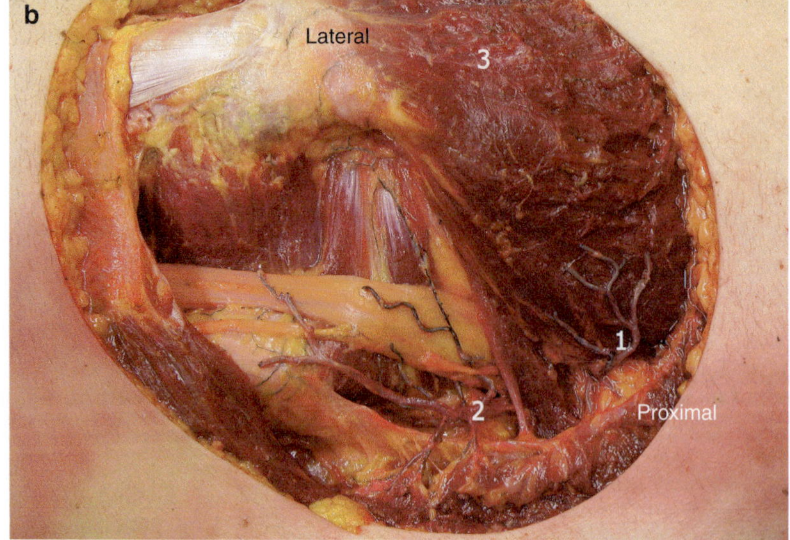

Fig. 1.15 (**a**) Sciatic nerve. Posterior view of a left hip. (1) Superior gluteal nerve, (2) superior gluteal artery, (3) piriformis, (4) ischial tuberosity, (5) sacrotuberous ligament, (6) inferior gluteal artery, (7) posterior femoral cutaneous nerve, (8) sciatic nerve, (9) quadratus femoris m., (10) gluteus medius resected, (11) obturator internus. (**b**) Sciatic nerve. Posterior view of a left hip. (1) Superior gluteal artery, (2) inferior gluteal artery, (3) gluteus medius

hamstrings like the inferior gluteal nerve and artery [19]. As it runs down, the nerve describes a wide curve cephalad to the ischial tuberosity. On reaching the lateral aspect of this prominence, the sciatic nerve changes direction to run almost vertically down toward the thigh. The sciatic nerve has a segmental arterial supply by branches of the inferior gluteal artery, medial circumflex femoral artery, and perforating arteries of the thigh (usually the first and second) [39–41], and the venous drainage is performed through the perforators to the femoral profunda system in the thigh and to the popliteal vein at the knee [42].

Under normal conditions, the sciatic nerve is able to stretch and glide in order to accommodate moderate strain or compression associated with joint movement. During a straight leg raise with knee extension, the sciatic nerve experiences a proximal excursion of 28.0 mm at 70–80° of hip flexion [43].

Function: Most sciatic neural fibers are destined to motor and sensory innervation distal to the knee. However, important branches arise from the nerve in the deep gluteal space and thigh. It provides knee flexion by innervation of the posterior thigh muscles and almost all sensory and motor functions below the knee. The tibial nerve provides all motor function to the posterior compartment of the leg and to the plantar muscles of the foot, while the common peroneal nerve provides motor function to the anterior and lateral compartments of the leg.

Anatomical studies have demonstrated that the sciatic nerve in adults is located at about 10 cm from the midline in the gluteal area [44]. The sciatic nerve enters the thigh deep to the biceps femoris muscle. In here, as opposed to the gluteal area, the position of the nerve with respect to the midline is influenced both by the degree of hip abduction as well as by the amount of fat accumulating in the inner thigh.

Posterior Femoral Cutaneos Nerve

The posterior femoral cutaneous (PFCN) arises from the dorsal branch of the first and ventral branches of the second and third sacral rami.

Also known as posterior femoral cutaneous nerve, it is not a branch of the sciatic nerve, although both have a close relationship in the midgluteal area. It exits the pelvis through the greater sciatic foramen, first medial and then superficial (more posterior in anatomic position) to the sciatic nerve. Somewhere caudal to the ischium, the posterior cutaneous nerve of the thigh pierces the deep fascia (fascia lata) and becomes a superficial nerve (Fig. 1.16). The perineal branch innervates the upper inner region of the thigh, curves forward across the hamstrings below the ischial tuberosity, and runs through the fascia lata alongside the superficial perineal fascia to reach the skin around the scrotum in men and the skin around the labia majora in women. It communicates with the inferior rectal and posterior scrotal branches of the perineal nerve. The perineal branch gives off numerous branches to the skin of the upper part of the back and inner portion of the thigh, the popliteal fossa, and the proximal area of the back of the leg [45]. It provides sensory innervation to the posterior thigh as far down as the popliteal fossa and upper leg. It also supplies the sensory innervation of the lower buttocks.

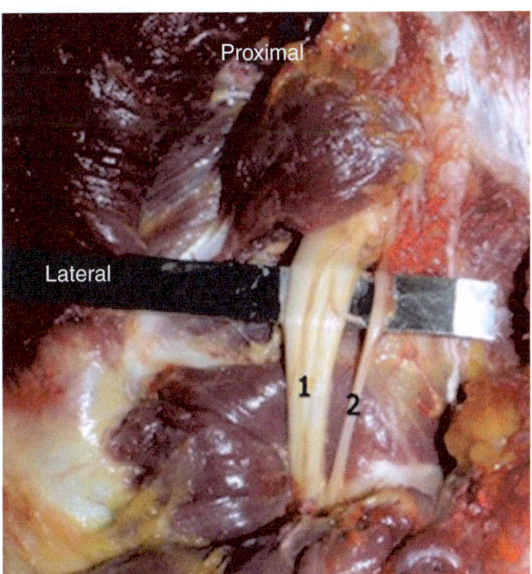

Fig. 1.16 Posterior femoral cutaneous nerve. This nerve is not a branch of the sciatic nerve, although both have a close relationship in the midgluteal area. (1) Sciatic nerve. (2) Posterior femoral cutaneous nerve

Therefore, at the level of the subgluteal fold, this sensory nerve is separated from the sciatic nerve by the thick fascia lata, explaining why a subgluteal approach to the sciatic nerve will not consistently anesthetize the posterior thigh [46]. The inferior gluteal artery descends within the thigh alongside the PCNT and distributes blood to the posterior surface of the thigh [47].

The Pudendal Nerve

The pudendal nerve arises from the sacral plexus. Subsequently, it passes around the ischial spine and reenters the pelvic cavity through the lesser sciatic foramen. It then courses under the levator ani muscle on top of the obturator internus muscle. Along its course in the ischiorectal fossa, the nerve gives off small inferior rectal branches and one or two perineal branches. The nerve coursed through the gluteal region between the sacrospinous and sacrotuberous ligaments and moved toward the inner surface of the obturator internus muscle [48] (Fig. 1.17).

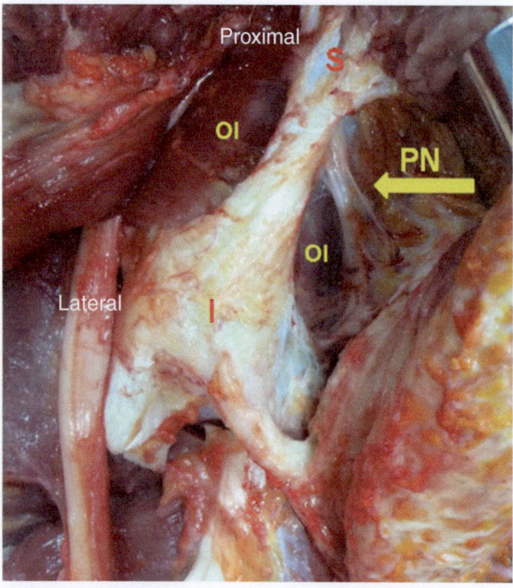

Fig. 1.17 Pudendal nerve. The nerve coursed through the gluteal region between the sacrospinous and sacrotuberous ligaments and moved toward the inner surface of the obturator internus muscle. *OI* obturator internus, *PN* pudendal nerve

The Vessels

The anatomic positions of the superior, inferior gluteal artery (IGA), and medial circumflex femoral artery (MCFA) are relevant within the deep gluteal space. Accompanying the respective nerves that exit the pelvis through the greater sciatic notch are the superior gluteal vessels, inferior gluteal vessels, and internal pudendal vessels. The gluteus maximus muscle is a class III muscle, having two dominant vascular pedicles (the superior gluteal artery or SGA and the inferior gluteal artery or IGA) and its additional contributions (the medial and lateral circumflex femoral arteries, the first perforating branch of the femoral artery, the internal pudendal artery, and the lumbar artery) from the surrounding area [49]. The SGA exits from the pelvic cavity to the gluteal region in the company of the superior gluteal nerve lying above the piriformis muscle in the greater sciatic notch. The IGA enters the deep gluteal space with the inferior gluteal nerve and supplies the gluteus maximus muscle (Fig. 1.18). This artery also gives a superficial arterial branch that crosses the sciatic nerve laterally between the piriformis and superior gemellus muscles. Another branch of the IGA is the descending branch, which runs along the posterior femoral cutaneous nerve in a frequency of 72% according to a cadaveric study [47].

The medial circumflex femoral artery follows the inferior border of the obturator externus and crosses over its tendon and under the external rotators and piriformis muscle [50] (Fig. 1.19). It has its origin medially from the femoral artery between the pectineus and iliopsoas tendons, along the inferior border of externus obturator muscle. The existence of an anastomosis between the inferior gluteal artery and the medial femoral circumflex artery is frequent [51]. The vascular supply of the femoral head is mainly provided by the medial femoral circumflex artery (MFCA) and its branches. The MFCA has its origin from the deep femoral artery (83%) or the femoral artery (27%) [51]. The MFCA has usually five branches: ascending, descending, acetabular, superficial, and deep. The deep branch of the

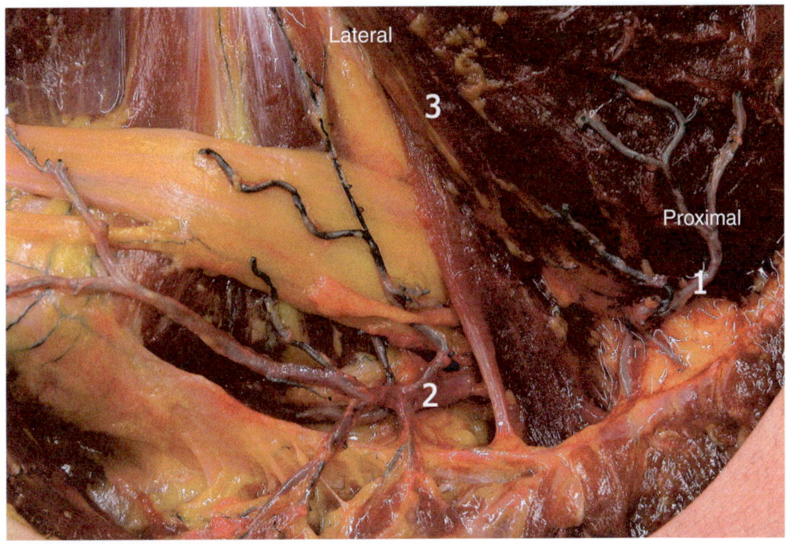

Fig. 1.18 Close detail of the superior and inferior gluteal arteries. The superior gluteal artery (1) exits from the pelvic cavity to the gluteal region in the company of the superior gluteal nerve lying above the piriformis muscle (3). The inferior gluteal artery (2) enters the deep gluteal space with the inferior gluteal nerve and supplies the gluteus maximus muscle

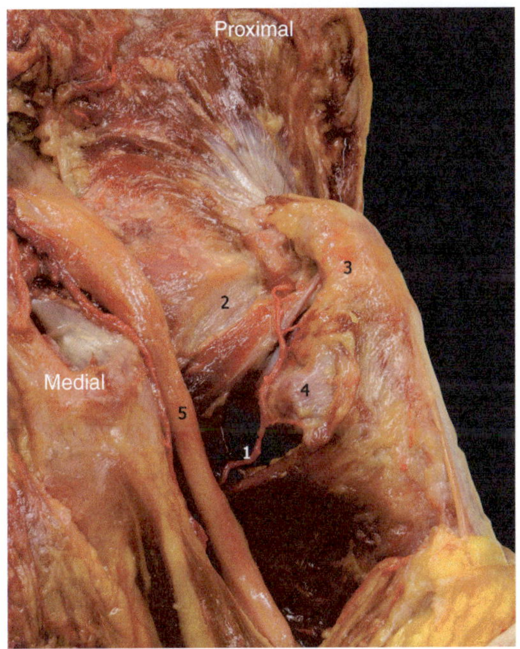

Fig. 1.19 Posterior view of the pelvitrochanteric muscles on a left hip. The quadratus femoris muscle has been partially removed to show the ascendant branch of the medial femoral circumflex artery. (1) Medial femoral circumflex artery. (2) Hip capsule. (3) Greater trochanter. (4) Lesser trochanter. (5) Sciatic nerve

MFCA is the most responsible for femoral head and neck vascularization and passes just deep to the external rotator muscles [52].

Surgical Technique and Normal Endoscopic Anatomy of the Deep Gluteal Space: Deep Gluteal Space Access

Careful preoperative planning, precise portal placement, a knowledge of the anatomy and potential complications, and a methodical sequence of endoscopic examination are essential for effective arthroscopy/endoscopy of any joint or space [53]. The deep gluteal space is a recently defined anatomic region for endoscopic access [1]. The deep gluteal space is the posterior extension of the peritrochanteric space so entrance into the deep gluteal space is accomplished by portals traveling through the peritrochanteric space, which is between the greater trochanter and the iliotibial band. In most cases, the procedure is performed in the supine position and may be performed concomitant to a hip arthroscopy of the central and/or peripheral compartments, if indicated.

Voos et al. [54]. described the arthroscopic anatomy of the hip in the peritrochanteric compartment: The borders of the peritrochanteric compartment consist of the tensor fascia lata and iliotibial band laterally, the abductor tendons superomedially, the vastus lateralis inferomedially, the gluteus maximus muscle superiorly, and its tendon posteriorly. Within the space exist the trochanteric bursae and the gluteus medius and minimus tendons at their attachment on the greater trochanter.

Different portals have been described to access the peritrochanteric space. Basically, we can divide these portals into two groups: (1) standard portals redirected to the peritrochanteric space (anterolateral, anterior, and posterolateral portals) and (2) portals described to access the peritrochanteric space [55] (proximal anterolateral accessory portal, distal anterolateral accessory portal, peritrochanteric space portal, and auxiliary posterolateral portal) (Fig. 1.20a, b). The peritrochan-teric space portal is established at the level of the modified mid-anterior portal 1 cm lateral to the anterior superior iliac spine and in the interval between the tensor fascia lata (laterally) and the sartorius (medially). This portal enters peritrochanteric space underneath IT band at level of vastus lateralis ridge. Entering at vastus lateralis ridge avoids inadvertent deep penetration of vastus lateralis or gluteus medius muscle. The proximal anterolateral accessory portal is placed directly posterior to the proximal mid-anterior portal 3–4 cm proximal. It perforates the junction of the gluteus maximus and tensor fascia lata to form the iliotibial band, entering into the peritrochanteric

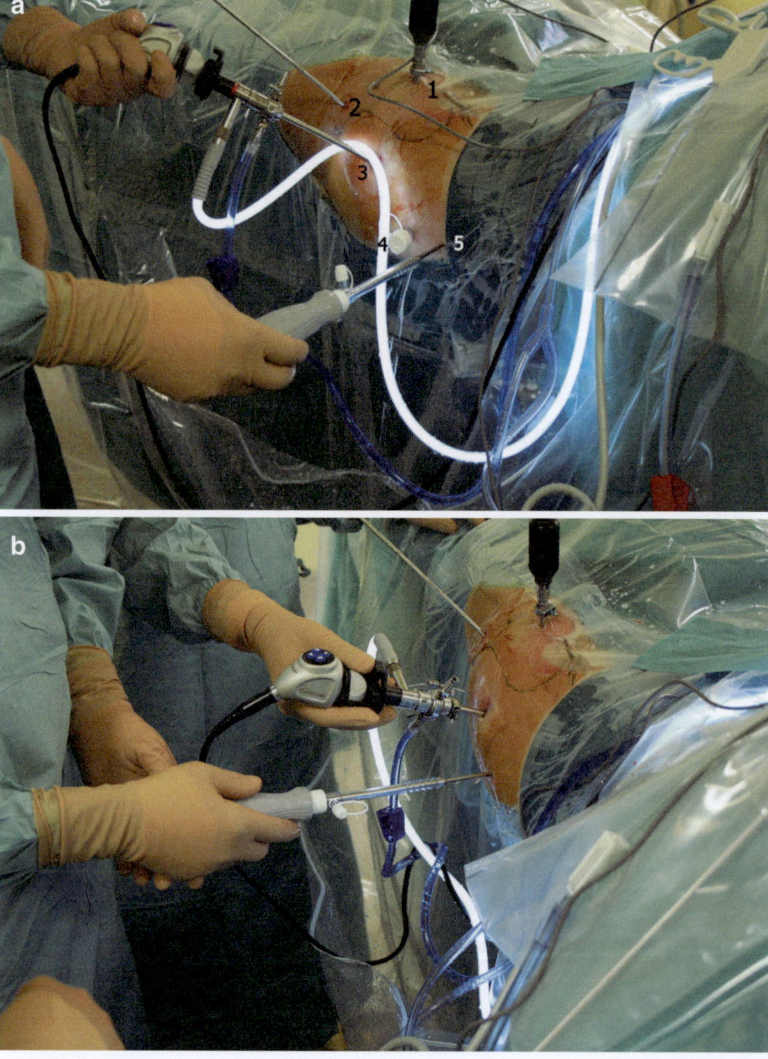

Fig. 1.20 (**a, b**) Left gluteal region showing portal placement for subgluteal endoscopy. (1) Midanterior portal. (2) Distal anterolateral accessory portal. (3) Anterolateral portal. (4) Posterolateral portal. (5) Auxiliary posterolateral portal placement

space. The distal anterolateral accessory portal is placed distally to the peritrochanteric space portal at the same distance that exists between the first two portals (proximal anterolateral accessory and peritrochanteric space portals). It penetrates into the peritrochanteric space just anterior to the iliotibial band. This portal is the only one which has a structure at risk, the transverse branch of lateral femoral circumflex artery. This artery courses in close proximity to the distal anterolateral accessory portal before going deep into the vastus lateralis muscle. Robertson et al. located this artery at a mean distance of 23.4 mm (range 17–40 mm) medially to the portal [55].

Technique: Following the completion of the central and peripheral work, any traction is discontinued, and the leg is abducted to about 15–20° in order to open the interval between the trochanter and the iliotibial band, and the leg is internally rotated 20–40°, for the same reason. We perform the procedure with the 70° arthroscope, and in some cases or larger patients, the use of an extra longer arthroscope is required (Fig. 1.21). First the peritrochanteric space portal is established. A 5.0-mm metallic cannula is positioned between the ITB and the lateral aspect of the greater trochanter, and the tip of the cannula can be used to sweep proximal and distal to ensure placement in the proper location. Fluoroscopy can also be used to confirm that the cannula is located immediately adjacent to the greater trochanter at the vastus ridge (Fig. 1.22).

The arthroscope is placed perpendicular to the patient, and look in a distal direction in order to identify the gluteus maximus tendon inserting into the linea aspera of the femur posteriorly. Then the peritrochanteric space is entered through the anterolateral accessory, distal anterolateral accessory, and posterolateral portals as working portals, and systematic inspection of this space is performed. Visualizing through the peritrochanteric portal, the examination begins at the gluteus maximus insertion at the linea aspera (Fig. 1.23a, b). Fibrous tissue bands may need to be removed from the space in this location to visualize the coalescence. Once this structure is identified, the area of the sciatic nerve can then be known. It lies directly posterior to this structure as it exits the deep gluteal space. Rotating proximally, the vastus lateralis fibers are identified and can be traced toward its insertion on the vastus tubercle. Rotating the arthroscope anterior and superior, the gluteus minimus tendon is visualized anteriorly. Moving anteriorly above the gluteus minimus lies the gluteus medius tendon and its attachment to the greater trochanter. Fibrous bands from the trochanteric bursa may need to be removed in order to best visualize the medius attachment to the greater trochanter (Fig. 1.24). The iliotibial band sits posteriorly

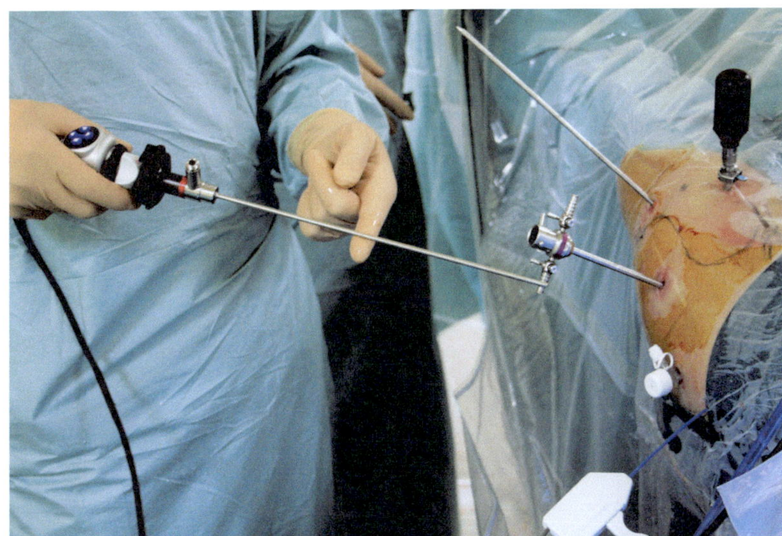

Fig. 1.21 Equipment. Perform the procedure with the 70° arthroscope, and in some cases or larger patients, the use of an extra longer arthroscope is required

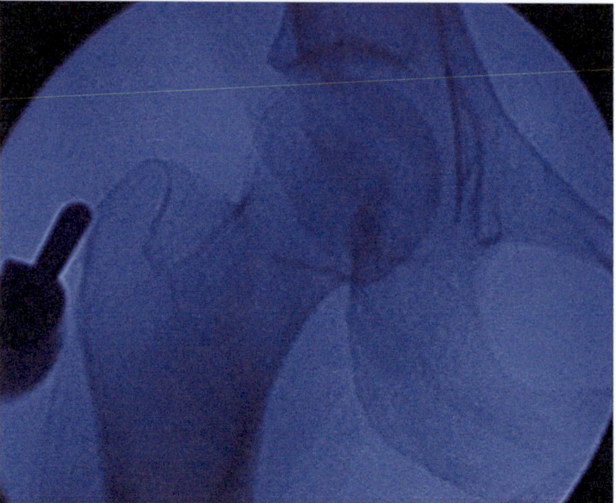

Fig. 1.22 Right hip. Entering at vastus lateralis ridge avoids inadvertent deep penetration of vastus lateralis or gluteus medius muscle

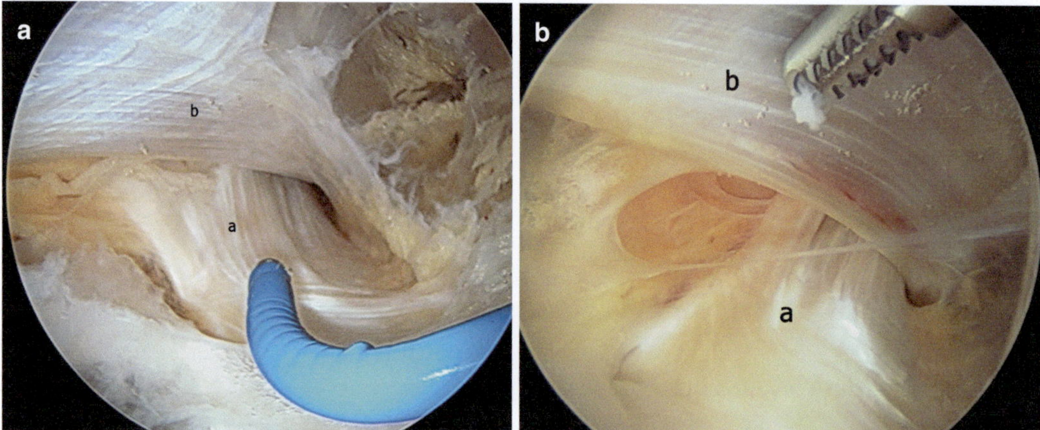

Fig. 1.23 Endoscopic view of the right hip. Visualizing through the peritrochanteric portal, the examination begins at the gluteus maximus insertion at the linea aspera. (a) Gluteus maximus insertion. (b) Vastus lateralis

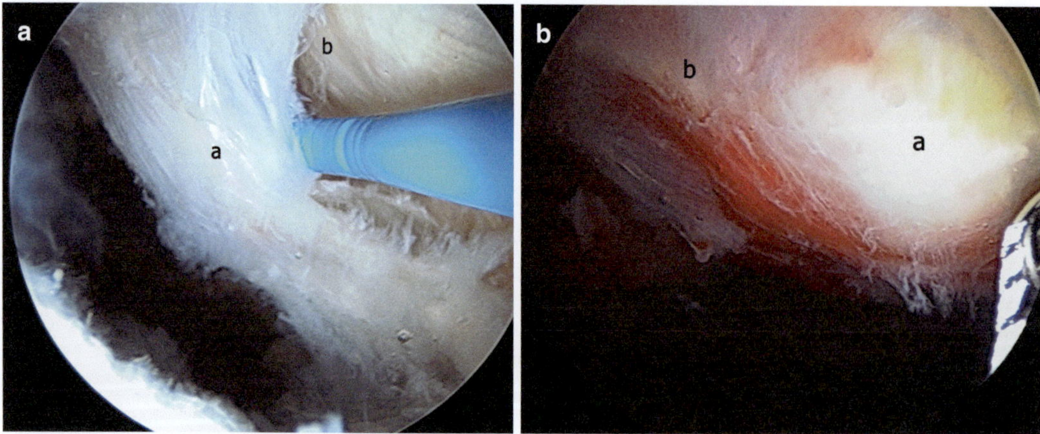

Fig. 1.24 (**a, b**) Endoscopic view of the right hip. Fibrous bands and bursa from the trochanteric bursa may need to be removed in order to best visualize the medius attachment to the greater trochanter. (**a**): (a) Fibrous bands and bursa, (b) vastus ridge. (**b**): (a) Greater trochanter, (b) gluteus medius

and can be seen with a small posterior maneuver of the arthroscope and rotation. For better sciatic nerve assessment, we switch the scope to the anterolateral portal and the procedure then continues by exposure of the bursa and resection of abnormal bursal tissue, and the sciatic nerve is identified. It lies 3–6 cm directly posterior to gluteus maximus tendon inserting into the linea aspera as it exits the deep gluteal space. Sciatic nerve assessment is carried out through the anterolateral and posterolateral portals in many cases, but sometimes we need an auxiliary posterolateral portal [1]. It is placed 3 cm posterior and 3 cm superior to the greater trochanter. It allows a better visualization of the sciatic nerve up to the sciatic notch. There is a significant risk of injury of the superior gluteal nerve if the gluteus medius muscle is perforated with the cannula by error.

Inspection of the sciatic nerve begins distal to the quadratus femoris (Fig. 1.25), just above the gluteal sling. Visualize the sciatic nerve as it courses posterior to the quadratus femoris, noting the color, epineural blood flow, and epineural fat. A normal sciatic nerve will have noticeable epineural blood flow and epineural fat, whereas an abnormal sciatic nerve will appear white, lacking epineural blood flow (Fig. 1.26). The epineural fat in many cases is diminished or completely obliterated. Take care to preserve as much of the epineural fat pad as possible during dissection [57]. A blunt probe or surgical dissector can then be employed to expose the sciatic nerve and determine the tension [56]. After the dissection at

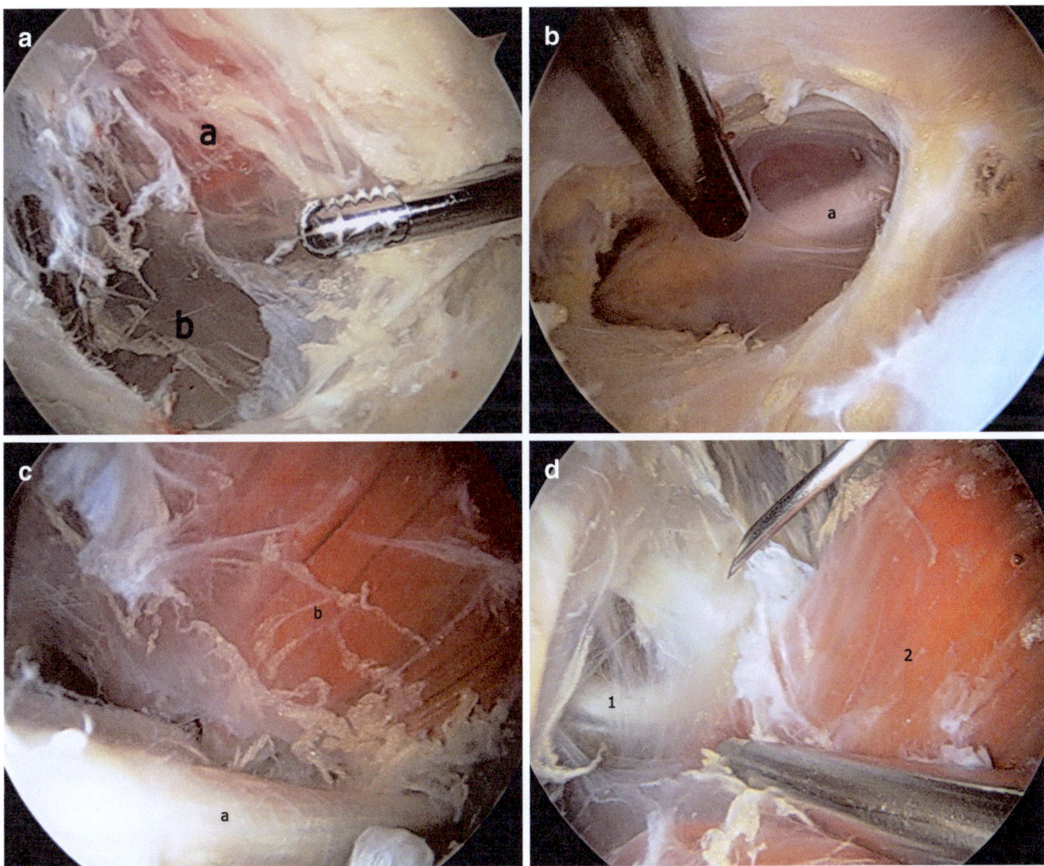

Fig. 1.25 (**a–f**) Endoscopic view of the left hip. Dissection at the level of the quadratus femoris. (**a**): (a) Quadratus femoris, (b) window to access the sciatic nerve. (**b**): (a) Sciatic nerve. (**c**): (a) Sciatic nerve, (b) quadratus femoris. (**d**): (1) First perforating femoral artery (distal to quadratus), (2) quadratus femoris. (**e, f**): (1) Quadratus femoris, (2) sciatic nerve

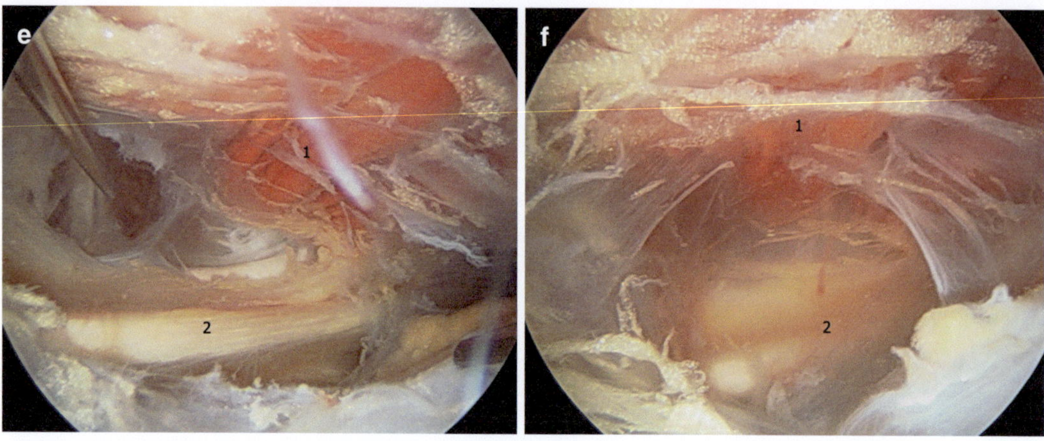

Fig. 1.25 (continued)

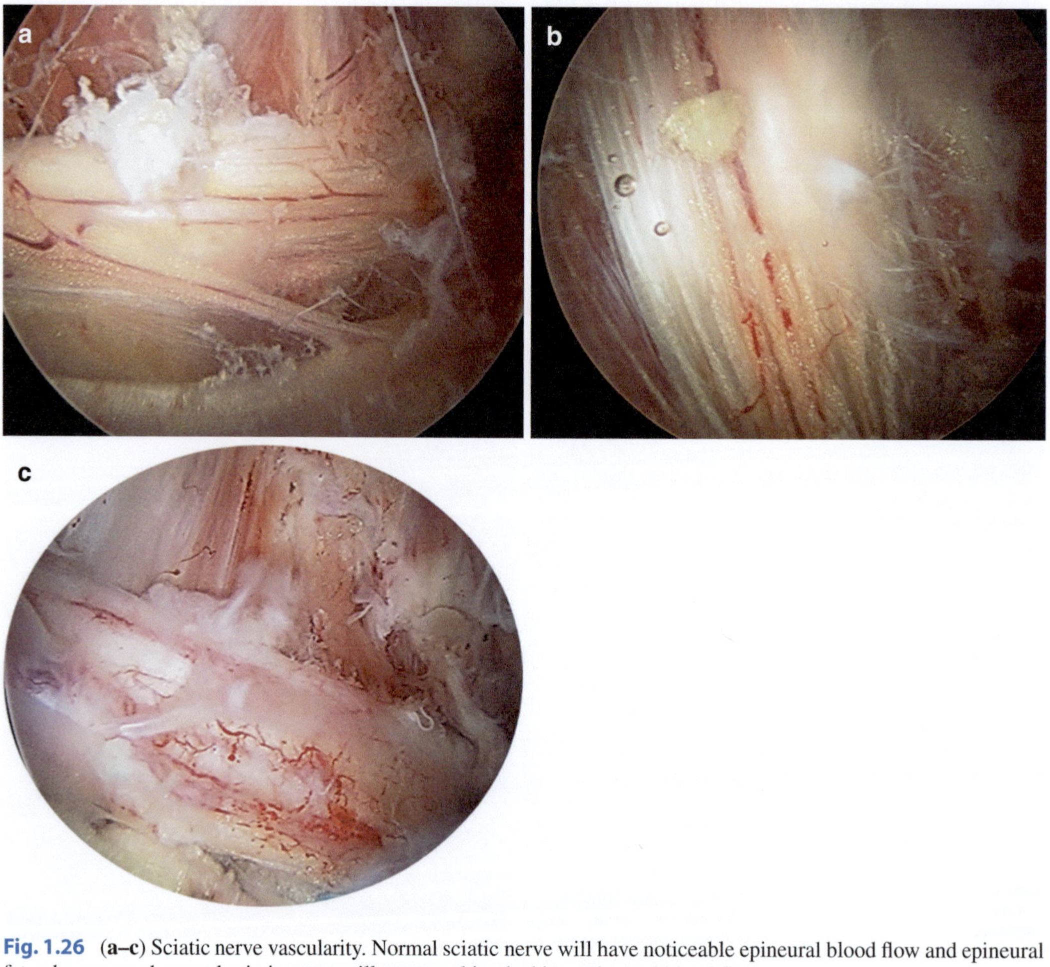

Fig. 1.26 (**a–c**) Sciatic nerve vascularity. Normal sciatic nerve will have noticeable epineural blood flow and epineural fat, whereas an abnormal sciatic nerve will appear white, lacking epineural blood flow

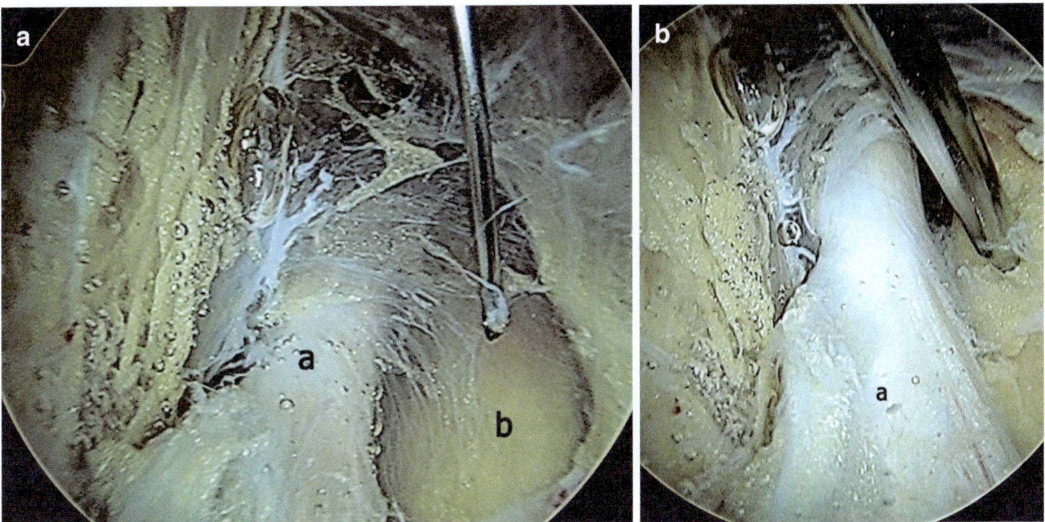

Fig. 1.27 (**a, b**) Endoscopic view of the right hip looking distally showing the ischial tunnel. (a) Sciatic nerve. (b) Hamstring tendons

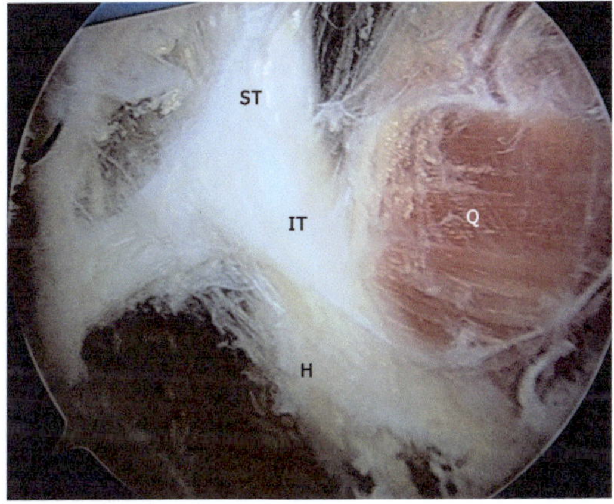

Fig. 1.28 Left hip. *H* hamstring origin, *IT* ischial tuberosity, *Q* quadratus muscle at the isquial tuberosity insertion, *ST* sacrotuberous ligament

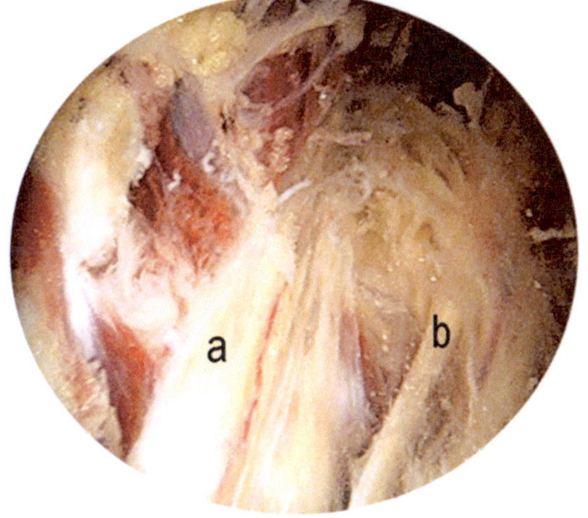

Fig. 1.29 Endoscopic view in a right hip looking distally. (a) Sciatic nerve. (b) Posterior femoral cutaneous nerve

the level of the quadratus femoris, turn the scope distal and perform all distal decompression before any proximal work. Inspect the ischial tunnel (Fig. 1.27), hamstring origin, and sacrotuberous ligament (Fig. 1.28), releasing any fibers from the sciatic nerve. Assess the lateral, medial, and retrosciatic borders of the sciatic nerve to ensure the distal release is complete. Identify the posterior cutaneous nerve (Fig. 1.29). After the distal dissection, move proximal for a trochanteric bursectomy, while paying attention to keep

the shaver blade directed away from the gluteus medius. The sciatic nerve should now also be possible to visualize proximally, and care must be taken to avoid nerve damage caused by the motorized instrument or excessive traction. When the piriformis tendon is identified (Fig. 1.30), it should be possible to identify the tendons of the gemellus and obturatorius internus muscles (Fig. 1.31). Clean any vascular scar bands over the quadratus femoris and the conjoint tendon of the gemelli and obturator internus. A blunt

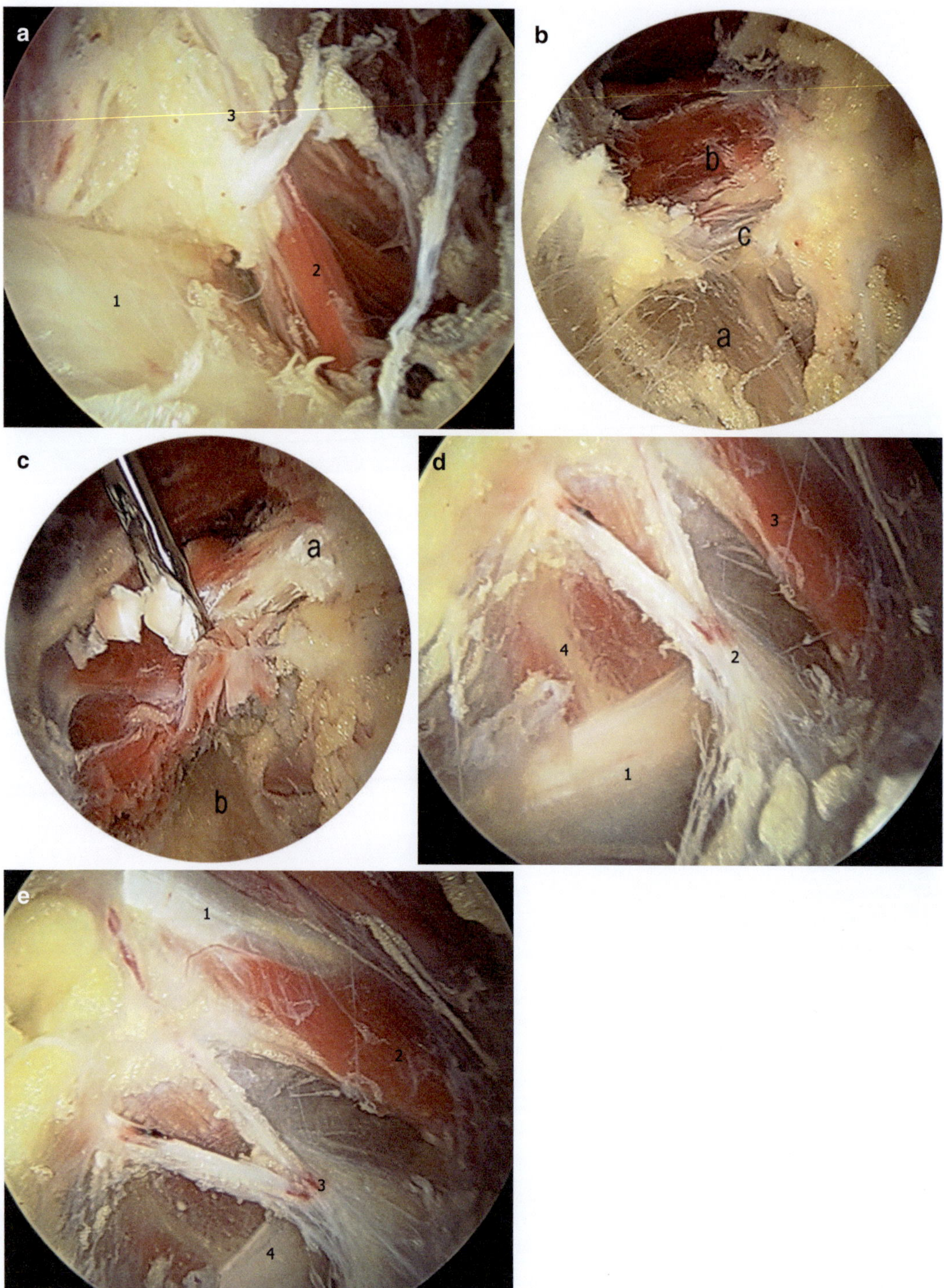

Fig. 1.30 (**a–e**) Piriformis tendon is identified proximally. (**a**): Left hip: (1) sciatic nerve, (2) piriformis muscle, (3) piriformis tendon. (**b**): Right hip: (a) sciatic nerve, (b) piriformis muscle, (c) piriformis tendon. (**c**): Right hip: (a) releasing the piriformis tendon, (b) sciatic nerve. (**d**): Left hip: (1) sciatic nerve, (2) branch of the inferior gluteal artery, (3) piriformis muscle (4). (**e**): (1) Piriformis tendon, (2) piriformis muscle, (3) branch of the inferior gluteal artery, (4) sciatic nerve

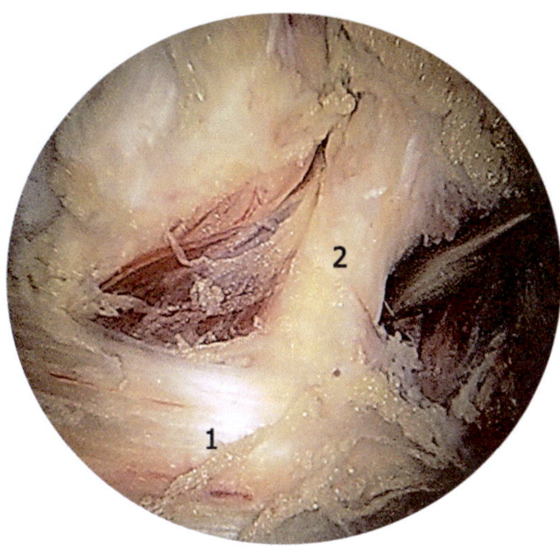

Fig. 1.31 Right hip: (1) sciatic nerve, (2) obturator internus

dissector, such as a switching stick, can be employed for release of scar bands. Fibrovascular tissue can also be cauterized with a radiofrequency probe (Fig. 1.32). The concept of fibrous bands playing a role in causing symptoms related to sciatic nerve mobility and entrapment represents a radical change in the current diagnosis of and therapeutic approach to DGS [10] (Fig. 1.33).

With the arthroscope visualizing the nerve, the hip can be flexed and rotated in any direction in order to assess not only the mobility but also for any evident of impingement. The kinematic excursion of the sciatic nerve is then assessed with the leg in flexion with internal/external rotation and full extension with internal/external rotation [1]. Finally, the piriformis muscle is located, and any abnormal anatomical variants

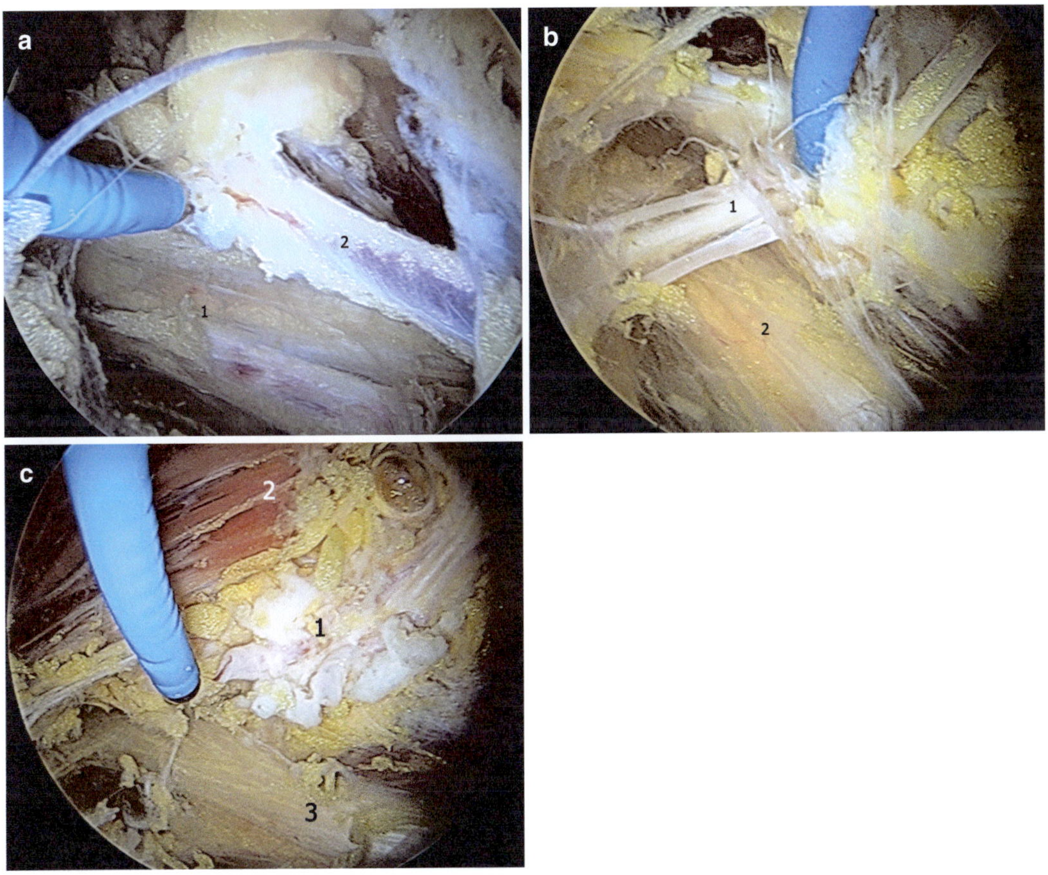

Fig. 1.32 (**a–c**) Vascular bands. (**a**): Right hip showing vascular tissue being cauterized with a radiofrequency probe. (1) Sciatic nerve. (2) Venous branch close to the nerve. (**b**) Right hip: (1) confluence of vessels, (2) sciatic nerve. (**c**) (1) Vessels after release, (2) piriformis (3) sciatic nerve

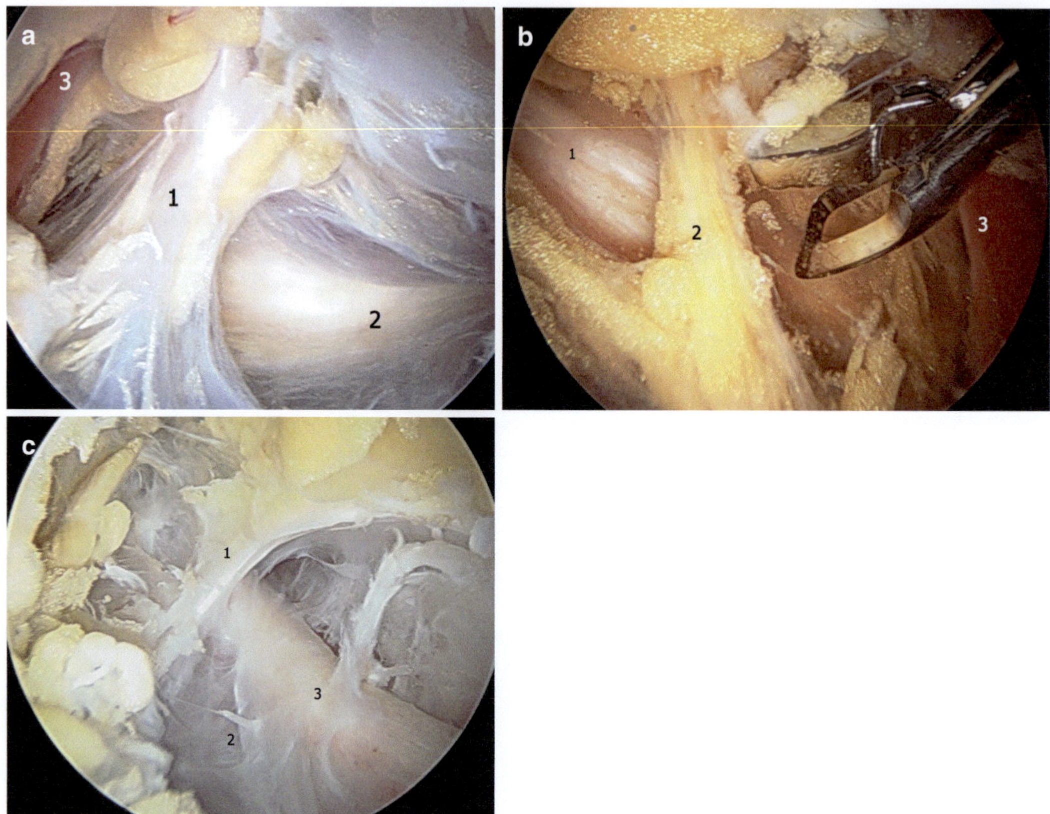

Fig. 1.33 (**a–c**) Fibrotic bands. (**a**): Right hip: (1) Fibrotic band. (2) Sciatic nerve. (3) Piriformis muscle. (**b**): Left hip: (1) Sciatic nerve. (2) Fibrofatty band. (3) Piriformis. (**c**): Right hip: (1) Proximal band. (2) Medial band. (3) Lateral medial band

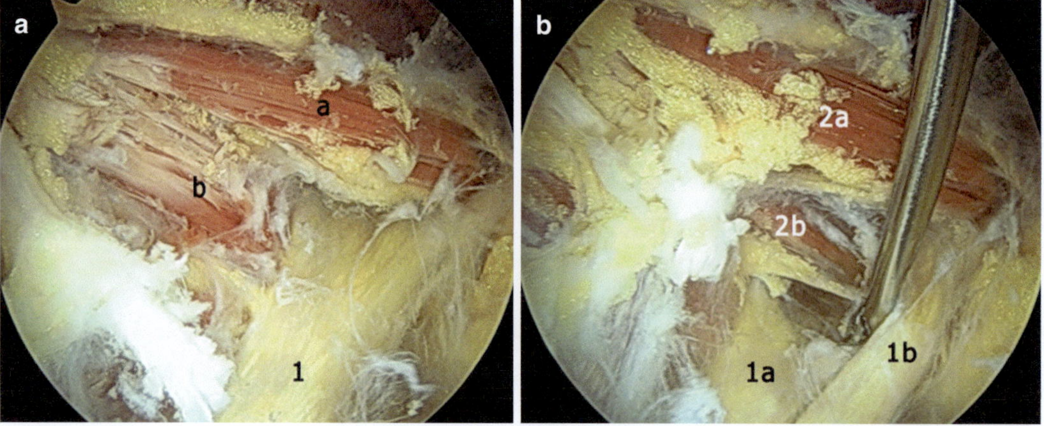

Fig. 1.34 (**a, b**) Anatomical variants of the sciatic. Endoscopic view showing a type B of Beaton. Left hip. (**a**): Before the identification of the sciatic branches, the sciatic nerve is passing through the piriformis muscle. (1) Sciatic nerve. (a) Superior piriformis. (b) Inferior piriformis. (**b**): After dissection, a divided sciatic nerve passing through and below the piriformis muscle is identified. (1a) Sciatic nerve: tibial branch. (1b) Common peroneal nerve pierces the piriformis. (2a) Inferior piriformis. (2b) Superior piriformis

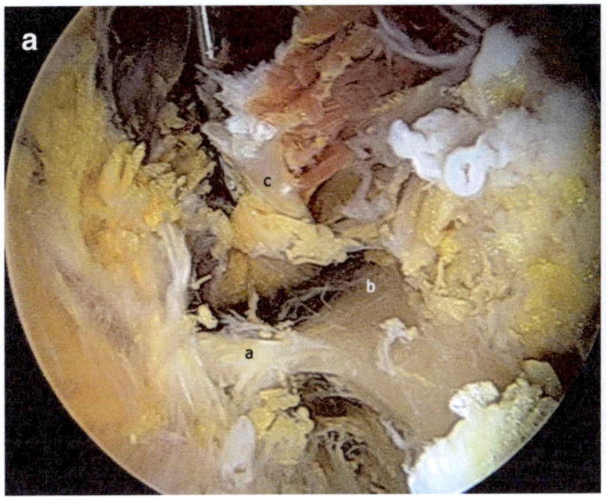
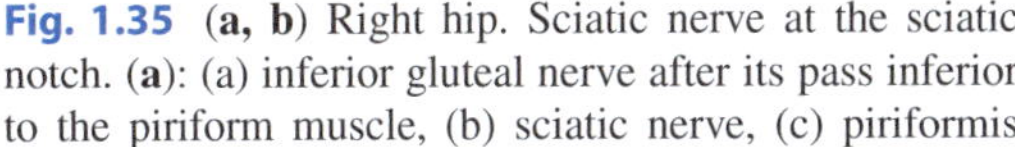
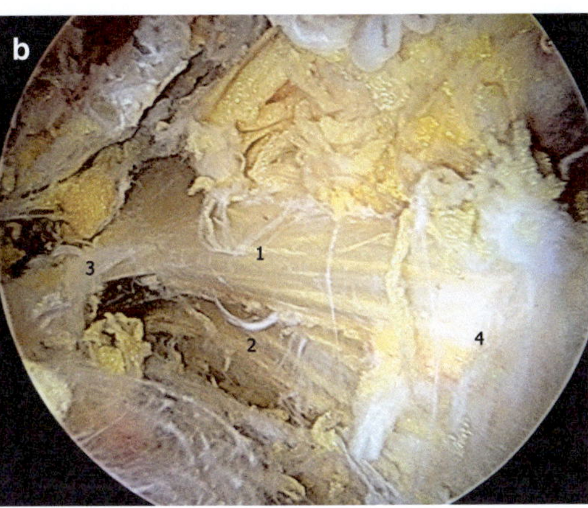

Fig. 1.35 (**a, b**) Right hip. Sciatic nerve at the sciatic notch. (**a**): (a) inferior gluteal nerve after its pass inferior to the piriform muscle, (b) sciatic nerve, (c) piriformis tendon after release. (**b**): (1) peroneal branch of the sciatic nerve, (2) tibialis nerve branch of the sciatic nerve, (3) inferior gluteal nerve, (4) sciatic nerve running distally

are identified (Fig. 1.34). Constant attention must be paid to the branches of the inferior gluteal artery lying in proximity to the piriformis muscle. Looking back proximal, in the region of the obturator internus, a superficial arterial branch of the inferior gluteal artery crosses the sciatic nerve laterally between the piriformis and superior gemellus muscles and must be cauterized and released prior to inspection of the piriformis with a radiofrequency probe. Some cases involve a large vessel or a confluence of vessels which may require ligation. The piriformis muscle can be classified as split, bulging split with the sciatic nerve passing through the body, split tendon with an anterior and posterior component, and split in two distinct components with one dorsally and one inferiorly going between a bifurcated sciatic nerve [1].

In many cases, a thick tendon can hide under the belly of the piriformis overlying the nerve. A rotatory shaver can be used to shave the distal border of the piriformis muscle to gain adequate access to the piriformis tendon. Carefully grasp the tendon with arthroscopic scissors and pull the scissors toward you to ensure only the tendon is released. The superior gluteal nerve and artery are in proximity and must be diligently avoided. Identify the inferior gluteal nerve after its pass inferior to the piriform muscle and possible anatomical variations of the sciatic nerve (Fig. 1.35).

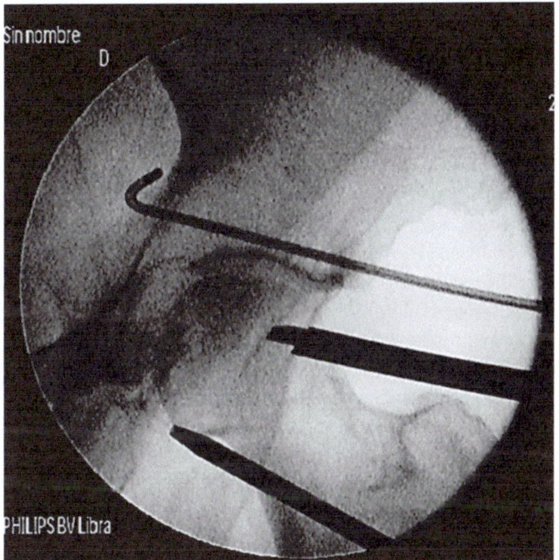

Fig. 1.36 Fluoroscopic view showing location of the scope and instruments in the deep gluteal space. Probe at the sciatic notch. Switching stick at the ischial tunnel

Finally probe the sciatic nerve up to the sciatic notch (Fig. 1.36).

Summary

Currently, there is unprecedented enthusiasm for hip arthroscopy, as this modality is transforming the management of hip injuries. The development of periarticular hip endoscopy has led to an understanding of the pathophysiological mechanisms underlying piriformis syndrome, which has supported its further classification. Careful preoperative planning, precise portal placement, a knowledge of the anatomy and potential complications, and a methodical sequence of endoscopic examination are essential for effective arthroscopy of any joint. A better knowledge of the deep gluteal space anatomy will help the surgeons to identify the different structures and treat their pathologies. The whole sciatic nerve trajectory in the deep gluteal space can be addressed by an endoscopic surgical technique, allowing the treatment of the diverse causes of sciatic nerve entrapment. The technique of endoscopic decompression of the sciatic nerve requires significant hip arthroscopy experience with familiarity with the gross and endoscopic anatomy.

References

1. Martin HD, Shears SA, Johnson JC, Smathers AM, Palmer IJ. The endoscopic treatment of sciatic nerve entrapment/deep gluteal syndrome. Arthroscopy. 2011;27(2):172–81.
2. Martin HD, Palmer IJ, Hatem MA. Deep gluteal syndrome. In: Nho S, Leunig M, Kelly B, Bedi A, Larson C, editors. Hip arthroscopy and hip joint preservation surgery. New York: Springer; 2014. p. 1–17.
3. Bierry G, Simeone FJ, Borg-Stein JP, Clavert P, Palmer WE. Sacrotuberous ligament: relationship to normal, torn, and retracted hamstring tendons on MR images. Radiology. 2014;271(1):162–71.
4. Martin HD, Savage A, Braly BA, et al. The function of the hip capsular ligaments: a quantitative report. Arthroscopy. 2008;24:188–95.
5. Hewitt JD, Glisson RR, Guilak F, et al. The mechanical properties of the human hip capsule ligaments. J Arthroplasty. 2002;17:82–9.
6. Loukas M, Louis RG Jr, Hallner B, Gupta AA, White D. Anatomical and surgical considerations of the sacrotuberous ligament and its relevance in pudendal nerve entrapment syndrome. Surg Radiol Anat. 2006;28:163–9.
7. Henry AK. Exposures in the lower limb. In: Extensile exposures. Baltimore: Williams & Wilkins; 1970. p. 180–97.
8. Testut L, Latarjet A. Anatomía humana. 4th ed. Barcelona: Salvat Editores SA; 1990. p. 660–76.
9. Pfirrmann CWA, Chung CB, Theumann NH, et al. Greater trochanter of the hip. Attachment of the abductor mechanism and a complex of three bursae – MR imaging and MR bursography in cadavers and MR imaging in asymptomatic volunteers. Radiology. 2001;221:469–77.
10. Hernando MF, Cerezal L, Pérez-Carro L, Abascal F, Canga A. Deep gluteal syndrome: anatomy, imaging, and management of sciatic nerve entrapments in the subgluteal space. Skeletal Radiol. 2015;44(7):919–34.
11. Shinohara H. Gemelli and obturator internus muscles: different heads of one muscle? Anat Rec. 1995;243:145–50.
12. Solomon LB, Lee YC, Callary SA, Beck M, Howie DW. Anatomy of piriformis, obturator internus and obturator externus: implications for the posterior surgical approach to the hip. J Bone Joint Surg Br. 2010;92:1317–24.
13. Hallin RP. Sciatic pain and the piriformis muscle. Postgrad Med. 1983;74:69–72.
14. Chen WS. Bipartite piriformis muscle: an unusual cause of sciatic nerve entrapment. Pain. 1994;58:269–72.
15. Beason LE, Anson BJ. The relation of the sciatic nerve and its subdivisions to the piriformis muscle. Anat Rec. 1937;70:1–5.
16. Pecina M. Contribution to the etiological explanation of the piriformis syndrome. Acta Anat. 1979;105:181–7.
17. Roche JJ, Jones CD, Khan RJ, Yates PJ. The surgical anatomy of the piriformis tendon, with particular reference to total hip replacement: a cadaver study. Bone Joint J. 2013;95-B:764–9.
18. Van der Made AD, Wieldraaijer T, Kerkhoffs GM, Kleipool RP, Engebretsen L, Van Dijk CN, Golano P. The hamstring muscle complex. Knee Surg Sports Traumatol Arthrosc. 2015;23:2115–22.
19. Miller SL, Gill J, Webb GR. The proximal origin of the hamstrings and surrounding anatomy encountered during repair. A cadaveric study. J Bone Joint Surg Am. 2007;89(1):44–8.
20. Garrett WE Jr, Rich FR, Nikolaou PK, Vogler JB 3rd. Computed tomography of hamstring muscle strains. Med Sci Sports Exerc. 1989;21(5):506–14.
21. Beck M, Sledge JB, Gautier E, et al. The anatomy and function of the gluteus minimus muscle. J Bone Joint Surg Br. 2000;82:358–63.
22. Gottschalk F, Kourosh S, Leveau B. The functional anatomy of tensor fasciae latae and gluteus medius and minimus. J Anat. 1989;166:179–89.
23. Bywaters EGL. The bursae of the body. Ann Rheum Dis. 1965;24:215–8.
24. Duparc F, Thomine JM, Dujardin F, et al. Anatomic basis of the transgluteal approach to the hip-joint by anterior hemimyotomy of the gluteus medius. Surg Radiol Anat. 1997;19:61–7.
25. Standring S. Gray's anatomy the anatomical basis of clinical practice. London: Churchill Livingstone Elsevier; 2008.
26. Akita K, Sakamoto H, Sato T. Arrangement and innervation of the glutei medius and minimus and the piriformis: a morphological analysis. Anat Rec. 1994;238:125–30.
27. Lavigne P, de Loriot Rouvray TH. The superior gluteal nerve. Anatomical study of its extrapelvic portion and surgical resolution by trans-gluteal

approach. Rev Chir Orthop Reparatrice Appar Mot. 1994;80:188–95.

28. Diop M, Parratte B, Tatu L, et al. Anatomical bases of superior gluteal nerve entrapment syndrome in the piriformis foramen. Surg Radiol Anat. 2002;24:155–9.

29. Thomine JM, Duparc F, Dujardin F, et al. Abord transglutéal de hanche par hémimyotomie antérieure du gluteus medius. Rev Chir Orthop. 1999;85:520–5.

30. Apaydin N, Bozkurt M, Loukas M, et al. The course of the inferior gluteal nerve and surgical landmarks for its localization during posterior approaches to hip. Surg Radiol Anat. 2009;31:415–8.

31. Ling ZX, Kumar VP. The course of the inferior gluteal nerve in the posterior approach to the hip. J Bone Joint Surg Br. 2006;88:1580–3.

32. Smoll NR. Variations of the piriformis and sciatic nerve with clinical consequence: a review. Clin Anat. 2010;23(1):8–17.

33. Natsis K, Totlis T, Konstantinidis GA, Paraskevas G, Piagkou M, Koebke J. Anatomical variations between the sciatic nerve and the piriformis muscle: a contribution to surgical anatomy in piriformis syndrome. Surg Radiol Anat. 2014;36(3):273–80.

34. Güvençer M, Iyem C, Akyer P, Tetik S, Naderi S. Variations in the high division of the sciatic nerve and relationship between the sciatic nerve and the piriformis. Turk Neurosurg. 2009;19(2):139–44.

35. Hollinshead WH. Anatomy for surgeons: the back and limbs. 3rd ed. Philadelphia: Harper & Row; 1982.

36. Sunderland S, Hughes ES. Metrical and non-metrical features of the muscular branches of the sciatic nerve and its medial and lateral popliteal divisions. J Comp Neurol. 1946;85:205–22.

37. Sunderland S, Ray LJ. The intraneural topography of the sciatic nerve and its popliteal divisions in man. Brain. 1948;71:242–73.

38 Moayeri N, Groen GJ. Differences in quantitative architecture of sciatic nerve may explain differences in potential vulnerability to nerve injury, onset time, and minimum effective anesthetic volume. Anesthesiology. 2009;111:1128–34.

39. Georgakis E, Soames R. Arterial supply to the sciatic nerve in the gluteal region. Clin Anat. 2008;21:62–5.

40. Karmanska W, Mikusek J, Karmanski A. Nutrient arteries of the human sciatic nerve. Folia Morphol (Warsz). 1993;52:209–15.

41. Ugrenovic SZ, Jovanovic ID, Vasovic LP, Stefanovic BD. Extraneural arterial blood vessels of human fetal sciatic nerve. Cells Tissues Organs. 2007;186:147–53.

42. Del Pinal F, Taylor GI. The venous drainage of nerves; anatomical study and clinical implications. Br J Plast Surg. 1990;43:511–20.

43. Coppieters MW, Alshami AM, Babri AS, Souvlis T, Kippers V, Hodges PW. Strain and excursion of the sciatic, tibial, and plantar nerves during a modified straight leg raising test. J Orthop Res. 2006;24:1883–9.

44. Franco CD. Posterior approach to the sciatic nerve in adults: is Euclidean geometry still necessary? Anesthesiology. 2003;98:723–8.

45. Standring S, editor. Gray's anatomy. 39th ed. Edinburgh: Elsevier; 2005. p. 1457.

46. Franco CD, Choksi N, Rahman A, et al. A subgluteal approach to the sciatic nerve in adults at 10 cm from the midline. Reg Anesth Pain Med. 2006;31:215–20.

47. Windhofer C, Brenner E, Moriggl B, et al. Relationship between the descending branch of the inferior gluteal artery and the posterior femoral cutaneous nerve applicable to flap surgery. Surg Radiol Anat. 2002;24:253–7.

48. Schraffordt SE, Tjandra JJ, Eizenberg N, et al. Anatomy of the pudendal nerve and its terminal branches: a cadaver study. ANZ J Surg. 2004;74:23–6.

49. Mathes SJ, Nahai F. Reconstructive surgery: principles, anatomy, and technique. New York: Churchill Livingstone; 1997. p. 501–35.

50. Kalhor M, Beck M, Huff TW, Ganz R. Capsular and pericapsular contributions to acetabular and femoral head perfusion. J Bone Joint Surg Am. 2009;91:409–18.

51. Gautier E, Ganz K, Krugel N, Gill T, Ganz R. Anatomy of the medial femoral circumflex artery and its surgical implications. J Bone Joint Surg Br. 2000;82:679–83.

52. Carliouz H, Pous JG, Rey JC. Les epiphysiolyses femorales superrieures. Rev Chir Orthop Reparatice Appar Mot. 1968;54:388–481.

53. Perez Carro L, Golano P, Fernandez EN, Ruperez VM, Victor Diego V, Cerezal L. Normal articular anatomy. In: Kim J, editor. Hip magnetic resonance imaging. Berlin: Springer; 2014. p. 57–72.

54. Voos JE, Rudzki JR, Shinkdle MK, et al. Arthroscopic anatomy and surgical techniques for peritrochanteric space disorders in the hip. Arthroscopy. 2007;23:1246.e1–5.

55. Robertson WJ, Kelly BT. The safe zone for hip arthroscopy: a cadaveric assessment of central, peripheral, and lateral compartment portal placement. Arthroscopy. 2008;24:1019–26.

56. Guanche CA. Hip arthroscopy techniques: deep gluteal space access. In: Nho SJ, et al., editors. Hip arthroscopy and hip joint preservation surgery. New York: Springer; 2015. p. 351–60.

57. Martin HD, Hatem MA, Champlin K, Palmer IJ. The endoscopic treatment of sciatic nerve entrapment/deep gluteal syndrome. Tech Orthop. 2012;27:172–83.

Hip-Spine Effect: Hip Pathology Contributing to Lower Back, Posterior Hip, and Pelvic Pain

Anthony Nicholas Khoury, Juan Gómez-Hoyos, and Hal D. Martin

Introduction

Low back pain is an epidemic with an estimated 80% of the global population complaining of symptoms [1]. The complex nature of the pathology and confounding variables that attribute to the pain are poorly understood. In the United States, more than 1.5 million lumbar magnetic resonance imaging studies are performed every year. Three hundred thousand MRIs report nerve root compression, and only 200,000 patients obtain relief from discectomies or surgeries directed at relieving pressure on the spinal roots [2]. Physicians who treat spinal-related complaints should recognize that other orthopedic diagnoses involving the hip or lower limb are present in approximately 86% of the cases [2].

The prevalence of low back pain in the population results in a high level of cost for treatment. Currently, the low back pain symptoms are the most frequent motive for consultation, generally treated by both orthopedic surgeons and neurosurgeons. Low back pain treatment varies depending on the surgical discipline consulted; however, the majority of patients display no abnormalities on MRI and do not achieve pain relief from procedures directed at alleviating pressure on the spinal roots [2]. Failure to diagnose the underlying pathology may result in opioid addiction.

The first description of a coexistence between lumbar pain and hip abnormalities was produced by Offierski in 1983 [3]. Lumbar pathology has been shown to explain hip pain, as hip pathology has been involved in the development of lumbar pain by the disruption of normal lumbopelvic kinematics. The classical definition of hip-spine syndrome proposed by Offierski considers a concomitant hip and spine pathology and differentiates presentation as "simple," "complex," and "secondary." Simple hip-spine syndrome is considered as only one source of pathology, whereas the complex is a dual hip and spine disability

A. N. Khoury, MS (✉)
Hip Preservation Center, Baylor University Medical Center, Baylor Scott and White Health, Dallas, TX, USA

Bioengineering Department, University of Texas at Arlington, Arlington, TX, USA
e-mail: Anthony.Khoury@bswhealth.org

J. Gómez-Hoyos, MD
International Consultant, Hip Preservation Center / Baylor Scott and White Research Institute, Baylor University Medical Center, Dallas, TX, USA

Department of Orthopaedic Surgery - Health Provider Clínica Las Américas / Clínica del Campestre, Medellin, Antioquia, Colombia

Professor - School of Medicine - Sports Medicine Program, Universidad de Antioquia, Medellín, Antioquia, Colombia

H. D. Martin, DO
Medical and Research Director, Hip Preservation Center, Baylor University Medical Center, Dallas, TX, USA

© Springer International Publishing AG, part of Springer Nature 2019
H. D. Martin, J. Gómez-Hoyos (eds.), *Posterior Hip Disorders*,
https://doi.org/10.1007/978-3-319-78040-5_2

without a clear pathologic source. The "secondary" classification recognizes a coexistent contribution of hip and spine pathology to pain [3–5]. This rudimentary classification requires updating based on current understanding of biomechanics. Hip pathologies that contribute to lumbar pain include flexion deformities [3], osteoarthritis [6, 7], developmental dysplasia of the hip [8], and limited hip range of motion [9, 10]. Recently, biomechanical studies have been developed to investigate the biomechanical relationship between abnormal hip pathology and lumbar spine kinematics. The biomechanical studies aim to address specific contributors to lumbar pathology arising in the hip, as opposed to the classical definition in which the disease occurs simultaneously. The authors of the biomechanical studies instead propose a unique categorization of flexion, extension, and flexion and extension hip-spine effect (Table 2.1).

Accurate assessment of the hip joint requires a multi-level approach that takes into consideration the numerous structures surrounding the hip. These levels include the (1) osseous, (2) capsulolabral, (3) musculotendinous, (4) neurovascular, and (5) kinematic chain (see Chap. 3). The kinematic chain level is the most critical level for advanced understanding of the hip-spine relationship because the hip is the center axis of body movement. Abnormalities in any of the levels of the hip joint

affect the overall kinematic chain motion and lead to disruptions in normal movement. Maintaining a registry that includes iHot, mHHS, and Oswestry Disability Index is recommended.

Structural anatomic orientation is a critical factor for proper body function. Any deviations from normal anatomy may have a profound impact on body motion through kinematic chain disturbances. The comorbidity of hip- and lumbar-related pain is especially observed in athletic activities including baseball and golf. Causation of pain during activity may be directly related to amplified mechanotransduction of forces and compensatory joint kinematics [11]. Cam impingement specifically is abundant in a younger athletic population in which large hip range of motion is required [12–16].

Current treatment methods for hip and lumbar spine pathologies have largely focused on the individual components without accounting for the global effects of the structures involved. The biomechanics of hip pathology must be studied in depth to provide a discreet knowledge of diseases. Advanced understanding will allow for more comprehensive surgical and conservative treatment planning, as well as the development of devices that correct the problem effectively and economically. Ben-Galim et al. reported improvement in low back pain symptoms following total hip arthroplasty [6]. Similar publications addressing low back pain relief after hip pathology treatment including arthroscopy [9] and physical therapy [10] have produced promising conclusions about the hip-spine relationship.

Osseous impingements that restrict normal hip motion include ischiofemoral impingement and femoroacetabular impingement. Femoroacetabular impingement is an abnormal osseous contact between the proximal femur and acetabular rim that occurs during end-range hip motion [13].

Recent investigations regarding the biomechanical interactions between hip pathologies including ischiofemoral impingement, femoroacetabular impingement, and femoral version have been conducted. Patients seeking treatment of these commonly diagnosed and treated hip pathologies have reported low back pain relief.

Table 2.1 Descriptive classification of the Hip-spine effect

1. *Limited hip motion in extension*
1.1 Ischiofemoral impingement
1.2 Anterior capsular hip contracture
1.3 Quadricep contracture
2. *Limited hip motion in flexion*
2.1. Anterior hip impingement
2.1.a. Pincer-type
2.1.b. Cam-type
2.1.c. Mixed-type
2.1.d. Subspinous
2.2 Posterior hip capsular contracture
2.3 Hamstring contracture
3. *Flexion and extension hip-spine*
3.1 Abnormal femoral neck version
3.2 Abnormal pelvic tilt
3.3 Hip osteoarthritis

To fully understand the relationships between these pathologies and lumbar pain, cadaveric models have been developed. The cadaveric model provides a scientifically reproducible medium for testing the intricate hip-spine interactions due to real-life conditions and variability within samples that reflect a more normal population. Regional deformation and load change in the lumbar region as a consequence of abnormal hip anatomy provides valuable information on how the hip affects the spine, and its converse.

This chapter will introduce the structural aspects of the complex biomechanical relationship between hip pathology, including ischiofemoral impingement, anterior hip impingement, and abnormal femoral anteversion, with the lumbar spine.

Ischiofemoral Impingement

Ischiofemoral impingement is characterized as decreased space between the lesser trochanter of the femur and ischium of the pelvis (Fig. 2.1). The smallest distance between these two osseous structures is commonly defined by magnetic resonance imaging, with the feet taped in the natural walking position to dynamically assess the pathology. An ischiofemoral space distance less than 17 mm is a diagnostic feature for ischiofemoral impingement [17]. Reports by Torriani et al. included subjects reporting low back pain symptoms resulting from ischiofemoral impingement restrictions in hip motion [18]. Gómez-Hoyos et al. introduced two clinically relevant examinations to diagnose ischiofemoral impingement with high sensitivity [19]. The ischiofemoral impingement test yielded a sensitivity of 0.82 and the long-stride walking test a sensitivity of 0.94. The reproduction of pain during these examinations suggests a significant cause-effect relationship with a terminal hip extension block. Secondary responses to the impingement can influence lumbopelvic kinematics.

Ischiofemoral impingement was utilized by Gómez-Hoyos et al. as a hip extension deficit model to simulate a primary hip-spine effect due to the limited terminal hip extension effect produced by the hip pathology [20]. The study was the first to develop a biomechanical cadaveric model for measuring a hip-spine interaction. Ischiofemoral impingement was simulated by creating a zero-space impingement between the lesser trochanter and lateral aspect of the ischial tuberosity using metallic washers (Fig. 2.2). The specimen was positioned laterally, and the leg was moved to 10° and 20° hip extension in neutral hip abduction (Fig. 2.3). The loading differential between the native ischiofemoral space state and simulated impingement state, measured in newtons (N), of the L3-L4 and L4-L5 spinal facet joints was used to assess the biomechanical relationship between the hip pathology and lumbar spine. The spinal facet joints were accessed through a direct posterior approach. An incision was created in the facet joint to allow placement of ultra-sensitive piezoresistive force sensors (Tekscan, Inc.) (Fig. 2.4). Resultant data described significant increase in lumbar facet joint loading during the impingement state, as compared to the native state for L3-L4 and L4-L5 spine segments. An average 30.81% increase in facet joint overload was observed between impinged state and native state.

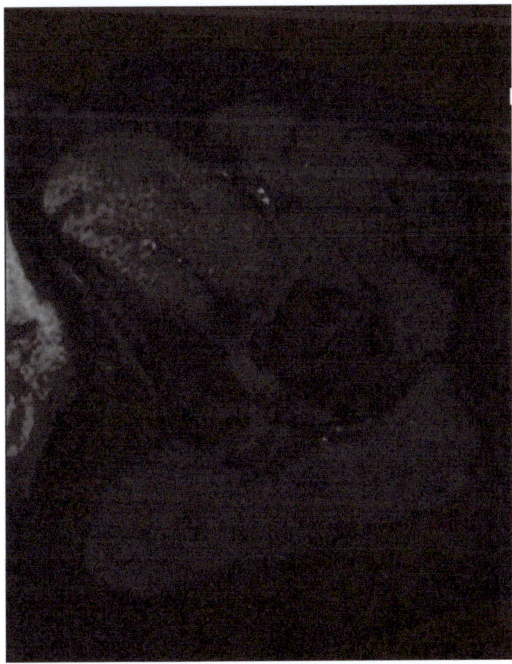

Fig. 2.1 Ischiofemoral impingement visualized with MRI

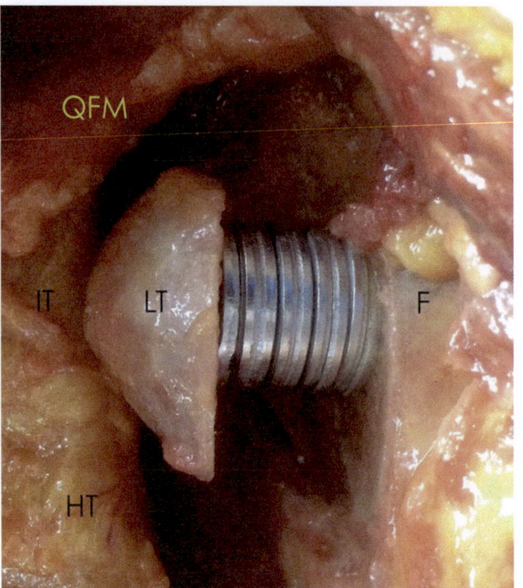

Fig. 2.2 Lesser trochanter osteotomy to simulate ischiofemoral impingement (*F* femur, *HT* hamstrings' tendon origin, *IT* ischial tuberosity, *LT* lesser trochanter, *QFM* quadratus femoris muscle)

The load-bearing properties of facet joints and intervertebral disks in response to frontal plane pelvic obliquity were recently investigated by Popovich et al. [21]. The characteristic patterns studied showed significant interactions in the load-sharing properties of the lumbar spine segments during various directional loading parameters commonly experienced. Cadaveric lumbosacral segments were subjected to flexion/extension, lateral bending, and axial rotation with the facet joints and intervertebral disks measured. The largest facet joint loading was observed during rotation moments, especially when combined with pelvic obliquity. Conversely, intradiscal pressure was found to be highest in flexion and lateral bending positions of the spine. Isolated lumbar spinal flexion resulted in the lowest value facet joint loading. This finding is relevant to ischiofemoral impingement and supports the biomechanical relationship observed in the study by Gómez-Hoyos et al. Ischiofemoral impingement

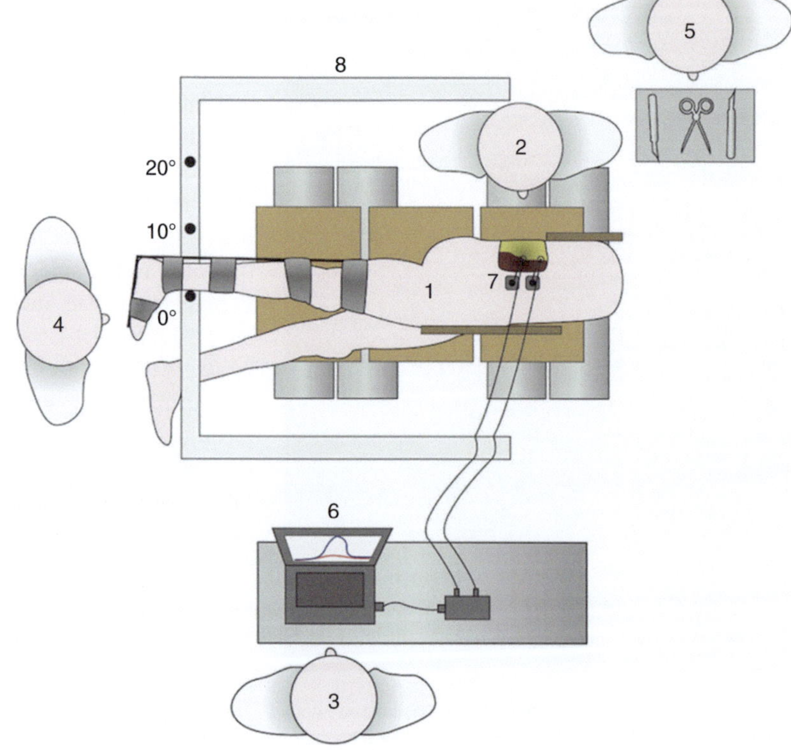

Fig. 2.3 Experimental setup and testing methods for ischiofemoral impingement and femoral version (1. Superior view of specimen positioned laterally on a dissection table with two fixated boards; 2. Surgical approach and sensor placement; 3. Engineer operating force sensor device; 4. Physical therapist manipulating leg positions for testing conditions; 5. Surgical assistant; 6. Computer software recording peak lumbar facet forces; 7. Sensor placement in facet joints; 8. Custom designed PVC frame)

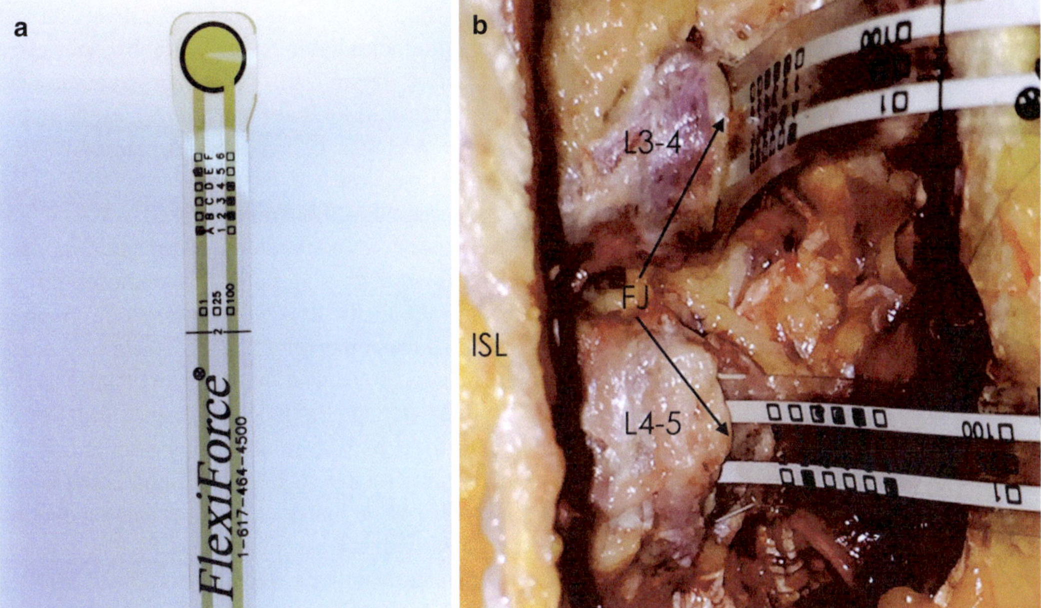

Fig. 2.4 Ultra-sensitive piezoresistive (**a**) force sensor and (**b**) placement in L3-L4 and L4-L5 lumbar facet joints. (*FJ* facet joint, *ISL* interspinous ligament)

causes a terminal block during hip extension. The resulting mechanism is a pelvic anterior tilt. Further consequences of the block result in lumbar spine extension and an increase in spinal facet joint loading due to premature coupling. Although intervertebral disk measurement were not reported in this study, one can safely assume a decrease in intervertebral disk loading, as the disk is unloaded in the spine extension state.

The presented studies addressing lumbar spine biomechanics in the presence of altered movement and impingement provide significant insight into possible low back pain and Sacroiliac joint mechanisms. Ischiofemoral impingement was shown to increase lumbar facet joint loading. Facet joints function to transmit applied loading to the spine in addition to directing motion [22–26]. These mechanotransduction properties inhibit potential overloading to not only the spinal segments but nerve roots and intradiscal tissue. A biomechanical study performed by Yang et al. describes facet joints bearing approximately 3–25% of compressive loads [23]. The facet joint capsule contains several mechanoreceptive, proprioceptive, and nociceptive nerve endings. The nerve endings can also be found in abundance

within the subchondral bone and synovium [24, 27–30]. The presented biomechanical studies describe significant increased loading profiles in response to hip movement. An untreated pathology, such as ischiofemoral impingement, causing consistent prominent joint loading can result in low back pain due to increased nerve ending activation. Secondary issues can influence central nervous system response and dysfunction [22].

Ischiofemoral impingement is but one of several factors that can contribute to abnormal hip and spine mechanics. A terminal hip extension block resulting from the impingement causes increased loading in the spinal facet joints. Further sections utilize the spinal facet joint to measure the impact of other hip pathologies.

Femoral Version and the Iliofemoral Ligament

Femoral neck version is the axial orientation of the femoral neck in relation to the horizontal axis of the posterior femoral condyles [31–33]. For males, average femoral neck version is anteriorly oriented in 10° and 20° for females [33, 34].

Patients presenting with abnormal femoral neck version have concomitant gait symptoms as a result of rotational misalignment of the lower extremities. Decreased femoral neck version occurs when the femoral neck version is less than 10° and the femoral head has a posterior projection into the acetabular cup. Femoral retroversion is considered as femoral neck version below 0°.

The vector ground reaction force changes through the gait cycle. Upon initial contact, heel strike, the ground reaction vector force is toward the anterior region of the hip joint. The vector then moves posteriorly as the gait cycle progresses [35]. Any alterations to the natural anatomy, whether osseous, musculotendinous, or capsulolabral, affect the normal transmission of the force vector during the gait cycle. Specifically, the axial orientation of the femoral neck affects the capsulolabral and musculotendinous structure of the hip and lumbar spine. Therefore, the ground reaction forces transmitted during gait may be interrupted by an abnormal femoral neck angle. Gómez-Hoyos et al. investi-

gated the effect of abnormal femoral version and the iliofemoral ligament on the lumbar spine, in a cadaveric model [36]. The authors hypothesized an increase in lumbar facet loading would occur in the presence of simulated decreased (−10°) femoral version.

Increased (+30°) and decreased (−10°) femoral version were simulated in cadaveric models. The femoral version values were chosen due to bony impingements causing a premature coupling block beyond the values. A transverse osteotomy was created distal to the lesser trochanter, and a lateral external fixator held the femoral segments. The distal portion of the femur was internally/externally rotated to achieve desired femoral version, based on native version measurements performed with CT imaging (Fig. 2.5). The hip was dynamically moved from 0° to 10° and 20° hip extension, with neutral abduction (Fig. 2.3). Ultra-sensitive piezoresistive force sensors were used to measure loading changes in the spine facet joints of L3-L4 and L4-L5 (Fig. 2.4). The increased/decreased femoral version state was

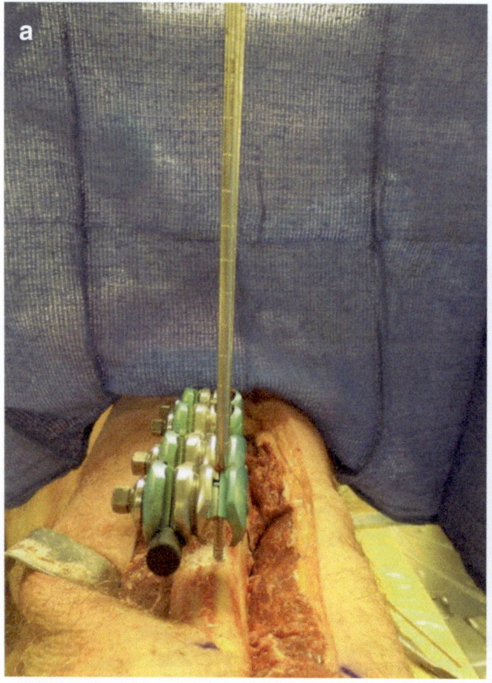
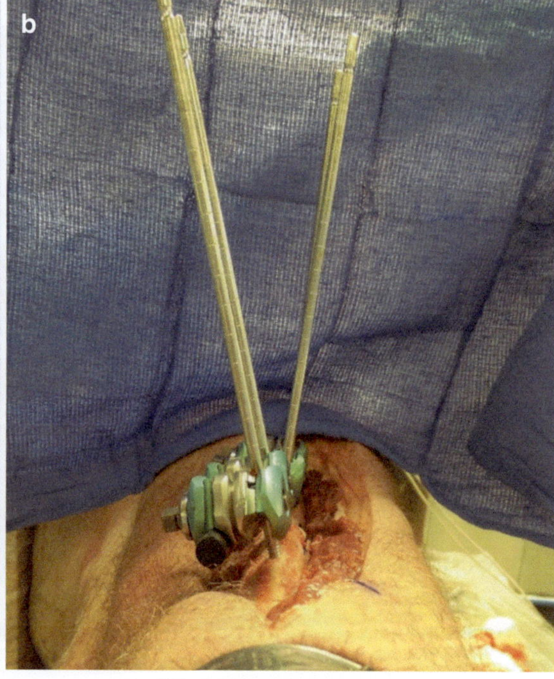

Fig. 2.5 Increased (+30°) and decreased (−10°) femoral version simulation. An osteotomy was performed prior to experimentation. The osteotomy was held in place with an external fixator (**a**). Femur distal to osteotomy was rotated to achieve increased or decreased femoral version with the foot in 0° rotation (**b**)

compared to the native state loading. Upon completion of version experiments, the medial and lateral arms of the iliofemoral ligament were released, at the mid-aspect of the ligament.

Contrary to the original hypothesis, the authors discovered a significant decrease in lumbar facet loading in the presence of decreased femoral version. Native version measures at 20° hip extension were reported to be 149.7 N in the L3-L4 facet joint and 147.9 N in the L4-L5 facet joint. In the simulated decreased femoral version (−10°) state, the measured loading was 74.3 N in the L3-L4 joint and 103.4 N in the L4-L5. The peak percent change between native and decreased femoral version was a 173.95% decrease for L3-L4 and 176.69% decrease for L4-L5. Increased femoral version, +30°, resulted in the largest mechanotransduction to the facet joints with reported values being 167.5 N in L3-L4 and 175.2 N in L4-L5.

Motivation to investigate the femoral version effect on lumbar facet loading is largely based on clinical observations. A recent case study by Martin et al. reported femoral de-rotational osteotomy to restore native femoral version resulted in relief of low back pain symptoms in all patients included in the cohort [37]. Mean Harris hip score postsurgery increased 24.5% from an average presurgery average of 70.7–88.0. Visual analog scale showed significant improvement, with patients reporting a 70.6% improvement postsurgery. The discrepancy between clinical observations and laboratory experiments for decreased femoral version concludes a profound impact on the lumbar spine resulting from abnormal hip anatomy.

Femoral version dictates the rotatory alignment of the long axis of the femur. Version of the femoral head, associated with inclination of the pelvis, allows for hip flexion to be transposed into rotatory movements of the femoral head [38]. Factors including muscle activity and kinetic direction are contributors to rotatory movements and are guided by pelvic tilt and rotation. Facet loading compensation can also be a factor of pelvic tilt. Femoral version dictates sacral slope, therefore inducing lumbar lordosis adaptations and consequent inhibitions of trunk flexion [39, 40]. In the case of +30° anteversion, the sacral slope is increased, therefore introducing lumbar hyperlordosis. The hyperlordosis inhibits trunk forward flexion [40]. These abnormalities may also be influenced by mal-aligned hip prostheses.

Iliofemoral ligament release in the −10° femoral version state resulted in decreased lumbar facet joint loading in L3-L4 and L4-L5. Specifically, a 245.7% decrease was observed in L3-L4 and a 257.3% decrease in L4-L5, in 20° terminal hip extension. The hip capsule functions to restrict medial rotation, followed by extension, abduction, and finally lateral rotation [41]. During mid-stance to pre-swing of the gait cycle, the leg rotates medially. Capsuloligamentous and muscular restrictions to hip extension and medial rotation force the lumbar spine to rotate increasingly as a compensatory mechanism. As previously mentioned, the facet joints function to inhibit axial rotation; therefore, axial lumbar rotation may cause increased compressive forces of the impacted facet joint.

Gait analysis for patients with decreased femoral version was performed by Schröder et al. Real-time gait analysis provides valuable information on joint kinematics resulting from hip pathologies. Significant findings from this study include a decreased in terminal hip extension in the decreased femoral version cohort and significantly increased anterior pelvic tilt throughout the gait cycle. Additionally, L5 markers demonstrated increased contralateral rotation during the gait cycle. The results support findings and explanations of hip-related pathologies contributing to abnormal lumbar kinematics.

Femoroacetabular Impingement

Anterior hip impingement, specifically femoroacetabular impingement, is increasingly observed in the population [13]. The pathology exists in two forms: cam impingement and pincer impingement. Cam impingement is characterized by a bony overgrowth along the superior portion of the femoral head, resulting in an increased radius of the femoral neck at the femoral head-neck junction [42]. The cam impingement produces shear forces which results in an "outside-in" acetabular cartilage damage and labral tears. Excessive hip flexion maneuvers place the anterosuperior femoral head within the acetabulum. The presence of a cam-type impingement amplifies the damage as the femoral head-neck junction rolls into the acetabulum [13]. Hip flexion may contribute to abnormal lumbopelvic kinematics. Kim et al. reported significantly decreased hip flexion in the seated position in subjects with low back pain and increased posterior pelvic tilt [43]. Pincer impingement is a bony overgrowth along the acetabular border and is a result of abnormal acetabular development. Similar to the pincer impingement, continued excessive hip movements contribute to labral damage and delamination of cartilage. Pain is associated with these degenerative mechanisms, and early onset of osteoarthritis is a significant factor [12]. Cam and pincer impingement can occur independently or as a combination of the two.

As previously described with ischiofemoral impingement, abnormal bony hip anatomy alters normal lumbopelvic function and transmits increased mechanotransduction through the pelvis and spine. Cam and pincer impingements have been described to contribute to increased sacroiliac and lumbar spine stresses [11, 44–47]. Khoury et al. conducted a study to investigate the effect of cam-type impingement on lumbar spine loading [48]. Cam impingement was simulated in cadaveric models based on previously published methods [42] (Fig. 2.6). Ultra-sensitive piezoresistive force sensors were placed directly into the anterior portion of L3-L4, L4-L5, and L5-S1 intervertebral disks (Fig. 2.7). Loading in the disks was measured in the native and impinged state during 90° and 120° hip flexion, as well as hip flexion plus internal rotation. The final movement was an impingement test, at which the hip was flexed, internally rotated, and adducted. Peak intradiscal loading was observed in the L5-S1 segment (116 N) compared to L4-L5 (101 N) and L3-L4 (51 N) ($p < 0.001$). Hip flexion to 120° as well as flexion plus internal rotation resulted in the largest intradiscal pressures, 110 N and 106 N, respectively. The presented study con-

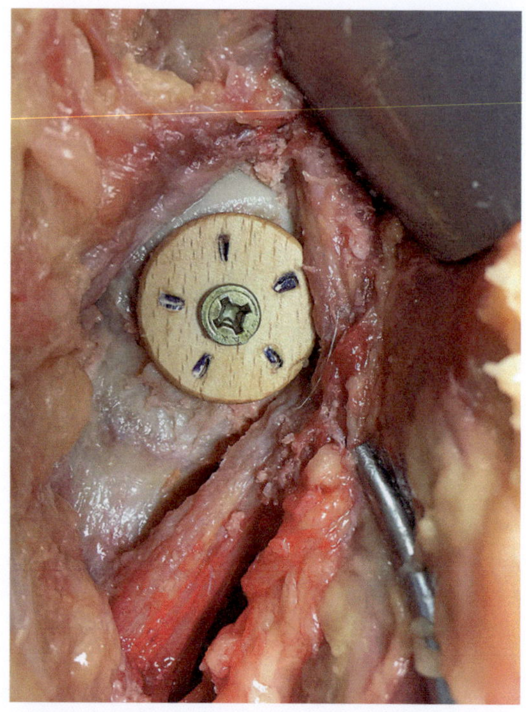

Fig. 2.6 Cam-type femoroacetabular impingement simulation. A fabricated wood was placed at the femoral head-neck junction

firmed a direct link kinematic chain relationship between simulated anterior hip impingement and lumbar intradiscal pressure during hip flexion and internal rotation.

Recent investigations regarding anterior hip impingement and lumbopelvic consequences have been conducted. Birmingham et al. introduced a simulated cam impingement to assess the impact of rotational motion at the pubic symphysis. Resultant data concluded cam impingement contributing to pubic symphysis rotation, an approximate 35% increase, after impingement occurs. Although pubic symphysis motion is common, premature contact as a result of abnormal bony hip parameters including cam impingement or decreased femoral version results in pathologic motion, especially during sports activity. Lamontagne et al. studied pelvic motion during maximal squat in subjects with cam impingement [12]. No differences in hip motion during the squat motion were observed in subjects with FAI compared to the control group; however the FAI group on average was not able to squat as low.

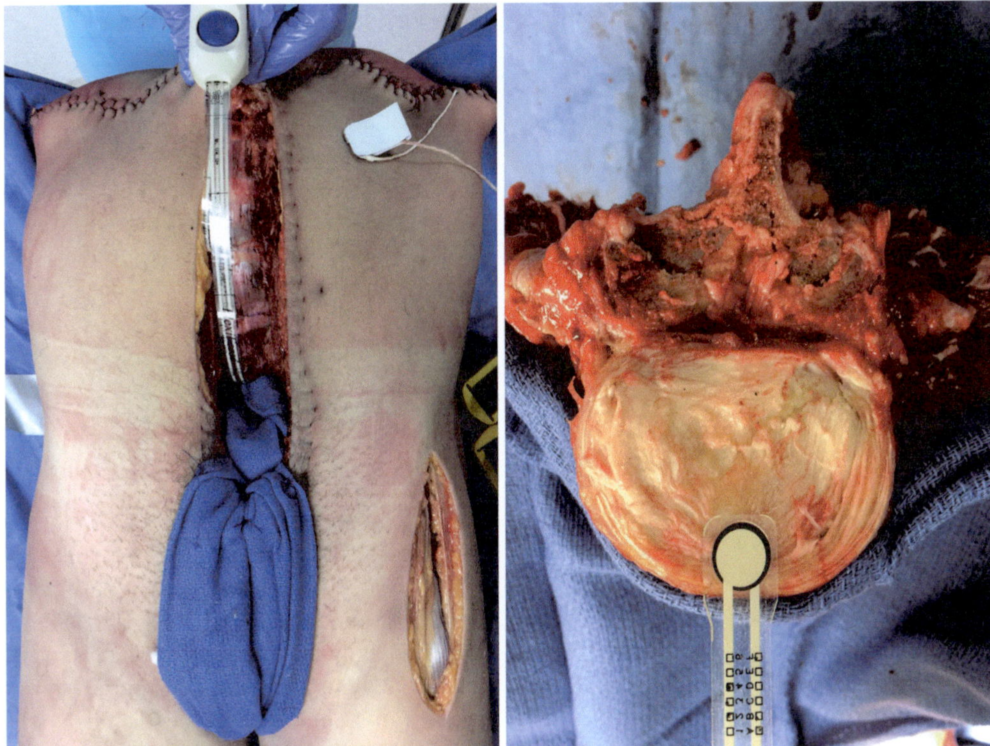

Fig. 2.7 Sensor placement in L3-L4, L4-L5, and L5-S1 intervertebral disk

A significant finding observed was a decrease in sagittal pelvic range of motion in the FAI group compared to the control group. The authors propose premature contact between the femur and acetabulum may occur with reduced sagittal pitch, however femoral torsion parameters were not controlled.

Nerve Kinematics and the Hip-Spine Effect

The presented three hip pathologies contribute to pelvic and spine symptoms through interruption of normal sciatic nerve kinematics. Nerve elongation, compression, and position are directly proportional to hip flexion and extension range of motion [49]. The location of the sciatic nerve within the deep gluteal space increases the likelihood of injury resulting from abnormal femoropelvic anatomy. The resultant nerve injuries are secondary effects of the hip pathology. In the case of ischiofemoral impingement, the sciatic nerve transverses through the ischiofemoral space. The decreased space may subject the nerve to increased compression forces as the lesser trochanter comes in contact with the ischium during hip extension (Fig. 2.8). Femoral version has been proven to influence sciatic nerve complications as well, independent of the lesser trochanter orientation and space. The increased femoral version can lead to greater trochanteric sciatic impingement (Fig. 2.9), in addition to hip flexion abduction and external rotation (FABER), and deviations from a normal kinematic track. Martin et al. described the effect of femoral version on nerve kinematics and proved the nerve relaxes with increasing abduction angles [50]. The posterior projection of the femoral head, observed with decreased femoral version, has been shown to elongate the sciatic nerve bedding during hip flexion [49]. Visual observations of the nerve during hip flexion revealed a torsional characteristic to the medial line [50]. The "spiraling" effect has not been proven in the literature; however anatomic descriptions of fiber band alignment exist

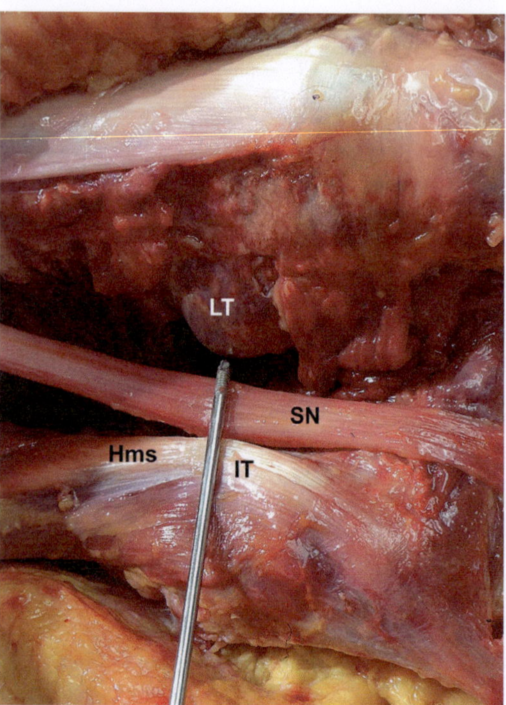

Fig. 2.8 Sciatic nerve impingement within the ischiofemoral space

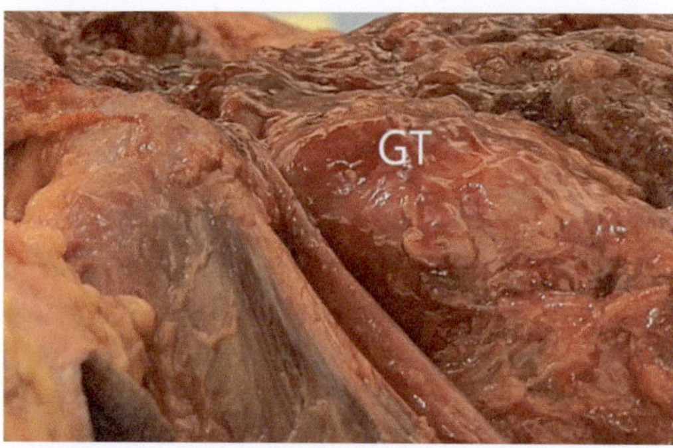

Fig. 2.9 Sciatic nerve impingement within the greater trochanter

and support this claim [51–53]. Lumbar spine and pelvic pain can be associated to increased mechanotransduction arising from abnormal femoral anatomy in addition to interruption of normal sciatic nerve kinematics.

The Pelvis and Sagittal Plane Balance

A critical factor within the hip-spine-pelvis core pathomechanics is sagittal plane imbalance. The impingements and bony abnormalities addressed affecting the mechanotransduction of load through the spine do so by influencing pelvic planes. Deviations in pelvic position alter spinal alignment [54]. The normal curvature of the lumbar spine allows for load to be uniformly distributed through the length of the spine.

Future Directions

Three-dimensional motion capture technologies provide an important medium to study hip-spine interactions. Studies including Schroder et al.'s not only act as research mediums for these interactions but also act as diagnostic tools for patients in a clinical setting. Simplified systems incorporating electromagnetic sensor systems are cost-efficient and provide ease of use for clinicians at any level. Primary investigations by the Hip Preservation Center regarding the lateral ischiofemoral impingement test describe a visualized anterior pelvic tilt during hip extension maneuvers. These findings support those determined by Schröder et al. and confirm anterior pelvic tilt occurs not only in the gait cycle but in a lateral position. Additional findings by the hip preservation group include the visualization of a hip-pelvis pathology in deep hip flexion with decreased femoral version subjects. The hip-pelvis interaction is a future direction of the overall hip-spine pathology. Premature coupling of the hip joint due to bony impingements and abnormal femoral version significantly impact normal lumbopelvic kinematics. Hip-spine-core abnormal kinematics directly influence kinematics opposite the plane of motion and affect all four levels of the human anatomy.

References

1. Huijbregts P. Lumbopelvic region: anatomy and bio-mechanics. In: Wadsworth C, editor. HSC 112 current concepts of orthopaedic physical therapy. LaCrosse, WI: Orthopaedic Section APTA; 2001.
2. Filler AG. Piriformis and related entrapment syndromes: diagnosis & management. Neurosurg Clin N Am. 2008;19(4):609–22.
3. Offierski CM, Macnab MB. Hip-spine syndrome. Spine (Phila Pa 1976). 1983;8(3):316–21.
4. Devin CJ, Mccullough KA, Morris BJ, Yates AJ, Kang JD. Hip-spine syndrome. J Am Acad Orthop Surg. 2012;20:434–42.
5. Buckland AJ, Miyamoto R, Patel RD, Slover J, Razi AE. Differentiating hip pathology from lumbar spine pathology: key points of evaluation and management. J Am Acad Orthop Surg. 2017;25(2):23–34.
6. Ben-galim P, Ben-galim T, Rand N, et al. Hip-spine syndrome the effect of total hip replacement surgery on low back pain in severe osteoarthritis of the hip. Spine (Phila Pa 1976). 2007;32(19):2099–102.
7. Fogel GR, Esses SI. Hip spine syndrome: management of coexisting radiculopathy and arthritis of the lower extremity. Spine J. 2003;3:238–41.
8. Matsuyama Y, Hasegawa Y, Yoshihara H, et al. Hip-spine syndrome: total sagittal alignment of the spine and clinical symptoms in patients with bilateral congenital hip dislocation. Spine (Phila Pa 1976). 2004;29(21):2432.
9. Redmond JM, Gupta A, Hammarstedt JE, Stake CE, Domb BG. The hip-spine syndrome: how does back pain impact the indications and outcomes of hip arthroscopy? Arthroscopy. 2014;30(7):872–81.
10. Lejkowski PM, Poulsen E. Elimination of intermittent chronic low back pain in a recreational golfer following improvement of hip range of motion impairments. J Bodyw Mov Ther. 2013;17(4):448–52.
11. Gebhart JJ, Weinberg DS, Conry KT, Morris WZ, Sasala LM, Liu RW. Hip-spine syndrome: is there an association between markers for cam deformity and osteoarthritis of the lumbar spine? Arthroscopy. 2016;32(11):1–6.
12. Lamontagne M, Kennedy MJ, Beaulé PE. The effect of cam FAI on hip and pelvic motion during maximum squat. Clin Orthop Relat Res. 2009;467(3):645–50.
13. Ganz R, Parvizi J, Beck M, Leunig M, Notzli H, Siebenrock KA. Femoroacetabular impingement: a cause for osteoarthritis of the hip. Clin Orthop Relat Res. 2003;417:112–20.
14. Goodman DA, Feighan JE, Smith AD, Latimer B, Buly RL, Cooperman DR. Subclinical slipped capital femoral epiphysis. Relationship to osteo-arthrosis of the hip. J Bone Joint Surg Am. 1997;79(10):1489–97.
15. Ito K, Leunig M, Ganz R. Histopathologic features of the acetabular labrum in femoroacetabular impingement. Clin Orthop Relat Res. 2004;429:262–71.
16. Murray RO, Duncan C. Athletic activity in adolescence as an etiological factor in degenerative hip disease. J Bone Joint Surg Am. 1971;53(B(3)):406–19.
17. Schröder RG, Reddy M, Hatem MA, et al. A MRI study of the lesser trochanteric version and its relationship to proximal femoral osseous anatomy. J Hip Preserv Surg. 2015;2(4):410–6.
18. Torriani M, Souto SCL, Thomas BJ, Ouellette H, M a B. Ischiofemoral impingement syndrome: an entity with hip pain and abnormalities of the quadratus femoris muscle. AJR Am J Roentgenol. 2009;193(1):186–90.
19. Gómez-Hoyos J, Martin RRL, Schröder R, Palmer IJ, Martin HD. Accuracy of two clinical tests for ischiofemoral impingement in patients with posterior hip pain and endoscopically confirmed diagnosis. Arthroscopy. 2015:1–6.
20. Gómez-Hoyos J, Khoury AN, Schröder R, Johnson E, Palmer IJ, Martin HD. The hip-spine effect: a biomechanical study of ischiofemoral impingement effect on lumbar facet joints. Arthroscopy. 2016;33(1):101–7.
21. Popovich JM, Welcher JB, Hedman TP, et al. Lumbar facet joint and intervertebral disc loading during simulated pelvic obliquity. Spine J. 2013;13(11):1581–9.
22. Jaumard NV, Welch WC, Winkelstein BA. Spinal facet joint biomechanics and mechanotransduction in normal, injury and degenerative conditions. J Biomech Eng. 2011;133(7):71010.
23. Yang KH, King AI. Mechanism of facet load transmission as a hypothesis for low-back pain. Spine (Phila Pa 1976). 1984;9(6):557–65.
24. Kalichman L, Hunter DJ. Lumbar facet joint osteoarthritis: a review. Semin Arthritis Rheum. 2007;37:69–80.
25. Elder BD, Vigneswaran K, Athanasiou KA, Kim DH. Biomechanical, biochemical, and histological characterization of canine lumbar facet joint cartilage NIH public access. Neurosurgery. 2010;66(4):722–7.
26. Haher TR, O'Brien M, Dryer JW, Nucci R, Zipnick R, Leone DJ. The role of the lumbar facet joints in spinal stability. Identification of alternative paths of loading. Spine (Phila Pa 1976). 1994;19(23):2667–70, discussion 2671.
27. McLain RF. Mechanoreceptor endings in human cervical facet joints. Spine (Phila Pa 1976). 1994;19(5):495–501.
28. Vandenabeele F, Creemers J, Lambrichts I, Lippens P, Jans M. Encapsulated Ruffini-like endings in human lumbar facet joints. J Anat. 1997;191:571–83.

29. McLain RF, Pickar JG. Mechanoreceptor endings in human thoracic and lumbar facet joints. Spine (Phila Pa 1976). 1998;23(2):168–73.

30. Chen C, Lu Y, Kallakuri S, Patwardhan A, Cavanaugh JM. Distribution of A-δ and C-fiber receptors in the cervical facet joint capsule and their response to stretch. J Bone Joint Surg Am. 2006;88(A):1807–16.

31. Miller F, Merlo M, Liang Y, Kupcha P, Jamison J, Harcke HT. Femoral version and neck shaft angle. J Pediatr Orthop. 1993;12:382–8.

32. Tonnis D, Heinecke A. Acetabular and femoral anteversion: relationship with osteoarthritis of the hip. J Bone Joint Surg Am. 1999;81(12):1747–70.

33. Gulan G, Matovinovi D, Nemec B, Rubini D, Ravli J. Femoral neck anteversion: values, development, measurement, common problems. Coll Antropol. 2000;24(2):521–7.

34. Murphy SB, Simon SR, Kijewski PK, Wilkinson RH, Griscom NT. Femoral anteversion. J Bone Joint Surg Am. 1987;69(8):1169–76.

35. Krebs DE, Robbins CE, Lavine L, Mann RW. Hip biomechanics during gait. J Orthop Sports Phys Ther. 1998;28(1):51–9.

36. Gomez-Hoyos J, Khoury A, Schroder R, Marquez-arabia W, Palmer I, Martin H. The hip-spine effect part II: a biomechanical study of abnormal femoral neck version and the iliofemoral ligament effect on lumbar facet joint load. Arthroscopy. 2016. Submitted.

37. Martin H, Khoury A, Gomez-Hoyos J, Helal A, Fincher C, Jones A. Outcomes of femoral derotational osteotomy for decreased femoral anteversion: a case series. Santiago: International Society for Hip Arthroscopy; 2017.

38. Levangie PK, Norkin CC. Joint structure and function: a comprehensive analysis. 5th ed. Philadelphia: F.A. Davis; 2011.

39. Lazennec JY, Rousseau MA, Riwan F, et al. Relations hanche rachis: consequences fonctionnelles; applications aux arthroplasties totales de hanche. *In: Le complexe lombo-pelvien De l'anatomie a la pathologie. Montpellier: Sauramps Medical*; 2005. p. 115–45.

40. Husson J-L, Mallet J-F, Huten D, Odri G-A, Morin C, Parent H-F. The lumbar-pelvic-femoral complex: applications in hip pathology. Orthop Traumatol Surg Res. 2010;96(4):S10–6.

41. Martin HD, Savage A, Braly BA, Palmer IJ, Beall DP, Kelly B. The function of the hip capsular ligaments: a quantitative report. Arthroscopy. 2008;24(2):188–95.

42. Birmingham PM, Kelly BT, Jacobs R, McGrady L, Wang M. The effect of dynamic femoroacetabular impingement on pubic symphysis motion: a cadaveric study. Am J Sports Med. 2012;40(5):1113–8.

43. Kim SH, Kwon OY, Yi CH, Cynn HS, Ha SM, Park KN. Lumbopelvic motion during seated hip flexion in subjects with low-back pain accompanying limited hip flexion. Eur Spine J. 2014;23(1):142–8.

44. Ellison JB, Rose SJ, Sahrmann SA. Patterns of hip rotation range of motion: a comparison between healthy subjects and patients with low back pain. Phys Ther. 1990;70(9):537–41.

45. Esola MA, McClure PW, Fitzgerald GK, Siegler S. Analysis of lumbar spine and hip motion during forward bending in subjects with and without a history of low back pain. Spine (Phila Pa 1976). 1996;21(1):71–8.

46. Sung PS. A compensation of angular displacements of the hip joints and lumbosacral spine between subjects with and without idiopathic low back pain during squatting. J Electromyogr Kinesiol. 2013;23:741–5.

47. Vad VB, Bhat AL, Basrai D, Gebeh A, Aspergren DD, Andrews JR. Low back pain in professional golfers the role of associated hip and low back range-of-motion deficits. Am J Sports Med. 2004;32(2):494–7.

48. Khoury A, Gomez-Hoyos J, Yeramaneni S, Martin HD. Biomechanical effect of anterior hip impingement on lumbar intradiscal pressure. Santiago: International Society for Hip Arthroscopy; 2017.

49. Shacklock M. Neurodynamics. Physiotherapy. 1995; 81(1):9–16.

50. Martin HD, Khoury AN, Schroder R, et al. The effects of hip abduction on sciatic nerve biomechanics during terminal hip flexion. J Hip Preserv Surg. 2017;4(2):178–86.

51. Merolli A, Mingarelli L, Rocchi L. A more detailed mechanism to explain the "bands of Fontana" in peripheral nerves. Muscle Nerve. 2012;46(4):540–7.

52. Clarke E, Bearn JG. The spiral nerve bands of Fontana. Brain. 1972;95(1):1–20.

53. Ushiki T, Ide C. Three-dimensional organization of the collagen fibrils in the rat sciatic nerve as revealed by transmission- and scanning electron microscopy. Cell Tissue Res. 1990;260(1):175–84.

54. Roussouly P, Nnadi C. Sagittal plane deformity: an overview of interpretation and management. Eur Spine J. 2010;19(11):1824–36.

Clinical Examination of the Patient with Posterior Hip Pain

Hal D. Martin

Clinical Examination of the Patient with Posterior Hip Pain

The diagnosis and treatment of patients with posterior hip pain has continued to evolve due to an increase in understanding of hip biomechanics, clinical anatomy, and treatment options available [1]. The hip has an intimate biomechanical relationship with the spine and lower limbs and an anatomic proximity with intra- and extrapelvic structures. Patients presenting with intra-/extra-articular posterior hip pain require a comprehensive history and physical examination with specific diagnostic tests to assess all structural levels comprising the hip joint. These structural levels are defined as the osseous, capsulolabral, musculotendinous, neurovascular, and the kinematic chain. The understanding of anatomy and biomechanics of each level is essential to the clinical examination of posterior hip pain. The establishment of a group of diagnostic tests as the background on which to cast the shadow of the pathologic condition is key to the recognition of any complex pattern. A comprehensive standardized battery of physical examination tests and techniques will provide reliability and lead to an accurate diagnosis in all layers of the hip.

H. D. Martin, DO
Medical and Research Director, Hip Preservation Center, Baylor University Medical Center, Dallas, TX, USA

The osseous level includes the femur, pelvis, and acetabulum which involve congruency, version, stability, and alignment. Traditionally, abnormalities of the osseous level are thought of as bony overcoverage or undercoverage of the hip joint when the source of pain is largely due to capsulolabral insult. However with posterior hip pain, consideration should also be given to how osseous abnormalities can directly (snapping hip, nerve impingement) or indirectly (contracture, instability) involve the musculotendinous, neurovascular, and kinematic levels of hip pain. The three planar geometry of the hip joint is complex and has a balanced interaction between soft tissue structures, neuromuscular activity, and range of motion [2]. Subtle alterations in osseous alignment can produce posterior hip pain both cephalic and caudal to the joint.

The capsulolabral level involves the hip ligaments, capsule, and labrum, which function primarily as hip joint stabilizers. The contribution to limiting range of motion for the ischiofemoral ligament, pubofemoral ligament, and medial and lateral arms of the iliofemoral ligament has been documented [3]. Recent research has shown the important role of the pubofemoral and teres ligaments in limiting hip rotation in hip flexion [4, 5]. Capsulolabral hip pain generators can occur concomitantly with posterior hip pain and should be sorted out accordingly. Lack of terminal hip extension is a major source of posterior hip pain and can be due to osseous, capsulolabral, and

© Springer International Publishing AG, part of Springer Nature 2019
H. D. Martin, J. Gómez-Hoyos (eds.), *Posterior Hip Disorders*,
https://doi.org/10.1007/978-3-319-78040-5_3

musculotendinous etiologies affecting each level including the neurovascular and kinematic chain.

The musculotendinous layer involves the musculature around the hip joint and functions as a dynamic stabilizer for hip, pelvis, and trunk motion. Pain and weakness of hip joint musculature can be the primary source of pain as a muscle tear, tendonosis, or tendonitis. Musculotendinous pathology can be a primary source of posterior hip pain (piriformis, obturator internus, or hamstrings) or secondary to osseous and capsulolabral pathology (a compensatory response to hip pain).

The neurovascular layer involves the neural and vascular structures of the hip joint. Pain, motor control, and proprioception contribute to hip joint kinematics and health. Neurovascular posterior hip pain can be illusive, however easily diagnosed with a comprehensive physical exam and thorough understanding of the neurovascular anatomy and biomechanics discussed in Chap. 2. Neurovascular generators of posterior hip pain can be extrapelvic and/or intrapelvic and therefore require a complete spine, urologic, and gynecologic history.

The kinematic chain encompasses the hip joint, lumbar spine, abdominal trunk, knee, and their interrelationship. The dynamic connection of the hip joint, lumbar spine, sacroiliac joint, and knee joint ultimately functions as a unit [6]. Any incongruity from all structural layers can result in a disruption of the kinematic chain. All structural levels of the hip joint and neighboring joints can affect the kinematic chain.

Independently, or in combination, DGS can be associated with distal etiologies, such as hamstring syndrome and ischiofemoral impingement (IFI). The presence of a scarred sciatic nerve to the hamstring tendon, in cases of hamstring syndrome, and sciatic nerve impingement between the ischium and the lesser trochanter are isolated causes of posterior hip pain that can be distinguished between intrapelvic and extrapelvic sciatic nerve entrapment [1, 7–11].

Ischiofemoral impingement and hamstring syndrome are two sources of posterior hip pain that can simulate symptoms of DGS. These two dynamic pathologic conditions are associated with physical activity, and the coexistence of both conditions cannot be excluded [1, 7]. To evaluate the etiology of posterior hip pain, it is necessary to understand, correlate, and assess the interaction between the osseous, capsulolabral, musculotendinous, neurovascular, and kinematic levels. The combination of a comprehensive history and physical examination with imaging and ancillary testing is critical to diagnose DGS precisely [1, 7, 12, 13].

Johnson first described the surgical treatment for IFI in 1977, when noticing a narrowing ischiofemoral space associated with posterior hip pain after a total hip implant. The case was successfully treated with resection of the lesser trochanter [14]. More recently, Martin et al. in a 2-year outcome study showed an improvement of the symptoms after partial lesser trochanterplasty in subjects diagnosed with IFI [15]. Surgical procedures to treat chronic hamstring tears and avulsions have reported positive outcomes in comparison with nonoperative treatment. Positive outcomes are also confirmed for surgical procedures to release scar tissue between the hamstring tendons and sciatic nerve [8, 16–18].

The goal of this chapter is to demonstrate how to recognize and diagnose the distal causes of DGS. Readers will be able to distinguish independent IFI or hamstring syndrome, which can exist with or without sciatic nerve impingement.

History and Physical Examination

The assessment of posterior hip pain requires a complete history, comprehensive physical examination, standardized radiographic exploration, and specific diagnostic tests as directed [1, 13]. A comprehensive history of the patient is obtained prior to the physical examination of the hip and should consider all hip levels, including the kinematic chain. The present condition is documented including the date of onset, presence or absence of trauma, and mechanism of injury. The pain features and presence or absence of popping will aid in the determination of intra-articular versus extra-articular causes. Related symptoms of the spine, abdomen, and lower extremity are documented. The following items must also be addressed: previous consultations, surgical interventions, past injuries, childhood or adolescent hip disease, ipsilateral knee disease, suggestive history of inflammatory arthritis, and risk factors for osteonecrosis. Treatments to date must be clearly defined, and current limitations are detailed.

Participation in sports and other activities is documented and can help determine the type of injury and help guide treatment planning considering the patient's goals and expectations. The hip pain and function can be scored utilizing one or more of the following questionnaires: Harris hip score (HHS) [19], modified HHS [20], international hip outcome tool (iHOT)-33 [21], and iHOT-12 [22].

Patients with DGS/sciatic nerve entrapment often have a history of trauma and symptoms of sit pain (inability to sit for >30 min), radicular pain of the lower back or hip, and paresthesias of the affected leg [23]. Hamstring syndrome and IFI have posterior hip pain that can be similar to the symptoms of DGS. Patients with hamstring syndrome and ischiofemoral impingement can present with radicular pain, and the coexistence of these conditions should be considered [1, 7].

The physical examination to diagnose DGS, hamstring syndrome, and IFI should be included in the standard hip joint evaluation protocol when posterior hip pain is a complaint (Table 3.1) [1, 7, 12, 13, 24, 25]. In the present work, a brief description of the key points and the main six tests previously validated to diagnose posterior hip pain will be given. All hip joint evaluations should assess of the three planar kinematic axes, comprising an analysis of gait and passive/active maneuvers in seated, supine, and lateral positions.

Posterior hip pain localized to proximal or distal regions producing distal SN impingement have different complaints from those who exhibit

Table 3.1 Steps for diagnosis and treatment of posterior hip pain

Condition	Diagnosis	Treatment
Ischiofemoral impingement	Assess structural contributing factors Distal pain lateral to the ischium Gait—long-stride walking (recreation of pain) versus short-stride (alleviated pain) Ischiofemoral impingement test	*Nonoperative*: – Abductor strengthening – Arch support – Injections – Limit stride length in sports and ADLs *Operative*: – Open resection of the LT – Distalization of the LT – Ischioplasty—associated semimembranosus tear – Ischioplasty + LT resection: recreate normal – THA—associated osteoarthritis – Femoral osteotomy – Endoscopic LT resection
Hamstring syndrome	Pain lateral to the ischium Gait—heel strike (recreation of pain) Active hamstring test—30° versus 90°	– Hamstring + IFI → ischioplasty + repair – Hamstring + sciatic nerve entrapment →open with neuromonitoring
DGS	Consider spine, SI, intrapelvis, and gluteal space pathologies Pain proximal at the level of the piriformis Passive piriformis stretch test Active piriformis test	*Nonoperative*: – Physical therapy—pelvic floor therapy – Guided injections – Steroids and neuromodulators *Operative*: – Open sciatic nerve decompression – Intrapelvic laparoscopic decompression – Endoscopic decompression

IFI ischiofemoral impingement, *LT* lesser trochanter, *SI* sacroiliac joint, *THA* total hip arthroplasty. Modified from [24]

pain with walking or sitting. An example of pain exacerbated by sitting can include driving; when the hip is in 30° flexion, the hamstrings (semimembranosus) have a different force vector angle in comparison with 90° activation. Activities with the hip in 30° hip flexion can reproduce SN complaints when the hamstrings are activated. Conversely, patients with IFI are more comfortable sitting and, however, have pain while walking at terminal hip extension. At terminal hip extension, the space between ischium and the lesser trochanter is diminished [1, 26]. Within this ischiofemoral space is the location of the sciatic nerve, and if the normal biomechanics of this space is disrupted, dynamic impingement of the SN is possible.

During the analysis of gait, the morphologic abnormalities of the hip joint, muscle weakness, pain patterns, and the long-stride walking test can provide important information to differentiate hamstring syndrome and IFI. IFI has been found to be more frequent in subjects with increased femoral version [26, 27]. An internal foot progression angle during gait can present an increased femoral version and consequently found with IFI [27]. A positive Trendelenburg sign can happen due to weakness of the gluteus medius muscle. A combination of hip adduction and pelvic tilt associated with rotational motion in axial load may contribute to lesser trochanteric impingement against the ischium, producing IFI symptoms [1, 26, 27]. The pattern of pain occurring during gait can be key to the diagnosis of posterior hip pain pathologies specifically long-stride walking versus short-stride walking. The long-stride heel strike test (LSHS) encourages dynamic hip flexion with knee flexion at heel strike (Fig. 3.1a and b). During initial heel strike, the hamstring muscles act eccentrically, followed by a concentric contraction with knee flexion. Subjects referring pain lateral to the ischium with hip flexion/knee flexion may present a positive sign for proximal chronic or acute hamstring tears [25]. Differentially, the long-stride walking (LSW) test for IFI encourages dynamic hip extension [7, 15]. The long-stride walking test is positive when the patient refers pain lateral to the ischium during *terminal extension* that is relieved with short steps [7, 15] (Fig. 3.1c and d). The LSW has a sensitivity of 0.94 and a specificity of 0.85 for the diagnosis of IFI [7].

In the seated position, palpation of the gluteal structures can also guide and distinguish sources of posterior hip pain [1] (Fig. 3.2). The physician palpates in three positions of the gluteal area using the ischial tuberosity as a reference point:

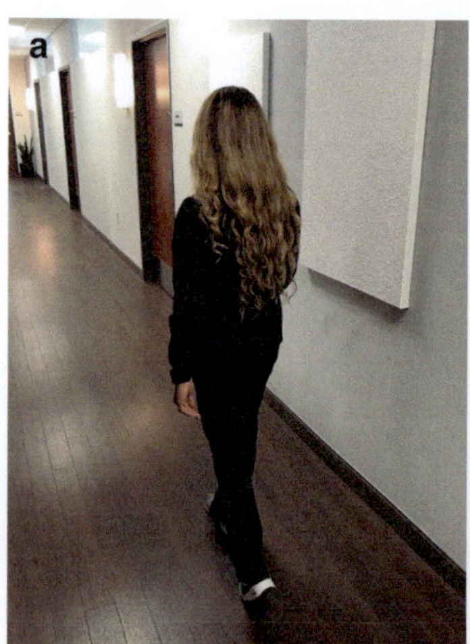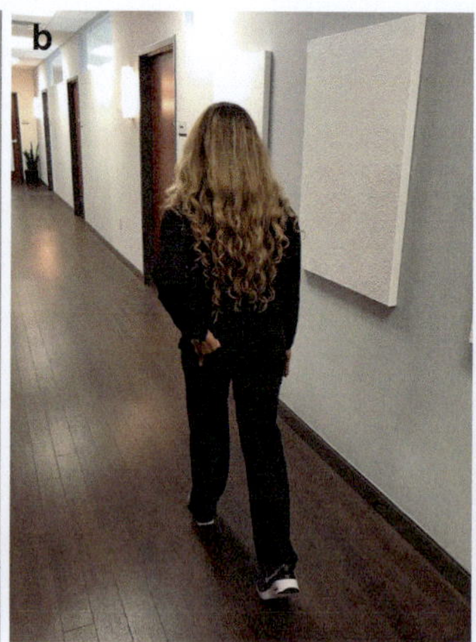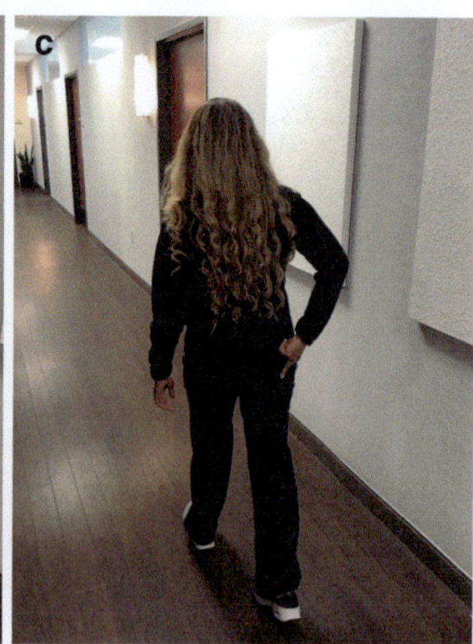

Fig. 3.1 Long-stride walking tests. (**a**) Long-stride heel strike (LSHS) test: the patient is instructed to walk at a self-select gait. (**b**) LSHS: the patient is instructed to perform a long-stride gait. A positive test is an immediate reproduction of pain proximal and lateral to the ischium with hip flexion at heel strike. Reprint with permission from [25]. (**c**) Long-stride walking (LSW) with extension, self-selected gait: no pain. (**d**) LSW, recreation of pain lateral to the ischium with terminal hip extension. Reprint with permission from [24]

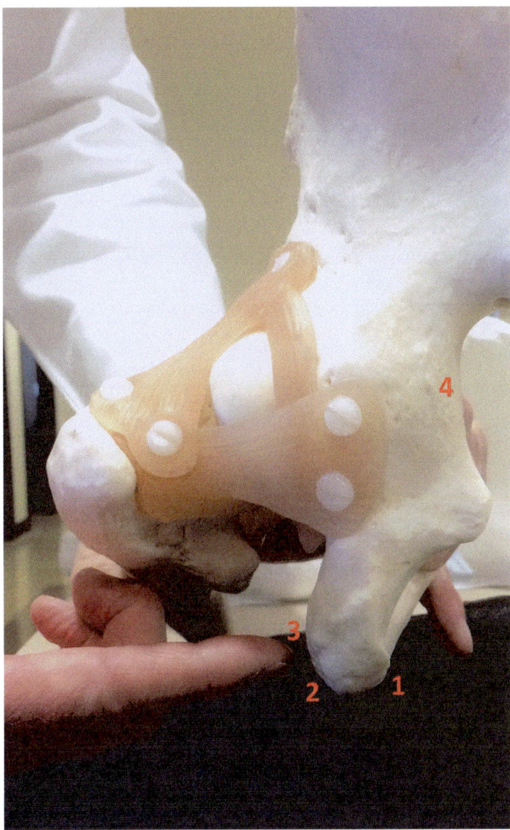

Fig. 3.2 Hand positioning for palpation of the deep gluteal space. From medial to lateral, the pudendal nerve entrapment is considered in cases of pain sensation medial to the ischium [1] in association with a tender sacrotuberous ligament, pain lateral to the ischium may represent hamstring syndrome [2] or ischiofemoral impingement [3], and finally pain sensation at the sciatic notch characterizes the piriformis muscle [4]. Reprint with permission from [24]

the piriformis (lateral/superior), at the level of the external rotators, and lateral to the ischium. If pain is localized at the ischium, rule out ischial tunnel syndrome, the hamstring bursa, or hamstring tears; and if the pain is lateral to the ischium, consider ischiofemoral impingement. If pain is more medial, one should evaluate the pudendal nerve. The seated palpation test can also be performed during the seated piriformis stretch test (Fig. 3.3a) which is a flexion, adduction with internal rotation test performed with the patient in the seated position [12, 23]. The examiner extends the knee (engaging the sciatic nerve) and passively moves the flexed hip into adduction

with internal rotation while palpating 1 cm lateral to the ischium (middle finger) and proximally at the sciatic notch (index finger). A positive test is the recreation of the posterior pain at the level of the piriformis or external rotators. The piriformis stretch test is performed (sensitivity of 0.52, specificity of 0.90) to diagnose DGS as the source of posterior hip pain rotators [12].

The active hamstring test at 30° (A-30) and at 90° (A-90) of knee flexion (Fig. 3.3b and c) is performed with the patient in the seated position while the examiner palpates the ischium, semimembranosus, and conjoint tendons. The patient is asked to actively flex the knee against resistance for 5 s with the knee in 30° flexion and again with the knee in 90° flexion. A positive test is recreation of the pain proximal and/or lateral to the ischium and/or weakness. Radicular complaints suggest sciatic nerve involvement. The use of both tests together yields a sensitivity of 0.84 and specificity of 0.97 [1, 25]. Proximal versus distal SN entrapment can be distinguished by the location of the symptomatic pain recreation.

Two tests to differentiate IFI and DGS are assessed in the lateral. The active piriformis test showed sensitivity of 0.78 and specificity of 0.80 to diagnose DGS and when used in association with the passive piriformis stretch test is a major contributor to diagnose sciatic nerve entrapment by the piriformis muscle. The patient is instructed to drive their heel into the examination table, initiating active hip abduction and external rotation against resistance from the examiner position (Fig. 3.4a). Similar to the piriformis stretch test, a positive test is the presence of posterior pain at the level of the piriformis or external rotators [12]. While the patient is in the lateral position, the IFI test is performed (Fig. 3.4b and c). The pain is produced when the examiner extends the hip in adduction or in neutral position. To confirm the suspicion of IFI, the examiner extends the hip in abduction with no symptom of pain, proving the presence of an impinging pathology. The IFI test showed a sensitivity of 0.82 and specificity of 0.85 and in combination with the long-stride walking is utilized to identify IFI [7].

Assessment of the biomechanical axis alignment will provide information of the pelvic

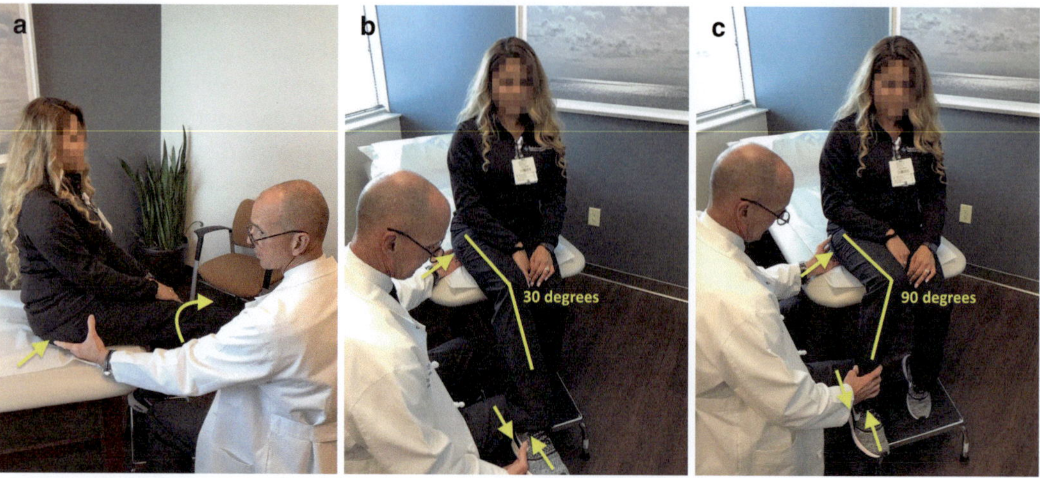

Fig. 3.3 Seated piriformis stretch test and seated hamstring active tests. (**a**) Piriformis stretch test, (**b**) active hamstring test at 30° knee flexion, (**c**) active hamstring test at 90° knee flexion. Reprint with permission from [24]

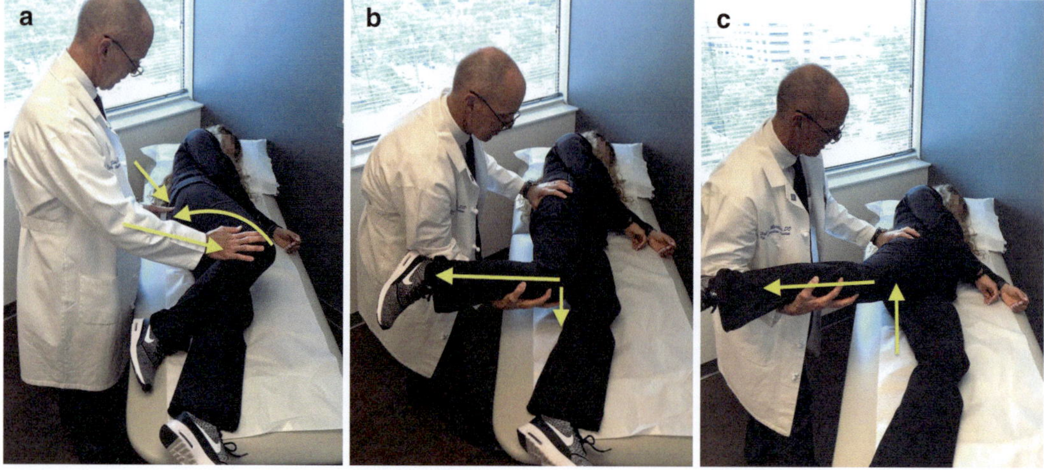

Fig. 3.4 Lateral tests for differentiation of distal causes of DGS. Lateral position test. (**a**) Active piriformis test: recreation of pain lateral to the piriformis muscle helps to distinguish proximal from distal involvement etiologies, (**b**) ischiofemoral impingement test (recreation of pain lateral to the ischium), (**c**) alleviation of the symptoms with hip abduction. Reprint with permission from [24]

positioning. In normal osseous morphologic conditions, the balance between hip flexors and extensors influences the pelvic positioning in the sagittal axis. An abnormal pelvic positioning, posteriorly or anteriorly, has been associated with weakness and/or stiffness of the hip muscles involved with pelvic positioning, and this factor may contribute to the development of DGS and IFI [28–31].

The influence of limited hip range of motion on spine mobility and function has been shown as one of the causes of chronic low back pain [32–36]. Patients with ischiofemoral impingement may present associated symptoms of low back pain due to the limited hip extension. This clinical observation was confirmed by Gomez-Hoyos in a cadaveric study [6]. Limiting hip extension by decreasing the ischiofemoral space resulted in increased intra-facet joint pressure of the lumbar spine (L3–L4 and L4–L5). A complete physical examination of the hip must include a lumbar spine evaluation and cases of low back pain should include a hip evaluation.

Differential Diagnosis

During the comprehensive history and physical examination, the examiner must be aware of DGS symptoms simulated by intra- and extra-pelvic structures. Cyclic pain with a history of urogynecologic conditions (endometriosis, bladder or bowel issues, and dysmenorrhea) may indicate an intrapelvic sciatic nerve entrapment [1, 37]. Pudendal nerve entrapment is an isolated condition that may be associated with DGS that can be differentiated by a pain location and typical characteristics. Patients with pudendal nerve entrapment present with pain medial to the ischium and sensations of burning, tearing, stabbing, lightning-like, electrical, and sharp shooting, and/or foreign body sensation, which is made worse with sitting (alleviated with toilet stool sitting) and reduced with standing [38]. The nerve can be entrapped in more than one location (piriformis, obturator internus muscles, sacrotuberous and sacrospinous ligaments, or the falciform process), and a pelvic floor manual test performed by a trained physical therapist will assist the diagnosis and relationship of these intrapelvic conditions [38].

Imaging and Ancillary Tests

The standard imaging studies include the standing AP pelvis, false profile, and lateral images. All intra-articular pathology is ruled out through a comprehensive history and physical examination assessing the five levels of osseous, capsulolabral, musculotendinous, neurovascular structures, and the kinematic chain. Specifically in posterior hip cases, the T3 MRI is performed to rule out intrapelvic sources of SN entrapment versus extrapelvic sciatic nerve entrapment. The extrapelvic MRI patient positioning is important for IFI assessment. The feet are secured in a neutral walking position, which will most closely simulate a dynamic assessment of the ischiofemoral space. If the feet are not secured in this functional position, a false impression of decreased ischiofemoral space could occur. The assessment of the semimembranosus and its orientation to the lateral ischium is best visualized on T2 axial or T2 coronal imaging. This view allows for the detection of a partial tear or undersurface tears of the semimembranosus. In cases of active subluxation of the semimembranosus, dynamic MRI testing and dynamic US are useful. In dynamic US, the patient is placed in the prone position and the patient performs a bicycling motion with active hamstring contraction. The activated semimembranosus will sublux into the ischial tunnel recreating the radicular pain of the SN. Scarring in this region can be assessed by T1 and T2 MRI in the axial and coronal planes. The T3 MRI of the intrapelvis is utilized for gynecologic and vascular entrapments of the SN and/or its roots. This type of partial tear with subluxation into the ischial tunnel can be correlated with the physical examination assessment with the knee extended and the hip abducted.

Ancillary testing can include EMG; however it has not been found to be useful. If EMG is utilized, the testing should be performed in a dynamic modality with the knee in extension and the hip in flexion and abduction, and the symptomatic side is compared with the non-symptomatic side looking at neural latency. Injection tests have been advocated for supporting the diagnosis of posterior extra- and intra-articular hip disorders. Guided injections utilizing CT, fluoroscopy, ultrasound, or MRI increase accuracy to the correct injection site. US, as described above, in addition to injection testing, is beneficial in the exact diagnosis of either IFI or HS tears involvement. Injection tests can include dynamic fluoroscopy to assess the IFS or visualizing the dynamic recreation of the IF pain with the hip in terminal hip extension. Fluoroscopy can also be helpful in recreating greater trochanteric sciatic nerve impingement, which can exist proximally. The ligamentous constraints of the hip do affect the overall kinematics of the hip and can affect the exact locations of impingement. This is evidenced through a multilayer effect, not just osseous but also capsulolabral, which can influence any of the other structures above or below the primary area of complaint.

Conclusion

In conclusion, posterior hip pain, with or without sciatic nerve involvement, is recognized through a comprehensive history and physical examination utilizing ancillary testing and three planar radiographic assessments. Differential diagnosis of DGS, IFI, hamstring syndrome, and pudendal nerve entrapment is dependent upon the understanding of the entire anatomy, biomechanics, and clinical presentation of posterior hip pain.

References

1. Martin HD, Reddy M, Gomez-Hoyos J. Deep gluteal syndrome. J Hip Preserv Surg. 2015;2(2):99–107.
2. Chambers HG, Sutherland DH. A practical guide to gait analysis. J Am Acad Orthop Surg. 2002;10(3):222–31.
3. Martin HD, Savage A, Braly BA, Palmer IJ, Beall DP, Kelly B. The function of the hip capsular ligaments: a quantitative report. Arthroscopy. 2008;24(2):188–95.
4. Martin HD, Hatem MA, Kivlan BR, Martin RL. Function of the ligamentum teres in limiting hip rotation: a cadaveric study. Arthroscopy. 2014;30(9):1085–91.
5. Martin HD, Khoury AN, Schroder R, Johnson E, Gomez-Hoyos J, Campos S, et al. Contribution of the pubofemoral ligament to hip stability: a biomechanical study. Arthroscopy. 2017;33(2):305–13.
6. Gomez-Hoyos J, Khoury A, Schroder R, Johnson E, Palmer IJ, Martin HD. The hip-spine effect: a biomechanical study of ischiofemoral impingement effect on lumbar facet joints. Arthroscopy. 2017;33(1):101–7.
7. Gomez-Hoyos J, Martin RL, Schroder R, Palmer IJ, Martin HD. Accuracy of 2 clinical tests for ischiofemoral impingement in patients with posterior hip pain and endoscopically confirmed diagnosis. Arthroscopy. 2016;32(7):1279–84.
8. Orava S. Hamstring syndrome. Oper Tech Sports Med. 1997;5(3):143–9.
9. Patti JW, Ouellette H, Bredella MA, Torriani M. Impingement of lesser trochanter on ischium as a potential cause for hip pain. Skelet Radiol. 2008;37(10):939–41.
10. Torriani M, Souto SC, Thomas BJ, Ouellette H, Bredella MA. Ischiofemoral impingement syndrome: an entity with hip pain and abnormalities of the quadratus femoris muscle. AJR Am J Roentgenol. 2009;193(1):186–90.
11. Young IJ, van Riet RP, Bell SN. Surgical release for proximal hamstring syndrome. Am J Sports Med. 2008;36(12):2372–8.
12. Martin HD, Kivlan BR, Palmer IJ, Martin RL. Diagnostic accuracy of clinical tests for sciatic nerve entrapment in the gluteal region. Knee Surg Sports Traumatol Arthrosc. 2014;22(4):882–8.
13. Martin HD, Palmer IJ. History and physical examination of the hip: the basics. Curr Rev Musculoskelet Med. 2013;6(3):219–25.
14. Johnson KA. Impingement of the lesser trochanter on the ischial ramus after total hip arthroplasty. Report of three cases. J Bone Joint Surg Am. 1977;59(2):268–9.
15. Hatem MA, Palmer IJ, Martin HD. Diagnosis and 2-year outcomes of endoscopic treatment for ischiofemoral impingement. Arthroscopy. 2015;31(2):239–46.
16. Dierckman BD, Guanche CA. Endoscopic proximal hamstring repair and ischial bursectomy. Arthrosc Tech. 2012;1(2):e201–7.
17. Gomez-Hoyos J, Reddy M, Martin HD. Dry endoscopic-assisted mini-open approach with neuromonitoring for chronic hamstring avulsions and ischial tunnel syndrome. Arthrosc Tech. 2015;4(3):e193–9.
18. Miller SL, Gill J, Webb GR. The proximal origin of the hamstrings and surrounding anatomy encountered during repair. A cadaveric study. J Bone Joint Surg Am. 2007;89(1):44–8.
19. Harris WH. Traumatic arthritis of the hip after dislocation and acetabular fractures: treatment by mold arthroplasty. An end-result study using a new method of result evaluation. J Bone Joint Surg Am. 1969;51(4):737–55.
20. Byrd JW, Jones KS. Prospective analysis of hip arthroscopy with 2-year follow-up. Arthroscopy. 2000;16(6):578–87.
21. Mohtadi NG, Griffin DR, Pedersen ME, Chan D, Safran MR, Parsons N, et al. The development and validation of a self-administered quality-of-life outcome measure for young, active patients with symptomatic hip disease: the international hip outcome tool (iHOT-33). Arthroscopy. 2012;28(5):595–605. quiz 6-10 e1.
22. Griffin DR, Parsons N, Mohtadi NG, Safran MR. Multicenter arthroscopy of the hip outcomes research N. A short version of the international hip outcome tool (iHOT-12) for use in routine clinical practice. Arthroscopy. 2012;28(5):611–6. quiz 6-8.
23. Martin HD, Shears SA, Johnson JC, Smathers AM, Palmer IJ. The endoscopic treatment of sciatic nerve entrapment/deep gluteal syndrome. Arthroscopy. 2011;27(2):172–81.
24. Martin HD, Khoury A, Schroder R, Palmer IJ. Ischiofemoral impingement and hamstring syndrome as causes of posterior hip pain where do we go next? Clin Sports Med. 2016;35(3):469–86.
25. Martin RL, Schröder SR, Gomez-Hoyos J, Khoury AN, Palmer IJ, McGovern RP, Martin HD. Accuracy of 3 clinical tests to diagnose proximal hamstrings tears with and without sciatic nerve involvement in patients with posterior hip pain. Athroscopy. 2017;34(1):114–21.
26. Schroder RG, Reddy M, Hatem MA, Gomez-Hoyos J, Toye L, Khoury A, et al. A MRI study of the lesser trochanteric version and its relationship to proximal femoral osseous anatomy. J Hip Preserv Surg. 2015;2(4):410–6.
27. Gomez-Hoyos J, Schroder R, Reddy M, Palmer IJ, Martin HD. Femoral neck anteversion and lesser trochanteric retroversion in patients with ischiofemoral

impingement: a case-control magnetic resonance imaging study. Arthroscopy. 2016;32(1):13–8.

28. Ekstrom RA, Donatelli RA, Carp KC. Electromyographic analysis of core trunk, hip, and thigh muscles during 9 rehabilitation exercises. J Orthop Sports Phys Ther. 2007;37(12):754–62.

29. Halbertsma JP, Goeken LN, Hof AL, Groothoff JW, Eisma WH. Extensibility and stiffness of the hamstrings in patients with nonspecific low back pain. Arch Phys Med Rehabil. 2001;82(2):232–8.

30. Neumann DA. Kinesiology of the hip: a focus on muscular actions. J Orthop Sports Phys Ther. 2010;40(2):82–94.

31. Sullivan MK, Dejulia JJ, Worrell TW. Effect of pelvic position and stretching method on hamstring muscle flexibility. Med Sci Sports Exerc. 1992;24(12):1383–9.

32. Cibulka MT, Sinacore DR, Cromer GS, Delitto A. Unilateral hip rotation range of motion asymmetry in patients with sacroiliac joint regional pain. Spine (Phila Pa 1976). 1998;23(9):1009–15.

33. Ellison JB, Rose SJ, Sahrmann SA. Patterns of hip rotation range of motion: a comparison between healthy subjects and patients with low back pain. Phys Ther. 1990;70(9):537–41.

34. Vad VB, Bhat AL, Basrai D, Gebeh A, Aspergren DD, Andrews JR. Low back pain in professional golfers: the role of associated hip and low back range-of-motion deficits. Am J Sports Med. 2004;32(2):494–7.

35. Van Dillen LR, Bloom NJ, Gombatto SP, Susco TM. Hip rotation range of motion in people with and without low back pain who participate in rotation-related sports. Phys Ther Sport. 2008;9(2):72–81.

36. Van Dillen LR, Gombatto SP, Collins DR, Engsberg JR, Sahrmann SA. Symmetry of timing of hip and lumbopelvic rotation motion in 2 different subgroups of people with low back pain. Arch Phys Med Rehabil. 2007;88(3):351–60.

37. Hibner M, Desai N, Robertson LJ, Nour M. Pudendal neuralgia. J Minim Invasive Gynecol. 2010;17(2):148–53.

38. FitzGerald MP, Kotarinos R. Rehabilitation of the short pelvic floor. II: treatment of the patient with the short pelvic floor. Int Urogynecol J Pelvic Floor Dysfunct. 2003;14(4):269–75.

Psychological Challenges in Treating Chronic Hip Pain

Timothy S. Clark

Effective evaluation of a patient's complaints of pain is enhanced if pain is understood as not only a reflection of patients' anatomy and biomechanics but also the patient's perceptions, emotions, history, and the psychosocial context in which their pain occurs. It is suggested that understanding of these factors enriches treatment planning, building compliance with treatment recommendations, and enhances treatment outcomes. This article provides a review of models and clinical research regarding patient's pain as well as recommendations for assessment and treatment so as to optimize outcomes.

The Complex Nature of Pain

Pain represents a complex biopsychosocial phenomena as summarized in the 2011 Institute of Medicine's comprehensive review [1]. Gate control theory suggests that input from both peripheral and central nervous system to the spinal "gates" can either enhance or inhibit transmission of pain signals [2]. The role of these factors applies to acute pain but become increasingly relevant as pain becomes chronic. Multiple psycho-logical factors impact the subjective experience of pain including attention, perception of control, understanding of the meaning of the experience, immediate emotional responses, and the situation in which the pain occurred. The thoughts associated with pain can trigger additional reactions, thoughts, and actions which can amplify and perpetuate pain and disability. Linton [3] has provided a clinically relevant review integrating the stages and factors impacting pain perception. Over time, some patients become preoccupied with persistent repeated efforts to escape all pain. Other patients and their social support networks begin to perceive them as disabled with the patient taking on a permanent "sick role."

These psychosocial models mirror changes in brain processing of pain signals. A recent study [4] compared brain functional magnetic resonance imaging (fMRI) of patients with back pain. First, they compared persons with acute/subacute pain to those with chronic (i.e., over 10 years). Second, they tracked changes in pain-related brain activity in patients longitudinally comparing findings of those for whom pain persisted to those for whom pain resolved. Research using results compared to meta-analytic probabilistic maps found that in acute/subacute pain response was limited to regions involving perception of pain. For those with chronic pain, activity was primarily involved with emotion-related circuitry. With longitudinal tracking, patients who recovered from back pain, demonstrated

T. S. Clark, PhD
Comprehensive Interdisciplinary Program, Baylor University Medical Center, Center for Pain Management, Dallas, TX, USA
e-mail: timothy.clark@BSWHealth.org

decreased brain activity in pain processing. In patients for whom pain persisted demonstrated increased involvement in emotion-related circuitry. Thus, brain representation of a constant percept underwent major shifts in brain activity as it became more chronic.

Factors Influencing Pain and Surgical Recovery

Limited literature has been published regarding the psychological and social factors impacting posterior hip disorders specifically. However, a rich literature exists regarding impact of psychological and social factors on back pain, outcomes of spine surgery, and outcomes of other orthopedic surgeries for joints such as hip, knee, and shoulder.

Back Pain and Spine Surgery

A number of studies have examined psychological factors impacting back pain. A study in 2002 [5] summarized 25 studies and determined that psychological distress/depression was the primary factor predicting chronicity and disability with secondary factors of somatization and some evidence of catastrophizing. In a large study of 1500 persons with low back pain treated in primary care settings, [6] multiple psychological measures were analyzed using an exploratory factor analysis, confirmatory analysis, and linear regression predicting pain and disability. Four factors were identified: pain-related distress, causal beliefs, coping cognitions, and perceptions of the future. Confirming the critical role of emotion, pain-related distress accounted for 34.6% of the variance in pain intensity and 51% of pain-related disability.

Factors adversely impacting outcome from spine surgery have been evaluated in multiple studies. Two excellent reviews by den Boer [7] and Block, Ben-Porath, and Marek [8] summarized a list of major factors found to adversely impact response to surgery or pain intervention (i.e., spinal cord stimulators, intrathecal narcotic pumps). Their listing included the following factors:

- Lower educational levels; higher levels of preoperative pain; less work satisfaction; longer sick leave; pre-existing psychopathology such as affective disorders or personality disorders; elevated emotional distress including depression, anxiety, fear, and anger; pain sensitivity and somatization; maladaptive coping or cognitive patterns such as passivity or catastrophizing; use of chronic opioid therapy; and interpersonal issues such as reinforcement of pain and disability behavior by a social support system.

Orthopedic Surgery

In addition, to the literature regarding back pain and surgery, research has been conducted regarding the impact of psychological factors on orthopedic surgery such as joint replacement or anterior cruciate ligament reconstruction. Factors evaluated have included depression, anxiety, optimism as a personality trait, expectations of outcomes, and maladaptive coping such as catastrophizing or pain fear. Outcomes have included functional improvement, patient satisfaction, and persistent postsurgical pain.

Depression/Anxiety

Findings are mixed, but some evidence indicates the negative impact of psychological factors such as affective distress on total hip arthroplasty (THA) and total knee arthroplasty (TKA) as well as other orthopedic procedures. A 2009 prospective study [9] of 6158 patients undergoing THA found that anxiety and depression as measured by the EQ-5D were a major predictor of patients' pain relief and satisfaction postoperatively. However, mixed findings were reported in a 2012 large systematic review [10] of the relationships of psychological factors on outcomes on TKA and THA. It was concluded that preoperative depression had no impact on postoperative function. However, lower preoperative mental health on global measures such as the SF-12 was associated with lower scores on function and pain. In a 2013 study [11] of joint replacement outcomes at 3 and 12 months postoperatively, levels of anxiety and depression were high prior to surgery and were reduced overall following surgery. However, patients with elevated preoperative anxiety and depression had worse patient-reported outcomes and had lower satisfaction. Another 2013 study [12] also found that presurgical pain and type of arthroplasty were primary predictors of persistent postsurgical pain, while patients' perception of illness and postsurgical anxiety contributed to persistent postsurgical pain. In a small study [13] of patients undergoing arthroscopic subacromial decompression, preoperative distress did not correlate with postoperative function or pain but did correlate with postoperative emotional distress.

Optimism/Hope

Evidence exists that optimism and positive expectation may positively impact outcomes. When 7000 patients undergoing TKA were classified as optimistic or pessimistic based on psychometric testing prior to surgery, those classified as pessimists were more likely to experience moderate to severe pain (odds ratio 2.2) and less improvement in knee function (odds ratio 0.53) but not at 5 years postsurgery. In another small study, [14], however, a measure of hope was not predictive of function or depression following TKA and THA, whereas higher self-efficacy predicted lower postsurgical depression.

Expectations

Patient expectations have also been examined. A 2002 study [15] of patients undergoing either THA or TKA found that patients who expected total pain relief had better physical function and improvement in pain level 6 months post surgery. In a more recent study in 2011 [16], THA patients with more preoperative positive functional expectations (such as walking further, doing housework, activities of daily living) had greater improvement 12 months postsurgery. For each additional individual expectation a patient endorsed, there was an associated 34% increase in improvement in outcomes. Another study [17] found evidence that behavioral outcome expectancies were stronger predictors of follow-up pain following TKA than response expectancies.

Self-Efficacy

A related construct to that of optimism or positive expectancy is that of self-efficacy. In a review of relevant literature, Brand and Nyland [18] concluded that self-efficacy, a patient's perception that they have the potential to carry out a task, is a factor impacting recovery from ACL reconstruction. In articles reviewed, patients with greater self-efficacy as measured by the knee self-efficacy scale were more likely to return to pre-injury physical activity intensity and frequency.

Catastrophizing

Catastrophizing is a construct that involves anxious preoccupation with pain, being overwhelmed by fear of pain, amplification or reactivity to pain, and feeling helpless in the face of pain. In a systematic review [19] of the relationships of pain catastrophizing to outcomes from TKA, variability was found in studies. However, moderate-level evidence was found for catastrophizing as an independent predictor of chronic post TKA pain.

Clinical Implications

We are unaware of any well-validated prospective study examining a broad array of psychological factors either in this patient population or as a predictor of outcome from posterior hip surgery. This research is also made more difficult by the heterogeneous causes and manifestations of hip pain. So the clinically relevant question is this: Are the findings regarding the role of psychological factors affecting pain generalizable or at least relevant to the problems of patients with posterior hip disorders? Based on our clinical experience providing presurgical evaluations to persons referred for evaluation from a tertiary hip preservation center, the answer is "yes" but with some caution.

First, the biopsychosocial model of illness and pain perception are relevant regardless of the nociceptive driver of the pain. Clinicians learn that they cannot measure pain but only pain behavior (e.g., verbal complaints, social withdrawal, nonverbal behavior, self-limitation). In other word measurement of pain is actually the measure of the unique responses of an individual to a subjective experience influenced by psychological and social factors. Thus, when pain is a primary indicator for necessity of surgery or when reduction of pain is a primary goal as an outcome, it may be helpful to see pain as the complex experience it is. Correspondingly, it has been found that both pain severity and unpleasantness can be dramatically altered by changes in cognitive and emotional processing. A study in 2011 [20] powerfully demonstrated that with brief training in mindfulness meditation, subjects were able to reduce pain unpleasantness by 57% and pain intensity by 40%. These changes in pain perception were mirrored by changes in the brain pathways triggered by the pain.

Second, as previously noted, over time pain begins to be a different experience and is processed differently in the brain. Chronic pain often becomes enmeshed in patients' unsuccessful attempts to escape, ignore, or fight pain resulting in demoralization. These old solutions which might have temporarily worked for acute pain become unsuccessful resulting in demoralization and disability. Ironically, the old solutions create a new problem.

Third, research identifying psychological processes impacting surgical outcome are likely to be relevant. Although not replicated at this time with patients specifically presenting with posterior hip disorders, research regarding models of pain perception and research predicting outcome of spine surgery, spinal cord stimulator implantation, or orthopedic surgeries such as TKA and THA are salient. Thus, a range of psychological factors to be assessed would include:

- Chronicity and severity of pain
- Chronic use of opioids especially in light of impact of opioid-induced hyperalgesia [21]
- Elevated emotional distress including depression, anxiety, and anger
- Pre-existing psychopathology including both affective disorder and persons with long-term maladaptive personality features

- Overwhelmed or inadequate coping evidenced by catastrophizing, demoralization, poor self-efficacy, fear of movement or pain, or negative expectations
- High levels of recent social stressors or a perception of inadequate resources to cope with stress
- Insufficient or maladaptive social support resulting either in low social resources, chronic conflict, or reinforcement by others of disability/pain behavior
- History of early life trauma impacting response to pain and stress as well as interpersonal support
- Current or past substance abuse

It is unclear if patients presenting at tertiary care clinics for posterior hip pain are similar to those presenting for spine or other joint replacement surgeries. Persons presenting at a tertiary center may not represent other patients with similar conditions who either did not have resources to obtain specialty care, it was not available to them, or they did not persist in seeking care. In other words, it is possible that persons in these clinics represent different socioeconomic status, gender, age, or class than general pain populations. We are unaware of research at this time to clarify these issues.

Recommendations

In light of the psychological factors impacting patients' perception of pain, a consistent and logical stepwise approach is recommended for assessment impacting treatment planning.

Physician Assessment

First, physicians may find it helpful to carry out a two-part screening for patients presenting for consultation. It is recommended that some psychosocial screening instrument be included as part of intake paperwork. In light of persistent research on the impact of depression, anxiety, and somatization on both patients' perception of pain and surgical outcomes, inclusion of screening instruments such as the Patient Health Questionnaire (PHQ-SADS) [22] may be considered. This instrument is free, easily available online with clear guidelines for scoring and interpretation, and well researched and has been used in a variety of medical settings. It measures and assists in diagnosis of four disorders: somatoform disorder, panic disorder, depression, and anxiety. An alternative is the Brief Battery for Health Improvement [23]. This instrument which can be purchased takes about 10 min and provides a more detailed evaluation of biopsychosocial factors impacting pain management.

In addition to a formal screening questionnaire, it is recommended that the physician and the medical team use both the clinical interview, brief psychosocial history, and clinical observation to review factors identified above which may impact patient coping. It may be useful for experienced clinicians to make referrals for additional evaluation when their "internal alarms" sound for unusual behavior and report.

Psychological Evaluation and Psychometric Testing

Second, formal psychological evaluation may be helpful for all patients or ones selected by the screening method above. Referral to a psychologist trained and experienced in health, medical, or rehabilitation psychology may be helpful both in identifying risk factors and also in identifying resources which could be used to reduce these risks and optimize outcome. Reviews [24] have found this type of approach to be helpful and not infrequently used [25, 26].

One of the earliest uses of presurgical psychological screening (PPS) was patient selection for spine surgery. That literature [25, 26] has expanded, and PPS is often required prior to permanent implantation of spinal cord stimulators and intrathecal narcotic pumps. Thus, the largest studies of prediction of outcomes have been carried out in this population. Using detailed interviewing, psychologists will inquire about the full range of factors identified in previous studies to

impact outcomes adaptation to pain and response to surgery. Some psychologists [27] have formalized these into an algorithm to quantify risk.

In addition to a detailed clinical interview, and review of the medical record, psychologists conduct standard psychometric testing. They may select instruments to measure a range of concepts found to impact adaptation. Domains and selected instruments are listed below:

- *Pain functioning*: The West Haven-Yale Multidimensional Pain Inventory [28]—measuring pain severity, interference by pain, affective distress, perception of control, social support, and responses of others to pain behavior and activity level
- *Depression and anxiety*: Beck Depression Inventory [29], Centers for Epidemiological Studies Depression Scale [30], and Beck Anxiety Inventory [31]
- *Adaptive and maladaptive coping*: Pain Catastrophizing Scale [32], Perceived Stress Scale [33], Coping Strategies Questionnaire [34], and Fear/Avoidance Behavior Questionnaire [35]
- *Disability*: Oswestry Disability Index [36]
- *Relationships*: Pain and Impairment Relationship Scale [37]
- *Risk factors for misuse of opioids*: Screener and Opioid Assessment for Patients with Pain (SOAPP) [38]

A more integrated assessment of these factors can be found in the Minnesota Multiphasic Personality Inventory-2 Restructured Form (MMPI-2-RF) [39] and its predecessors (MMPI, MMPI-2). Summarized in a recent study [8], studies with the MMPI-2 revealed poorer outcomes from surgery or spinal cord stimulator in persons with elevated depression, (scale 2), anxiety and fear (scale 7), anger (scale 4), and somatic preoccupation and reactivity (scales 1 and 3). In a 2013 study, Block, Ben-Porath, and Marek [8] found that certain scores on the MMPI-2-RF were associated with other psychological measures associated with negative surgical outcomes. In a recent study [40] of 172 men and 210 women who underwent spine surgery, scores on the MMPI-

2-RF were found to add 11% more unique variance in postoperative disability and negative over other medical/psychosocial factors. Scales most relevant were those measuring internalizing especially that of somatoform dysfunction, demoralization, and interpersonal difficulties. Similarly, in 2015, a study [41] was carried out of 319 patients undergoing implantation of spinal cord stimulators. They found that patients with scales associated with interpersonal problems, emotional dysfunction, and somatic and cognitive problems had higher pain and distress 5 months after implantation of the stimulator.

Physicians may have some concerns about the impact on the clinical relationship if they request a psychological evaluation. They may be concerned that patients will feel they are being seen as "a psych case" or that the physician thinks "it is in my mind." In our experience, explanations provided after the referral have already been made may raise patient concerns. Similarly, patients tend to react negatively if they are told they must undergo testing to see if they "pass" and can get surgery. As a result, it is recommended that patients be educated through materials presented prior to consultation and at the outset of the consultation. Patients are often less resistant if the consultation is introduced as a "mind/body/spirit" approach in which the goal is to assess all factors which could impact care. Patients often appreciate medical attention which also attends to the psychosocial and emotional impact of their pain. Education on the ways in which chronic pain begins to change the brain's assessment and response to pain often will be understood by patients. Finally, patients tend to appreciate when an evaluation is introduced as part of a routine comprehensive patient-centered approach to improve medical outcomes and provide all possible resources.

Intervention

Often assessment of psychosocial factors will result in one of three plans of actions. First, should no factors or only minimal factors be noted, the physician may proceed without additional psychological or psychiatric recommendations. Second, the levels of psychosocial factors may be such that the physician will choose nonsurgical approaches. This will occur rarely and would generally occur in the presence of severe psychiatric problems, personality disorder which could adversely impact cooperative with treatment, litigation and secondary gain issues, substance abuse, or other cognitive/psychological problems which could prevent cooperation in the recovery process and rehabilitation.

Third, not uncommonly, factors will be identified which might impact postoperative pain and recovery. In these cases, it may be helpful to initiate interventions either prior to surgery orc in addition to surgery to address the identified issues. These interventions can include initiation of medications for depression or anxiety or referral for behavioral medicine training by a mental health professional trained in health or rehabilitation psychology. Interventions could include cognitive behavioral therapy to improve coping and reduce emotional distress, biofeedback or self-regulation training to reduce physiological stress response, psychotherapy to reduce or cope with psychosocial stressors or impacts of early trauma, or simply education about appropriate expectations and to allay patients' anxiety about surgery. Often this intervention may be time limited (6–8 sessions), but more treatment may be needed depending on the level and chronicity of problems. Referral to a structured interdisciplinary pain program [42] may be appropriate for patients who have developed a chronic pain syndrome with high levels of pain behavior, elevated disability or inactivity, high somatic preoccupation or reactivity, elevated emotional distress, or marked deconditioning. These programs provide integrated goal-directed treatment by a coordinated team of clinicians (i.e., physician, psychologist, nurse, case manager, occupational therapist, physical therapist). Extensive research had documented both clinical effectiveness and cost effectiveness.

Summary

Patients present for assessment and treatment of musculoskeletal problems for both functional limitations and for pain. Current literature suggests that optimal evaluation and treatment planning consider the psychological and social aspects of patients' experience and lives. This literature not only suggests that these factors contribute to patients' complaints but also may impact outcome of medical treatment. All experienced clinicians have noted the impact of these factors as they treat patients. This chapter suggests that formal assessment and integration of these factors may assist physicians to optimize patient outcomes, satisfaction, and compliance with treatment plans. In the well-known words of the father of modern medicine, Sir William Osler, "The good physician treats the disease; the great physician treats the patient who has the disease" [43].

References

1. Institute of Medicine (US) Committee on Advancing Pain Research, Care, and Education. Relieving pain in America: a blueprint for transforming prevention, care, education, and research [Internet]. Washington (DC): National Academies; 2011. [cited 2015 Nov 9]. http://www.ncbi.nlm.nih.gov/books/NBK91497/.
2. McGrath PA. Psychological aspects of pain perception. Arch Oral Biol. 1994;39(Suppl):55S–62S.
3. Linton SJ, Shaw WS. Impact of psychological factors in the experience of pain. Phys Ther. 2011;91(5):700–11.
4. Hashmi JA, Baliki MN, Huang L, Baria AT, Torbey S, Hermann KM, et al. Shape shifting pain: chronification of back pain shifts brain representation from nociceptive to emotional circuits. Brain. 2013;136(9):2751–68.
5. Pincus T, Burton AK, Vogel S, Field AP. A systematic review of psychological factors as predictors of chronicity/disability in prospective cohorts of low back pain. Spine. 2002;27(5):E109–20.
6. Campbell P, Bishop A, Dunn KM, Main CJ, Thomas E, Foster NE. Conceptual overlap of psychological constructs in low back pain. Pain. 2013;154(9):1783–91.
7. den Boer JJ, Oostendorp RAB, Beems T, Munneke M, Oerlemans M, Evers AWM. A systematic review of bio-psychosocial risk factors for an unfavourable outcome after lumbar disc surgery. Eur Spine J. 2006;15(5):527–36.
8. Block AR, Ben-Porath YS, Marek RJ. Psychological risk factors for poor outcome of spine surgery and spinal cord stimulator implant: a review of the literature and their assessment with the MMPI-2-RF. Clin Neuropsychol. 2013;27(1):81–107.
9. Rolfson O, Dahlberg LE, Nilsson J-A, Malchau H, Garellick G. Variables determining outcome in total hip replacement surgery. J Bone Joint Surg Br. 2009;91(2):157–61.
10. Vissers MM, Bussmann JB, Verhaar JAN, Busschbach JJV, Bierma-Zeinstra SMA, Reijman M. Psychological factors affecting the outcome of total hip and knee arthroplasty: a systematic review. Semin Arthritis Rheum. 2012;41(4):576–88.
11. Duivenvoorden T, Vissers MM, Verhaar JAN, Busschbach JJV, Gosens T, Bloem RM, et al. Anxiety and depressive symptoms before and after total hip and knee arthroplasty: a prospective multicentre study. Osteoarthr Cartil. 2013;21(12):1834–40.
12. Pinto PR, McIntyre T, Ferrero R, Almeida A, Araújo-Soares V. Risk factors for moderate and severe persistent pain in patients undergoing total knee and hip arthroplasty: a prospective predictive study. PLoS One. 2013;8(9):e73917.
13. Thomas FM, Yeoman CAW. The effect of psychological status on pain and surgical outcome in patients requiring arthroscopic subacromial decompression. Int J Surg. 2011;9(5):1–5.
14. Hartley SM, Vance DE, Elliott TR, Cuckler JM, Berry JW. Hope, self-efficacy, and functional recovery after knee and hip replacement surgery. Rehabil Psychol. 2008;53(4):521–9.
15. Mahomed NN, Liang MH, Cook EF, Daltroy LH, Fortin PR, Fossel AH, et al. The importance of patient expectations in predicting functional outcomes after total joint arthroplasty. J Rheumatol. 2002;29(6):1273–9.
16. Judge A, Cooper C, Arden NK, Williams S, Hobbs N, Dixon D, et al. Pre-operative expectation predicts 12-month post-operative outcome among patients undergoing primary total hip replacement in European orthopaedic centres. Osteoarthr Cartil. 2011;19(6):659–67.
17. Sullivan M, Tanzer M, Reardon G, Amirault D, Dunbar M, Stanish W. The role of presurgical expectancies in predicting pain and function one year following total knee arthroplasty. Pain. 2011;152(10):2287–93.
18. Brand E, Nyland J. Patient outcomes following anterior cruciate ligament reconstruction: the influence of psychological factors. Orthopedics. 2009;32(5):335.
19. Burns LC, Ritvo SE, Ferguson MK, Clarke H, Seltzer Z, Katz J. Pain catastrophizing as a risk factor for chronic pain after total knee arthroplasty: a systematic review. J Pain Res. 2015;8:21–32.
20. Zeidan F, Martucci KT, Kraft RA, Gordon NS, McHaffie JG, Coghill RC. Brain mechanisms supporting modulation of pain by mindfulness meditation. J Neurosci. 2011;31(14):5540–8.
21. Lee M, Silverman SM, Hansen H, Patel VB, Manchikanti L. A comprehensive review of opioid-induced hyperalgesia. Pain Physician. 2011;14(2):145–61.
22. Kroenke K, Spitzer RL, Williams JBW, Löwe B. The patient health questionnaire somatic, anxiety, and depressive symptom scales: a systematic review. Gen Hosp Psychiatry. 2010;32(4):345–59.
23. Bruns D, Disorbio JM. The psychological evaluation of patients with chronic pain: a review of BHI 2 clinical and forensic interpretive considerations. Psychol Inj Law. 2014;7(4):335–61.

24. Siqueira JLD, Morete MC, Siqueira JLD, Morete MC. Psychological assessment of chronic pain patients: when, how and why refer? Rev Dor. 2014;15(1):51–4.
25. Presurgical psychological screening: understanding patients, improving outcomes [Internet]. http://www.apa.org. [cited 2016 Feb 7]. http://www.apa.org/pubs/books/4317298.aspx.
26. Young AK, Young BK, Riley LH, Skolasky RL. Assessment of presurgical psychological screening in patients undergoing spine surgery: use and clinical impact. J Spinal Disord Tech. 2014;27(2):76–9.
27. Block A, Ohnmeiss D, Ben-Porath Y, Burchett D. Presurgical psychological screening: A new algorithm, including the MMPI-2-RF, for predicting surgical results. The Spine Journal. 2011;11(10): S137–8.
28. Kerns RD, Turk DC, Rudy TE. The west haven-yale multidimensional pain inventory (WHYMPI). Pain. 1985;23(4):345–56.
29. Beck AT, Ward CH, Mendelson M, Mock J, Erbaugh J. An inventory for measuring depression. Arch Gen Psychiatry. 1961;4:561–71.
30. Radloff LS. The CES-D scale a self-report depression scale for research in the general population. Appl Psychol Meas. 1977;1(3):385–401.
31. Fydrich T, Dowdall D, Chambless DL. Reliability and validity of the beck anxiety inventory. J Anxiety Disord. 1992;6(1):55–61.
32. Osman A, Barrios FX, Kopper BA, Hauptmann W, Jones J, O'Neill E. Factor structure, reliability, and validity of the pain catastrophizing scale. J Behav Med. 1997;20(6):589–605.
33. Cohen S. Perceived stress in a probability sample of the United States. In: Spacapan S, Oskamp S, editors. The social psychology of health. Thousand Oaks: Sage; 1988. p. 31–67.
34. The coping strategies questionnaire and chronic pain adjustment: a conceptual and empirical reanal-

ysis. Clin J Pain [Internet]. LWW. [cited 2016 Feb 14]. http://journals.lww.com/clinicalpain/Fulltext/1994/06000/The_Coping_Strategies_Questionnaire_and_Chronic.3.aspx.
35. Waddell G, Newton M, Henderson I, Somerville D, Main CJ. A fear-avoidance beliefs questionnaire (FABQ) and the role of fear-avoidance beliefs in chronic low back pain and disability. Pain. 1993;52(2):157–68.
36. Fairbank JC, Pynsent PB. The oswestry disability index. Spine. 2000;25(22):2940–52. discussion 2952.
37. Riley JF, Ahern DK, Follick MJ. Chronic pain and functional impairment: assessing beliefs about their relationship. Arch Phys Med Rehabil. 1988;69(8):579–82.
38. Butler SF, Budman SH, Fernandez K, Jamison RN. Validation of a screener and opioid assessment measure for patients with chronic pain. Pain. 2004;112(1–2):65–75.
39. Tellegen A, Ben-Porath YS. The Minnesota multiphasic personality inventory-2 restructured form (MMPI-2-RF): technical manual. Minneapolis: University of Minnesota Press; 2008.
40. Marek RJ, Block AR, Ben-Porath YS. The Minnesota multiphasic personality inventory-2-restructured form (MMPI-2-RF): incremental validity in predicting early postoperative outcomes in spine surgery candidates. Psychol Assess. 2015;27(1):114–24.
41. Block AR, Marek RJ, Ben-Porath YS, Kukal D. Associations between pre-implant psychosocial factors and spinal cord stimulation outcome: evaluation using the MMPI-2-RF. Assessment. 2017;24(1):60–70.
42. Gatchel RJ, McGeary DD, McGeary CA, Lippe B. Interdisciplinary chronic pain management: past, present, and future. Am Psychol. 2014;69(2):119–30.
43. Centor RM. To be a great physician, you must understand the whole story. MedGenMed. 2007;9(1):59.

Moisés Fernández Hernando, Luis Pérez-Carro,
and Luis Cerezal

Introduction

Posterior hip pain in the adult, associated or not with sciatica, is among the most common diagnostic and therapeutic challenges for orthopedists and radiologists [1]. Over the past decade, much has changed with the approach to diagnosing and treating hip pathology based on development of imaging techniques and further advances in hip arthroscopy [2–4]. Because of the ever-increasing use of advanced magnetic resonance neurography (MRN) and the excellent outcomes of the endoscopic treatment, radiologists and orthopedists must be aware of the anatomy and pathologic conditions of the posterior hip. Extra-articular pathologies of the posterior hip comprise a wide range of injuries. MR imaging is the diagnostic procedure of choice for assessing posterior hip pain and may substantially influence management of these patients [5].

In one way or another, pathologies of the posterior hip are often associated with sciatic nerve involvement. Throughout this chapter we will describe many causes of hip pain associated with the involvement of this nerve, although they can obviously trigger posterior hip pain by themselves.

Similarly, in this chapter we will describe the main imaging techniques that are useful for the assessment of the posterior hip as well as their strengths and weaknesses. We also describe two of the main causes of posterior hip pain, deep gluteal syndrome and ischiofemoral impingement, both unfamiliar and poorly developed entities until now. Regarding the pathophysiology, diagnosis, classification, and treatment of these entities, there have been great advances in the last two years, which will be discussed from the point of view of the image.

Through the description of etiological factors and pathophysiological mechanisms involved in subgluteal and ischiofemoral impingement syndromes, we will also review little-known and specific pathologies that may be independently behind the posterior hip pain, even if they are not associated with these syndromes.

Finally, we will briefly evaluate the role of the image in the assessment of other well-known but equally important conditions of the posterior hip including fractures of the posterior acetabulum, neural pathology, bursae diseases, gluteal disorders, or hamstring conditions.

M. F. Hernando, MD (✉) · L. Cerezal, MD, PhD
Diagnóstico Médico Cantabria (DMC),
Musculoskeletal Radiology,
Santander, Cantabria, Spain

L. Pérez-Carro, MD, PhD
Clínica Mompia, Orthopedic Surgery Department,
Santa Cruz de Bezana, Cantabria, Spain

© Springer International Publishing AG, part of Springer Nature 2019
H. D. Martin, J. Gómez-Hoyos (eds.), *Posterior Hip Disorders*,
https://doi.org/10.1007/978-3-319-78040-5_5

Imaging Methods to Evaluate the Posterior Hip

Imaging plays a key role in the workup of unexplained hip pain. Plain radiography, ultrasound (US), computed tomography (CT), and magnetic resonance imaging (MRI) have all been used to assess posterior hip anatomy and pathologies.

Plain Radiography

Plain radiography is the initial imaging exam obtained for suspected hip diseases as it may demonstrate obvious causes of pain such as avascular necrosis, dysplasia, femoroacetabular impingement, degenerative joint disease, stress fracture, or tumors. Although this is the first diagnostic test that should be performed, most of the diseases occurring on the posterior hip are not visible radiographically. Standard hip radiographic series include an anteroposterior (AP) view of the pelvis, coned-down AP, and frog leg lateral views of the symptomatic hip. This series may be augmented with 45° and 90° Dunn views, cross table lateral, and false profile views. Oblique or Judet views are typically used in the setting of trauma to better depict acetabular fractures [6, 7].

Ultrasound

The adult hip poses several challenges to ultrasound evaluation. The structures to analyze in posterior hip are deeply situated requiring the use of relatively low-frequency transducers, thereby limiting resolution. Further, it is heavily operator dependent and does not provide the global overview and comprehensive information about the supporting soft tissues of the hip, nerves located deep within the hip, intra-articular structures, and bone marrow. These are the reasons why US does not play an important diagnostic role in patients with posterior hip pain [8, 9].

Despite these limitations, ultrasound can display several pathologic conditions about the hip. The real-time capability allows the assessment of conditions elicited by provocative maneuvers, playing an increasingly important role in "dynamic disorders," such as posterior "snapping hip." Moreover, ultrasound is well suited for image-guided interventional procedures including injection of the joint, tendon sheaths, or bursa, aspiration of ganglion cysts, drainage of para-articular fluid collections, and treatment of calcifying tendinosis. Furthermore, ultrasound is not subject to artifact introduced by indwelling metallic hardware. In addition, sonography is noninvasive and lacks ionizing radiation [10, 11].

The ESSR identified in 2012 the field of clinical indications for musculoskeletal ultrasound of the hip supported by expert knowledge. According to the clinical guidelines for musculoskeletal ultrasound (MSKUS), it is highly recommended only for fluid detection, extra-articular snapping hip, synovitis/effusion/synovial cysts, sports hernias, Morel-Lavallee lesions, high-grade muscle injuries, lateral femoral cutaneous nerve, and femoral nerve. Musculoskeletal ultrasound is deemed not indicated for intra-articular snapping hip, osteoarthritis, labral tears, low-grade muscle injuries, psoas tendon problems, trochanteric pain, sciatica, external rotator conditions, and growing pain [10].

Computer Tomography

Computed tomography (CT) is the gold standard for detecting osseous deformities of hip and pelvic pathologies. CT scans are useful for evaluating a variety of hip and pelvic conditions including femoroacetabular impingement (FAI), acetabular dysplasia, malalignment syndromes, traumatic hip instability, avulsions, fractures, and the component positioning after total hip arthroplasty. Surface rendering techniques have also helped to better define subtle osseous abnormalities at the proximal femur and acetabulum [12]. In addition, the lower cost, rapidly acquired high-resolution images with multiplanar 2D and 3D reconstructions with the added benefits of shortened exam time, and new lower radiation dose scanning techniques make CT an ideal modality for imaging the osseous structures of hip and pelvis. Finally, although MRI is much better able to demonstrate bone marrow and soft tissue abnormalities, CT can be used in the setting of proximal femur, acetabular, or sacral neoplasm to further characterize tumor matrix and to depict cortical destruction and breakthrough [13]. Additionally, contrast-enhanced CT is also the technique of choice for the assessment of vascular diseases of pelvis, hip, and deep gluteal space although MRI can also perform angiographic sequences.

Magnetic Resonance

MRI provides an excellent noninvasive means of assessing pathology of the posterior hip. It is the established secondary imaging exam of choice in the evaluation of unexplained hip pain for most clinical presentations. MRI provides exquisite anatomical detail and unique information regarding soft tissue and marrow abnormalities not seen on plain radiographs, CT, or nuclear medicine exams. Moreover, it is very effective in demonstrating intra-articular and extra-articular pathology, often identifying the source of pain and thus helping guide the appropriate management. MRI readily depicts many sources of extra-articular hip pathology including bursitis, myotendinous injury, occult fractures, sacroiliitis, and pelvic or subgluteal conditions [5, 14, 15]. The addition of 3T MRI has provided a significant improvement in image resolution, increasing our ability to visualize articular cartilage, posterior labral abnormalities, pelvic neuropathies and extra-articular causes of hip pain, including fibrovascular bands that are involved in the deep gluteal space [5, 16]. Specific protocols and the current and future state of the RM will be evaluated in this chapter in detail.

Radiological Anatomy of the Posterior Hip

The deep gluteal space is the main space of the posterior hip. It is the cellular and fatty tissue located between the middle and deep gluteal aponeurosis layers [2, 3, 5] (Fig. 5.1). These aponeuroses are not clearly visible on MRI since they are closely linked to muscle fasciae. Its posterior limit is the gluteus maximus muscle. At its inferior margin, it continues into and with the posterior thigh. Laterally it is demarcated by the linea aspera and the lateral fusion of the middle and deep gluteal aponeurosis layers extending up to the tensor fasciae latae muscle via the iliotibial tract. The posterior border of the femoral neck, the greater and lesser trochanters, and the posterior surface of the acetabulum form the anterior limit. Within the space superior to inferior, piriformis, superior gemellus, obturator internus, inferior gemellus, and quadratus femoris are included [2, 5]. The medial margin is comprised of the greater and minor sciatic foramina (Fig. 5.2). The greater sciatic foramen is bounded by the outer edge of the sacrum, the greater sciatic notch (superior and anterior), and the sacrospinous ligament (inferior). The limits of the lesser sciatic foramen are the lesser sciatic notch (external), sacrospinous lower border (superior), and the upper edge of the sacrotuberous ligament (inferior) [2, 3]. The sacrospinous ligament is a triangular-shaped structure, with its base attached to the anterior sacrum (S2–S4) and coccyx and apex attached to the ischial spine [17]. The sacrotuberous is a strong support ligament with an attachment similar to the sacrospinous ligament medially that reaches distal and inferiorly to the ischial tuberosity [18] (Figs. 5.1 and 5.2). The falciform process is an expansion that extends off this ligament and fuses with the fascia of the obturator internus [3] (Fig. 5.1c).

The greater sciatic foramen contains the piriformis muscle as a satellite structure. The superior gluteal artery and nerve run within the suprapiriform space; the inferior gluteal artery/nerve, sciatic, posterior femoral cutaneous, obturator internus/SG, and quadratus femoris/gemellus inferior nerves run within the infrapiriform space [3, 5]. It is important to differentiate these normal neurovascular bundles and isolated nerves that normally run along the deep gluteal space and not to confuse them with pathologic fibrovascular bands [5]. The lesser sciatic foramen contains the obturator internus muscle (Figs. 5.3, 5.4, and 5.5).

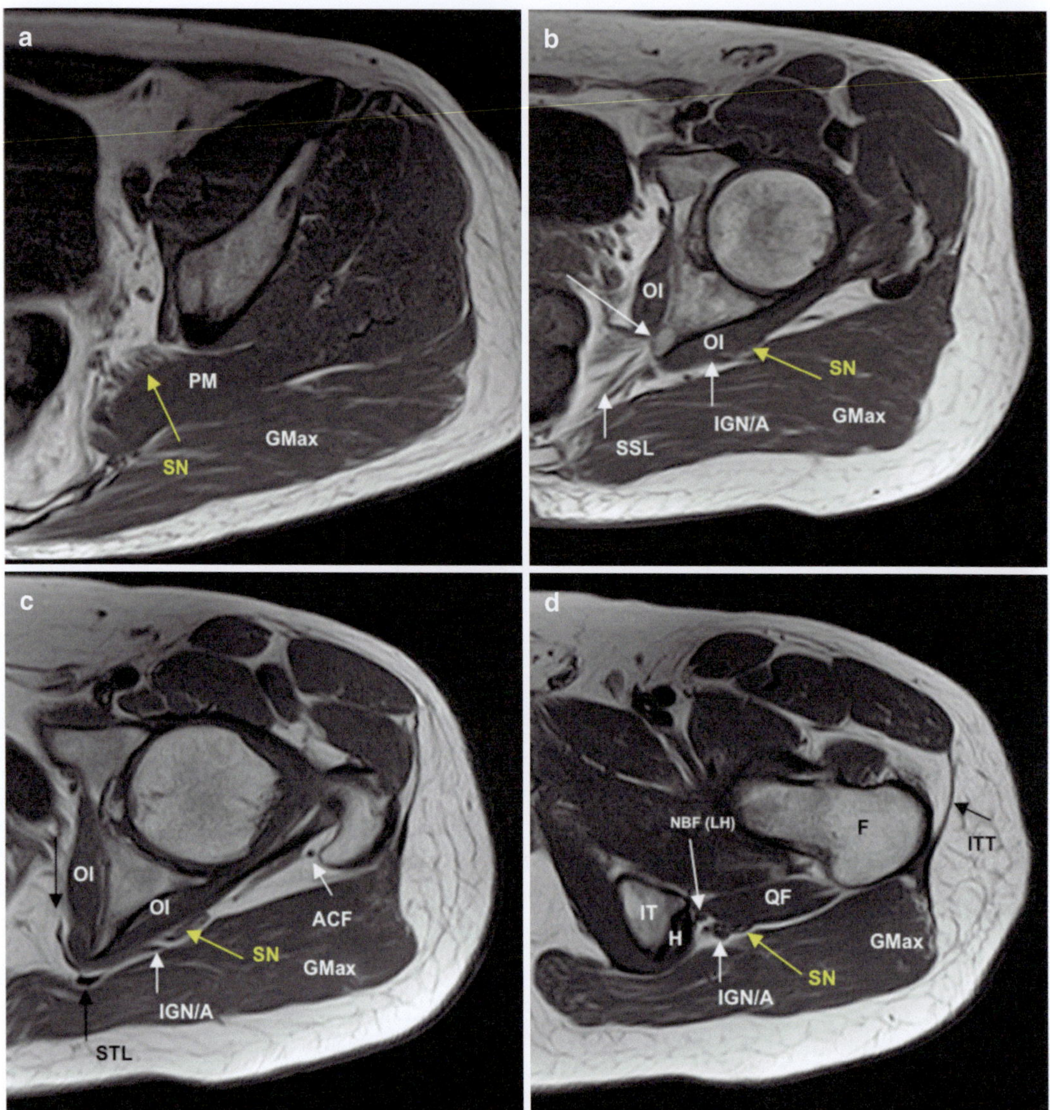

Fig. 5.1 Normal anatomy of the deep gluteal space. Consecutive from cranial to caudal axial T1-weighted MR images illustrating the main anatomic relationship in the deep gluteal space. (**a**) Level of the piriformis muscle (PM). (**b**, **c**) Level of the obturator internus muscle (OI). (**d**) Level of the quadratus femoris muscle (QF). Sciatic nerve (SN, arrow), *GMax* gluteus maximus muscle, *OI* obturator internus muscle, *ACF* ascending circumflex femoral artery, ischial spine (large arrow in **b**), *SSL* sacrospinous ligament, *STL* sacrotuberous ligament, *IT* ischial tuberosity, *H* hamstring tendons, *ITT* iliotibial tract, *ING/A* inferior gluteal nerve/artery, *NBF(LH)* long head of the biceps femoris nerve(arrowhead), *F* femur. Falciform process = black arrow

Muscles and Tendons

The piriformis muscle inserts into the ventrolateral aspect of the sacrum (S2–S4) and into the medial, superior, and posterior aspect of the greater trochanter (Fig. 5.5). Distinct fascial planes separate the piriformis muscle from the gluteal group of muscles posteriorly and from the retroperitoneal structures anteriorly. Identification of these fascial planes is important when searching pathology in the deep gluteal space originating from parasacral and retroperitoneal spaces. The fascial plane ante-

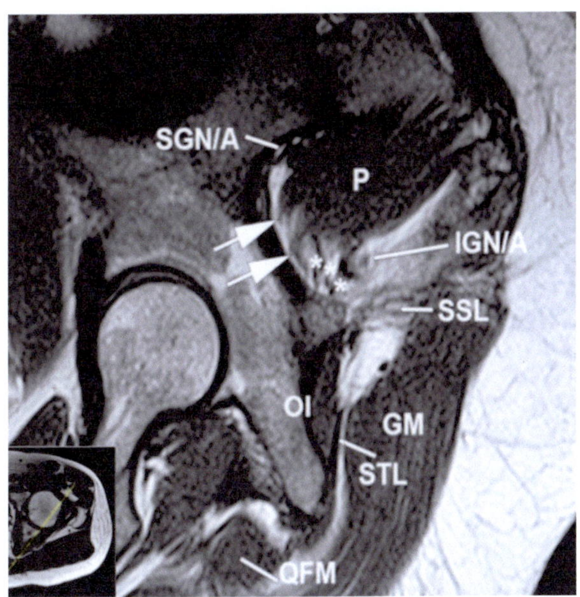

Fig. 5.2 Normal anatomy of the medial limit of deep gluteal space. Sagittal-oblique T1-weighted MR image shows the greater and minor sciatic foramina and its contents, including piriformis muscle (P), obturator internus-gemelli complex (OI), and quadratus femoris muscle (QFM). The superior gluteal nerve and artery (SGN/A) run within the suprapiriform space; the inferior gluteal nerve/artery (IGN/A), tibial and peroneal components of the sciatic nerve (arrows), and posterior femoral cutaneous, obturator internus/superior gemellus, and quadratus femoris/gemellus inferior nerves (asterisks from cranial to caudal) run within the infrapiriform space. *GM* gluteus maximus muscle, *SSL* sacrospinous ligament, *STL* sacrotuberous ligament

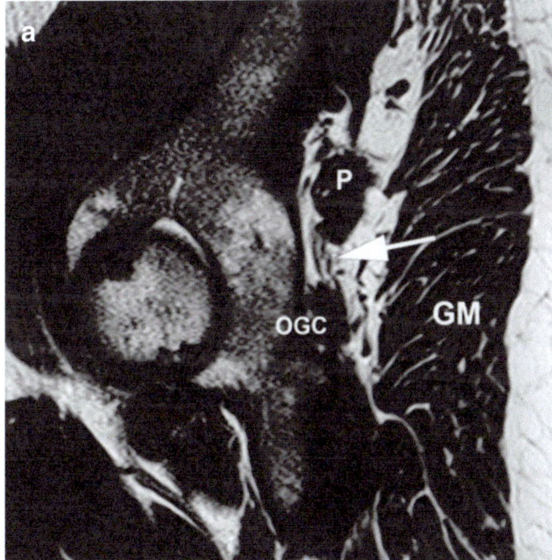

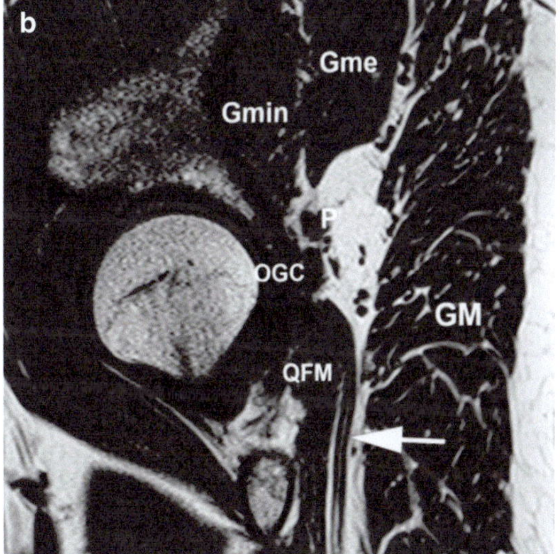

Fig. 5.3 Normal anatomy of the deep gluteal space. Consecutive from medial (**a**) to lateral (**b**) sagittal T1-weighted MR images show the piriformis muscle (P), the obturator internus-gemelli complex (OGC), the quadratus femoris muscle (QFM), the gluteus minimus muscles (Gmin), the gluteus medium muscle (Gme), and the gluteus maximus muscle (GM) and its relation with the sciatic nerve (arrows) in the middle area of the deep gluteal space and in the ischial tunnel

rior to the piriformis muscle communicates with the presacral space and thus with the opposite side (Fig. 5.1a). Unlike the anterior fascial plane, the fascial plane posterior to the piriformis does not cross the midline and ends medially at the lateral border of the sacrum (Fig. 5.1a). Prominent fascial planes also surround the sacrospinous ligament anteriorly and posteriorly. The space anterior to the ligament is the same space that contains the sacral plexus more superiorly. The space posterior to the ligament containing the sciatic nerve is limited medially by the sacrum [19] (Fig. 5.1b).

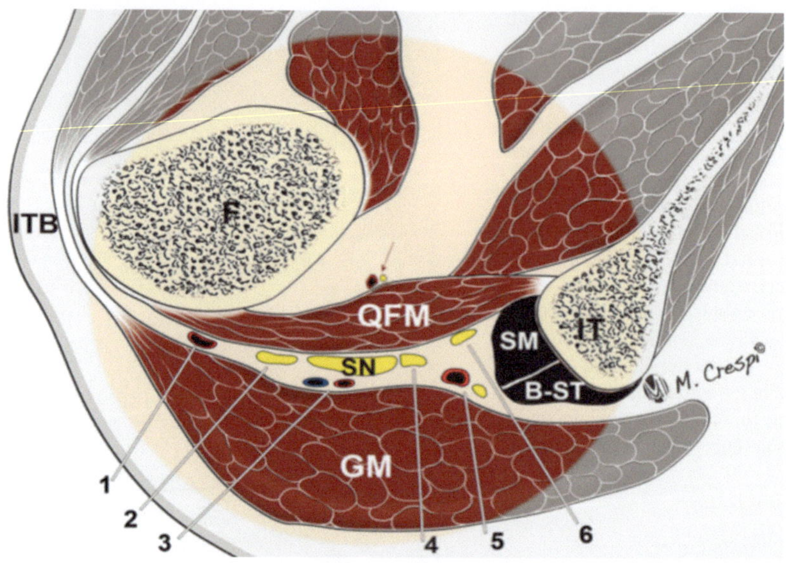

Fig. 5.4 Normal anatomy of the deep gluteal space. Diagram illustrates the most important neurovascular, muscular, tendinous, and osseous structures within the IFS. *GM* gluteus maximus muscle, *QFM* quadratus femoris muscle, *SN* sciatic nerve, *SM* semimembranosus tendon, *B-ST* conjoint tendon of biceps femoris-semitendinosus, *ITB* iliotibial band, *1* ascending posterior circumflex femoral artery, *2* nerve to the short head of the biceps femoris, *3* vasa vasorum of the sciatic nerve, *4* posterior cutaneous nerve of the thigh, *5* inferior gluteal artery and nerve, *6* nerve to the long head of the biceps femoris. Note the QFM nerve entering the muscle through its anterior surface (red arrow). Reprinted with permission from Massimiliano Crespi

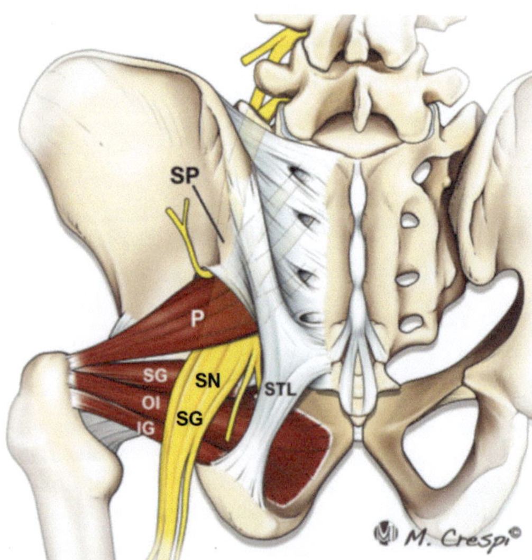

Fig. 5.5 Normal anatomy of the deep gluteal space. The diagram illustrates the main bone, ligament, muscle, and tendon structures located in deep gluteal space in a back view. *SP* sacral plexus, *SN* sciatic nerve, *STL* sacrotuberous ligament, *P* piriformis muscle, *SG* superior gemellus muscle, *OI* obturator internus muscle, *IG* inferior gemellus muscle. Reprinted with permission from Massimiliano Crespi

The obturator internus arises from the inner surface of the anterolateral wall of the pelvis and exits the pelvis through the lesser sciatic foramen (Figs. 5.1b and 5.5). The superior gemellus arises for the outer surface of the ischial spine and the inferior gemellus arises from the ischial tuberosity. The gemelli blend with the tendon of the obturator internus and insert on the anterior portion of the medial surface of the greater trochanter (Figs. 5.1c and 5.5). Often, the piriformis tendon is partially blended with the common tendon of the obturator/gemelli complex [20, 21].

The quadratus femoris muscle (QFM) is a flat, quadrilateral muscle that is situated within the deep gluteal space of the hip. This muscle has a somewhat striated appearance. The fibers run along the axial plane and are more closely opposed along the femoral end of the muscle. Along the ischial aspect, the fibers are more loosely arranged and have more interspersed fat [22, 23]. The quadratus femoris nerve arises from the ventral surface of (L4), L5, and S1 in 79.4% of the population. This nerve exits the pelvis through the greater sciatic notch, travels inferiorly along the anterior surface of the gemellus and obturator internus muscles, and enters the quadratus muscle through its anterior surface [24–26] (Figs. 5.6 and 5.7).

The obturator externus muscle is a triangular muscle, which covers the outer surface of the anterior wall of the pelvis. It arises from the margin of bone immediately around the medial side of the obturator foramen, the inferior ramus of the pubis, the ramus of the ischium, and the medial two-thirds of the outer surface of the obturator membrane. The fibers converge and pass posterolaterally and upward, ending in a tendon which runs across the back of the neck of the femur and the lower part of the capsule of the hip joint. It is finally inserted into the trochanteric fossa, which is located medial to the posterior aspect of the greater trochanter [27] (Figs. 5.7 and 5.8).

The blended iliopsoas muscle inserts distally on the lesser trochanter of the femur. The psoas major tendon is the main tendon and inserts into the apex of the lesser trochanter. The iliacus tendon is located more lateral, receives the most medial iliacus muscular fibers, and fuses with the main tendon. The most lateral fibers end up without any tendon on the anterior surface of the lesser trochanter and in the infratrochanteric

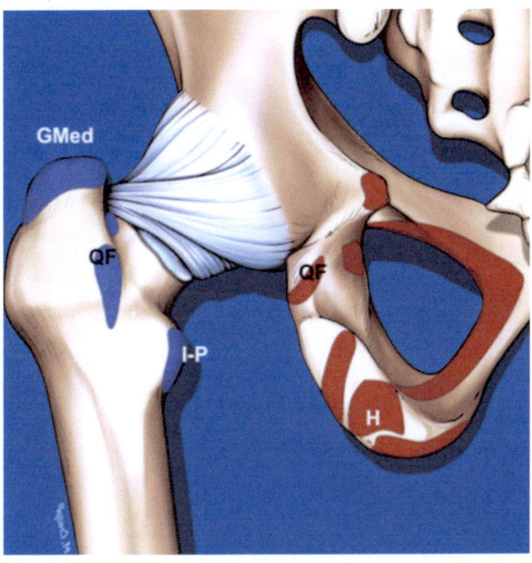

Fig. 5.6 Normal anatomy of the deep gluteal space. The diagram illustrates the most important tendon footprints within the deep gluteal space. *GMed* lateral gluteus medius footprint, *QF* quadratus femoris insertions, *I-P* iliopsoas footprint, *H* hamstring

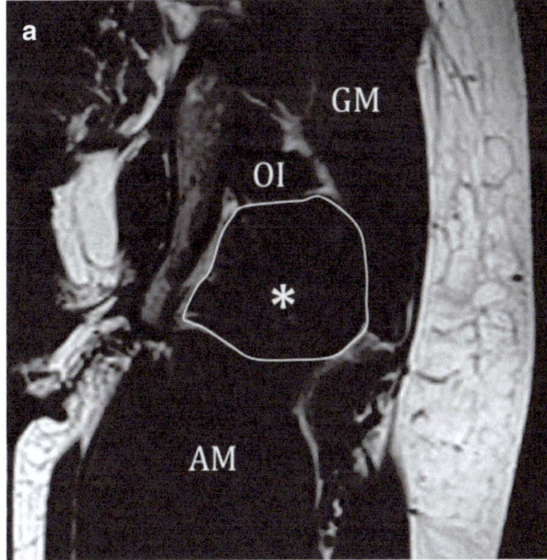

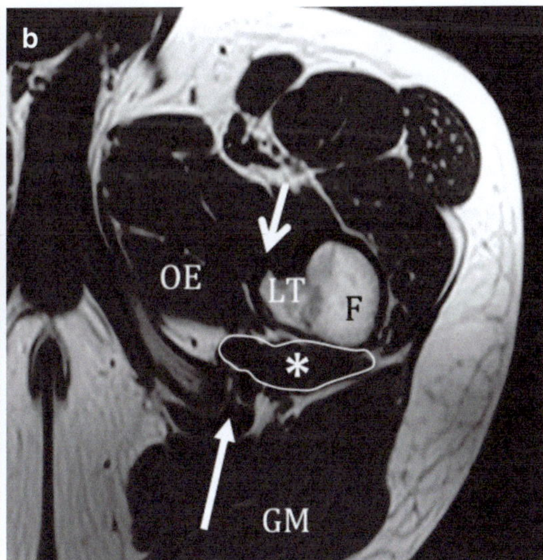

Fig. 5.7 Normal anatomy and relationships of the QFM. Coronal (**a**) and axial (**b**) T1-weighted MR images illustrating the main anatomic relationship of the QFM. *GM* gluteus maximus, *AM* adductor magnus, *OE* obturator externus, *LT* lesser trochanter. Short arrow = ilio-psoas tendon, long arrow = hamstring tendons. The QFM (white line and asterisk) is often best evaluated on axial images, where the origin, insertion, and relations can be assessed. Because of the muscle's orientation in the coronal plane, the abnormal signal may be difficult to visualize on routine coronal images, particularly if the field of view is large

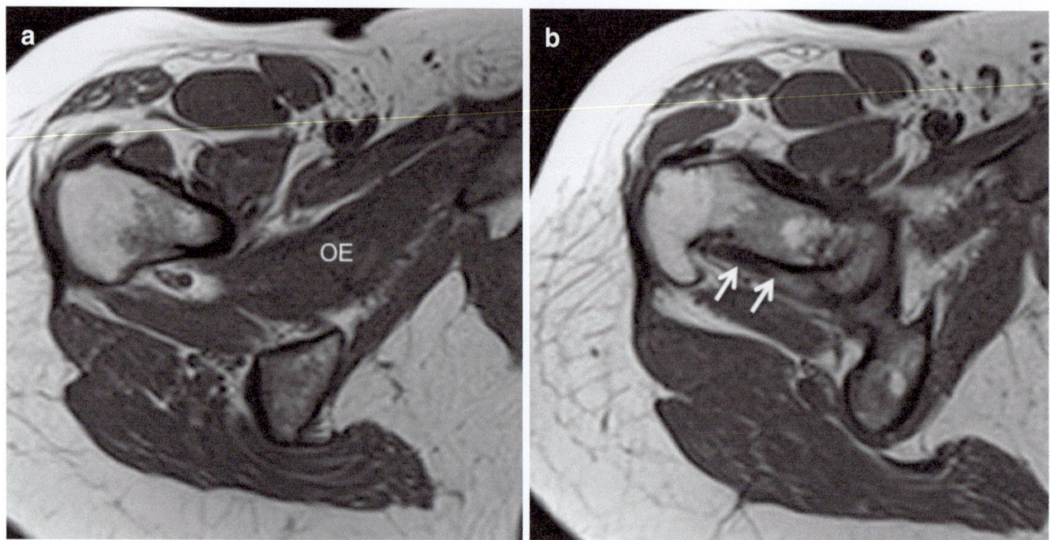

Fig. 5.8 Normal anatomy of the obturator externus muscle (OE). Axial T1-weighted MR images show its medial (**a**) and lateral (**b**) insertion (arrows)

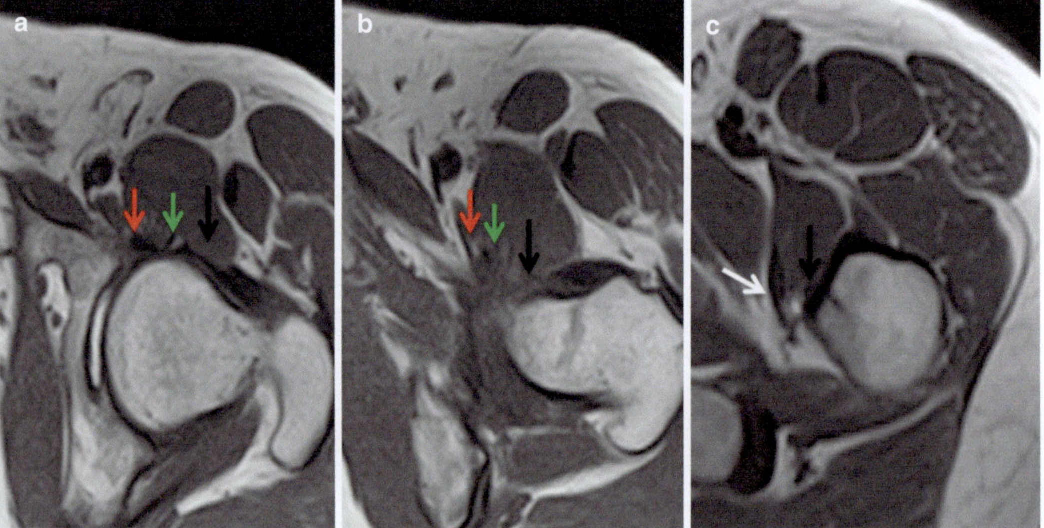

Fig. 5.9 Normal anatomy of the iliopsoas muscle-tendon complex. Consecutive from cranial to caudal axial T1-weighted MR images (**a–c**) illustrating its three components. Red arrows = psoas major tendon, green arrows = iliacus tendon, black arrow = blended iliacus-psoas tendon (inserting distally into the lesser trochanter), white arrows = lateral fibers of the iliacus tendon (ending up without any tendon on the anterior surface of the lesser trochanter and in the infratrochanteric region)

region. The most inferior muscular fibers of the iliacus join the principal tendon of the psoas passing around it by its ventromedial surface [28] (Fig. 5.9).

The hamstrings (HS) are a muscle group formed by long head of the biceps femoris, the semitendinosus (ST), and the semimembranosus (SM) muscles; all originate from the ischial tuberosity and innervate by the tibial branch of the sciatic nerve. The SM footprint is lateral and anterior to the crescent-shaped footprint of the common insertion of the ST and long head of the biceps femoris. The medial portion of the adductor magnus arises from the tuberosity of the ischium, which is located medial to the hamstring footprints. Sacrotuberous ligament (STL) shows continuity with both ischium and BF-ST tendon but not SM tendon. In HS rupture, tendon retraction is significantly less when STL remains attached to BF-ST tendon [29, 30] (Figs. 5.10 and 5.11).

Bursae

About 20 types of bursae have been described in the literature around the hip and pelvic areas, with variable extents and prevalences. The obturator externus, ischiogluteal, gluteofemoral, iliopsoas, obturator internus, piriformis, and trochanteric bursae are the most commonly affected by disease (Fig. 5.12). The anatomy and pathology of these bursae will be developed in a separate section at the end of this chapter.

Vascular Anatomy

The superior and inferior gluteal arteries (Figs. 5.1, 5.2, and 5.4) branch off of the internal iliac artery within the pelvis (lumbosacral region). The superior gluteal artery descends out of the pelvis through the upper greater sciatic notch, and the inferior gluteal artery descends out of the pelvis through the lower greater sciatic notch. The superior gluteal artery and nerve divides 1–2 cm above the superior border of the piriformis and fans out in a course anterior and distal to the greater sciatic foramen between the gluteus minimus and gluteus medius supplying the gluteus medius, gluteus minimus, and tensor fascia lata. The inferior gluteal nerve and artery enter the pelvis at the greater sciatic notch medial to the sciatic nerve passing between the piriformis muscle and coccygeus muscles. It descends along with the sciatic nerve and posterior femoral cutaneous nerve between the greater trochanter and ischial tuberosity. The inferior gluteal artery gives rise to two branches underlying the external rotators contributing to the perfusion of the acetabulum and capsule. A superficial arterial branch of the inferior gluteal artery crosses the sciatic nerve laterally between the piriformis and superior gemellus muscle [31] (Figs. 5.1, 5.2, and 5.4).

The medial and lateral femoral circumflex arteries (M/L-FCA) supply the metaphysis and the epiphysis of the femur forming an extracapsular arterial ring surrounding the base of the femoral neck. The MFCA arises from the femoral artery. It passes in a posterior direction between the iliopsoas and pectineus muscles and then between the medial capsule and the obturator externus muscle.

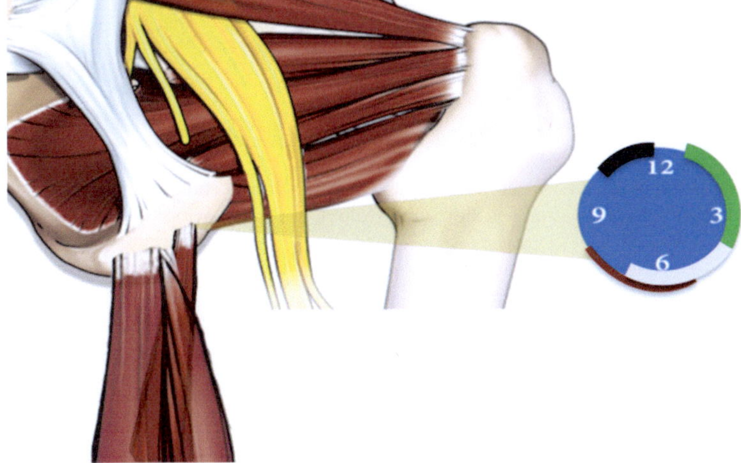

Fig. 5.10 Normal anatomy of the hamstring tendon complex. The diagram illustrates the footprint of the right hamstring tendons on the ischium.
Green = semimembranosus footprint, white = common insertion of the ST and long head of the biceps femoris, black = medial portion of the adductor magnus, red = sacrotuberous ligament insertion

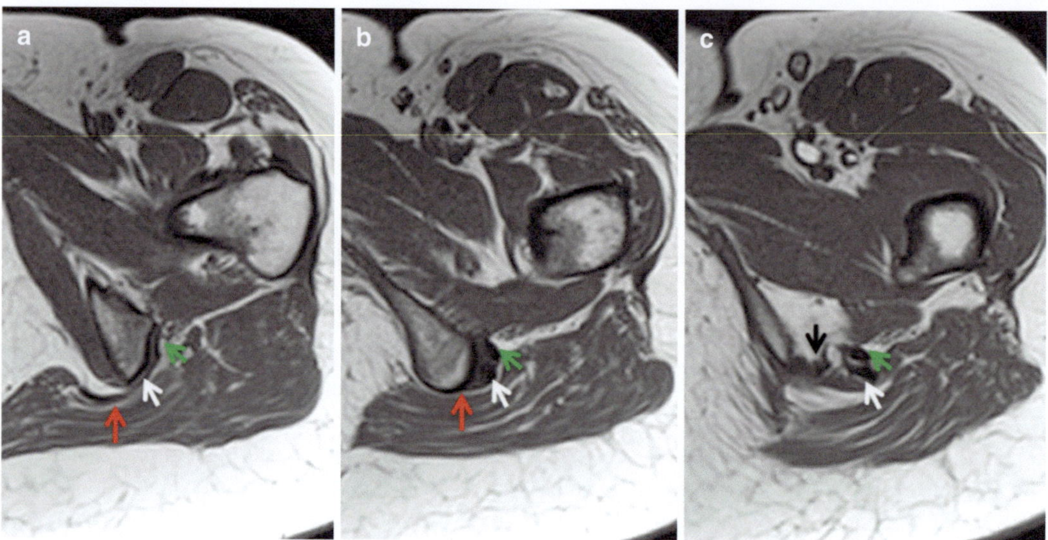

Fig. 5.11 Normal anatomy of the proximal hamstring tendon complex. Consecutive from cranial to caudal axial T1-weighted MR images (**a–c**) illustrate hamstring insertion onto the ischial tuberosity. Green arrows = semimembranosus footprint, white arrows = common insertion of the ST and long head of the biceps femoris, black arrow = medial portion of the adductor magnus, red arrows = sacrotuberous ligament insertion. The colors used in this image correspond to the colors used in Fig. 5.10 for a better understanding of the different tendon insertions

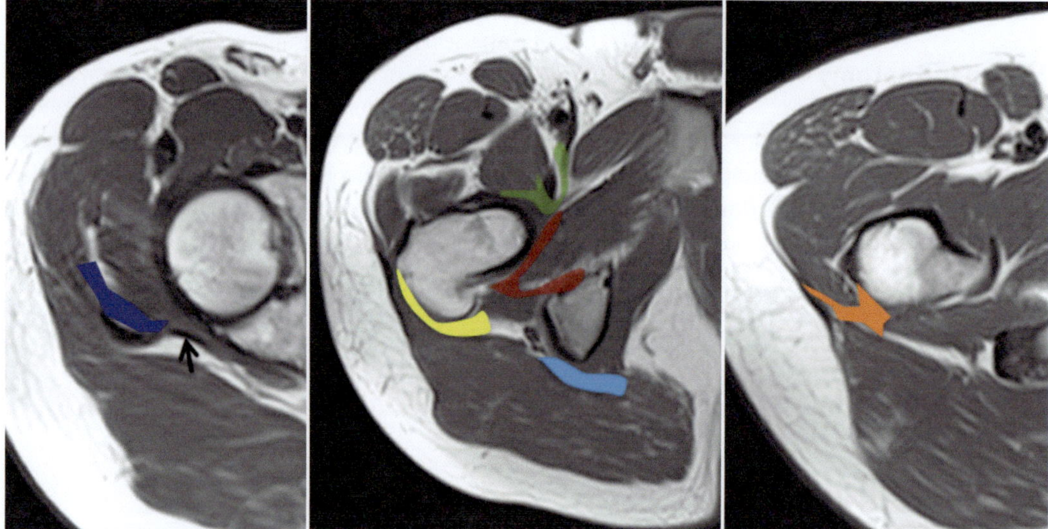

Fig. 5.12 Normal bursae around the posterior hip joint. Obturator externus (red), ischiogluteal (blue), gluteofemoral (yellow), iliopsoas (green), piriformis (dark blue), and gluteofemoral bursae are the most frequent bursae of the posterior hip that may be affected by disease

It then gives rise to the medial ascending cervical branches, muscular branches to supply the obturator externus muscle, and posterior ascending cervical arteries at the posterior aspect of the extracapsular region at the intertrochanteric line.

The termination of the MFCA traverses the lateral capsule in the posterior trochanteric fossa (lateral ascending cervical branches) providing most of the arterial supply to the femoral head, neck, and trochanter. The LFCA arises from the "profunda" artery; runs laterally, anterior to the iliopsoas; and ascends laterally and superiorly being the source of the anterior ascending cervical branches. All cervical ascending arteries traverse the capsule from the base and progress subsynovially up the femoral neck [32, 33] (Figs. 5.13 and 5.14).

Nerves

The lumbar plexus is composed of the ventral rami of L1–L4 and is anatomically located behind or less commonly within the psoas muscle, making it difficult to identify on CT and MRI [34]. The sacral plexus is derived from the anterior rami of spinal nerves L4, L5, S1, S2, S3, and S4 (Fig. 5.15). A minor branch of L4 combines with the ventral ramus of L5 to form the lumbosacral trunk (Fig. 5.16a). It descends over the sacral ala and combines with the ventral rami of S1, S2, and S3 (and a branch of S4) to form the sacral

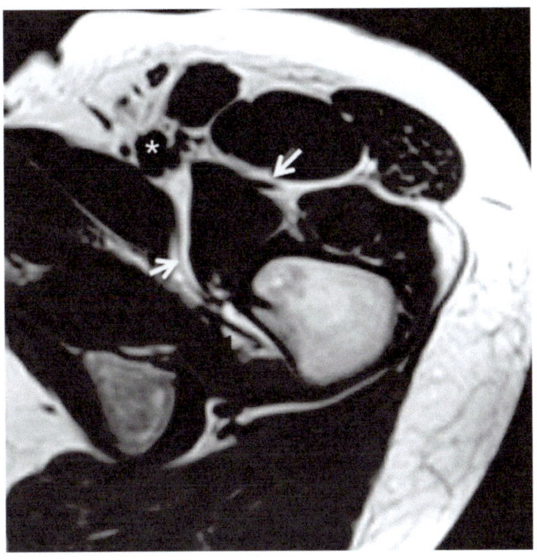

Fig. 5.13 Normal anatomy of the posterior and anterior ascending femoral arteries. Axial T1-weighted MR image shows both arteries (black arrows) originating from the medial and lateral circumflex femoral arteries, respectively (white arrows). Asterisk = femoral artery and profundus femoral artery

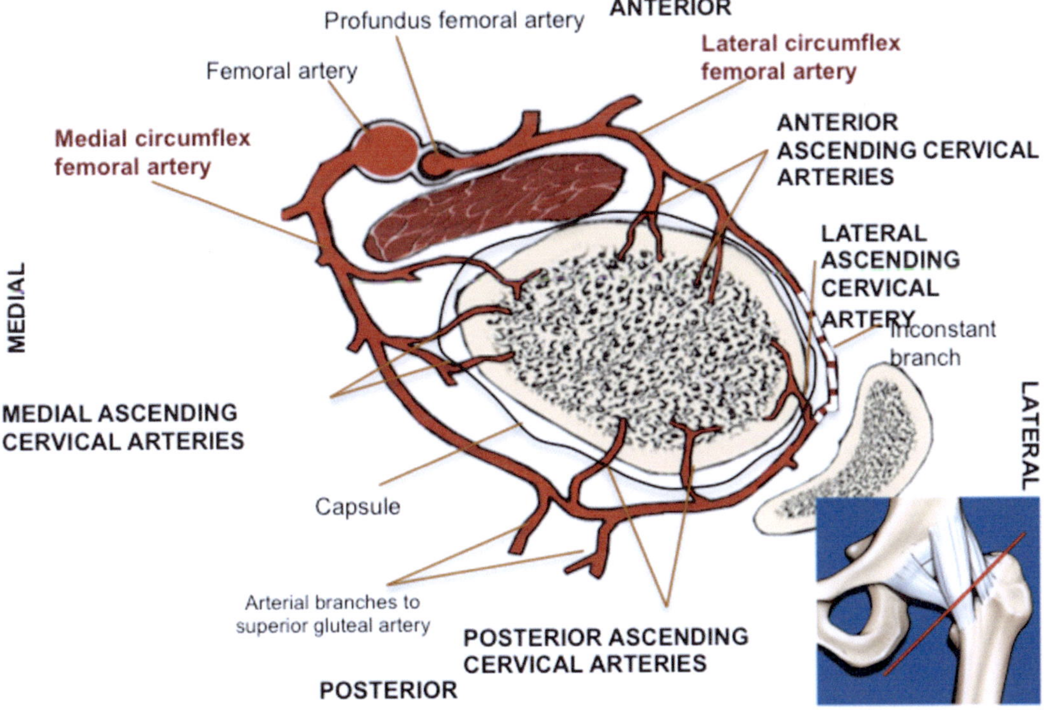

Fig. 5.14 Normal anatomy of vascular structures around the femur. The diagram illustrates the main vascular structures around the femur (right side). This anatomy must be kept in mind during imaging-guided injections to provide a less difficult, less painful, and free-risk path to the desired point of injection

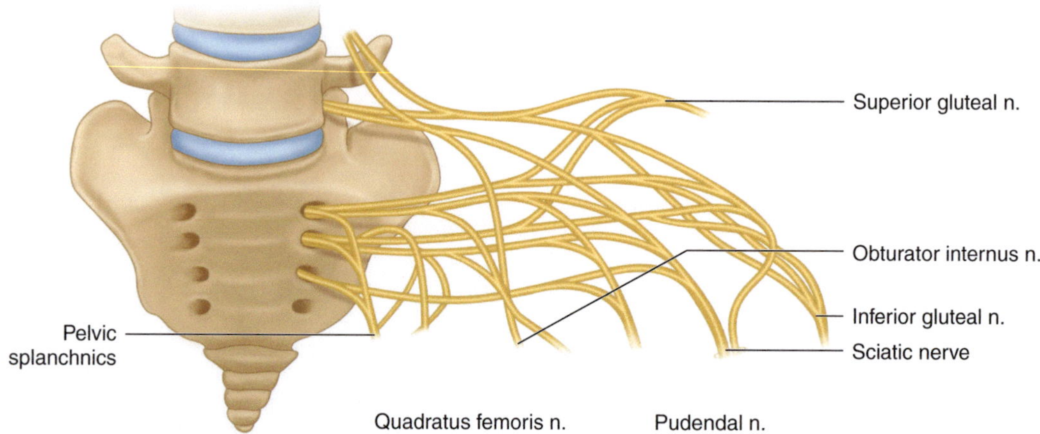

Fig. 5.15 Normal anatomy of the lumbosacral plexus. The diagram illustrates the main nerves arising from L4 through S3 at the lumbosacral enlargement

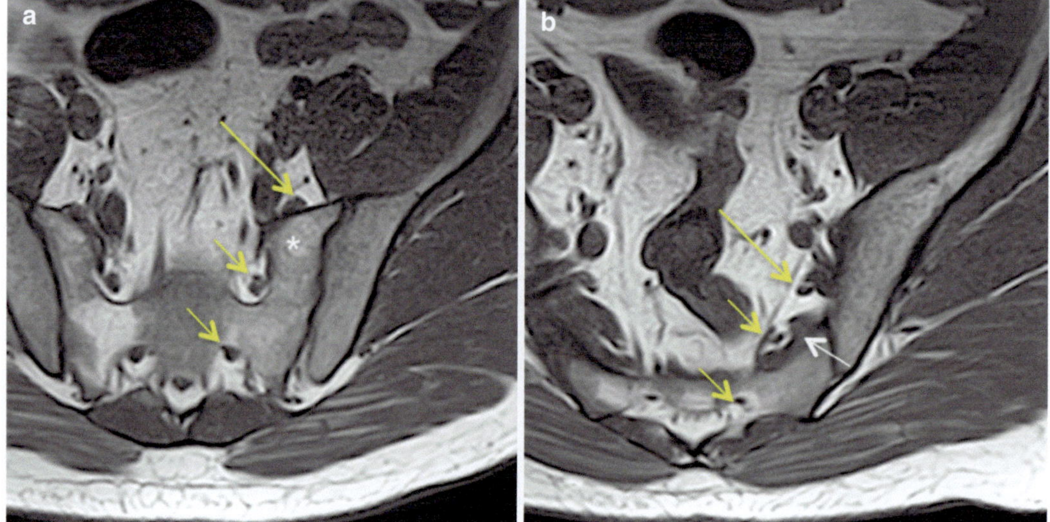

Fig. 5.16 Normal anatomy of the sacral plexus. Consecutive from cranial to caudal axial T1-weighted MR images illustrate the main anatomic relationship of the sacral plexus roots. (**a**) Level of the sacrum. (**b**) Level of the supra-piriformis space. (**c**, **d**) Level of piriformis muscle. Sacral roots = yellow arrows, large arrow = lumbosacral trunk, white arrow = piriformis muscle, asterisk = sacral ala

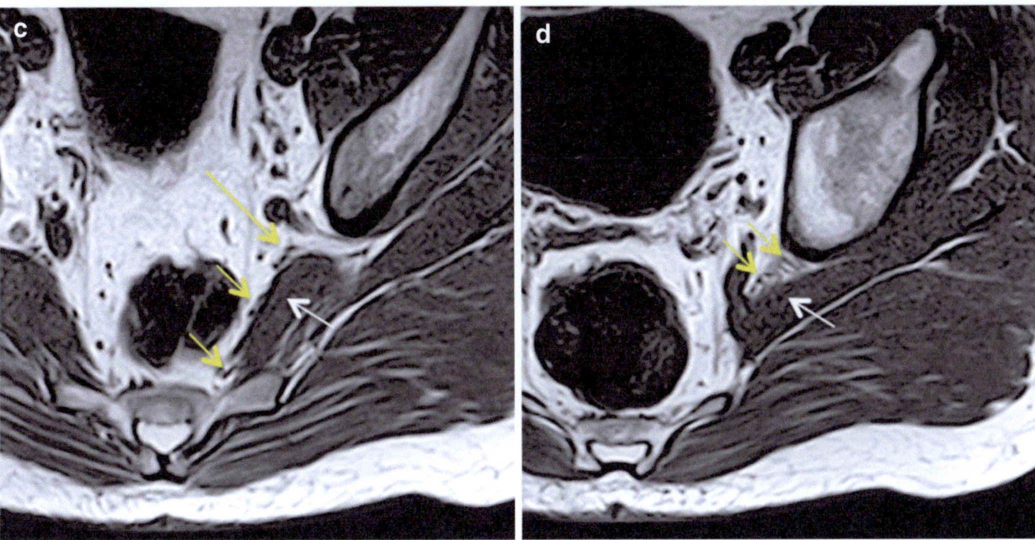

Fig. 5.16 (continued)

plexus. These branches decrease in thickness from top to bottom [35]. The first branch obliquely crosses the upper edge of the piriformis, the second running ahead of this muscle, and the third branch passes through its lower edge (Fig. 5.16). Smaller field-of-view coronal-oblique images aligned with the sacrum and sagittal images centered on the sacrum allow the sacral plexus to be seen [36]. The lumbosacral trunk and the anterior divisions of the sacral plexus combine to form the medial and anterior component of the sciatic nerve (tibial nerve), while the posterior divisions merge to form the lateral and posterior component (peroneal nerve). Both pass through the anterior third of the greater sciatic foramen enclosed in a common sheath and supported in the piriformis muscle arrangement perpendicular to its long axis, just behind the sacrospinous ligament insertion into the ischial spine (Figs. 5.1a, 5.2, 5.3, and 5.16). Within the superior deep gluteal space, sciatic nerve runs inferiorly and laterally ahead of the pyramidal (Figs. 5.2 and 5.3). After curves it takes the longitudinal direction of the thigh, behind the obturator internus-gemelli complex and quadratus femoris and lateral, in intimate contact, to the conjoined tendon of the long head of biceps and semitendinosus, lying near the posterior capsule of the hip joint [37] (Figs. 5.1, 5.2, 5.3, 5.4, 5.5,

5.16, and 5.17). At this level the sciatic nerve is located in the middle third and least frequently in the inner third of the line between the ischium and the greater trochanter, at a mean of 1.2–0.2 cm from the most lateral aspect of the ischial tuberosity. At the level of the sacrospinous ligament insertion, the sciatic nerve can be identified as a robust and circular structure with a diameter of between 0.9 and 1.2 cm [38]. Throughout its course the nerve is covered by the gluteus maximus [2, 3, 8]. There is no artery after a similar course because the chief blood supply to the thigh is through the anterior femoral artcry. With hip flexion, the sciatic nerve experiences a proximal excursion of 28.0 mm [39] (Figs. 5.17 and 5.18).

Imaging Assessment in "Deep Gluteal Syndrome"

Deep gluteal syndrome (DGS), also named subgluteal syndrome, is an underdiagnosed entity characterized by pain and/or dysesthesias in the buttock area, hip, or posterior thigh and/or radicular pain, due to a non-discogenic sciatic nerve entrapment in the deep gluteal space.

In a prospective MRI study of the lumbar spine in asymptomatic patients, 20% of theme

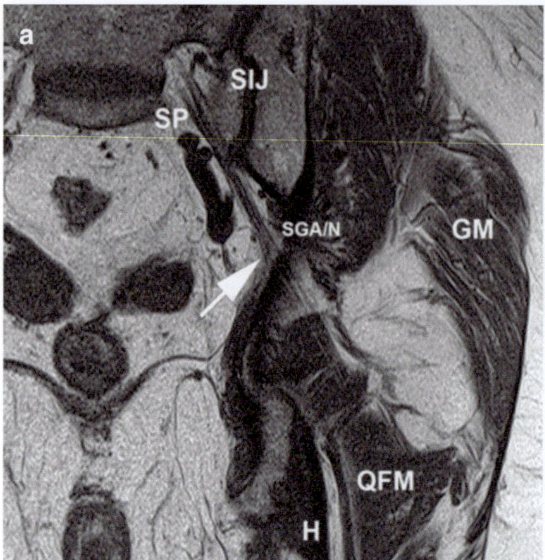

Fig. 5.17 Normal anatomy of the deep gluteal space. Consecutive from anterior (**a**) to posterior (**b**) coronal T1-weighted MR images illustrating the main anatomic relationship in the deep gluteal space. Sciatic nerve (arrow), *SP* sacral plexus, *SGA/N* superior gluteal artery and nerve, *GM* gluteus maximus muscle, *QFM* quadratus femoris muscle, *H* hamstring tendons, *SIJ* sacroiliac joint, *OI* obturator internus muscle, *P* piriformis muscle

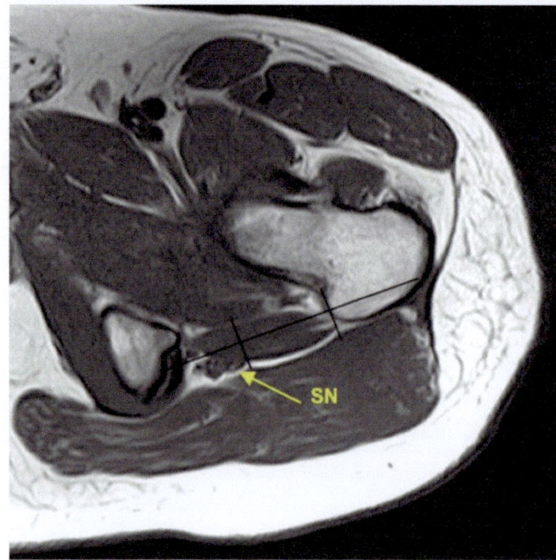

Fig. 5.18 Normal location of the sciatic nerve. Axial T1-weighted MR image shows the location of the sciatic nerve in the inner third of the line between the ischium and the greater trochanter, at a mean of 1.2–0.2 cm from the most lateral aspect of the ischial tuberosity

between 20 and 59 years of age had a herniated disc and 57% of the 60- to 80-year-old group had evidence of a herniated disc or canal stenosis. Moreover, in 20% of cases, the sciatica is of both discogenic and non-discogenic origin [40].

However, in practice, causes of non-discogenic entrapment are often overlooked, partly due to the high sensitivity of lumbar spine MRI. It is known that sacral plexus and sciatic nerve entrapments may be a result from a high spectrum of extrapelvic (within the deep gluteal space) or intrapelvic pathology. Due to the variation of anatomical entrapment, the term "deep gluteal syndrome" may be a more accurate description of this non-discogenic sciatica [2].

Multiple orthopedic and non-orthopedic conditions may manifest as a DGS [5, 35, 40]. A broad spectrum of known pathologies may nonspecifically be located in the deep gluteal space and can therefore trigger DGS. These entities can be found in any other body area affecting other nerves and can be classified as traumatic, iatrogenic, inflammatory/infectious, vascular, gynecologic, and tumors/pseudotumors. On the other hand, there are specific entrapments of this anatomical area. These entrapments within the deep gluteal space include fibrous bands, piriformis syndrome, obturator internus/gemellus syndrome, quadratus femoris and ischiofemoral pathology, hamstring conditions, gluteal disorders, or orthopedic causes [5] (Table 5.1).

Table 5.1 Potential etiologies of DGS according to the pathophysiological mechanisms

Specific entrapments
Fibrous and fibrovascular bands
Piriformis syndrome
Hypertrophy of the piriformis muscle
Dynamic sciatic entrapment by piriformis
Anatomical variations of sciatic-piriformis complex
Anomalous attachment of the piriformis muscle
Fibrosis after classic open surgery
Trauma- or overuse-related conditions (avulsions, tendinosis, strains, calcifying tendinosis, and spasm)
Gemelli-obturator internus syndrome
Hypertrophy of the obturator internus muscle
Dynamic sciatic entrapment by obturator internus
Anatomical variations of sciatic-piriformis complex
Scissor-like piriformis-obturator internus entrapment
Trauma- or overuse-related conditions (avulsions, tendinosis, strains, calcifying tendinosis, and spasm)
Quadratus femoris and ischiofemoral pathology
Trauma- or overuse-related conditions
Ischiofemoral impingement
Hamstring conditions
Gluteal disorders
Orthopedic and other causes
Nonspecific entrapments
Traumatic
Iatrogenic
Inflammatory/infectious
Vascular
Gynecological
Pseudotumors and tumors

Specific Entrapments

Fibrous and Fibrovascular Bands

The concept of fibrous bands, which may or may not contain blood vessels, playing a role in causing symptoms related to sciatic nerve entrapment represents a radical change in the current diagnosis and therapeutic approach for the all-inclusively used term "piriformis syndrome." Typically constricting fibrous bands are present in many cases of sciatic nerve entrapment during endoscopy [2, 3]. Under normal conditions, the sciatic nerve is able to stretch and glide in order to accommodate moderate strain or compression associated with joint movement [41]. Diminished or absent sciatic mobility during hip and knee movements due to these bands is the precipitating cause of sciatic neuropathy (ischemic neuropathy) [5, 42] (Figs. 5.19 and 5.20).

From the point of view of its macroscopic structure, there are three primary types of bands: pure fibrous bands (Fig. 5.21), without identifiable macroscopic vessels by MRN imaging and endoscopy; fibrovascular bands, with vessels macroscopically identifiable by MRN (Fig. 5.22); and pure vascular bands, exclusively formed by a vessel without surrounding fibrous tissue [5].

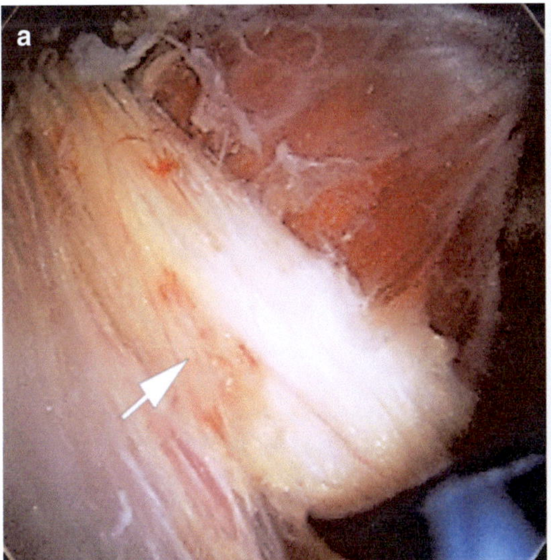
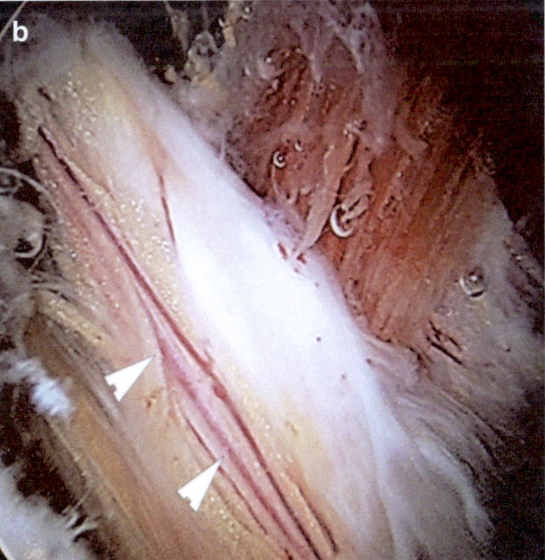

Fig. 5.19 Endoscopic view showing the pathogenic mechanism of DGS. (**a**) Edematous and flattened sciatic nerve due to fibrovascular entrapment (arrow) in a patient with ischemic neuritis. (**b**) Normal vascularization recovery (arrowheads) after nerve neurolysis

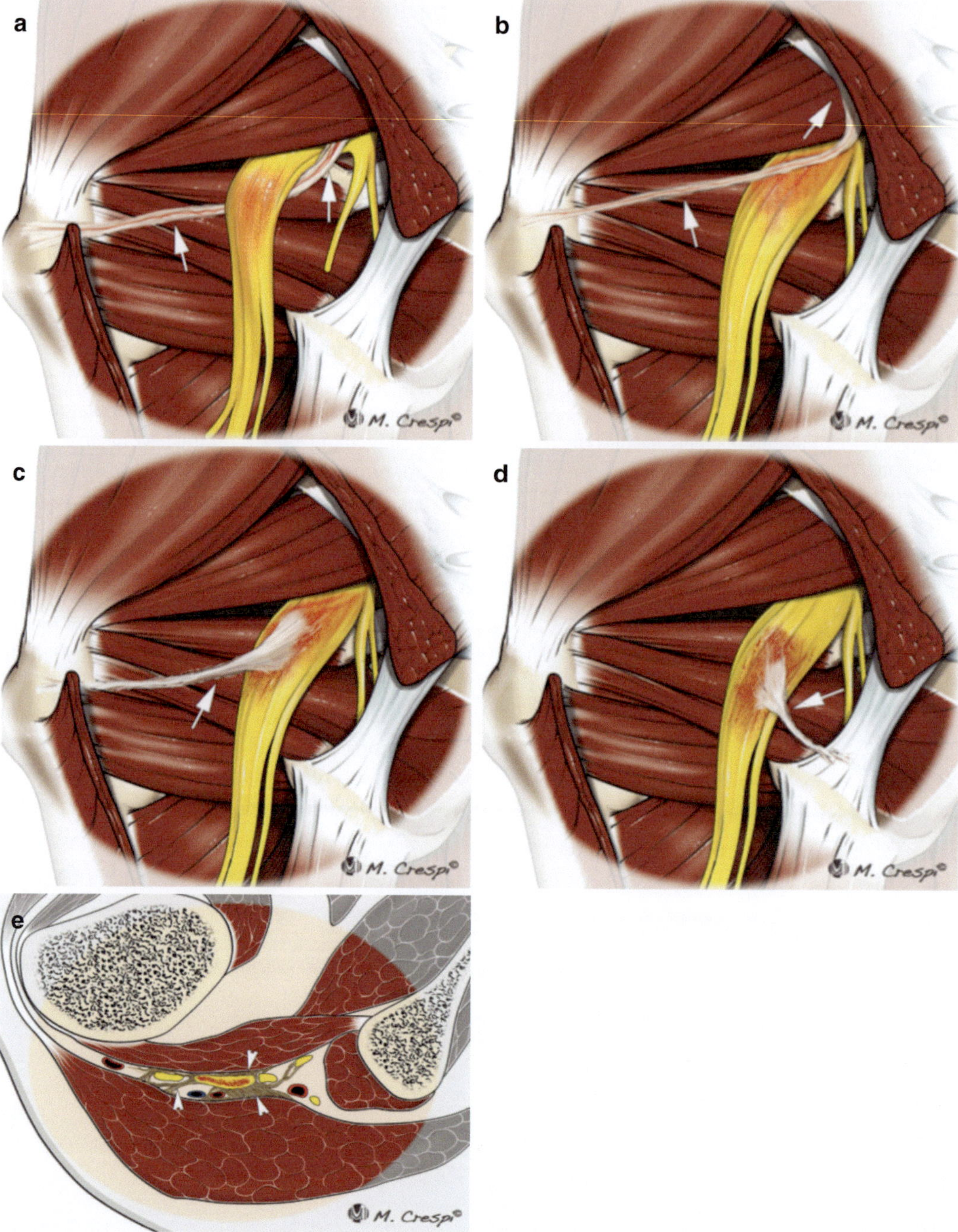

Fig. 5.20 Pathogenic classification of fibrous/fibrovascular bands. (**a**, **b**) Compressive or bridge-type bands limiting the movement of the sciatic nerve from anterior to posterior (type 1A) or from posterior to anterior (type 1B). (**c**, **d**) Adhesive bands or horse-strap bands (type 2), which bind strongly to the sciatic nerve structure, anchoring it in a single direction. They can be attached to the sciatic nerve laterally (type 2A) or medially (type 2B). (**e**) Bands anchored to the sciatic nerve with undefined distribution (type 3). Reprinted with permission from Massimiliano Crespi

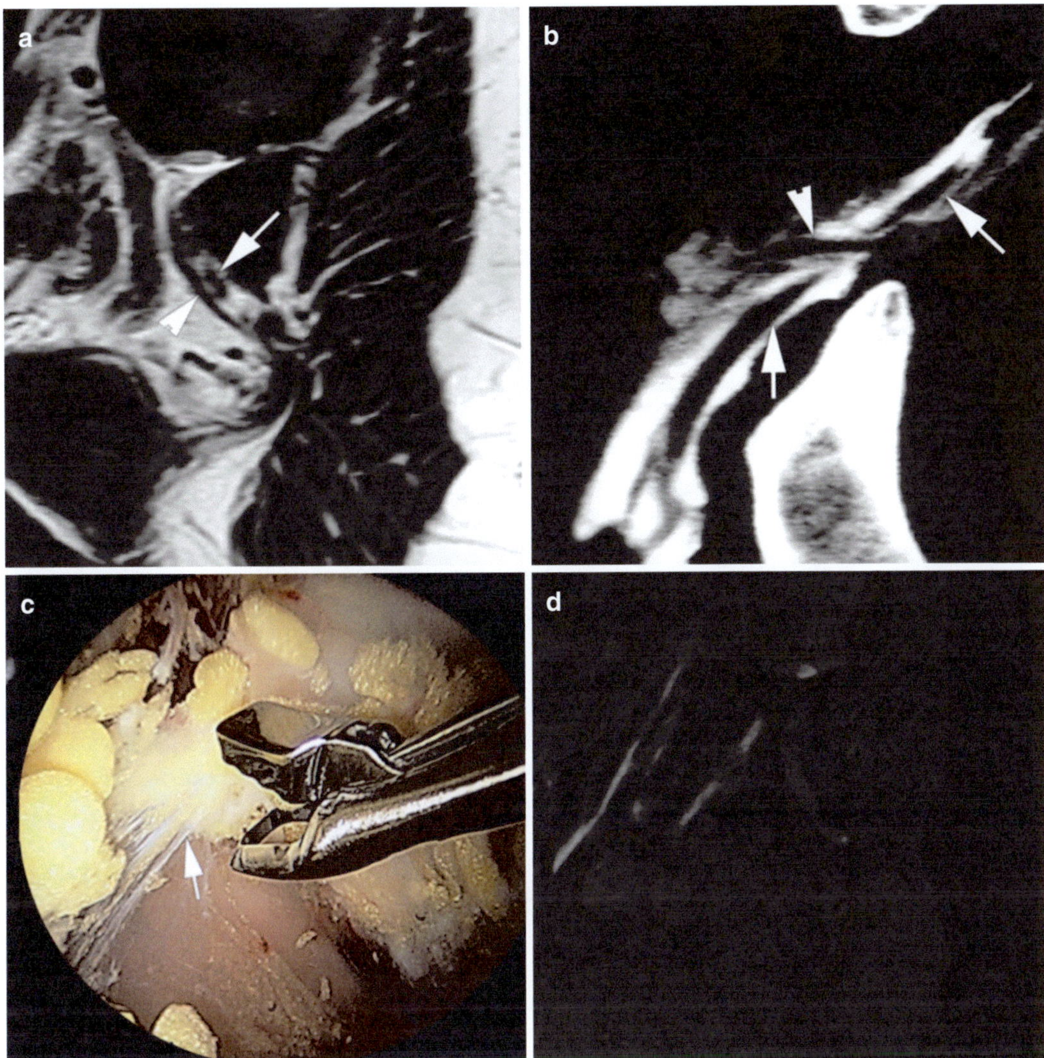

Fig. 5.21 Purely fibrotic proximal type-1A band in a 39-year-old woman with DGS. (**a**) Double sagittal-oblique PD-weighted MR image shows a compressive or bridge-type band (arrowhead) limiting the movement of the sciatic nerve (arrow) from anterior to posterior. (**b**) Coronal-oblique MDCT reconstruction of the same band (arrowhead) after infiltration test. The iodinated contrast around the sciatic nerve (arrow) allows better delineation of this band. (**c**) Endoscopic image shows the sciatic nerve decompression through resection of this band (arrowhead). (**d**) Double sagittal-oblique fat-saturated PD-weighted MR image shows a compressive or bridge-type band (arrowhead) limiting the movement of the sciatic nerve (arrow) from anterior to posterior. Note the signal hyperintensity of the sciatic nerve indicative of neuritis

Based on their location, they can be classified as proximal, which affects the sciatic nerve in the vicinity of the greater sciatic notch, and distal, which affects the ischial tunnel region, between the quadratus femoris and proximal insertion of the hamstrings and middle bands, located at the level of the piriformis and obturator internus-gemelli complex (piriformis-obturator space). In each of these three locations, these bands can be located medial or lateral to the sciatic nerve [5] (Fig. 5.5).

Depending on the pathogenic mechanism, bands can be classified as (Fig. 5.20):

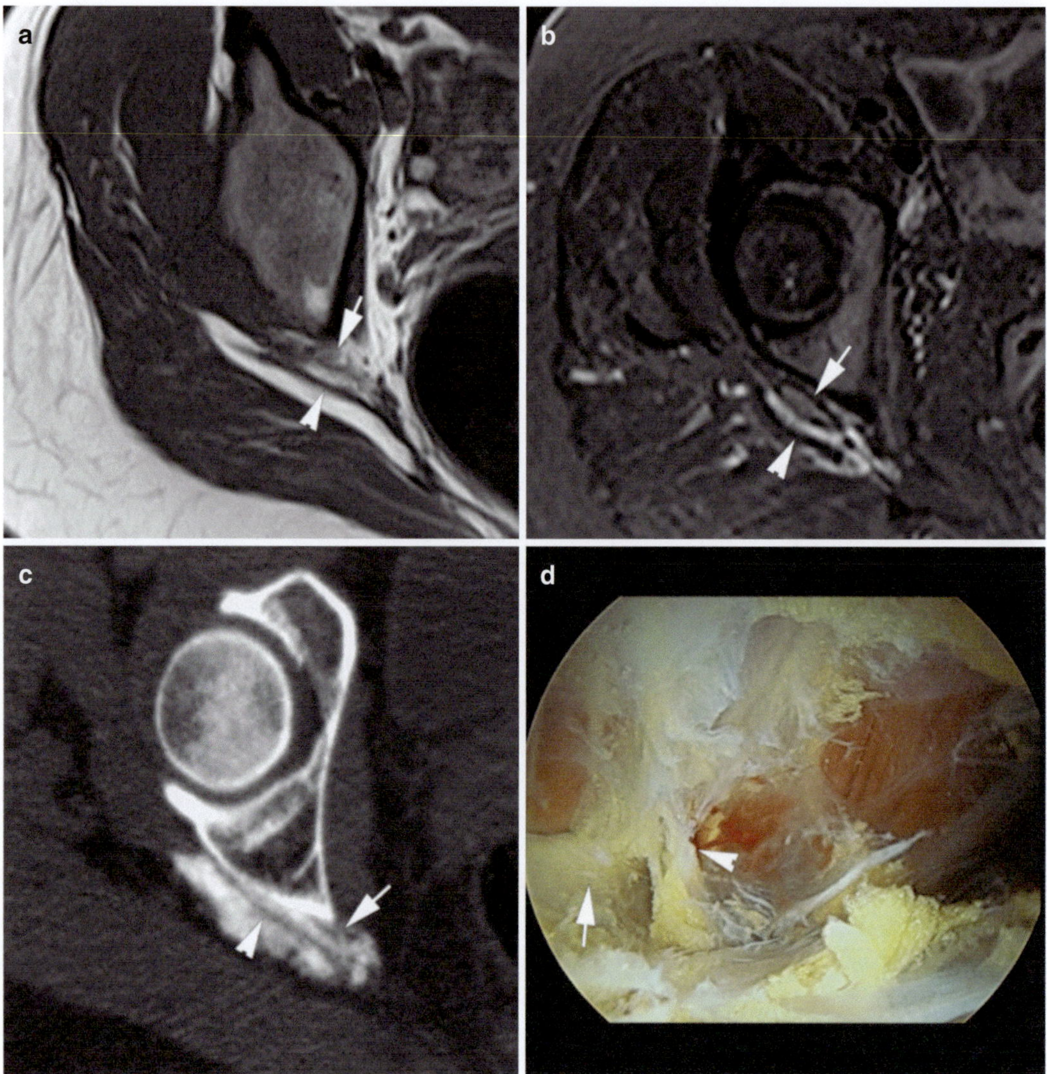

Fig. 5.22 Proximal fibrovascular type-1B band in a 44-year-old woman with DGS. (**a**) Axial-oblique T1-weighted MR image and (**b**) axial PD fat-suppressed MR image show a fibrovascular band with an artery macroscopically identifiable (arrowheads) located behind the sciatic nerve (arrows). (**c**) Axial-oblique MDCT reconstruction of the same fibrovascular band after the infiltration test performance. The iodinated contrast around the nerve allows better delineation of this band. (**d**) Endoscopic image shows the sciatic nerve (arrow) compression by a fibrovascular band (arrowhead). Note the bleeding vessel during resection of the band. Resection of the band resulted in complete resolution of symptoms

(a) Compressive or bridge-type bands (type 1), which limit the movement compressing the nerve from anterior to posterior (Type 1A) (Figs. 5.20a and 5.21) or from posterior to anterior (Type 1B) (Figs. 5.20b and 5.22). The former is located in front of the sciatic nerve. These fibrous bands usually extend from the posterior border of the greater tro-chanter and surrounding soft tissues (distal insertions are variable) to the gluteus maximus onto the sciatic nerve and extend up to the greater sciatic notch [5].

(b) Adhesive bands or horse-strap bands (type 2), which bind strongly to the sciatic nerve structure, anchoring it in a single direction and not allowing to perform its normal excursion during the hip movements. These bands can be attached to the sciatic nerve laterally, from the major trochanter (type 2A), or medially, from the sacrospinous ligament (type 2B). Lateral bands are the most common. Among those classified as medial bands, proximal location is more frequent [5] (Figs. 5.20c and 5.23).

(c) Bands anchored to the sciatic nerve with undefined distribution (type 3). These kinds of bands, with an erratic distribution, are characterized by anchoring the nerve in multiple directions (Figs. 5.20e and 5.24). As type-2 bands, they are secondary to a broad spectrum of musculoskeletal and extraskeletal pathology [5].

Radiologists and orthopedics should be aware of this bands classification as it provides useful information enabling the surgeon to choose the appropriate instruments, patient positioning, endoscopic portals, and intraoperative management. Any band found should be classified within these three groups. Because of its higher frequency, special attention must be given to branches of the inferior gluteal artery (IGA) nourishing fibrous bands in the proximity of the piriformis muscle [5] (Figs. 5.2 and 5.4).

Piriformis Syndrome

The development of periarticular hip endoscopy and MRI techniques has allowed for the understanding of the pathophysiological mechanisms underlying piriformis syndrome and DGS, and, therefore, it has supported further its classification. Thereby, piriformis syndrome can be classified as a subgroup of DGS but not all DGS are piriformis syndrome [3].

Reported incidence rates for piriformis syndrome among patients with low back pain vary widely from 5% to 36% [43, 44]. Actual prevalence is difficult to determine accurately because it is often underdiagnosed or confused with other conditions. Until now piriformis syndrome has probably been underdiagnosed, rather than overdiagnosed [45]. Filler et al. did publish an investigation of 239 patients with sciatica who had either failed spine surgery (46%) or a failure to determine the exact cause of their sciatica. After performing MR neurography and interventional MR imaging, the final rediagnosis was piriformis syndrome in 67.8% of patients. None of the studies published to date include the concept of fibrous bands or other causes that are discussed in this chapter. Therefore, the pain attributed to piriformis muscle could have other not evaluated causes.

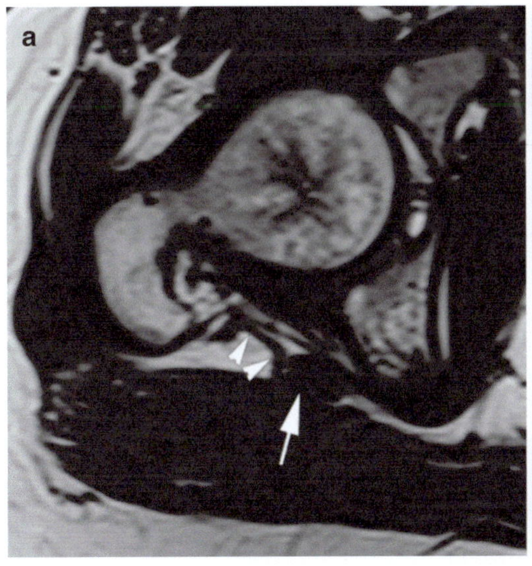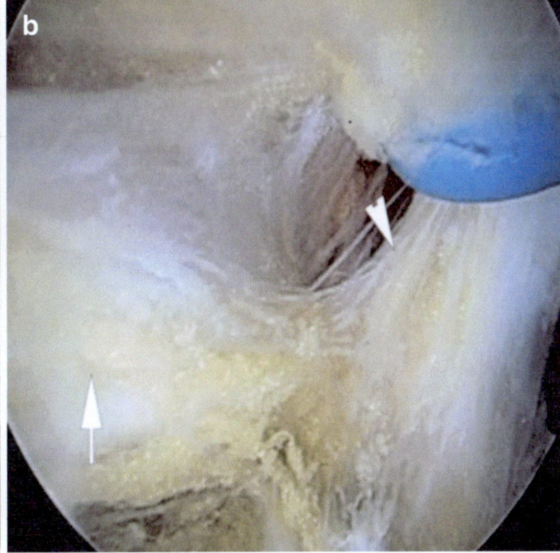

Fig. 5.23 Adhesive and lateral type-2A fibrous band in a 31-year-old woman with DGS. Axial PD-weighted MR image (**a**) and endoscopic view (**b**) show a fibrous band (arrowheads) attached to the sciatic nerve (arrow), laterally from the major trochanter (type 2A)

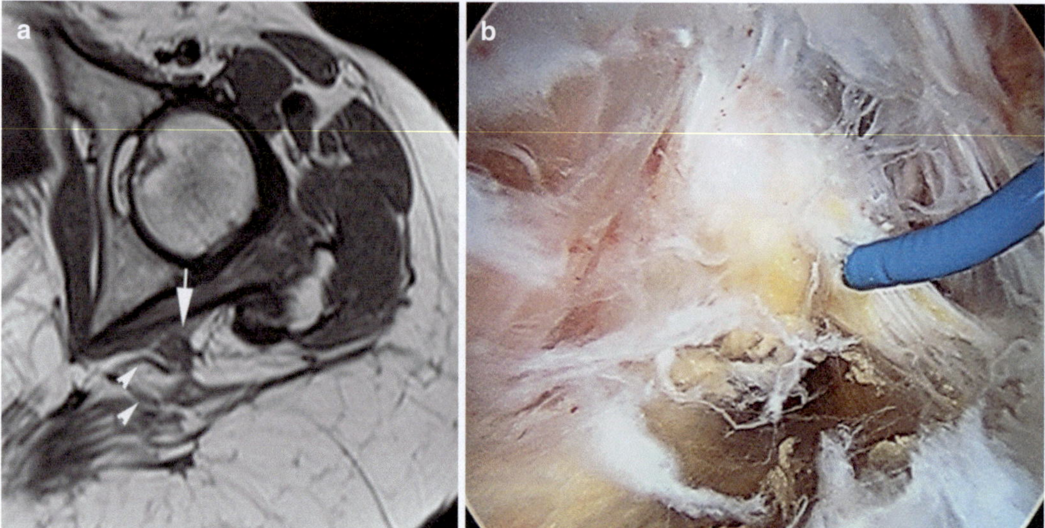

Fig. 5.24 Type-3 scarred bands in a 51-year-old woman with DGS. (**a**) Axial T1-weighted MR image shows fibrous irregular bands (arrowheads) with undefined distribution in the perisciatic fat, anchoring the sciatic nerve (arrow) in multiple directions. (**b**) The endoscopic image shows the sciatic nerve decompression, more complex when this type of bands is resected

Radiographic studies have limited application to the diagnosis. Until now, MRI and CT were to be reserved for ruling out disc and vertebral pathologic conditions and were limited to assess the presence of piriformis muscle enlargement. Advances in the knowledge of the deep gluteal space pathology, the dynamics of the sciatic nerve, and technical improvement of MRI make the latter a required test to assess piriformis syndrome [5].

There are two types of piriformis syndrome, primary and secondary. Primary piriformis syndrome has an anatomic cause (anatomical variations or anomalous attachments). Secondary piriformis syndrome occurs as a result of a precipitating cause. Fewer than 15% of cases have a purely primary cause [46].

Potential sources of pathology related to the piriformis muscle can be classified into six types [5].

Hypertrophy of the Piriformis Muscle

Asymmetric enlarged piriformis muscle with anterior displacement of the sciatic nerve may be a cause of DGS. According to Russell, muscle size asymmetry of 2 mm is present in 81% of patients with no history or clinical suspicion of piriformis syndrome. Moreover, none of the patients with asymmetry of 4 mm or more had symptoms suggestive of piriformis syndrome in his study [47]. Muscle asymmetry singly has only a specificity of 66% and a sensitivity of 46% during identification of patients with muscle-based piriformis syndrome. Asymmetry associated with sciatic nerve hyperintensity at the sciatic notch reveals a specificity of 93% and a sensitivity of 64% in patients with piriformis syndrome distinct from that which had no similar symptoms [5] (Fig. 5.25).

First-line treatment consists of conservative measures, including rest, anti-inflammatories, muscle relaxants, and physical therapy for a 6-week period. The CT-guided infiltration test is valid for diagnosis and treatment [5]. The improvement of symptoms after image-guided infiltration confirms the diagnosis. In refractory cases, Botox infiltration is the next step. Botulinum toxin blocks presynaptic conduction, thereby creating a temporary paresis, and induces a denervative process and atrophy of the piriformis muscle. In a few cases, piriformis endoscopic resection is ultimately necessary [3, 48, 49].

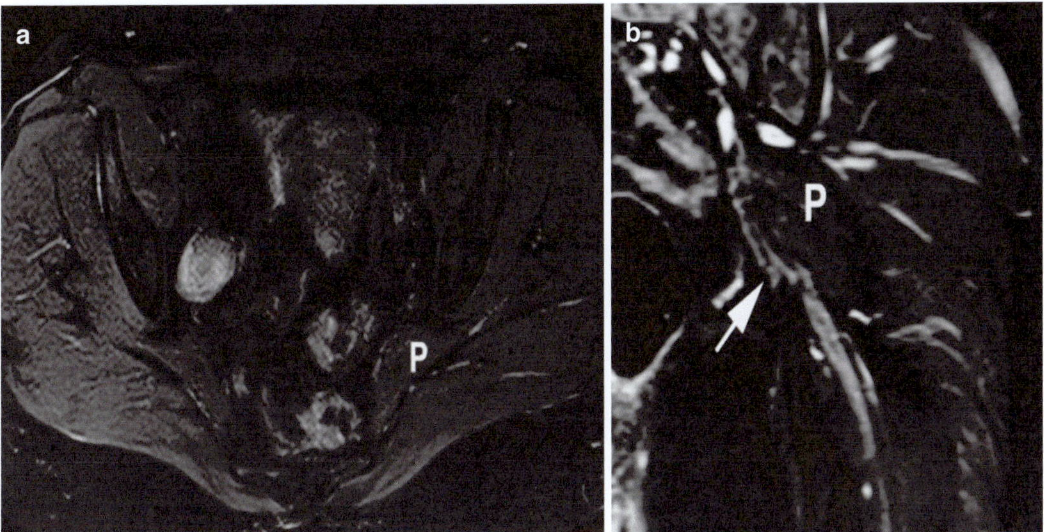

Fig. 5.25 DGS secondary to hypertrophy of the piriformis muscle in a 34-year-old woman with DGS. Axial (**a**) and coronal (**b**) PD-weighted fat-saturated MR images show a left hypertrophic piriformis muscle (P) and associated sciatic neuritis (arrow in **b**)

Dynamic Sciatic Nerve Entrapment by Piriformis Muscle

Dynamic entrapment of the sciatic nerve by piriformis is not uncommon. Often the only finding at imaging that can be shown is nerve signal hyperintensity in edema-sensitive sequences at the level of the greater sciatic notch [5] (Fig. 5.26). Similarly as in the previous case, the CT-guided infiltration test has an important not only diagnostic but also therapeutic function, as healing is achieved multiple times (over 80% in our experience). In many cases trapping is only temporary; therefore, MRI cannot show neuritis if just before its implementation exercise has not been done or the position that produces the symptoms has not been adopted. Undergo a provocative test for several minutes just before performing MRI is helpful for the detection of sciatic neuritis secondary to piriformis dynamic entrapment [5]. Definitive diagnosis is sometimes endoscopic, demonstrating the entrapment during dynamic maneuvers. Endoscopic piriformis release, initially reported by Dezawa et al. [50], and subsequent verification of correct nerve mobility is required. Because some cases are transient, an infiltration test is always the first step in the treatment sequence, which leads to diagnosis, and facilitates a high percentage of healing without resorting to surgery, which is reserved for recurrent cases or cases that do not improve with physical therapy [3, 5, 48, 51].

Anomalous Course of the Sciatic Nerve (Anatomical Variations)

Descriptions of variations concerning the relationship between the piriformis muscle and sciatic nerve have been limited. The prevalence of sciatic-piriformis complex variations has been 16.9% in a meta-analysis of cadaveric studies and 16.2% in published surgical case series. Variants are usually bilateral. What is rare is to find two different types of high divisions on both sides in same patient. Normally, the sciatic nerve passes through the greater sciatic foramen below the piriformis muscle. However, it may divide into its common fibular and tibial nerve components within the pelvis [52–55].

Six categories of anatomical variations of the relationship between the piriformis muscle and sciatic nerve were originally reported in 1937 by Beaton and Anson [52] (Fig. 5.27):

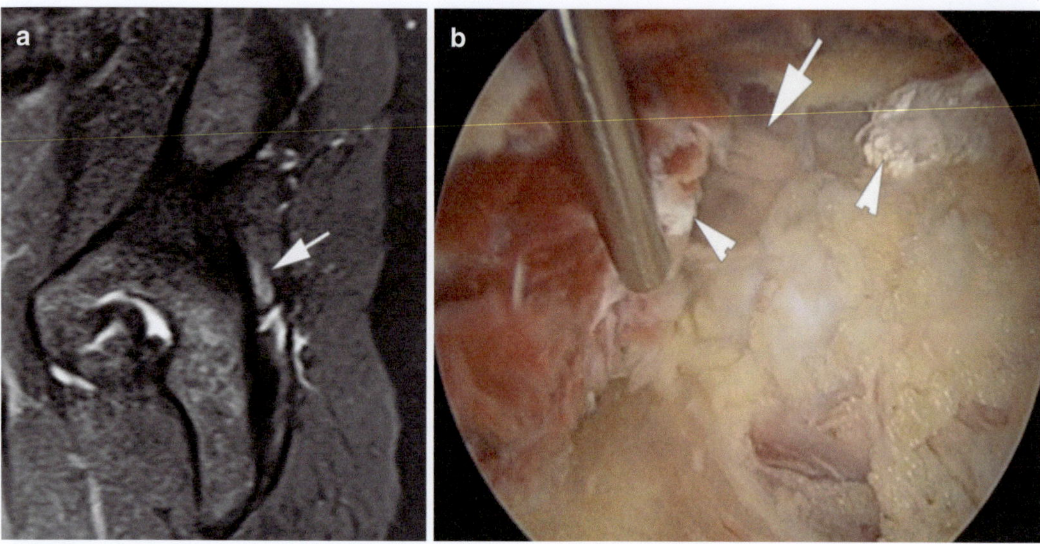

Fig. 5.26 Dynamic entrapment of the sciatic nerve by piriformis muscle in a 45-year-old man with DGS. (**a**) Double sagittal-oblique fat-suppressed PD-weighted MR image shows sciatic neuritis (arrow) with no other associated abnormalities. The definitive diagnosis in this patient was endoscopic, demonstrating the sciatic nerve entrapment. (**b**) Endoscopic piriformis release (arrowheads) resulted in sciatic nerve decompression (arrow) and complete relief of symptoms

- Type A, undivided nerve comes out below the piriformis muscle.
- Type B, a divided sciatic nerve passing through and below the piriformis muscle (Fig. 5.28).

We have described a subset additional type-B variation; in this variation, the sciatic nerve appears to pass below the piriformis muscle but a smaller accessory piriformis muscle, with its own separate distal tendon, passing between the common fibular and tibial portions of the sciatic nerve. This variation can also be seen in patients without high division of the sciatic nerve (Fig. 5.29a). These variants, in the same way as the other types, are easily identifiable by MR imaging [5] (Fig. 5.29b).

- Type C, a divided nerve passing above and below undivided muscle.
- Type D, an undivided sciatic nerve passing through the piriformis muscle.
- Type E, a divided nerve passing through and above the muscle heads.
- Type F, undivided sciatic nerve passing above undivided muscle.

Smoll presented the overall reported incidence of these six variations in over 6000 dissected limbs. Relationships A, B, C, D, E, and F occurred in 83.1%, 13.7%, 1.3%, 0.5%, 0.08%, and 0.08% of limbs, respectively [53]. Therefore, with the exception of the relationship A (normal course), B-type piriformis-sciatic variation is the most commonly found (Fig. 5.28).

The fact that these piriformis-sciatic nerve anomalies exist is important for the surgeon to recognize; however, the anomaly itself may not always be the etiology of DGS symptoms as some asymptomatic patients present these variations and some symptomatic patients do not. A subsequent event such as any etiology reported in this paper or prolonged sitting, direct trauma to the gluteal region, fibrous bands, prolonged stretching, overuse, pelvic/spinal instability, or orthopedic conditions may then precipitate sciatic nerve neuropathy [5].

The CT-guided infiltration test is helpful in many cases to achieve the improvement or resolution of symptoms. During this procedure, radiologist should be ensured that the solution is distributed along the portion of the nerve that lies between the muscle bellies to have diagnostic validity and potential therapeutic effect [5] (Fig. 5.30).

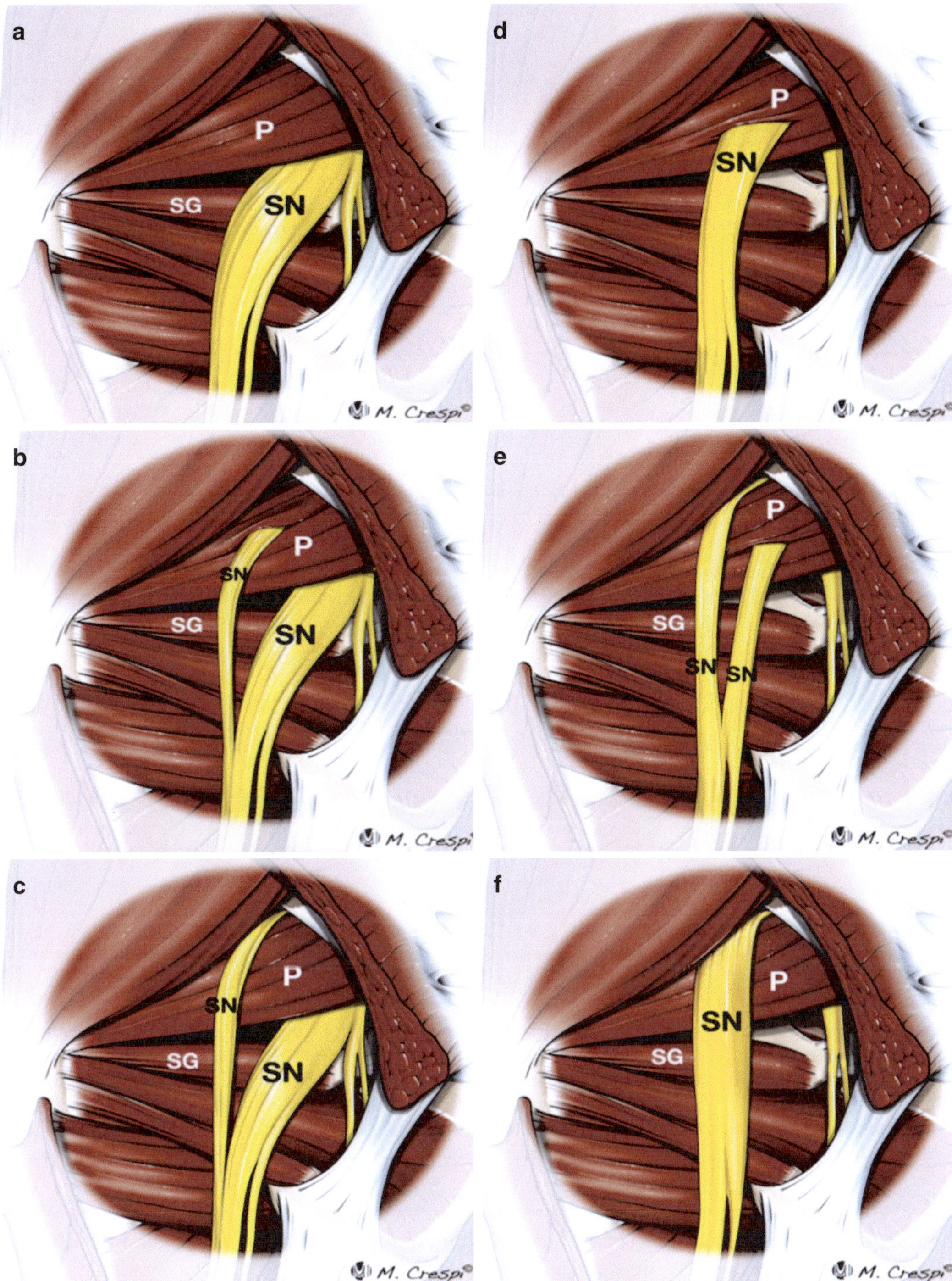

Fig. 5.27 Anatomical variations of the relationship between piriformis muscle and sciatic nerve. (**a–f**) Diagrams illustrate in a posterior view the six variants, originally described by Beaton and Anson. (**a**) An undivided nerve comes out below the piriformis muscle (normal course). (**b**) A divided sciatic nerve passing through and below the piriformis muscle. (**c**) A divided nerve passing above and below undivided muscle. (**d**) An undivided sciatic nerve passing through the piriformis muscle. (**e**) A divided nerve passing through and above the muscle heads. (**f**) An undivided sciatic nerve passing above undivided muscle. *SN* sciatic nerve, *P* piriformis muscle, *SG* superior gemellus muscle

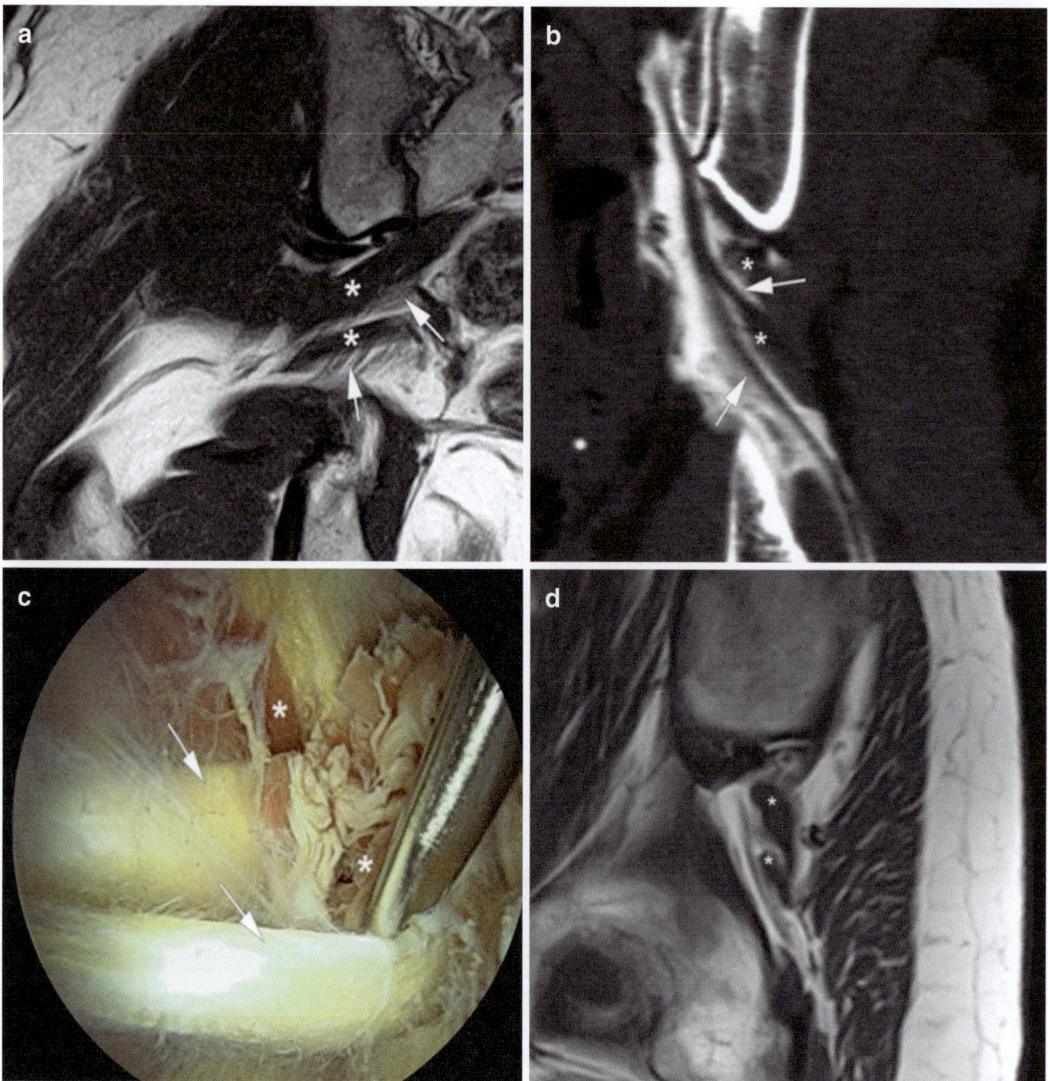

Fig. 5.28 Right type B of Beaton and Anson piriformis-sciatic complex variation in a 34-year-old woman with DGS. (**a**) Coronal and (**d**) sagittal PD-weighted MR image shows a high sciatic nerve division (arrows) with its two branches passing through and below the piriformis muscle bellies (asterisks). (**b**) Sagittal-oblique MDCT reconstruction after performing the infiltration test shows in negative the same anatomical variant. The contrast medium placed in the perineural space facilitates the visualization of the variant. (**c**) The endoscopic image confirmed this sciatic nerve variation easily identified by MRI

If it does not get resolution of symptoms, endoscopic tenotomy of the piriformis muscle is indicated but must be performed both proximal and distal to the variant, because if only the distal portion is tenotomized, retraction of the muscle may drag the nerve medially, resulting in clinical worsening [5]. Many patients do not improve of their symptoms because piriformis tenotomy is performed by open surgery without considering this fact (Fig. 5.31).

Anomalous Attachments

Anomalous attachments include variations in proximal or distal insertions [56] (Fig. 5.32). Described variants of the origin of the piriformis muscle are not frequent but have added many cases in our series.

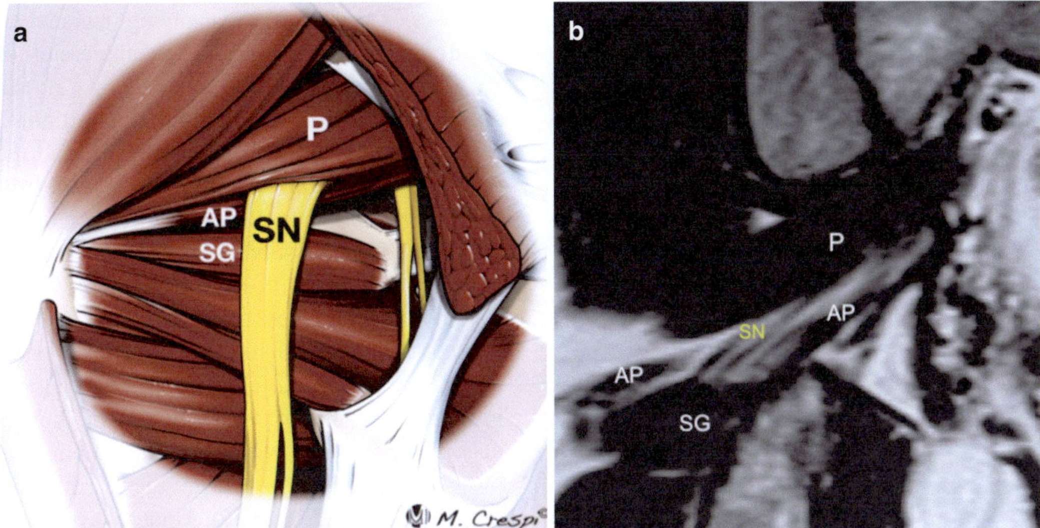

Fig. 5.29 Non-Beaton and Anson piriformis-sciatic complex variation in a 45-year-old woman with DGS. (**a**) Diagram illustrates the variant, not originally described by Beaton and Anson. (**b**) Coronal PD-weighted MR image shows a normal sciatic nerve (SN) passing between the piriformis muscle (P) and an accessory muscle belly (AP). *SG* superior geminus. Reprinted with permission from Massimiliano Crespi

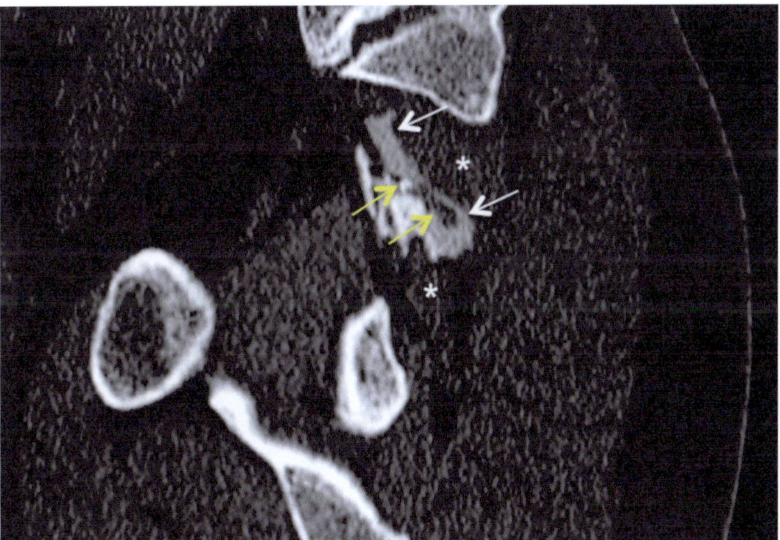

Fig. 5.30 Double injection of anesthetic and corticosteroid technique (infiltration test) in a 28-year-old patient with a B-type piriformis muscle. Sagittal MDCT image shows the final result of CT-guided infiltration of the periasciatic space through the piriformis muscle. The solution contains a small amount of iodinated contrast to assess the location of injection more accurately. During the procedure, radiologist should be ensured that the solution (white arrows) is also distributed along the peroneal nerve (yellow arrow) that lies between the muscle bellies of piriformis muscle (asterisks) to have diagnostic validity and potential therapeutic effect

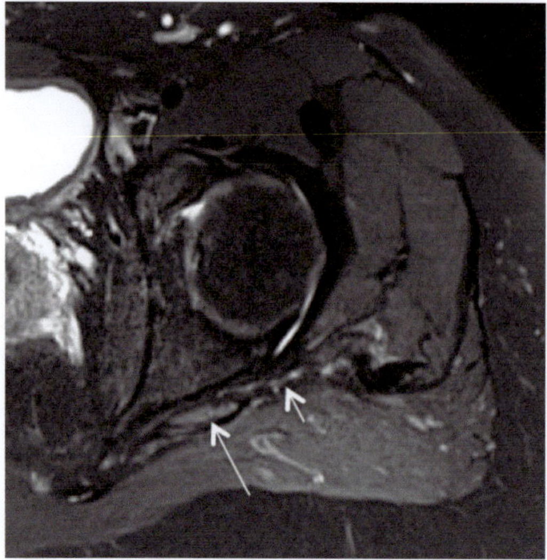

Fig. 5.31 DGS secondary to retraction of the type-B piriformis tendon (left side) after tenotomy in a 29-year-old man. Axial PD-weighted fat-saturated MR image shows sciatic neuritis (large arrow) and the tendon retraction (short arrow). Endoscopic tenotomy of a type-B piriformis muscle must be performed both proximal and distal in this variant, because if only the distal section is tenotomized, retraction of the muscle may drag the nerve medially, resulting in clinical worsening

Cases with proximal involving include an intraforaminal insertion causing compression of the corresponding sacral root (Fig. 5.32), the presence of a larger than normal insertion, a wider insertion than normal and finally, and the existence of an intrapelvic (Fig. 5.32c) or extrapelvic accessory muscle belly. The presence of an extrapelvic accessory belly of piriformis muscle is not uncommon. It is inserted into the posterior and superior aspect of the iliac blade, next to the sacroiliac joint, and fuses with the distal myotendinous junction of the piriformis muscle. Proximally it sometimes attaches to the gluteus maximus. The innervation of this anomalous muscle is usually derived from the inferior gluteal nerve [57] (Fig. 5.32). Underlying pathophysiological mechanisms are based on disturbance of normal alignment of the axis contraction of the muscle or the direct impingement of the roots of the sacral plexus [5].

On the other hand, most of the distal anomalous insertions include full/partial insertion onto the obturator internus or conjoint piriformis/obturator distal attachment onto the greater tuberosity of the

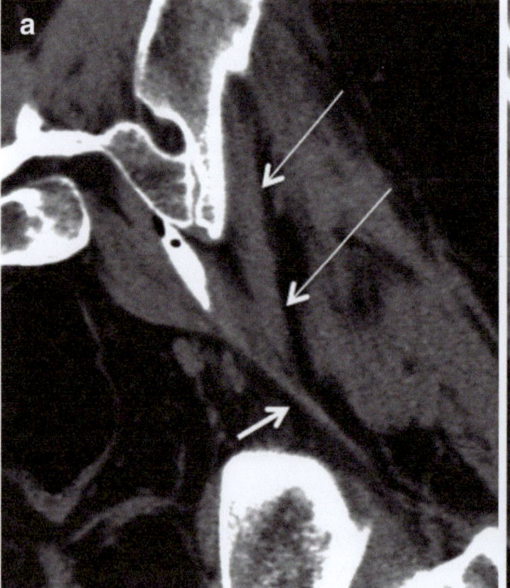
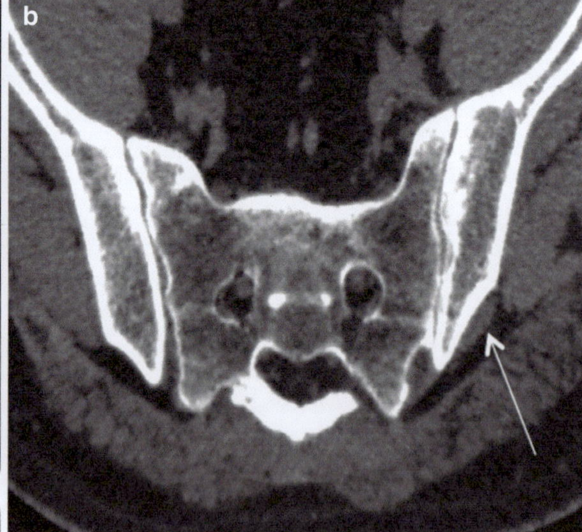

Fig. 5.32 Anomalous attachments of the piriformis muscle. (**a**, **b**) Sagittal-oblique and axial MDCT reconstruction in a 35-year-old woman, after performing botulinum toxin infiltration, shows an anomalous extrapelvic accessory muscle belly of piriformis muscle (large arrow) that fuses distally with the distal myotendinous junction (short arrow). (**c**) Coronal-oblique MDCT reconstruction in a 44-year-old man shows an anomalous intrapelvic accessory muscle belly of piriformis (arrow). (**d**) Axial-oblique MDCT reconstruction in a 42-year-old woman reveals an intraforaminal insertion of the piriformis muscle (arrow) entrapping a sacral root (arrowhead)

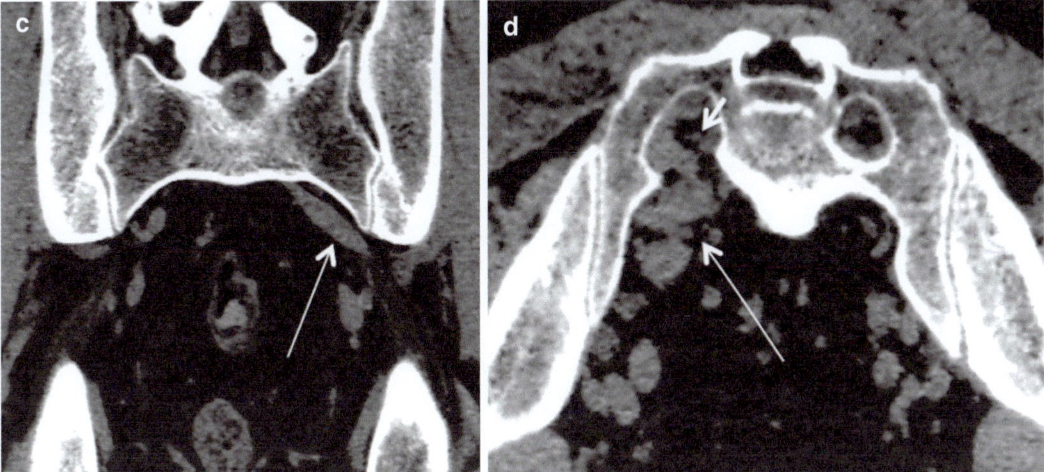

Fig. 5.32 (continued)

femur. These abnormalities in the distal insertion could not have been associated clearly with symptoms of nerve entrapment.

The treatment in these cases initially consists of conservative measures such as physical therapy program. Intramuscular botulinum toxin injection may be a useful treatment in some cases if the infiltration test does not relieve pain. However, endoscopic resection of the muscle is frequently required [5].

Sciatic Nerve Entrapment Secondary to Fibrosis After Classic Open Surgery of Piriformis Syndrome

This kind of surgery has a relatively high rate of postoperative fibrosis with subsequent entrapment of the sciatic nerve by the retracted stump of the muscle belly (type-3 bands). The endoscopic neurolysis of the sciatic nerve is the treatment of choice. Endoscopic release of the nerve in these cases is complex and tedious. Infiltration test shows very poor results in this situation [5] (Fig. 5.33).

Trauma- or Overuse-Related Conditions

Avulsions, tendinosis, strains, calcifying tendinosis, or spasm, as may occur in any other tendon (Figs. 5.34, 5.35, 5.36, and 5.37). Treatment usually consists of physical therapy.

MR imaging is required to detect complications, inflammatory changes, or the formation of fibrous bands, in which case infiltration or endoscopic debridement of the sciatic nerve may be required. Piriformis spasm is a diagnosis of exclusion that should be only distinguished from transient dynamic entrapment not associated with neuritis on MR imaging. In both cases treatment of choice is an infiltration test or intramuscular injection of Botox if there is no improvement [5]. The spasm is easily detectable during the perineural infiltration test. If the muscle shows a significant resistance to the passage of the needle, a diagnosis of spasm can be made. The solution should be located at the perineural space, but a part of it should also be instilled into the muscle. Muscle drill may also be effective if spasm exists but always guided by an imaging method as surrounding arteries are located in the vicinity and bleed easily, which can complicate the case with hematomas and hence fibrous bands formation. In addition, and similarly to shoulder, calcifying tendinosis can be solved by ultrasound-guided percutaneous evacuation with saline solution and local anesthetic (barbotage technique). Tendinosis can be treated with image-guided peritendinous infiltration with local anesthetic and steroid [58].

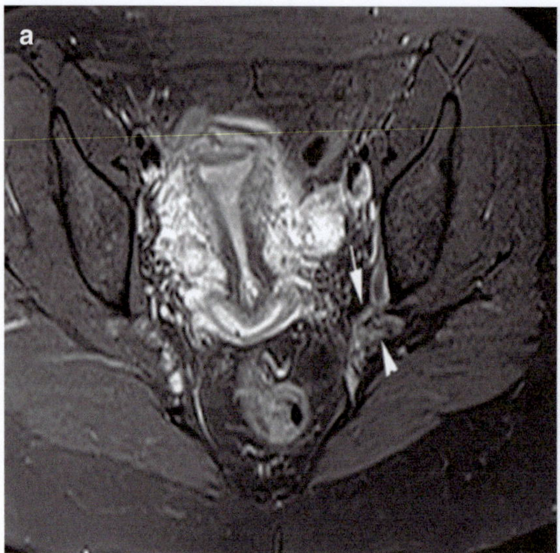 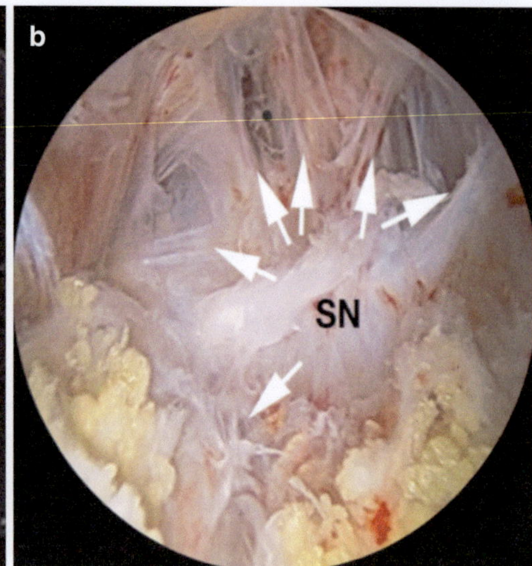

Fig. 5.33 Recurrence of DGS after classic open tenotomy of piriformis muscle in a 37-year-old woman. (**a**) Axial fat-suppressed PD-weighted MR image shows a sciatic neuritis (arrow) due to the entrapment by postsurgical fibrosis around the retracted stump of the resected and atrophic piriformis (arrowhead). (**b**) Endoscopic view of sciatic nerve (SN) entrapment by type-3 fibrous bands (arrows) in the same patient. Resection of these bands resulted in complete resolution of symptoms

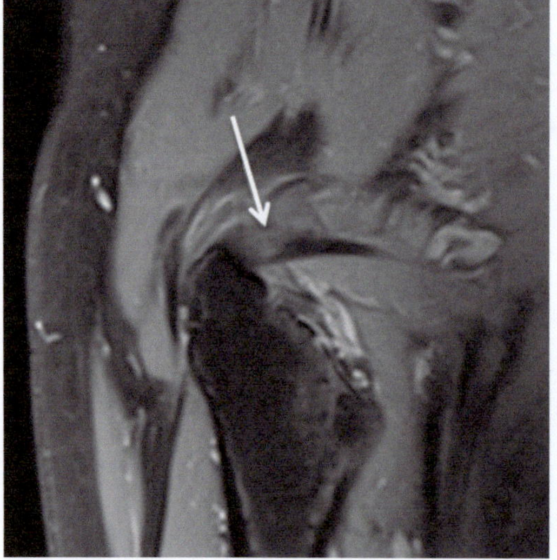 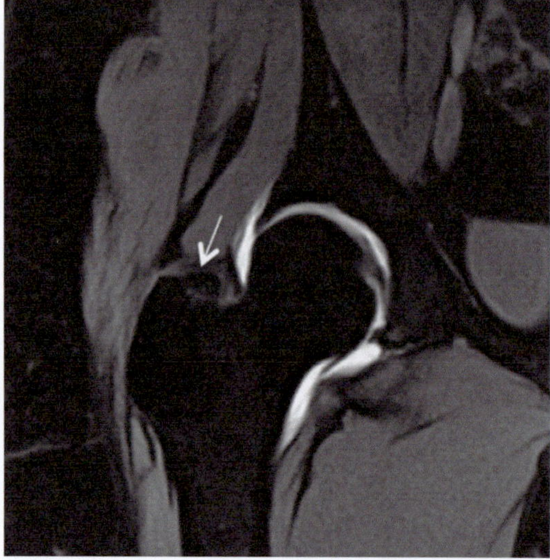

Fig. 5.34 DGS secondary to distal piriformis tendinosis in a 35-year-old man. Coronal-oblique fat-suppressed PD-weighted MR image shows a moderate thickening and fraying of piriformis tendon at the level of the distal enthesis on the medial side of the greater trochanter (arrow)

Fig. 5.35 DGS secondary to distal insertional piriformis avulsion in a 46-year-old woman. Coronal-oblique fat-suppressed PD-weighted MR arthrogram image shows a chronic avulsion of the piriformis tendon at the level of the distal enthesis on the medial side of the greater trochanter. No other abnormalities were seen in this study

Gemelli-Obturator Internus Syndrome

Obturator internus/gemelli complex pathology is rare and commonly overlooked in patients suffering from posterior hip pain associated o nor to sciatica. Because of its proximity and similarity in both structures and function, most treatments for piriformis syndrome also affect the internal obturator [59]. Dynamic compression of the sciatic nerve caused by a stretched or altered dynamic of the obturator internus muscle should be included as a possible diagnosis for DGS [60] (Fig. 5.38). Additionally to this simple entrapment a scissor-like effect between the piriformis an the obturator internus can be also the source of entrapment as the sciatic nerve passes under the belly of piriformis and over superior gemelli/obturator internus complex [5, 61]. The MR diagnosis of this entity is based on detection of neuritis not in prepiriformis area but in the obturator-piriformis space (Fig. 5.39). Insertional pathology and variations concerning the sciatic nerve and obturator internus/gemelli are also possible, the most frequent being an obturator internus penetrating the nerve [5]. The latter is easily identifiable by MRI (Fig. 5.40). In contrast to the first type of piriformis syndrome, an hypertrophied obturator internus is rarely found, usually in body builders (Fig. 5.41). In a study of six patients who underwent surgery for suspected piriformis syndrome, all were observed intraoperatively to have increased obturator internus muscle tension, hyperemia, and hypertrophy [43]. Furthermore, the obturator internus muscle was observed impinging on the sciatic nerve during an intraoperative Lasègue maneuver. Because of this proximity, similar pathway, and similar function,

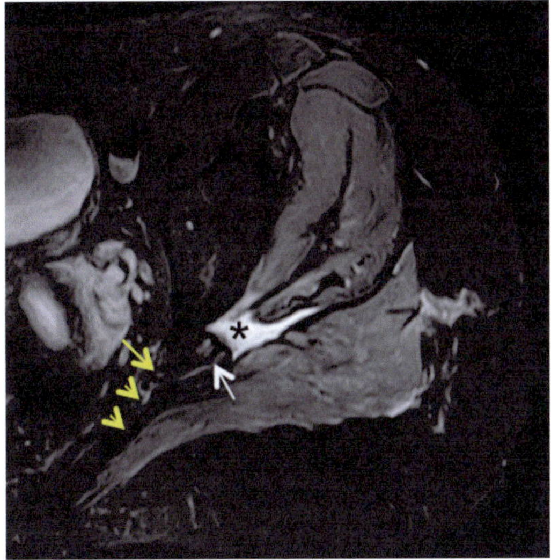

Fig. 5.36 DGS secondary to piriformis retraction in a 35-year-old woman. Axial-oblique fat-suppressed PD-weighted MR image shows a chronic retraction of the piriformis tendon after previous complete myotendinous tear. Note the sacral roots hyperintensity suggestive of neuropathy secondary to a fibrous entrapment as a result of the retraction. Acute inflammatory changes and a fluid collection added to chronic changes are also visible (asterisk)

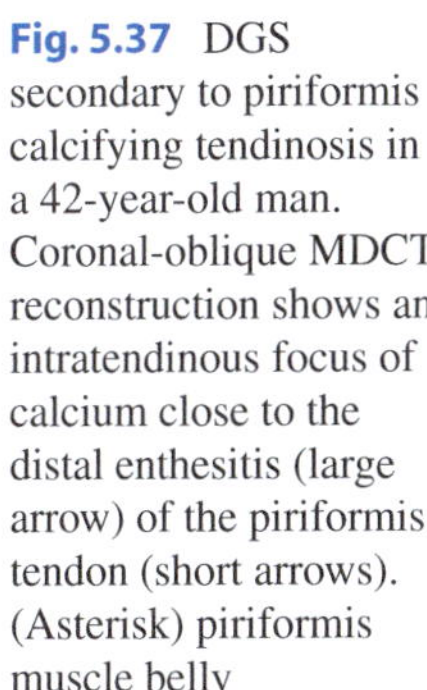

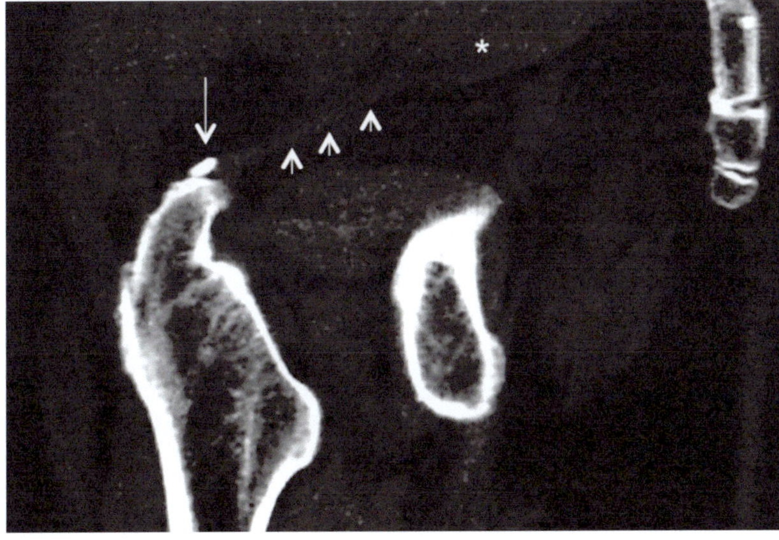

Fig. 5.37 DGS secondary to piriformis calcifying tendinosis in a 42-year-old man. Coronal-oblique MDCT reconstruction shows an intratendinous focus of calcium close to the distal enthesitis (large arrow) of the piriformis tendon (short arrows). (Asterisk) piriformis muscle belly

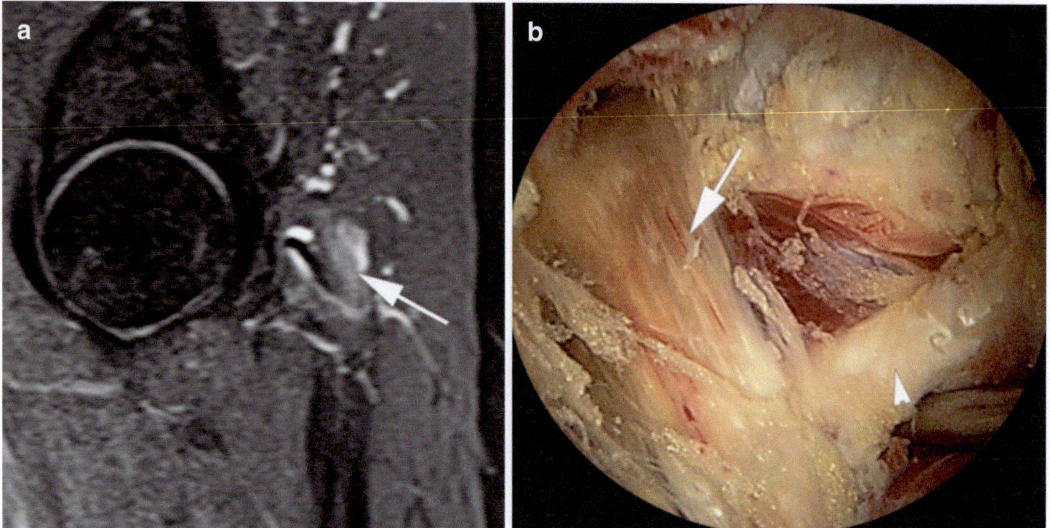

Fig. 5.38 Dynamic entrapment of the sciatic nerve by the obturator internus (OI) in a 48-year-old man with clinical diagnosis of DGS. (**a**) Double sagittal-oblique fat-suppressed PD-weighted MR image shows sciatic neuritis (arrow). (**b**) Endoscopic view confirms the dynamic entrapment of the sciatic nerve (arrow) by the obturator internus muscle (arrowhead). The OI muscle was found very tight and slightly hyperemic

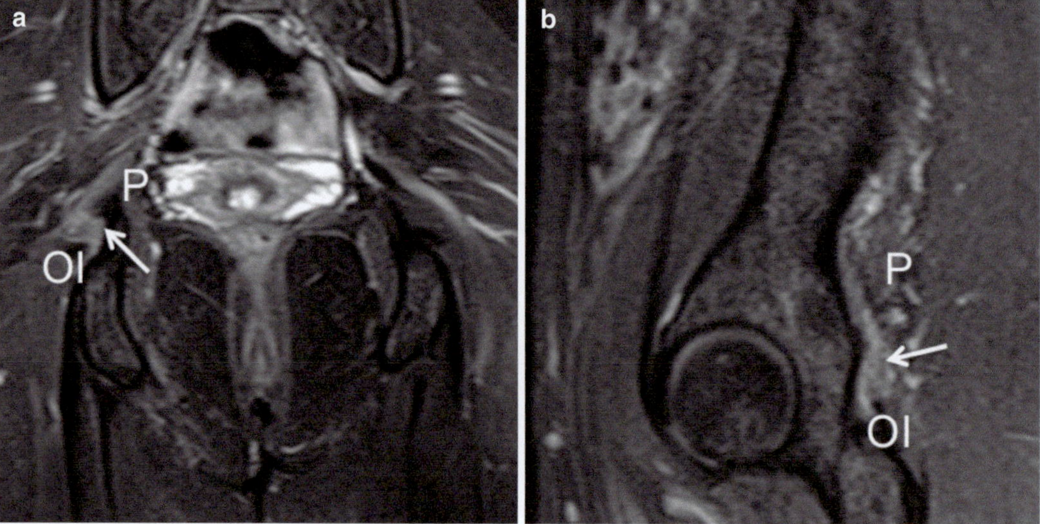

Fig. 5.39 Dynamic entrapment of the sciatic nerve by the obturator internus (OI) and the piriformis muscles (P) in a 42-year-old man with clinical diagnosis of DGS. (**a**) Coronal and (**b**) double sagittal-oblique fat-suppressed PD-weighted MR image shows sciatic neuritis (arrows) due to a scissor-like effect between the two muscles endoscopically confirmed

most treatments for patients with piriformis syndrome would affect the internal obturator muscle as well. Moreover, Cox et al. argued that the gemelli-obturator internus muscles and its associated bursa should be regarded as possible sources of retro-trochanterically located DGS [5]. Finally, MRI can also identify avulsions, tendinosis, calcifying tendinosis, or tears (Fig. 5.42). Management of these pathologies is identical to the different types of piriformis syndrome [3, 5].

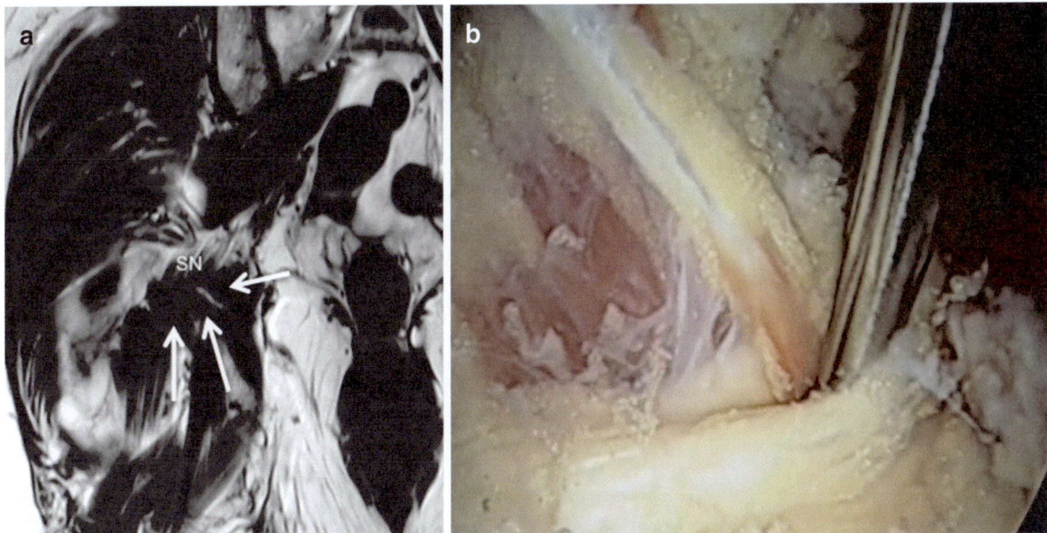

Fig. 5.40 Dynamic entrapment of the sciatic nerve by the obturator internus (OI) in a 38-year-old man with clinical diagnosis of DGS. (**a**) Coronal-oblique PD-weighted MR image shows the sciatic nerve (SN) passing through the obturator internus muscle (arrows). (**b**) Endoscopic view confirms the dynamic entrapment of the sciatic nerve by the variant of the sciatic-obturator internus complex during movements of the hip

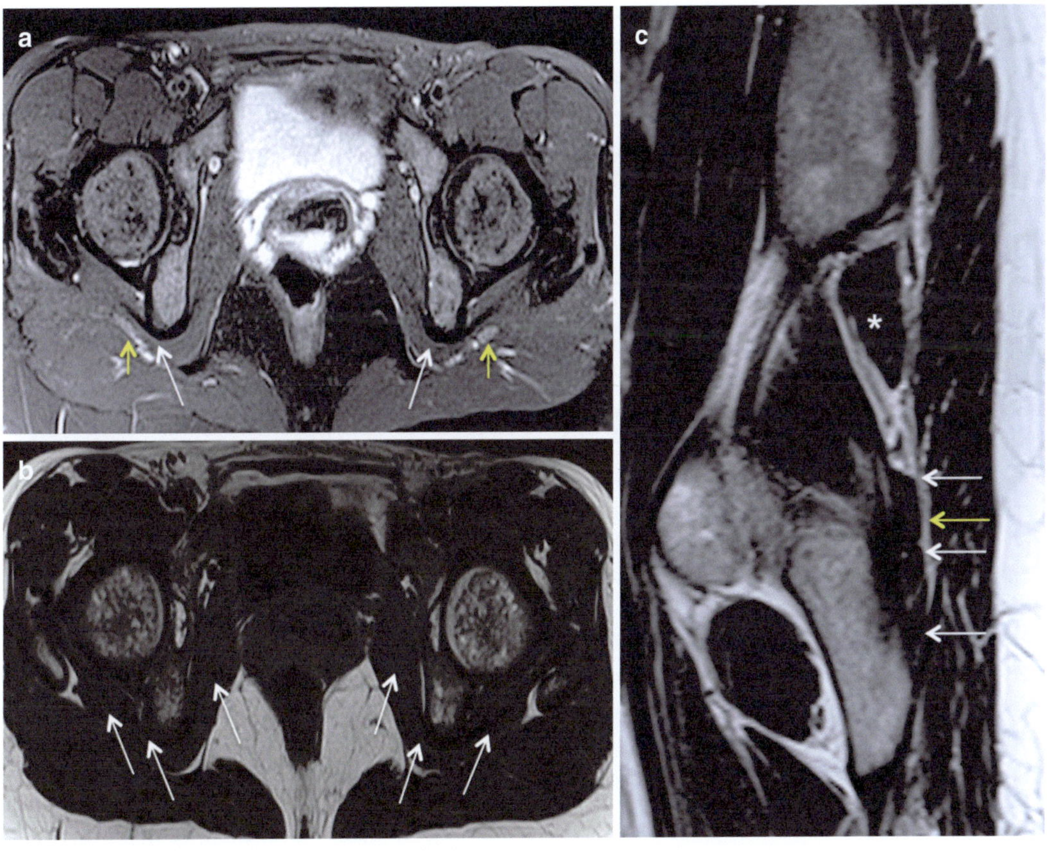

Fig. 5.41 DGS secondary to hypertrophy of the obturator internus muscle in a 27-year-old patient who practiced bodybuilding. Axial (**a**, **b**) and sagittal (**c**) PD-weighted MR images show bilateral hypertrophic obturator internus muscles (white arrow) and associated sciatic neuritis (yellow arrows) in the area of maximum space conflict

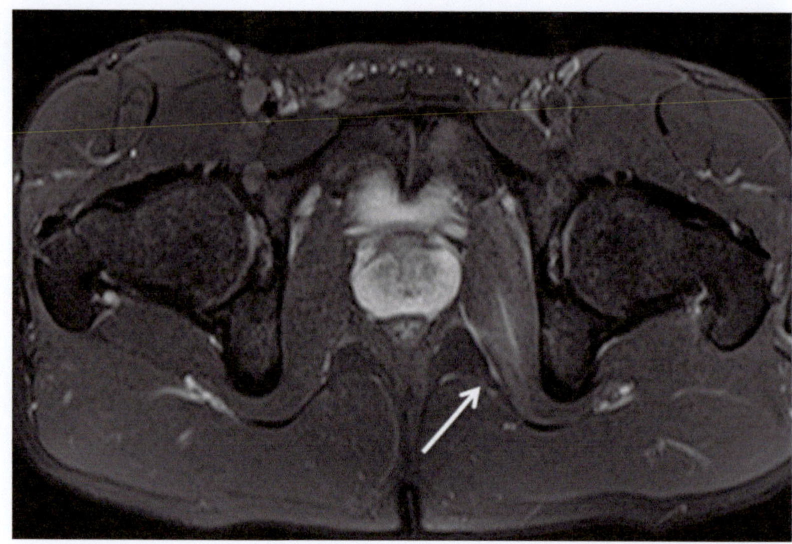

Fig. 5.42 DGS secondary to acute, isolated intramuscular and myofascial tear of the intrapelvic belly of the obturator internus in a 25-year-old patient. Axial fat-suppressed PD-weighted MR image shows edema and acute intramuscular hemorrhage (arrow) in this patient after an extreme movement in forced external rotation

Quadratus Femoris and Ischiofemoral Pathology

Strains and tears of quadratus femoris muscle (QFM) are infrequently reported in the medical literature [23]. Patients may present with acute or chronic hip, groin, and/or posterior gluteal pain. QFM tears appear as an area of intramuscular fluid signal intensity with surrounding muscle edema (Fig. 5.43c, d). Published cases of QFM tears usually involve the distal myotendinous junction, at the posteromedial aspect of the proximal femur, although tear at the femoral tendon insertion has also been reported. STIR, fat-suppressed PD, or fat-suppressed T2-weighted images are required to detect muscle edema. A grade I strain appears as muscle edema and may occur at the ischial origin of the QFM or as central or diffuse muscle edema, indistinguishable from that seen with IFI. A preserved ischiofemoral space facilitates the diagnosis. Isolated QFM strains or tears are uncommon. With severe edema, irritation of the adjacent sciatic nerve may cause DSG [62]. Chronic inflammatory changes and adhesions causing scar tissue between the muscle and the sciatic nerve result in entrapment during hip motion. In these cases endoscopic neurolysis of the sciatic nerve is required [5, 62].

Isolated dynamic entrapment of the sciatic nerve by the quadratus femoris muscle, spasm, or anatomical variants has not been reported.

In addition, exercise-induced edema of QFM has been described as a cause of retro-trochanteric pain with or without sciatica and must be taken into account [23].

Finally, narrowing of the ischiofemoral space leads to muscular, tendon, and neural changes in the ischiofemoral impingement [62–64]. The syndrome may occur acutely because of inflammation/edema (Fig. 5.44) or chronically because of fibrous tissue formation that traps the nerve [62] (Fig. 5.45). Ischiofemoral impingement will be broadly discussed in this chapter.

Hamstring Conditions

The sciatic nerve can be affected by a wide spectrum of hamstring origin enthesopathies appearing either isolated or in combination: partial/complete hamstring strain (acute, recurrent, or chronic), tendon detachment, avulsion fractures (acute or chronic/nonunited), apophysitis, nonunited apophysis, proximal tendinopathy, calcifying tendinosis, and contusions [5, 65]. Calcifying tendinosis is in our experience a not uncommon cause of DGS (Fig. 5.46). In the acute phase, edema predominates as a characteristic imaging finding resulting in sciatic nerve irritation. Chronic inflammatory changes and adhesions causing scar tissue between tendons or muscles and sciatic nerve result in entrapment during hip motion (ischial tunnel syndrome) [5, 65] (Fig. 5.47). Congenital fibrotic

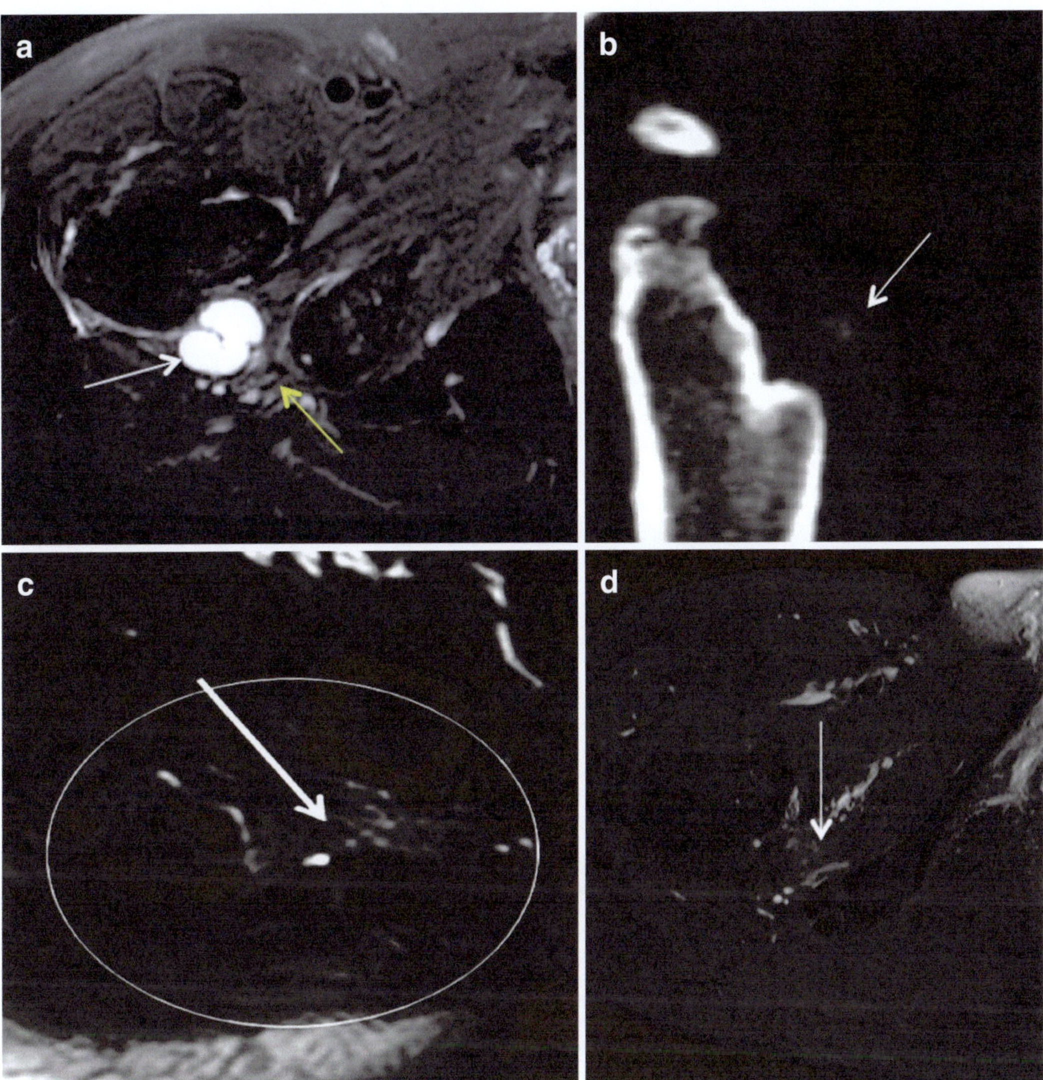

Fig. 5.43 Acute and chronic DGS secondary to quadratus femoris muscle pathology. (**a**) Axial fat-suppressed PD-weighted MR image shows sciatic neuritis (yellow arrow) in a patient with chronic partial tear of the QFM, intratendinous delamination, and secondary intramuscular cyst (white arrow). (**b**) Axial-oblique MDCT reconstruction shows an acute and distal QFM avulsion (arrow). (**c, d**) Axial fat-suppressed PD-weighted MR images show partial tears of the QFM appearing as an area of intramuscular fluid signal intensity with surrounding muscle edema

bands have also been reported. Imaging findings are specific to each injury and MR imaging is essential to select the appropriate treatment. Hamstring pathology will be discussed more extensively in this chapter.

Gluteal Disorders

The most common gluteus disorder causing sciatic nerve entrapment is gluteal contracture [5, 62]. It occurs in school-age children, with lifetime sequelae, and follows multiple intramuscular injections in the buttocks. Although the diagnosis is clinical, MRI may be requested for evaluation of the extent of fibrosis and degree of muscle atrophy. Gluteal contracture manifests characteristic features on MR imaging, including diffuse intramuscular fibrotic cords extending to the thickened distal tendon with atrophy of the

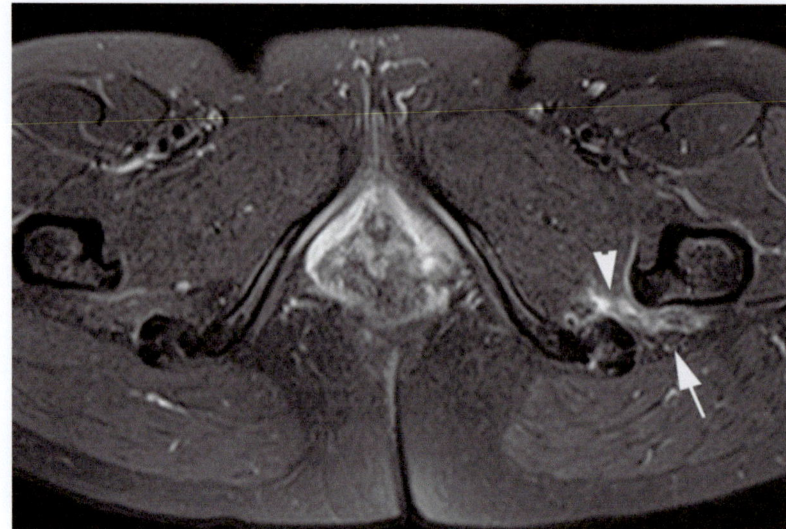

Fig. 5.44 DGS secondary to acute ischiofemoral impingement in a 57-year-old woman. Axial fat-suppressed PD-weighted MR image shows a narrowing ischiofemoral space causing impingement of the quadratus femoris muscle with secondary muscle edema (arrowhead). Sciatic neuritis is also shown (arrow)

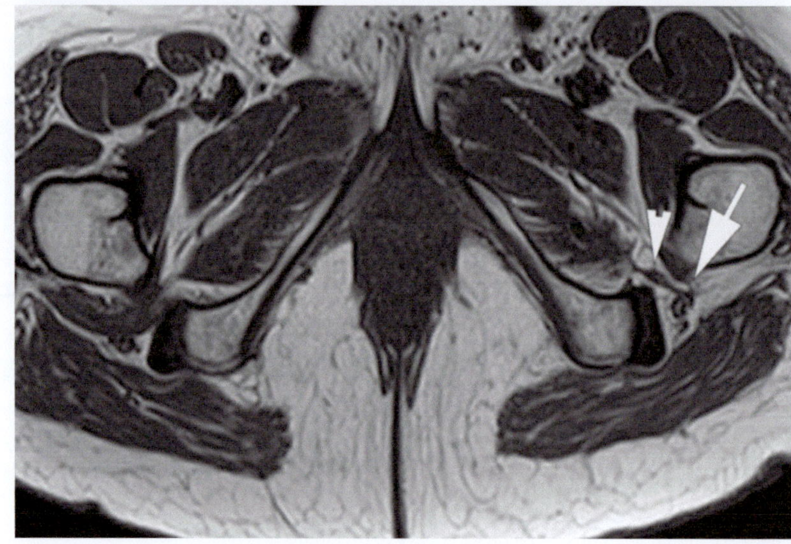

Fig. 5.45 Left DGS secondary to chronic ischiofemoral impingement in a 53-year-old woman. Axial PD-weighted MR image shows bilateral narrowing of the ischiofemoral space. On the left side, quadratus femoris muscle atrophy and a residual fibrous type-2 band (arrowhead) anchored to the sciatic nerve (arrow) are seen

gluteus maximus muscle and posteromedial displacement of the iliotibial tract. Perineural fibrosis is quite often the cause of DGS (Fig. 5.24). In advanced cases, medial retraction of the muscle and its tendon results in a depressed groove at the muscle-tendon junction and external rotation of the proximal femur [66]. Entrapment syndrome often occurs years later in patients suffering from gluteal contracture as a result of formation of fibrous bands type 3 [5, 62]. A constitutional fibrogenic diathesis has also been reported as an important factor [66]. Additionally, regardless of whether this is traumatic or not, any other gluteal pathology can be a cause of perisciatic fibrosis and DGS. The differential diagnosis includes disuse, denervation, chronic inflammatory myopathy, chronic compartment syndrome, fibromatosis, or posttraumatic hemosiderin deposition. Conservative measures such as passive stretching are usually not helpful. In cases of severe contracture or for cosmetic reasons, however, surgery is the only way to correct the deformity [66]. Endoscopic neurolysis does not always allow for the resection of all fibrous bands, and in severe cases (Fig. 5.24), open surgery may sometimes be required [5].

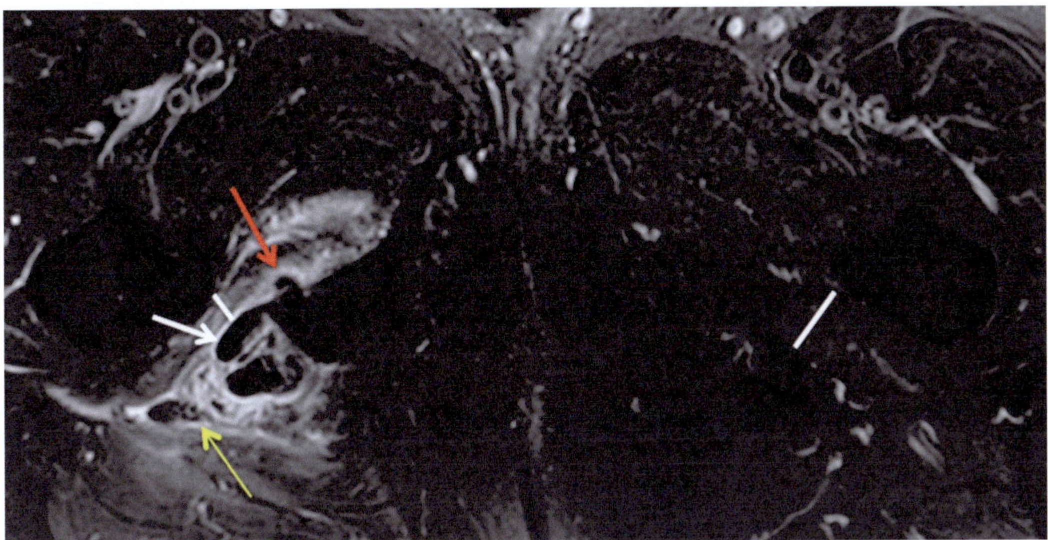

Fig. 5.46 Right DGS secondary to chronic calcifying tendinosis of the hamstring tendons causing ischiofemoral impingement in a 53-year-old woman. Axial PD fat-suppressed MR image shows a severe degenerative calcifying (red arrow) tendinopathy of hamstring tendons (white arrow) with reactive sciatic neuritis (yellow arrow). Note the significant narrowing of right ischiofemoral space compared to the left side (white lines)

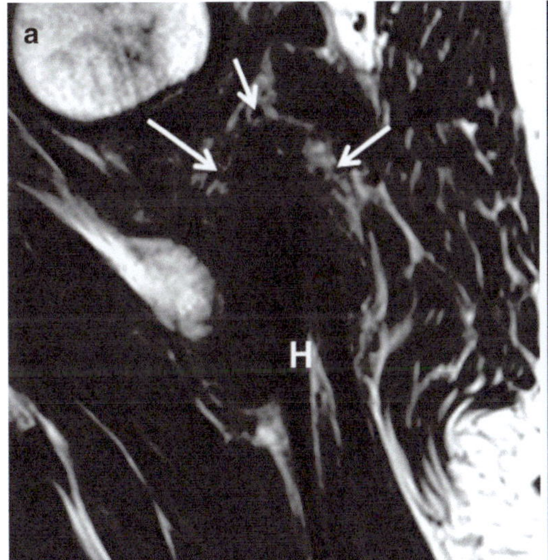
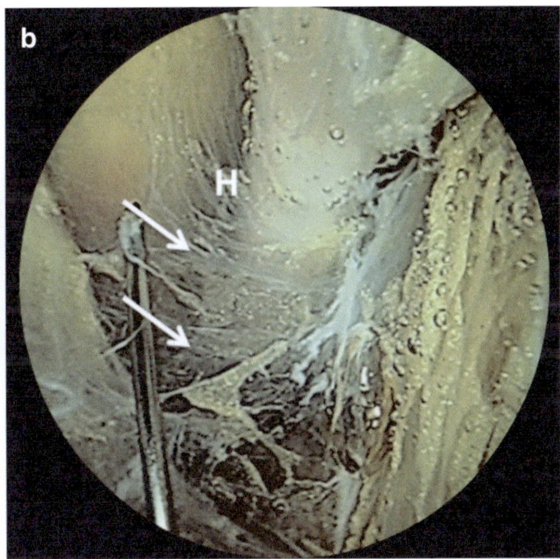

Fig. 5.47 DGS secondary to ischial tunnel syndrome in a 61-year-old woman. Axial PD-weighted MR (**a**) and endoscopic (**b**) images show a chronic fibrous entrapment of the sciatic nerve (arrows) within the distal subgluteal region due to previous proximal tear of the hamstring tendons

Orthopedic and Other Causes

Makhsous has confirmed using dynamic MRI that the soft tissue overlying the ischial tuberosity (IT) was found to be significantly thinner in a seated posture than it is in a supine posture even when there is no sitting load. These findings indicate that hip flexion alone can bring forth a significant decrease in soft tissue thickness underneath IT. Furthermore, the decrease is not uniform among the tissue layers in area around IT. Fat tissue experienced a significant decrease in thickness from non-weight-bearing sitting to weight-bearing sitting. Skin and subcutaneous tissue thickness was significantly smaller than the fat and muscle thicknesses in all postures. During flexion, internal rotation, and adduction, nerve changes its position and experiencing a slight lateralization and marked anterior excursion [67]. This would explain sciatic nerve signal changes in patients with pathology close to but not clearly in direct contact with the nerve.

Changes in osseous alignment of the pelvis, femur, and spine may affect normal sciatic nerve excursion and trigger DGS [68]. The excursion of the sciatic nerve with straight leg hip flexion performed by Coppieters et al. [39] did not indicate the osseous parameters of the hip, such as femoral version, which raises the question of how the sciatic nerve excursion may be affected by them. The femoral neck is normally anteverted to the bicondylar femoral plane at an angle of 35° to 50° at birth; this angle gradually decreases by 1.5° per year and reaches an approximate value of 16° at 16 years of age and 10° in the adult [69]. Together with other disorders, orthopedic conditions account for the few cases of DGS in which there are no image or

other evident endoscopic findings excluding sciatic neuritis that is, after all, the consequence. Pelvic instability and alterations of the sagittal balance of the spine are other poorly studied orthopedic causes that may trigger or predispose to the syndrome. The approach to these disorders will be discussed later.

Nonspecific Entrapments

Traumatic

Traumatic nerve injury may vary from disruption of axonal conduction with preservation of anatomical continuity to complete loss of continuity of the nerve trunk. Injury may be caused in the early period by laceration, stretching, or compression or later on by scar tissue, fibrous bands, or heterotopic ossification encasing the nerve [35].

Fractures Quite often, DGS develops following fracture of the sacrum (Fig. 5.48). In addition, the sciatic nerve may be injured in cases of acetabulum fractures, femur fractures, or femoral head dislocation. Other sources of sciatic nerve

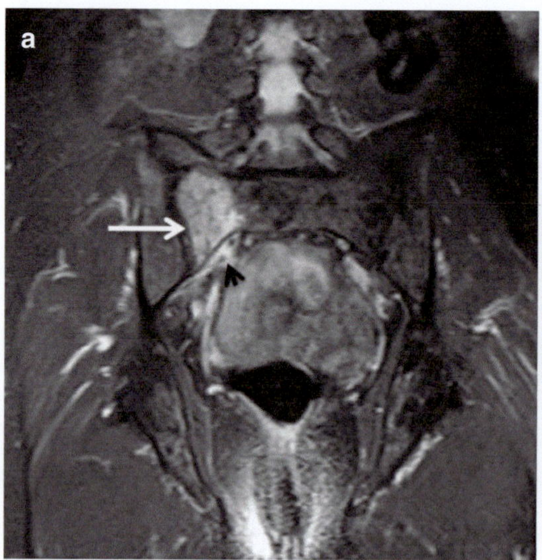
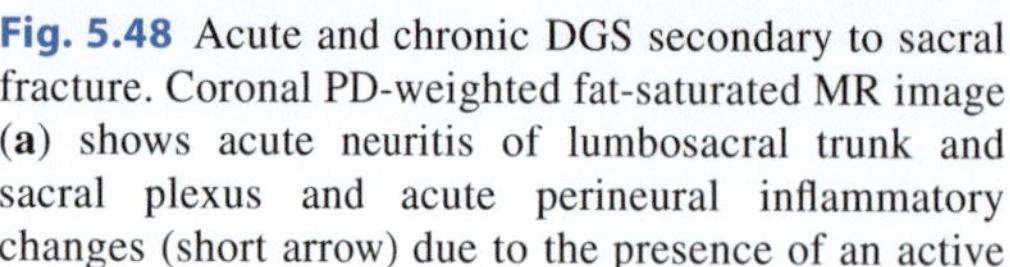
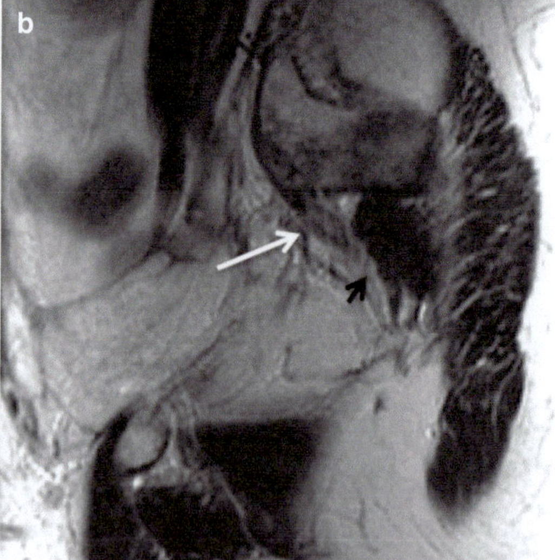

Fig. 5.48 Acute and chronic DGS secondary to sacral fracture. Coronal PD-weighted fat-saturated MR image (**a**) shows acute neuritis of lumbosacral trunk and sacral plexus and acute perineural inflammatory changes (short arrow) due to the presence of an active chronic stress fracture of the sacral ala (large arrow). Sagittal PD-weighted MR image (**b**) shows chronic type-3 fibrous bands (large arrow) trapping sciatic nerve proximally (short arrow) months later in the same patient

entrapment include malunion or healed of the ischium avulsions and lesser/greater trochanter fractures [70] (Fig. 5.49).

Hematomas Gluteal hematomas are usually related to trauma, hip surgery, and hemophilia or anticoagulation therapy. Hematomas can damage the nerve either directly (increased pressure on the nerve) or indirectly (ischemia as a result of vasa vasorum compression or fibrous bands formation that trap subgluteal nerves. Fibrous bands formed due to healing hematomas are among the most frequent causes of DGS and correspond to those formerly published cases with piriformis-syndrome-like pain and history of trauma. The MRI signal characteristics of the mass vary according to its contents of hemoglobin degradation products. Acute hematomas (1–4 days) have low signal intensity in all sequences and are surrounded by edema. In its early subacute (2–7 days) and late subacute (1–3 weeks) phases, they are hyperintense on T1-weighted images owing to its methemoglobin content. Signal intensity on T2-weighted images is low during the early subacute period but high during the late subacute period. The wall of a chronic hematoma has a hypointense signal on both sequences owing to hemosiderin accumulation. A mass that appears following trauma, follows the described stage-related pattern of signal changes, and is reduced in size over time is pathognomonic [35] (Fig. 5.50).

Direct Traumatic Neuropathy or Contusions During traumatic compressions nerves injured by contact with bone structures due to its deep location (acetabulum in the case of the sciatic nerve). MR neurography usually revealed mild enlargement and focal T2 hyperintensity of the sciatic nerve without macroscopic pathology (Fig. 5.51). Direct sciatic neuropathy rarely presents in non-penetrating trauma because of protection of the nerve by the pelvis, the gluteal muscles, and the tissues in the posterior thigh [34].

Traumatic Stump Neuroma In patients undergoing proximal lower limb amputations, MR neurography often reveals a low-signal-intensity mass within the sciatic nerve on T1-weighted

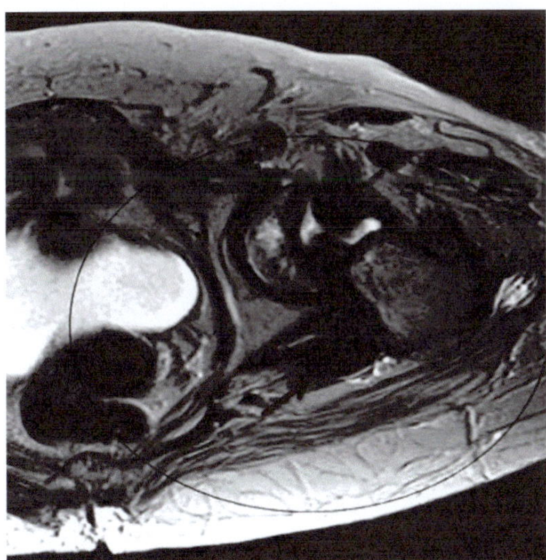

Fig. 5.49 DGS secondary to fibrous malunion of the left femoral neck. Axial PD-weighted MR image shows a sciatic nerve entrapment (black arrow) in the deep gluteal space due to the presence of a fibrous conglomerate as a result of inflammatory changes scarring in a patient with a nonunion and displaced fracture of the femoral neck

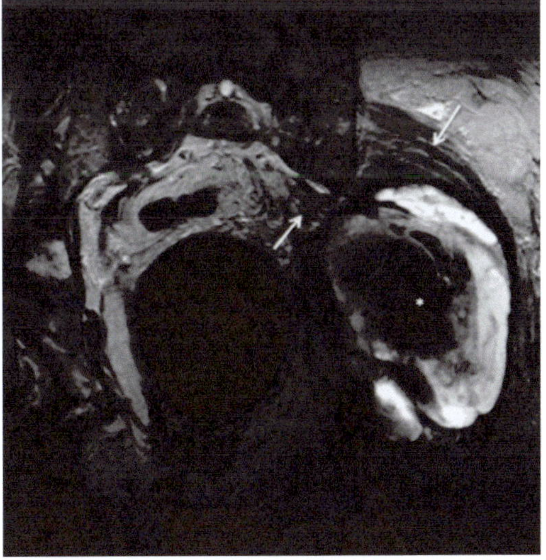

Fig. 5.50 DGS secondary to subacute subgluteal hematoma. Coronal T2-weighted MR image shows a subgluteal hematoma with partial extension through the sciatic foramen in a patient who has underwent hip prosthetic surgery. Note the hematic clots within the collection (asterisk) and the sciatic compromise (arrow)

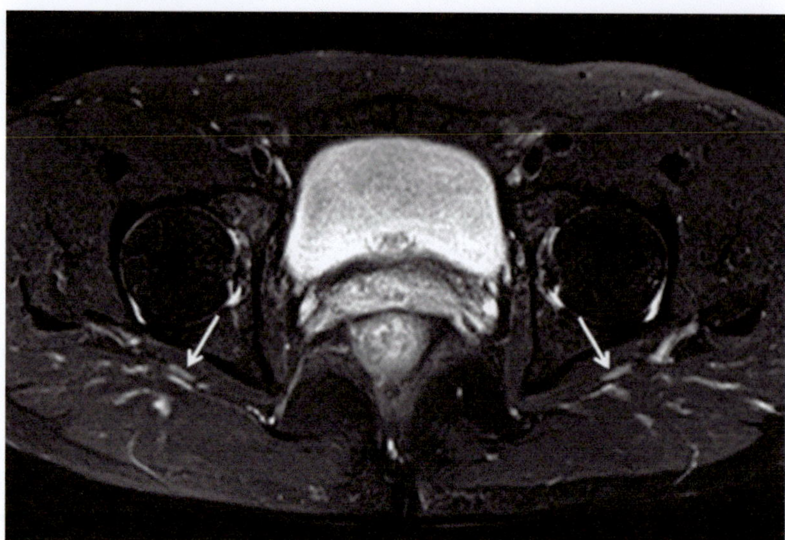

Fig. 5.51 Bilateral DGS secondary to subgluteal contusion. Axial T2-weighted MR image shows an increased endoneurial signal intensity of both sciatic nerves (arrows) without any other associated pathological finding in a patient with clinical diagnosis of deep gluteal syndrome after bilateral trauma. It is necessary a careful analysis of the signal intensity of the nerve to detect isolated neuritis since it is often the only imaging finding

spin-echo images that shows mild enhancement following intravenous administration of gadolinium. Proximal to these neuromas, the sciatic nerve often is enlarged with marked focal fascicular enlargement and abnormal increased T2 hyperintensity that must be correctly understood in the clinical setting because it is sometimes painful [37, 71].

Iatrogenic

Surgery The most common cause of neuropathy at the hip is iatrogenic and is associated with total hip replacement for primary osteoarthritis, related to stretching or direct trauma of the nerve. Excessive retraction, inadvertent resection during total hip replacement, and a poor positioning of the patient are the most well-recognized causes of superior gluteal nerve injury [72]. The inferior branch of the nerve is vulnerable during the direct lateral approach of Hardinge, and branches to the tensor fascia lata are at risk during the anterolateral or anterior approach. The high variability in the branching pattern and course of the nerve makes it even more susceptible to injury at surgery. Inferior gluteal entrapment neuropathy is rarely reported but is recognized as a complication of the posterior approach to hip arthroplasty [73]. Subclinical electromyographic abnormalities of both superior and inferior gluteal nerves have

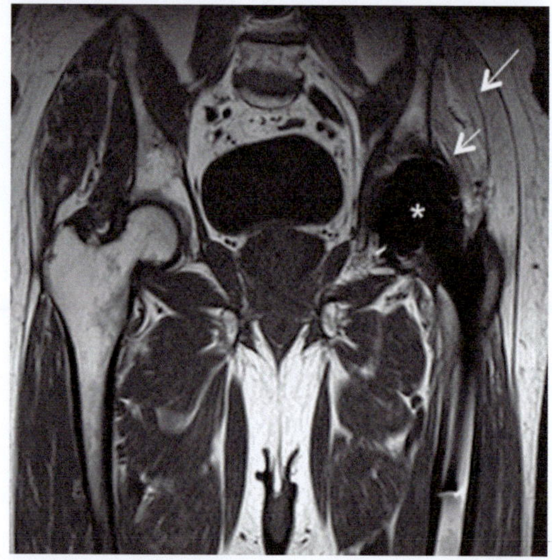

Fig. 5.52 DGS secondary to hip surgery. Coronal T1-weighted MR image shows atrophy of the left gluteus medium (large arrow) and minor (short arrow) muscles due to injury of gluteal nerves after prosthetic surgery of the hip (asterisk)

been described by Abitbol et al. in up to 77% of patients after total hip replacement, regardless of the surgical approach. Injury to the superior gluteal nerve is also a well-recognized complication of percutaneous placement of iliosacral screws. The pattern of muscular atrophy, a characteristic sign of neural entrapment, reveals the affected nerve and the level of injury [74] (Fig. 5.52).

Intramuscular Injections Nerve injury may be caused by accumulation of injected drugs within the perineural space, direct needle trauma, secondary to a compression by scar tissue or direct nerve fibers damage caused by neurotoxic chemicals included in the injected drug (Fig. 5.53).

Radiotherapy Postradiation neuropathy myositis is a rare condition most frequently observed following higher doses of radiation (5000 rads). Sciatic nerve may be damaged following radiotherapy either directly (by the harmful effects of radiation itself) or indirectly (by diffuse fibrosis of tissues surrounding the nerve). Imaging reveals a diffuse nerve thickening with no observable mass. Rarely, however, focal mass-like lesions similar to tumor recurrences may be observed, being hypointense on T1-weighted and hyperintense on T2-weighted MR images. Contrast enhancement following intravenous administration of gadolinium may also be observed [35] (Fig. 5.54).

Foreign Bodies Foreign bodies of any nature can injure or compress the subgluteal nerves, usually after high-energy trauma, surgery, or due to iatrogenic causes (Fig. 5.55).

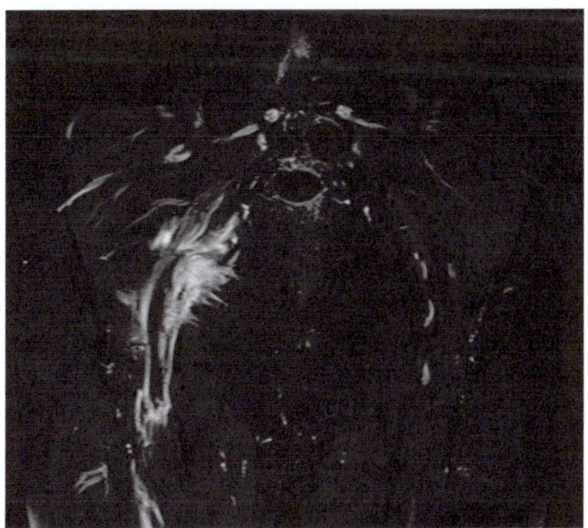

Fig. 5.53 DGS secondary to intramuscular injection. Coronal DP-weighted fat-saturated MR image shows sciatic neuritis in a patient immediately after a gluteal injection. Note the accumulation of the injected drug along the perineural space

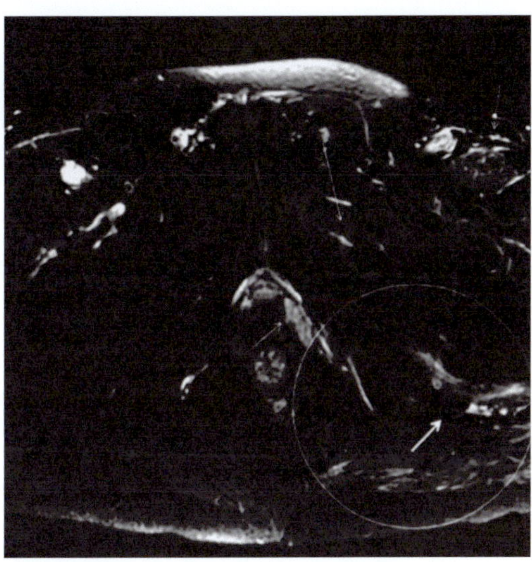

Fig. 5.54 DGS secondary to radiotherapy. Axial T1-weighted fat-saturated contrast-enhanced MR image shows diffuse nerve thickening with no observable mass suggestive of postradiation neuropathy in a patient with transitional cell carcinoma following higher doses of radiation (8000 rads). Edema and scar tissue around the nerve (arrow) caused DGS. Note the signal hyperintensity of several muscles included in the radiation field suggestive of postradiation myositis

Inflammatory/Infectious

Sacroiliitis Noninfectious sacroiliitis is a frequently encountered finding among seronegative spondyloarthropathies. Posterior hip pain and/or sciatica may be the result of referred pain or the inflammatory changes in the immediate neighborhood of the sacroiliac joint directly affecting the nerve [75]. In addition, septic sacroiliitis is a well-known cause of sacral and sciatic pyogenic neuritis (Figs. 5.56 and 5.57).

Osteoarthritis DGS can be seen as a result of mechanical compression of the sciatic nerve related to degenerative changes (osteophyte formation) in the hip joint especially in elderly patients although is not a frequent etiology of DGS.

Abscesses Gluteal and pelvic region abscesses are seldom encountered. They are usually related to gastrointestinal and urinary tract infections

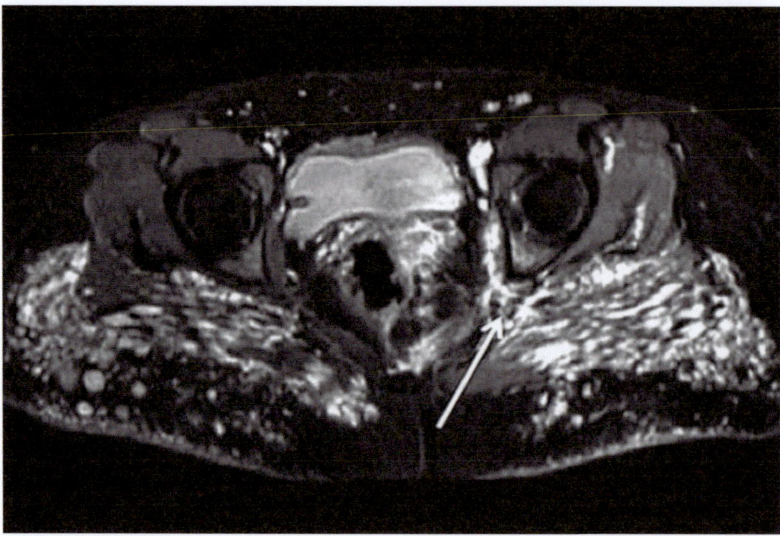

Fig. 5.55 DGS secondary to foreign bodies. Axial DP-weighted fat-suppressed MR image shows silicone injections not contained in a prosthesis trapping the sacral plexus and sciatic nerves, mainly on the left side. Siliconomas spread through the presacral, parasacral, and ischiorectal spaces and left obturator internal muscle. Scar tissue and edema are seen around the left sacral plexus, sciatic nerve, and pudendal nerve causing entrapment (arrow)

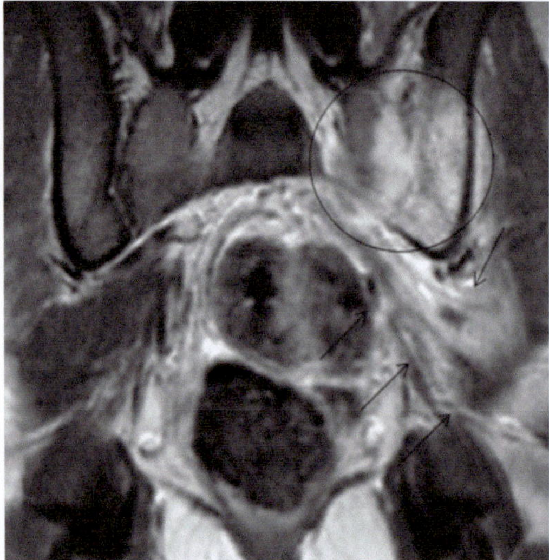

Fig. 5.56 DGS secondary to septic sacroiliitis. Coronal T2-weighted MR image shows edema around the left sacroiliac joint (circle) and purulent fluid in the presacral and prepiriformis spaces. The sciatic nerve and superior/inferior gluteal nerves have increased size and signal intensity, findings suggestive of pyogenic neuritis (arrows)

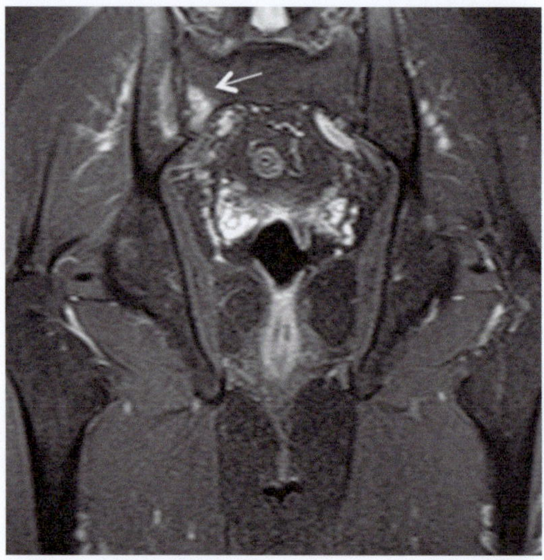

Fig. 5.57 Noninfectious active sacroiliitis simulating a right subgluteal syndrome in a patient with ankylosing spondylitis

and may affect the sacral plexus by spreading via normal anatomical routes. A gluteal and presacral abscess also related to sacral osteomyelitis may directly affect the lumbosacral plexus and sciatic nerve [35].

Myositis Myositis is a rare muscle infection, with the most commonly implicated bacteria being Staphylococcus and Streptococcus. When it affects gluteal or pelvic-trochanteric muscles, it may cause DGS. Piriformis myositis has been rarely reported in the literature. Recognized predisposing factors for the condition are mainly previous viral or parasitic infections, rheumatic disease, and HIV infection [76]. *Brucella* spp. is also a known bacterium identified as a cause of myositis [77]. It is also important to address the fact that muscle infections will finally extend to the retrofascial compartment and can become a source of confusion for the clinician, as the problem would seem worse at a more distant location than at the status of origin. Chiedozi described three distinct phases concerning myositis. During the first phase, inflammation is minimal. The muscle becomes hardened, with mild leukocytosis and no evidence of pus. After 2–3 weeks of the initial symptoms, the inflammation increases with evidence of purulence. Signs of systemic toxicity characterized the third phase [78] (Fig. 5.58).

On the other hand, inflammatory myopathies must be present in our differential diagnoses. The most common inflammatory myopathies are dermatomyositis, polymyositis (which rarely occurs as an isolated entity, more often associated with other features of connective tissue disease), and inclusion body myositis (Fig. 5.59).

Bursitis Distention of periarticular bursae of the hip is a recognized cause of DGS. Most commonly, bursitis has an inflammatory origin, secondary to degenerative tendinopathy of adjacent tendons but may be pyogenic, traumatic, etc. (Fig. 5.60).

Sciatic Nerve Sarcoidosis Sciatic nerve MR neurography may reveal a mildly enhancing mass centered within the sciatic nerve. The mass is hypointense on T1-weighted and T2-weighted imaging reveals fascicular enlargement proximal and distal to the mass. On the basis of homoge-

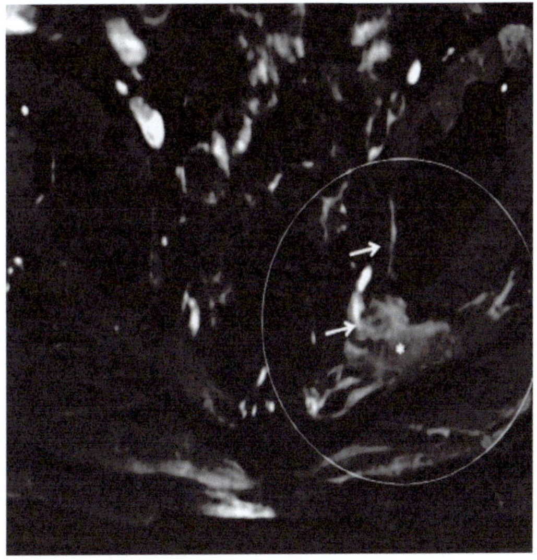

Fig. 5.58 DGS secondary to myositis. Axial PD-weighted fat-suppressed contrast-enhanced MR image shows a moderate and diffuse thickening of the left piriformis (asterisk) with regional soft tissue edema and a predominantly peripheral contrast enhancement in a patient suffering from piriformis myositis with incipient abscessification signs (circle). Note the diffuse hyperintensity of the sacral plexus due to the inflammatory infiltration and its extension anteriorly along the obturator internus space (arrows)

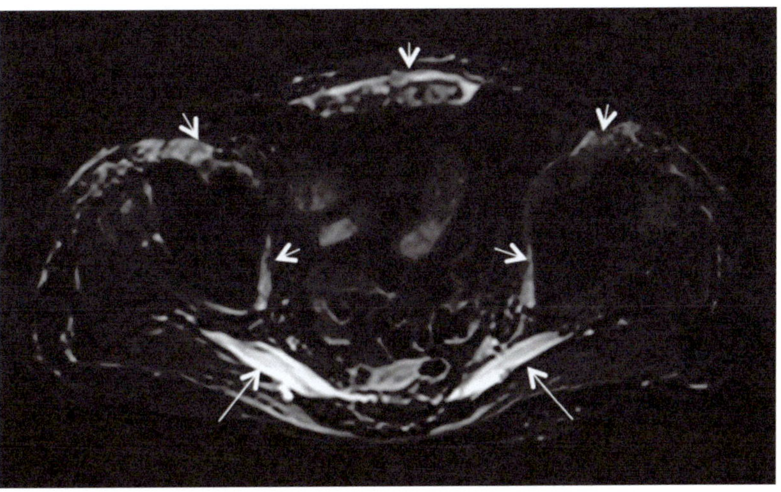

Fig. 5.59 DGS secondary to active myositis in a 67-year-old patient with a chronic, autoimmune inflammatory myopathy of the pelvic girdle musculature. Note the bilateral signal alteration of the rectus femoris, obturator internus, or iliopsoas muscles (short arrows) and both piriformis muscles (large arrows) in this patient with muscle weakness and active subgluteal pain

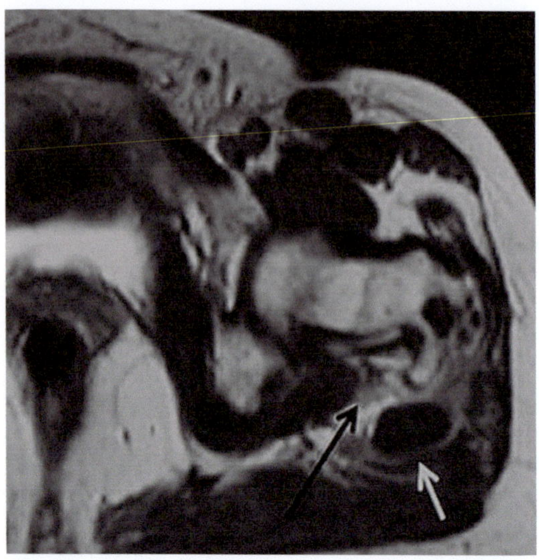

Fig. 5.60 DGS secondary to pyogenic bursitis. Axial PD-weighted MR image shows a moderate to severe distention of the trochanteric bursa (black arrow) associated with left sciatic nerve compromise (white arrow) in a patient with tuberculous trochanter bursitis. Signs of osteitis in the great trochanter may also be seen

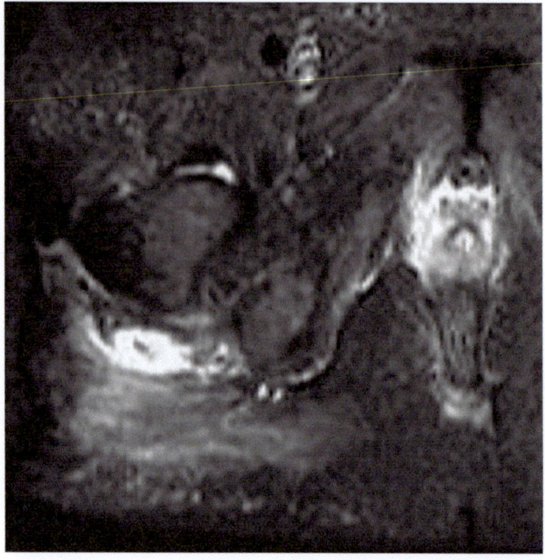

Fig. 5.61 DGS secondary to paraneoplastic syndrome. Axial STIR MR image shows a severe thickening of the sciatic nerve associated with significant perineural inflammatory changes in the deep gluteal space in a 56-year-old patient with lung carcinoma and well-characterized paraneoplastic antibodies (anti-Hu, anti-Yo, anti-Ri, antiamphiphysin, anti-CV2)

neous loss of normal fascicular architecture at the mass level and enhancement characteristics, a preoperative diagnosis of neurofibroma is often made. Surgical internal neurolysis and biopsy are necessary to demonstrate chronic inflammatory changes and multinucleated giant cells with noncaseating granulomas, characteristic of sarcoidosis [79].

Paraneoplastic, Autoimmune, and Other Infrequent Neuritis In cancer patients the development of peripheral neuropathies usually represents a side effect of therapy, infiltration of nerves or spinal roots by the tumor, or metabolic and nutritional deficits. A neuropathy is defined as paraneoplastic when none of the above causes are detected or when cancer-related immunological mechanisms are involved. At least 15% of cancer patients develop a paraneoplastic sensorimotor neuropathy, which is usually mild and develops during the terminal stage of the disease. There is another group of paraneoplastic neuropathies that often precede the diagnosis of the tumor and can be more debilitating than the cancer itself (Fig. 5.61). On the other hand, certain toxic substances such as lead, arsenic, and mer-

cury may produce a generalized poisoning of the peripheral nerves, with tenderness, pain, and paralysis of the limbs. Finally, other causes of generalized neuritis include alcoholism, vitamin-deficiency diseases such as diabetes mellitus, thallium poisoning, some types of allergy, and some viral and bacterial infections, such as diphtheria, syphilis, and mumps [80].

Vascular

Persistent Sciatic Artery The persistent sciatic artery (PSA) is a rare congenital anomaly with an incidence ranging from 0.025% to 0.04% of the population. This artery is prone to atherosclerotic change and is associated with aneurysmal change in 46.1% of the cases. The most frequent symptoms associated with PSA aneurysm are a painful pulsatile buttock mass, sciatic neuropathy caused by sciatic nerve compression, and lower limb ischemia caused by thrombosis or distal embolization [81]. According to Pris et al., sciatica is found in 36%. The aneurysms complications are embolism, thrombosis, rupture, fissuring, and sciatic nerve compression, because the course of the persistent sciatic artery through the thigh is varied but always close to the sciatic nerve [82]. Radiological investigations are important to identify, classify, and aid in performing endovascular intervention. Treatment of persistent sciatic artery includes open-surgery (graft interposition and femoropopliteal bypass, ilio-popliteal transobturator bypass, etc.) or endovascular intervention [83].

Aneurism or Pseudoaneurysm of Iliac Artery The lumbosacral trunk is anterior to the sacrum and posterior to the iliac vessels. Any aneurysmal or pseudoaneurysmal expansion of the iliac artery, especially affecting the internal iliac artery, may compress pelvic or subgluteal nerves. The basic mechanism of aneurysm-related sciatica is compression to the nerve. Although nerves are fairly resistant to ischemia and the lumbosacral plexus is rich in vascular supply, ischemia may play an additional role (vasa vasorum compression) [84].

Arteriovenous Malformation or Arteriovenous Fistula Although quite rarely, direct pressure on pelvic nerves by an arteriovenous malformation or arteriovenous fistula may also cause sciatica [85].

Thrombosis of Gluteal Arteries This is a cause of buttock claudication, occurring consistently after 150 m walking and disappearing after a short rest. Contrast-enhanced CT and magnetic resonance angiography (MRA) are the imaging tests of choice to demonstrate this condition. Selective angiography of iliac arteries is often requests, which clearly identifies a tight stenosis of the onset of the artery. Percutaneous angioplasty together with stenting of this artery induced a prompt and complete relief of pain [86] (Fig. 5.62).

Varicosity-Caused Deep Gluteal Syndrome Gluteal vascular compressive neuropathy coursing with intractable DGS, which was not elicited by posture change or cough, should add value to the presence of varicosities. Sitting on the affected side causes more pain than standing or walking. Magnetic resonance imaging reveals compression of the gluteal portion of the sciatic

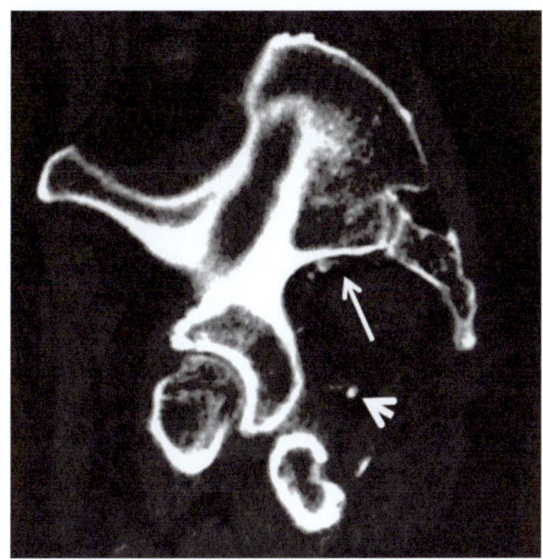

Fig. 5.62 DGS secondary to thrombosis of the superior gluteal artery. Sagittal-oblique MDCT contrast-enhanced reconstruction shows the lack of contrast filling of the superior gluteal artery (large arrow) as opposed to the normal contrast filling of the inferior gluteal artery (short arrow) in a 67-year-old patient suffering from intermittent gluteal claudication

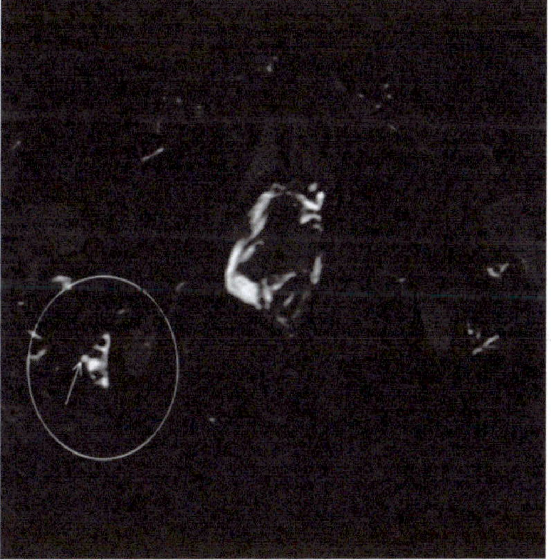

Fig. 5.63 DGS secondary to subgluteal varicosities. Axial PD-weighted fat-suppressed MR image shows focal varicosities compressing sciatic nerve (arrow) on the right side in this patient with deep gluteal pain which did not improve by postural changes

nerve by varicotic gluteal veins. Ligation and resection of varicotic vein result in relief of the patient's pain [5, 87] (Fig. 5.63).

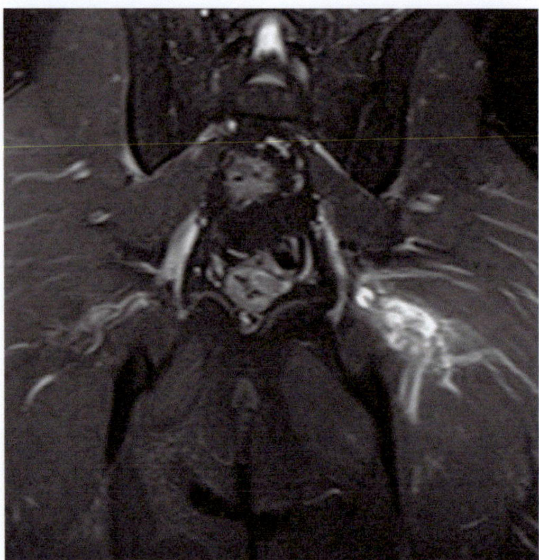

Fig. 5.64 DGS secondary to traumatic venous varix. Coronal PD-weighted fat-suppressed MR image shows focal varicosities of the inferior gluteal veins around the left sciatic nerve in this patient who suffered from a fall onto the buttock 4 months before

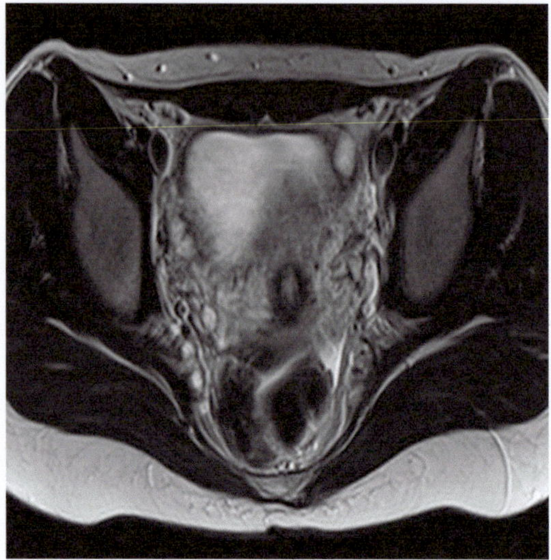

Fig. 5.65 DGS secondary to pelvic congestion syndrome. Axial T2-weighted MR image shows bilateral pelvic varicosities in this 41-year-old patient with a noncyclical pain that lasted more than 6 months and worsened by sitting and standing at the end of the day

Traumatic Venous Varix Development of traumatic venous varix of the inferior gluteal vein, usually formed after a fall onto the buttock, may cause sciatic neuropathy. Gradient echo and two-dimensional time-of-flight MRI sequences confirm the vascular lesion usually originating from the gluteal veins. Surgical resection is successful in obliterating the lesion and relieving the symptoms [5, 88] (Fig. 5.64).

Pelvic Congestion Syndrome The diagnosis of pelvic congestion syndrome is established by the demonstration of multiple dilated, tortuous parauterine veins with a width greater than 4 mm or an ovarian vein diameter greater than 5–6 mm (Fig. 5.65). Treatment options include coil embolization of the gonadal vein or laparoscopic ligation of the ovarian vein in selected cases [89, 90].

Gynecological

Multiple cases of posterior hip pain related to gynecological and obstetrical diseases or complications have been reported. Pathologic conditions in the pelvis and gynecological diseases must be borne in mind, especially when the right side is affected. Furthermore, it has been suggested that the sigmoid colon plays a role in preventing pressure on sacral plexus on the left side. It is recommended that women in their late 30s or premenopausal period presenting with DGS should have a thorough gynecological examination before back surgery or deep gluteal space arthroscopy is attempted, even where radiological imaging suggests a herniated intervertebral disc. Paying attention to gynecological pathology is essential to avoid false negatives cases, which lead the patient to unnecessary and ineffective treatments.

Adenomyosis DGS caused by adenomyosis of the uterus has been reported. As occurs with all intrapelvic pathology, in most cases lumbosacral trunk is the most frequently affected root. This condition is a benign invasion of the myometrium by the endometrium usually affecting women over the age of 30 and found in approximately 20% of removed uteri. It is otherwise known to manifest itself classically by progressive menstrual bleeding, increasingly painful dysmenorrhea, and a gradually enlarging, tender uterus [91] (Fig. 5.66b).

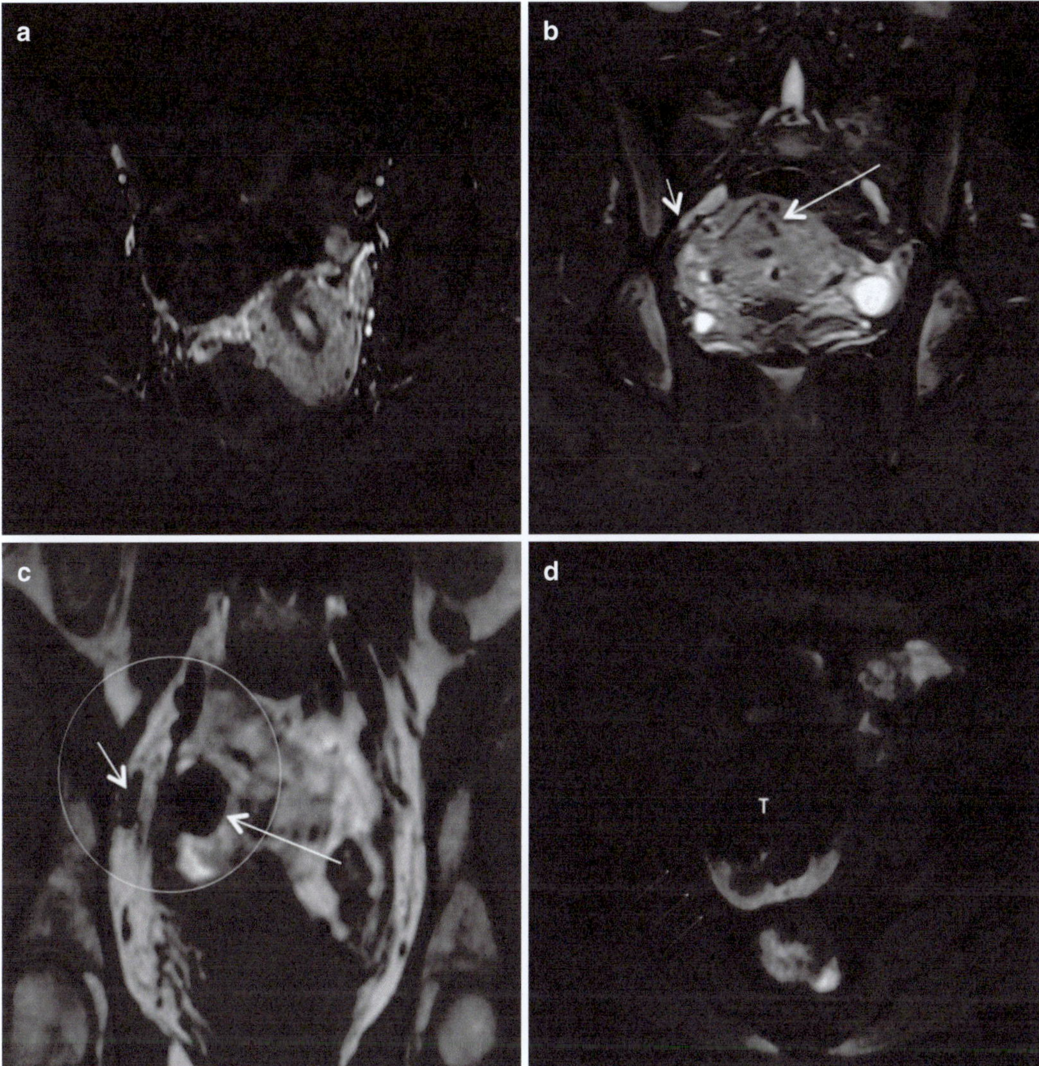

Fig. 5.66 DGS secondary to gynecological pathology. (**a**) Axial PD-weighted fat-suppressed MR image shows a retroverted uterus in a young patient with intermittent deep gluteal pain highly dependent on positions. (**b**) Coronal PD-weighted fat-suppressed MR image shows an extensive and diffuse enlargement of junctional zone (large arrow) with submucosal microcyst and ill-defined contours signaling diffuse adenomyosis trapping the right sciatic nerve (short arrow) in a 28-year-old woman with chronic dysmenorrhea. (**c**) Coronal T1-weighted fat- suppressed MR image shows a right endometrioma with a low-signal-intensity appearance due to hemosiderin deposits combined associated with the fibrous nature of the cyst wall (large arrow) as well as chronic fibrosis around the sciatic nerve at the level of the greater sciatic notch (short arrow). (**d**) Axial PD-weighted fat-suppressed MR image shows a mature cystic teratoma (T) that depends on the right ovary and sacral plexus neuritis (arrows)

Retroversion of the Uterus This is one of the most frequent and undervalued gynecological causes of DGS in our experience [5, 92] (Fig. 5.66a).

Tumors Hysteromyomas, tubo-ovarian abscess, ovarian cysts, and teratomas have also been reported to be a cause of lumbosacral plexopathy [92] (Fig. 5.66d).

Ectopic Endometriosis Endometriosis has been reported several times as a source of cyclic sciatica and subgluteal pain. It may compress the sciatic nerve within the pelvis, sciatic notch, or deep gluteal space being most frequent at the level of the sciatic notch and on the right. Sciatic pain typically starts a few days before menstruation, intensifies progressively, and shows some relief a week after menstruation is over. A focal mass is classically seen as high signal intensity on both T2- and T1-weighted images, suggesting acute bleeding; however, signal intensities can vary depending on the nature of the hemoglobin breakdown products. Endometriosis is the most frequently encountered benign mass causing sciatic nerve entrapment [93] (Fig. 5.66c).

Pregnancy Pregnancy-related DGS may be caused by the direct compression of the nerve roots or secondary to the possible ischemia of the neural elements caused by compression of the abdominal aorta and/or inferior vena cava by the gravid uterus. L5 root irritation, with unilateral foot drop in some cases, may occur through injury of the lumbosacral trunk by the fetal head or forceps during delivery. Up to 50% of women report back pain at some stage during pregnancy and in one-third the severity of the pain is such that it interferes with daily life. Although in many cases backache resolves shortly after delivery, in some it continues for months; in others it begins postpartum. Furthermore, during pregnancy, "piriformis syndrome" is more likely to occur. The pregnant woman begins to secrete the hormone "relaxin" which increases pelvic stretch and can potentially open up the space in the sacroiliac joints. Their spine also increases in lordosis -the curvature going anterior which tilts the pelvis forward moving it into increased flexion. The combination of all these pathophysiological mechanism precipitates the gluteal muscle group of the hip/pelvis to become elongated and strained, especially the deep and small muscles of the hip. Massage therapy can be used as a preventative measure and to relieve symptoms when aggravated [94].

Pseudotumors and Tumors

Primary Lesions of the Sciatic Nerve
Hypertrophic Neuropathy In this pathologic condition, MR neurography reveals an enhancing

sciatic nerve mass centered within the nerve that is isointense to muscle and that displaces several mildly swollen fascicles to the nerve peripherally. More distally an abnormal T2 hyperintensity with preserved fascicular morphology usually reflects a compressive neuropraxic injury. Biopsy reveals fibrosis and the characteristic "onion bulb" lesions. Surgical internal neurolysis must be performed. By their characteristic, preoperative diagnosis of schwannoma is common [95]. Current theories suggest that the breakage of the perineural barrier related or not to surgery during surgery is a predisposing or precipitating factor of focal hypertrophic neuropathy [96, 97] (Fig. 5.67).

Congenital Hypertrophic Neuropathies Dejerine-Sottas disease and other hereditary motor and sensory polyneuropathies are neurological disorders characterized by damage to the peripheral nerves, progressive muscle wasting, and diffuse neuritis of the sciatic nerve and/or the sacral plexus on imaging [98] (Fig. 5.68).

Schwannomas and Neurofibromas Schwannoma is the most common primary tumor of the sciatic nerve. It originates from the Schwann cells forming the sheath of the nerve. Schwannomas of the pelvis and posterior hip are quite rare. The imaging features of schwannoma overlap those of a solitary neurofibroma (originating from nerve fibers), and often they are indistinguishable (Fig. 5.69).

Lipomatosis and Intraneural Lipomas Lipomatosis, also known as fibrolipomatous hamartoma or fibrofatty proliferation, is a rare benign tumorlike lesion that most often affects the median nerve or its branches [99]. Rarely, involvement of the nerves of the lower extremities has been reported. Over 50% of patients are symptomatic because of mass sensation or focal compressive neuropathy. Several serpentine intralesional soft tissue attenuation structures that have a spaghetti-like appearance in longitudinal section and a coaxial cable-like appearance in cross section are considered pathognomonic. Differential diagnostic considerations of pelvic lipomatosis of nerve

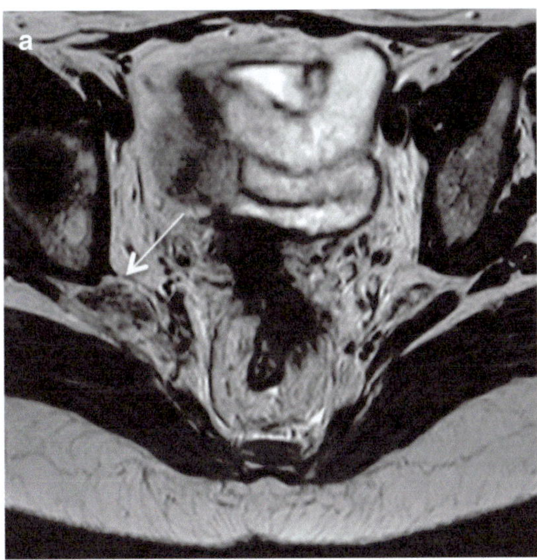

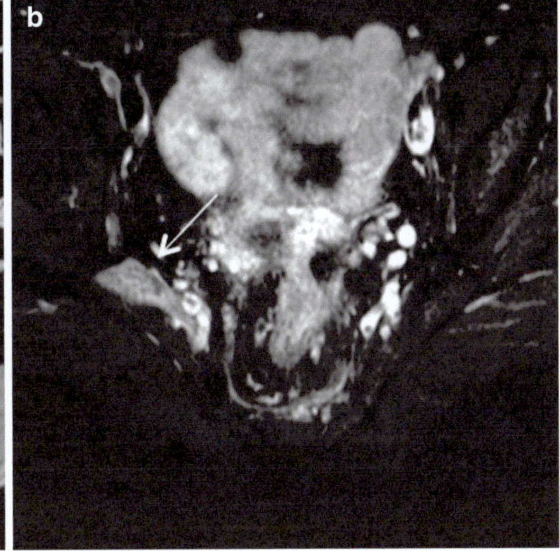

Fig. 5.67 DGS secondary to localized hypertrophic neuropathy. Axial PD-weighted (**a**) and axial PD-weighted fat-suppressed (**b**) MR images show a significant enlargement of sciatic nerve (arrows) in the right piriformis space in a patient with painless neurological deficit in the sciatic nerve territory two months after colorectal surgery

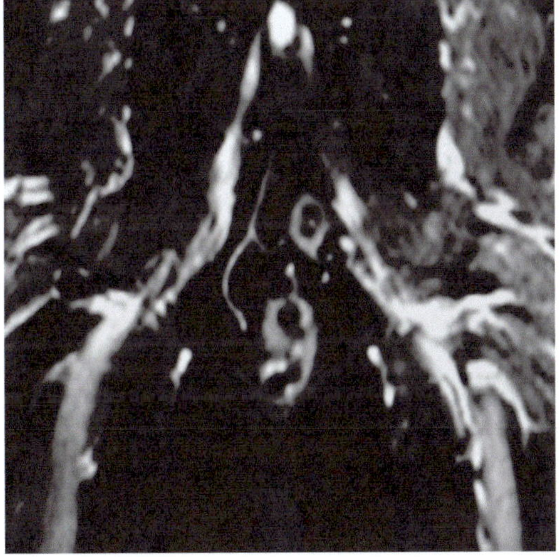

Fig. 5.68 Bilateral DGS secondary to Dejerine-Sottas disease. Coronal T1-weighted fat-suppressed contrast-enhanced MR image shows a significant abnormal thickening, clumping, and enhancement of the lumbosacral roots in a 3-year-old child with lower extremities weakness and loss of sensation

include intraneural lipoma and well-differentiated liposarcoma. Intraneural lipomas are focal encapsulated tumors located within the nerve sheath that do not involve individual nerve bundles. They appear as focal round or oval lesions of homogeneous or nearly homogeneous fat attenuation with crowding of adjacent normal nerve bundles. Conversely, lipomatosis of nerve tends to involve nerves diffusely [100].

Malignant Neurogenic Neoplasms They account for 7–8% of all malignant soft tissue neoplasms. Neurofibroma, rarely neurilemoma, and malignant peripheral neural sheath tumors (PNST) may arise in association with NF1. Patients present with pain and neurologic symptoms of motor weakness and sensory deficits more frequently than do patients with benign PNSTs. In patients with NF1, sudden increase in size of a previously stable neurofibroma suggests malignant transformation [101] (Fig. 5.70).

Benign and Malignant Tumors or Pseudotumoral Lesions

Many benign tumors and pseudotumoral lesions may appear along the course of the sacral plexus and sciatic nerve involving or trapping its components. Lipoma, osteochondroma, ganglion cyst, and pelvis lymph nodes are in our experience the most common benign tumors causing DGS [35] (Fig. 5.71). However, a wide range of other benign tumors and pseudotumoral lesions has been reported in the literature as a cause of posterior hip pain. Although the appearance of many of them is nonspecific, some offer imaging characteristics that suggest the exact diagnosis. We describe below some of them with special relevance.

Heterotopic Calcifications Infrapiriform canal syndrome related to ossification of the sacrospi-nous ligament secondary to pelvic balance abnormalities has been described as a cause of DGS [102] (Fig. 5.72).

Massive Periarticular Calcinosis This is a rare benign disease previously known as tumoral calcinosis and characterized by the presence of calcified, soft, and periarticular masses, variable in size, and with slowly progressive growth. It is

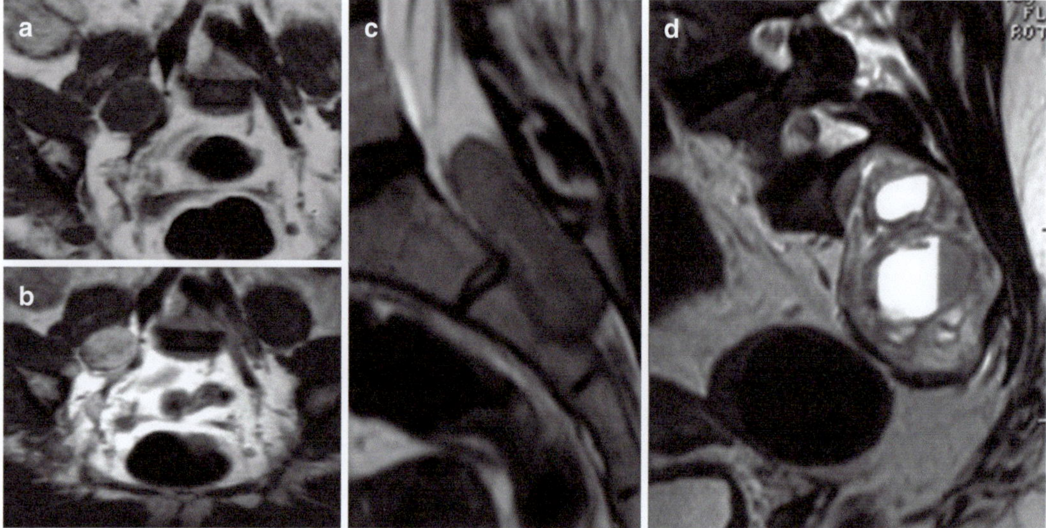

Fig. 5.69 DGS secondary to schwannomas of the sciatic nerve (**a**, **b**), the cauda equine (**c**), and anterior sacral roots (**d**)

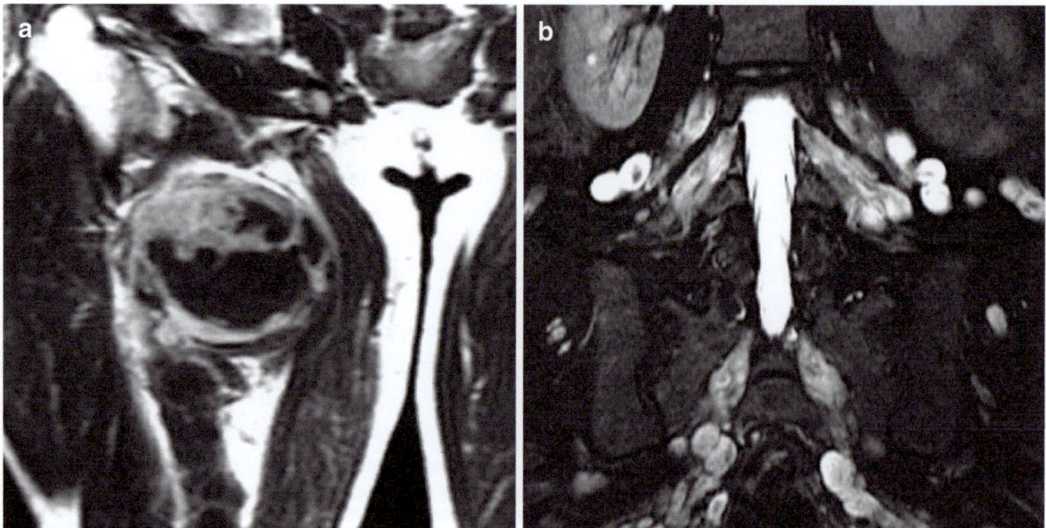

Fig. 5.70 DGS secondary to malignant neurofibroma (**a**), diffuse neurofibromatosis (**b**), plexiform neurofibroma (**c**), and malignant neurilemoma (**d**)

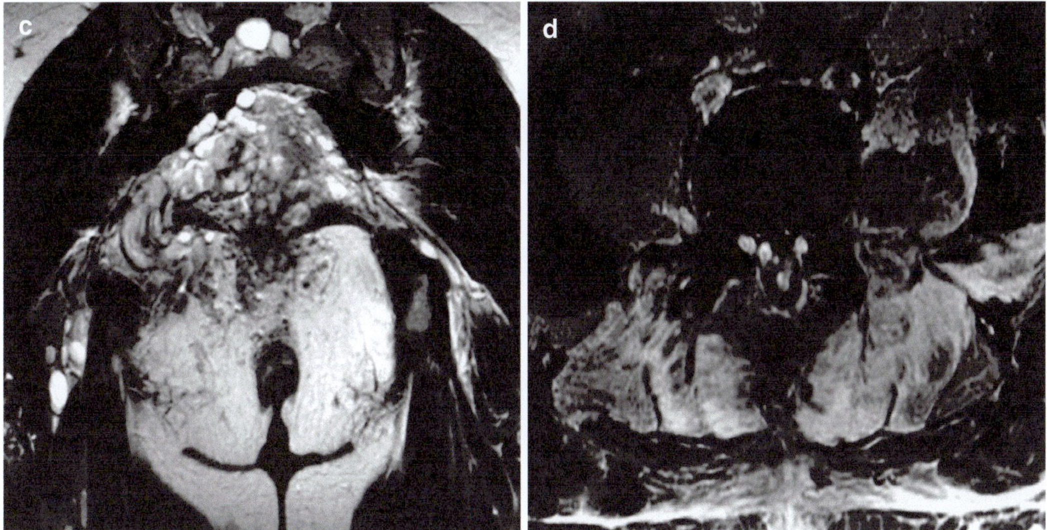

Fig. 5.70 (continued)

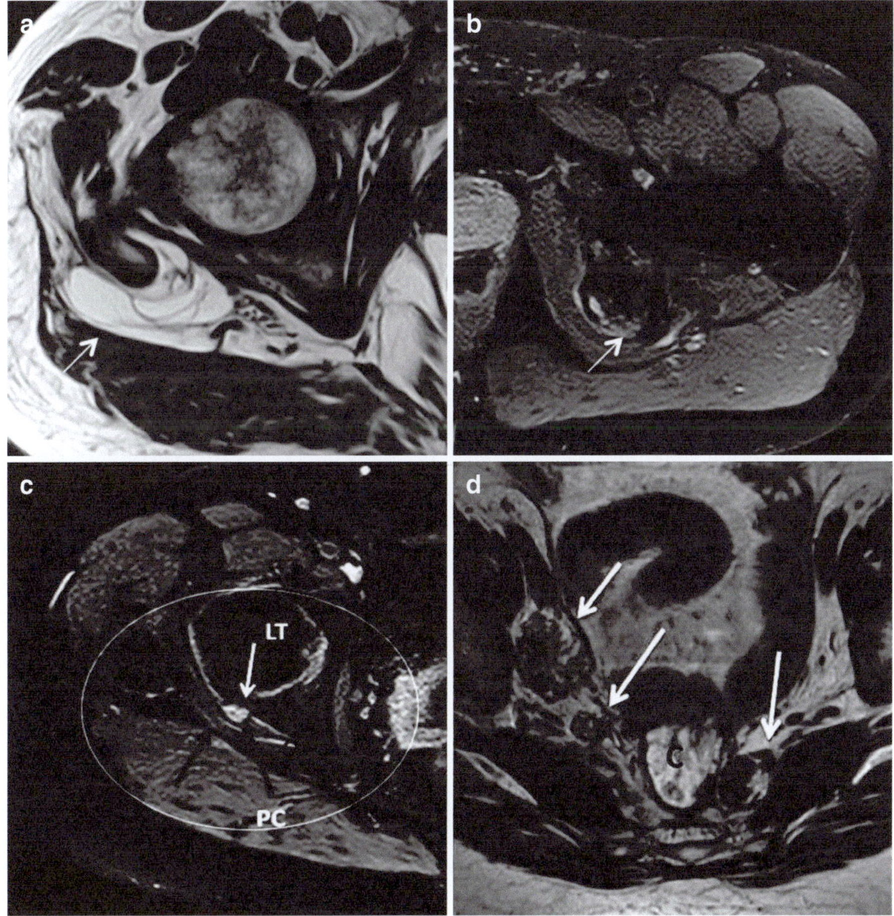

Fig. 5.71 DGS secondary to lipoma of the deep gluteal space (arrow in **a**), osteochondroma of the ischial tuberosity (arrow in **b**), paralabral cyst of the posterior labrum in a patient with femoroacetabular impingement (**c**), and calcified pelvis lymph nodes in a patient with colitis ulcerative (**d**)

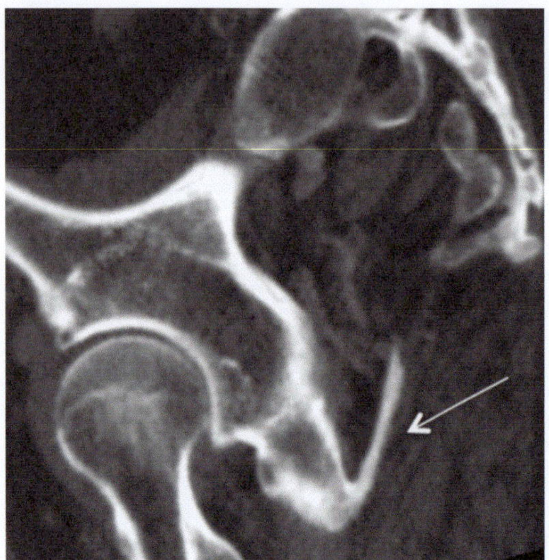

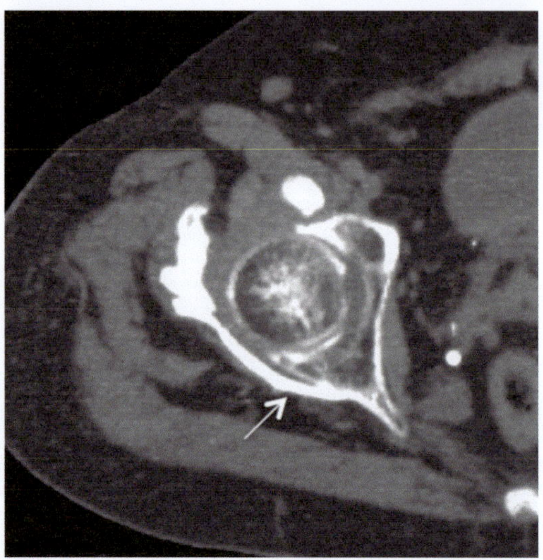

Fig. 5.72 Infrapiriformis canal syndrome. Sagittal-oblique MDCT reconstruction shows the ossification of the sacrotuberous ligament causing sciatic pain because of lack of mobility of the proximal sciatic nerve in a 32-year-old female patient with DGS

Fig. 5.73 DGS secondary to massive periarticular calcinosis. Axial-oblique MDCT reconstruction shows well-demarcated calcifications around the hip. Dynamic ultrasound study showed a continuous friction of the sciatic nerve over the posterior calcification and MRI showed moderate sciatic neuritis (not shown)

secondary to diffuse calcium phosphate deposition into soft tissue and may be seen in the setting of uremia, hyperparathyroidism, or vitamin D intoxication [103]. The soft tissue lesions are typically lobulated and well-demarcated calcifications that are most often distributed along the extensor surfaces of large joints [104] (Fig. 5.73). There are many conditions with similar appearances, including calcinosis of chronic renal failure, calcinosis universalis, calcinosis circumscripta, calcifying tendonosis, synovial osteochondromatosis, synovial sarcoma, osteosarcoma, myositis ossificans, tophaceous gout, and calcifying myonecrosis. Although surgical intervention can often provide symptomatic improvement, this lesion tends to recur in the presence of elevated calcium phosphate levels, and its management therefore requires a combined multidisciplinary surgical and medical approach [103, 105].

Soft Tissue Sarcomas Similar to intramuscular metastases, soft tissue sarcomas are seen as isohypointense T1-weighted and hyperintense T2-weighted MRI lesions (Fig. 5.74). However, necrosis, peritumoral edema, and lobulation are less frequently encountered in soft tissue sarcomas than in metastatic lesions. Histopathological examination is mandatory for a definitive diagnosis [106].

Intramuscular Metastasis Metastatic disease involving muscles of the posterior hip is not rare. The frequency of muscle metastasis is reported to be 0.8–16% in autopsy studies. Lung carcinomas are usually the primary source of metastasis, and involvement of muscles neighboring the sciatic nerve may also be observed. Intramuscular metastases are seen as low-attenuation masses in contrast-enhanced CT images, often demonstrating peripheral contrast attenuation. They are isohypointense on T1-weighted and hyperintense on T2-weighted MRI images when compared with surrounding muscle tissues. They usually cause expansion of the involved muscle, and accompanying peritumoral edema may be noticeable. In addition, hemorrhage, necrosis, and calcification within the mass may be observable. The variety of metastases that can be found affecting muscles or bones is as wide as the variety of malignant tumors [107] (Fig. 5.75).

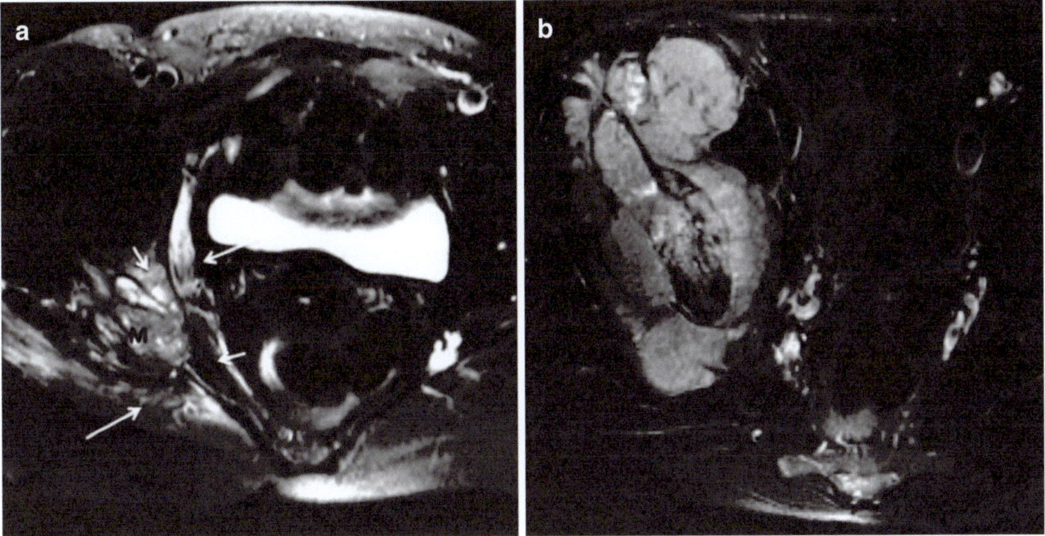

Fig. 5.74 DGS secondary to soft tissue sarcomas. Axial PD-weighted fat-suppressed MR images show a metastatic vaginal carcinosarcoma (M) (**a**) and Ewing sarcoma (**b**) affecting the deep gluteal space and sciatic nerve (arrow in a)

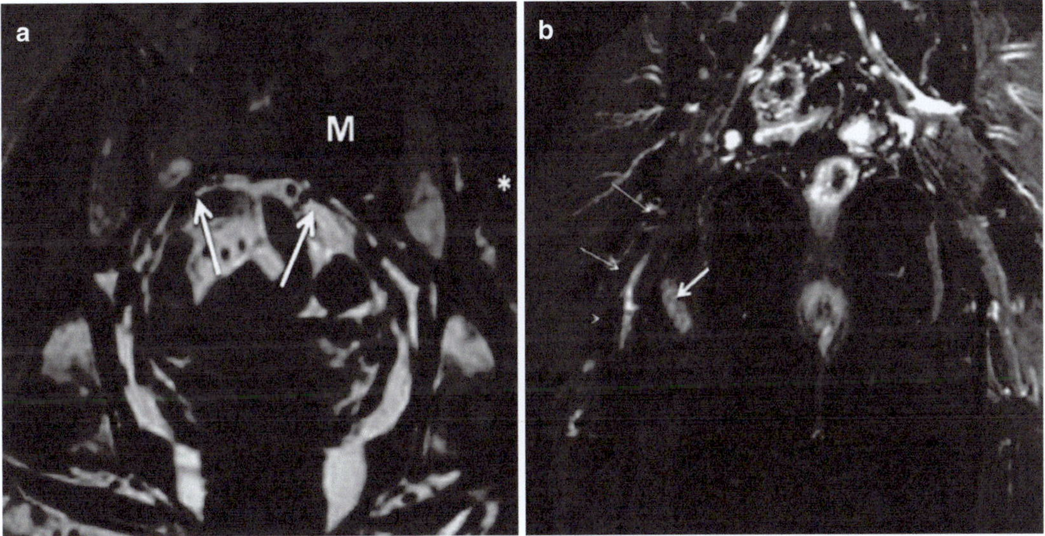

Fig. 5.75 DGS secondary to metastases. (**a**) Coronal T1-weighted MR image shows a sacral metastasis (M) from colorectal carcinoma affecting the left lumbosacral trunk (arrow). (**b**) Coronal PD-weighted fat-suppressed MR images show an ischial metastasis of lung carcinoma causing soft tissue edema and sciatic neuritis

Intra-abdominal and Intrapelvic Tumors The lumbosacral plexus and pelvic nerve may be affected as a result of compression or invasion by intra-abdominal or intrapelvic masses. Colorectal carcinoma is the most frequently encountered malignant tumor followed by the uterine, prostatic, and ovarian tumors. In addi-

tion, masses extending through the sciatic foramina may cause sciatic nerve entrapment in the deep gluteal space [35].

Lymphomas deserve special attention. There are three ways in which it may affect the sciatic nerve. The most frequent cause of lymphoma-related DGS is compression of the nerve by the enlarged lymph nodes. Secondly, extranodal involvement of soft tissues such as muscle (e.g., piriformis and gluteus muscles) may affect the sciatic nerve. In such cases, asymmetrical muscle expansion, heterogeneous/low focal density on CT images, or focal/diffuse low T1-weighted signal intensity and high T2-weighted signal intensity on the MRI images are radiologically observed. A uniform or ring-form contrast attenuation may be seen although the lesion may not attenuate contrast. Lastly, although very rare, direct lymphoma invasion of the sciatic nerve has also been reported [108] (Fig. 5.76).

Value of Imaging in Subgluteal Syndrome: Present and Future of MRI

Stewart argued that piriformis syndrome has been overdiagnosed and proposed that a definitive diagnosis would require surgical exploration to identify compression of the sciatic nerve by the piriformis muscle or by an associated fibrous band [5, 109]. However, MR neurography in a recent study demonstrated focal signal abnormalities within the sciatic nerve in the buttock in all patients with unexplained sciatica [45]. Filler

et al. recently reported similar findings in a larger series. These outcomes associated with advances in MRI hardware and development of new imaging techniques allowing detection of anatomical variations and fibrovascular bands that restrict mobility to nerve suggest that until now deep gluteal syndrome has probably been underdiagnosed rather than overdiagnosed and MR neurography is the diagnostic procedure of choice [5].

Explicit indications for ordering an MR neurography study and selection criteria for patients who might benefit from MR neurography after negative results of routine MR imaging of the lumbar segments of the spinal cord are beyond the scope of discussion. Good management of specific clinical tests by specialists is essential [37].

Although the primary goals of MR neurography are to localize the site of a nerve injury/fixation and to depict the lesions causing nerve entrapment or impingement, MRN has also been successfully used to assess the extent of the abnormality, to exclude the diagnosis of neuropathy by showing normal nerves and regional muscles, to detect incidental pathologies that mimic neuropathy symptoms, and to provide imaging guidance for perineural medication injections.

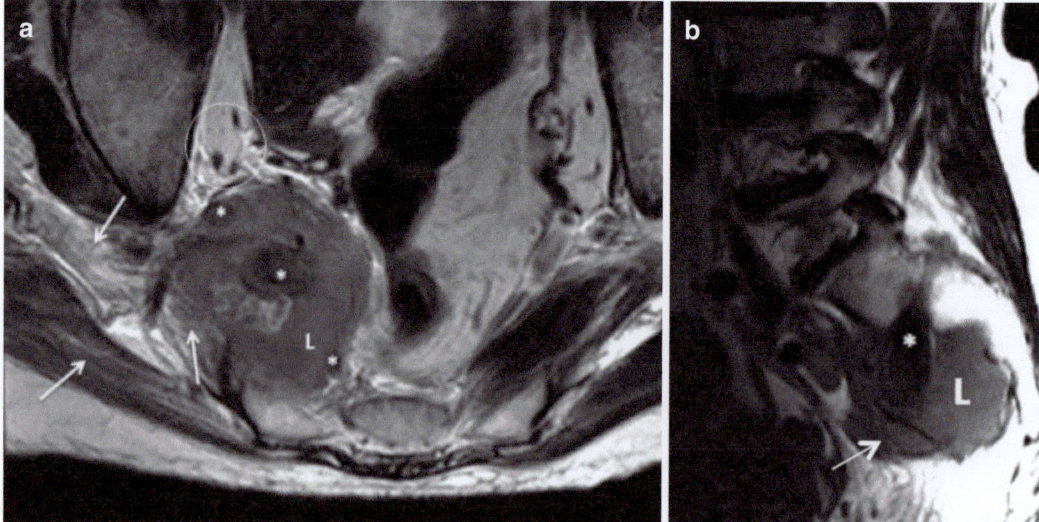

Fig. 5.76 DGS secondary to lymphoma. (**a**) Axial T1-weighted MR image shows direct infiltration of the piriformis muscle (arrows) and its extension through the prepiriformis space. (**b**) Sagittal T1-weighted MR images show direct lymphoma invasion of the sacral roots (asterisk)

Thus the performance of MRI has significant implications in treatment decisions [110].

Thoracic wraparound phased-array coil placed over the pelvis or thighs provides optimal coverage of the lumbosacral plexus and sciatic nerve. Pelvic phased-array coils are inadequate for examining the sciatic nerve in most patients. Imaging coverage from L3 through the ischial tuberosity centered in the midline is most suitable.

The normal sciatic nerve is a well-defined and easily identified oval structure with discrete fascicles (40–60 fascicles) isointense to adjacent muscle tissue on T1-weighted images. Normal nerve fascicles should be of uniform size and shape. Perifascicular and perineural high signal intensity from fat makes nerves conspicuous on T1-weighted images. Bone structure must be present normally in the perineural fat. On T2-weighted or fast spin-echo inversion recovery images, the normal sciatic nerve is isointense or mildly hyperintense to muscle and hypointense to regional vessels, with clearly defined fascicles separated by interposed lower signal connective tissue (Figs. 5.1, 5.2, 5.3, 5.16, and 5.17). Normal endoneurial fluid, when protected by an intact perineurial blood-nerve barrier, is thought to be primarily responsible for the normal signal intensity pattern of nerves at T2-weighted. A little to moderate amount of fat is contained within the nerve. The fluid-attenuated inversion recovery sequence is sensitive to increased water content, as seen with edema or other pathological processes. It also has inherent fat suppression. This makes STIR sequences ideal for imaging of sacral plexus and sciatic nerve entrapments [5].

Neural enlargement, loss of the normal fascicular appearance, and blurring of the perifascicular fat are morphologic changes that suggest neural injury (Figs. 5.22, 5.23, 5.24, 5.25, 5.26, 5.31, 5.33, 5.36, 5.38, 5.42, 5.43, 5.44, 5.45, 5.46, 5.48, 5.49, 5.50, 5.51, 5.52, 5.53, 5.54, 5.55, 5.56, 5.58, and 5.66). Size differentials and fascicular appearance are more difficult to discern in smaller nerves such as the inferior and superior gluteal nerves. Increased perifascicular and endoneurial signal intensity on T2-weighted images reflects a nonspecific response of the nerve to injury. This phenomenon has been explained by various hypothesized mechanisms, such as vascular congestion and blockade of axoplasmic flow, leading to abnormal proximal accumulation of endoneurial fluid and distal Wallerian degeneration changes. However, increased signal intensity in the nerve does not always indicate underlying disease. The magic angle effect is a well-recognized artifact in lumbosacral plexus and sciatic nerve imaging. Unlike in tendons, however, where the magic angle artifact can be overcome with longer echo times (>40 ms), spurious high nerve signal intensity related to the magic angle can persist at higher echo times (66 ms) as well as on short inversion time inversion recovery images. These angle-specific signal changes must be kept in mind, particularly when increased nerve signal intensity is the sole abnormality. Mild T2 hyperintensity within the nerve can often be observed in asymptomatic subjects, probably related to this effect or subclinical neuropathies. Because normal nerve and plexus are slightly hyperintense on fluid-sensitive images, high signal intensity that is focal or similar to that of adjacent vessels is more likely to be significant [19] (Fig. 5.51).

Double sagittal-oblique PD-weighted MR images, with and without fat suppression, acquired through thin slices and with no or a minimal gap between the slices, oriented with the long and perpendicular axis of the piriformis muscle (Fig. 5.77), are specially recommended to recognize fibrous bands, anatomical variants, and sciatic neuritis [5] (Figs. 5.2, 5.3, 5.21a, d, 5.26a, 5.28d, 5.38a, 5.39b, 5.42c, 5.47a, and 5.48b).

In addition muscle SI changes can indicate or can further confirm the presence of neuropathy. These denervation-related MR signal abnormalities have been shown to be a relative shift between intra- and extracompartmental fluid components and do not reflect real edema. Muscles may show acute denervation changes (edema-like SI) as early as 24 h from the onset of neuropathy; subacute changes (edema-like SI and minimal fatty replacement), weeks to months after injury; or chronic changes (fatty replacement and atrophy), months to years after nerve injury [110] (Fig. 5.52).

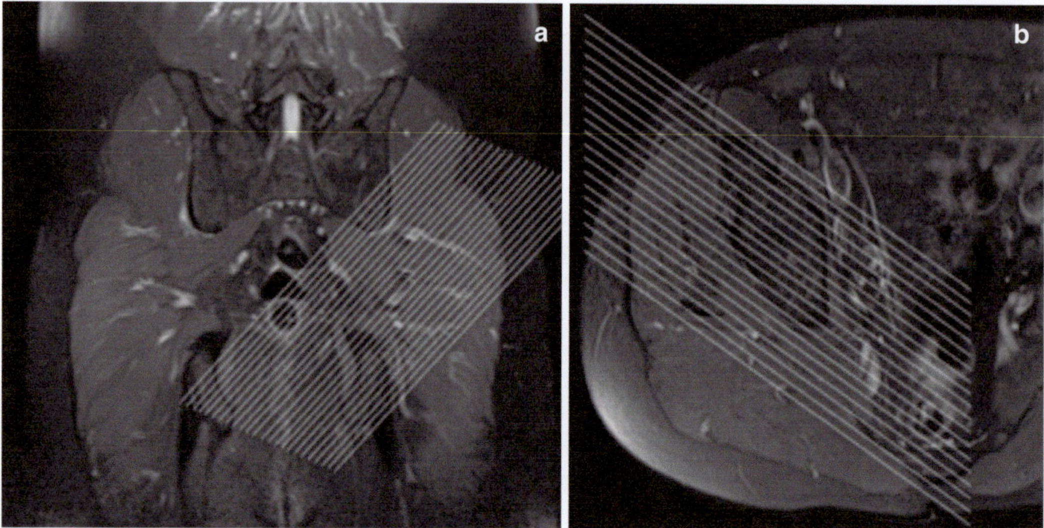

Fig. 5.77 Coronal (a) and sagittal (b) RM localizers and orientation of the planes to obtain the double sagittal-oblique PD-weighted MR image. This plane is perpendicular to the plane oriented with the long axis of the piriformis muscle and is highly recommended to recognize fibrous bands and anatomical variants of the sciatic-piriformis complex

Fig. 5.78 Acute pattern of partial denervation of the right gluteus maximus muscle

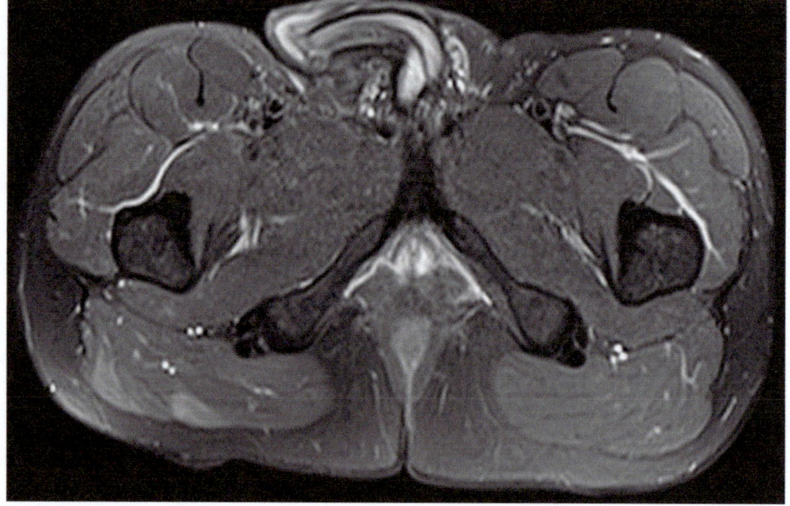

Sciatic nerve denervation involves hamstring muscles and the hamstring component of the adductor magnus. Signs of denervation of the gluteal muscles are common. In the early stage, the T1 signal of muscle remains normal. There are no abnormalities of the subjacent fascia or subcutaneous tissues; the normal architecture and size of the muscle are preserved. These features help distinguish denervation from other causes of increased muscle signal intensity, such as muscle strain, tear, infection, or infarct. The increased T1 signal indicates denervation-related muscle atrophy. With prolonged denervation, the bulk of the muscle will decrease and be completely replaced by fat. This process indicates irreversible end-stage disease and muscle atrophy. Although denervation often results in stereotypic muscle involvement, aberrant or cross-innervation can produce atypical denervation patterns [19] (Fig. 5.78).

Through the increasing use of 3T MR scanners, new phased-array surface coils, and parallel imaging aids in the acquisition of high-resolution and high-contrast images in short imaging times, it is possible to discriminate which particular small elements of the lumbosacral-sacral plexus are involved in tumors or neuropathies [110].

Focal alterations in nerve contour, course, fascicular pattern, size, caliber, or presence of perineural fibrovascular bands are best depicted on longitudinal high-contrast isotropic 3D images reconstructed along the course of the nerve using multiplanar reconstruction (MPR) or curved planar reconstruction. T2-weighted SPAIR images provide more homogeneous fat suppression than frequency-selective T2 fat-suppressed images in off-center areas (Fig. 5.72).

Contrast-enhanced fat-saturated T1-weighted images are only required when infections, inflammations, diffuse peripheral nerve lesions, tumors, and postoperative scar are suspected to be the cause of symptoms (Figs. 5.54 and 5.58). Enhancement in denervated muscles can be seen in these images [5].

Between 8 and 10 weeks after open neurolysis, signal is normalized. However, there is no experience when signal increased normalizes after arthroscopic release, since it is a recent developed technique. Persistent nerve enlargement, abnormal T2 hyperintensity approaching the SI of adjacent vessels, encasing perineural fibrosis, and fascicular abnormality suggest re-entrapment although preliminary data suggest this is not frequent.

Three-dimensional STIR, SPIR, and SPAIR sequences are powerful techniques for fat suppression that must be included in the MRN protocol to assess neuritis, neural tumors, and neural lesions (Fig. 5.79).

Finally, diffusion tensor imaging and especially diffusion tensor tractography of the sciatic nerve in the near future will bring more physiologic information in patients with sciatic nerve entrapment. Sacral plexus and sciatic nerve normative quantitative diffusion data such as apparent diffusion coefficient (ADC) and fractional anisotropy (FA) should be collected as a reference in these patients [111, 112] (Figs. 5.80 and 5.81).

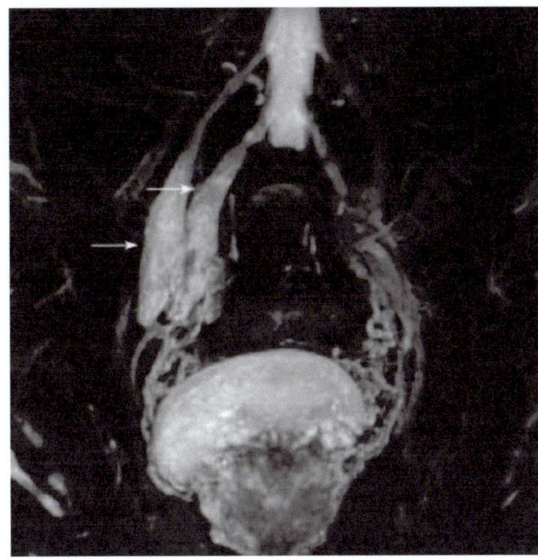

Fig. 5.79 Spectral attenuated inversion recovery (SPAIR) sequence for the assessment of the lumbosacral plexus and the sciatic nerve

Diagnostic and Therapeutic Injection Test

The injection test is a useful tool to treat this syndrome, enabling diagnosis and excluding articular pathology or disorders within other spaces. Guided injections with the patient lying prone, utilizing ultrasound, CT, or open MR imaging, have been used. A variant of the double-injection technique of an anesthetic and corticosteroids reported by Pace and Nagle with CT guidance and high volume injection through the piriformis muscle into the perineural sciatic fat or within the nerve sheath using a 22-gauge spinal needle is recommended. The solution is injected at a single point under the ischial spine, which distributes easily along the perisciatic fat with hip movements. Care should be taken not to infiltrate a sciatic nerve split, the pudendal bundle, or inferior gluteal vessels, as this may produce abundant bleeding. Most patients experience a significant immediate postinjection decrease in the symptoms. In case of partial improvement or lack of improvement, it can be repeated twice. Intramuscular infiltration with Botox (using the same procedure to guide infiltration) can be a temporary solution prior to surgery, especially in patients with piriformis muscle

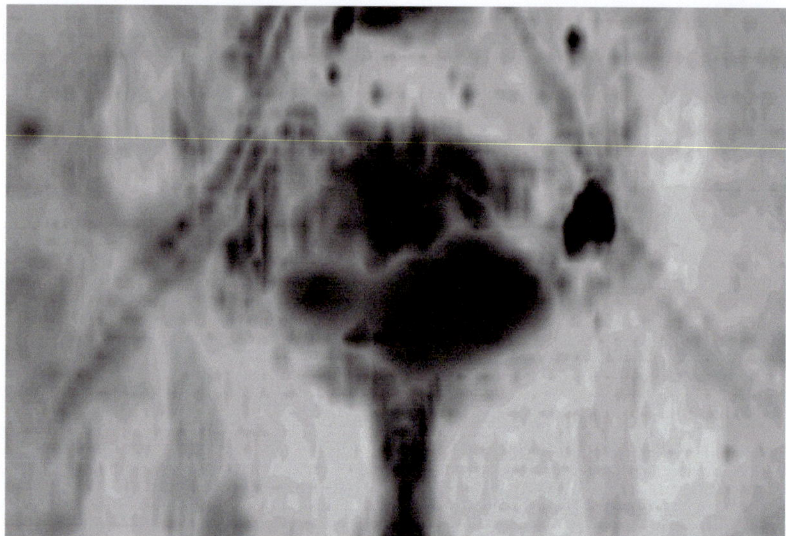

Fig. 5.80 Diffusion tensor imaging (DTI) to evaluate compressed nerve roots of the sacral plexus and sciatic nerve

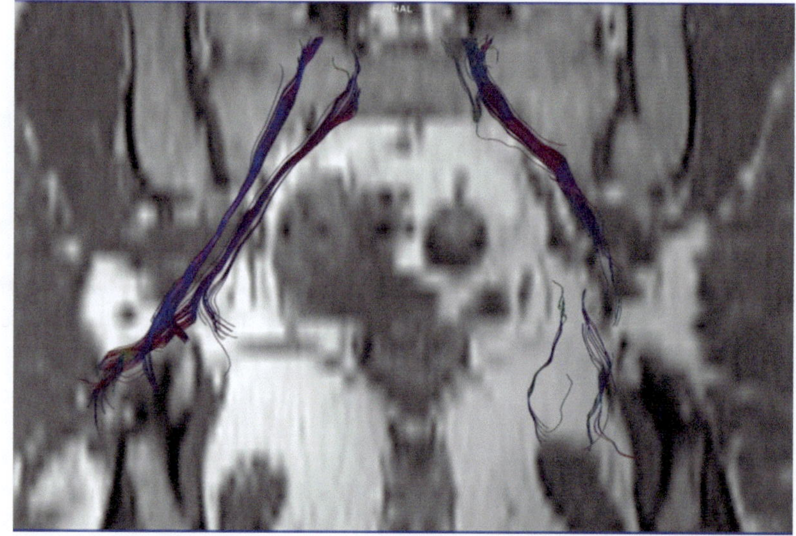

Fig. 5.81 Diffusion tensor tractography (DTT) image. DTT is useful for the visualization of abnormal nerve tracts, providing vivid anatomic information and localization of probable nerve compression. It also has great potential utility for evaluating variants of the sciatic-piriformis complex. Note in this case a clear high division of the sciatic nerve (type-B piriformis muscle)

abnormalities (dynamic entrapment, insertional variants, anatomical abnormalities, or spasm) [5, 62] (Fig. 5.82).

Imaging Assessment in "Ischiofemoral Impingement"

Ischiofemoral impingement syndrome (IFI) is a more frequent than expected form of extra-articular hip impingement defined by hip pain related to the narrowing of the space between the ischial tuberosity (IT) and the femur [22, 113–116] (Fig. 5.83). Although IFI is increasingly being discussed in the medical literature, it remains a poorly recognized condition because symptoms are often nonspecific. Hence, imaging plays an important role in its diagnosis and treatment [22, 63].

The incidence of IFI is unknown and the diagnosis generally depends on both clinical and imaging evidence. The dominant findings of studies related to IFI are focused on the narrowing of the mentioned space and the abnormalities of the QFM [22, 114]. However, it is increasingly better known the etiology and also the predisposing factors of this syndrome [62].

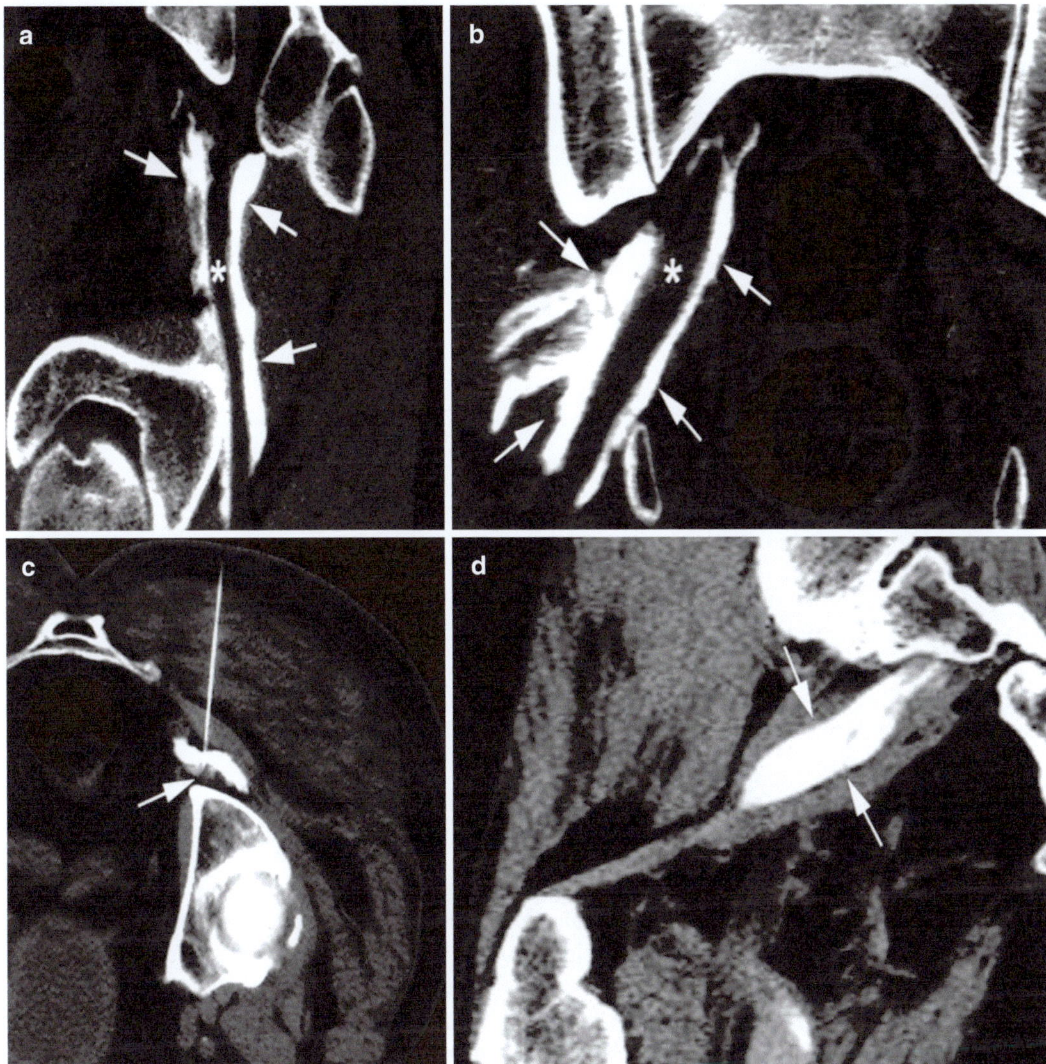

Fig. 5.82 Double injection of anesthetic and cortico-steroids technique (infiltration test). Sagittal-oblique (**a**) and coronal-oblique (**b**) MDCT reconstructions after performing the infiltration test show the final distribution of the solution (arrows) which is arranged around the sciatic nerve (asterisk) throughout its length along the deep gluteal space. The solution contains a small amount of iodinated contrast to assess more accurately the location of injection. Axial MDCT image (**c**) shows the sectional plane chosen for CT-guided infiltration of the perisciatic space (arrow) through the piriformis muscle. Botox infiltration. Sagittal-oblique MDCT reconstruction after performing botulinum toxin infiltration (**d**) shows the final distribution of the solution (arrows) centered on the thickness of the muscle belly to avoid extra-muscular extension

Diagnostic Imaging Criteria

The presence of narrowed IFS and QFM space (QFS) as well as QFM edema represents the most significant indicators for IFI [114, 116]. Observing findings consistent with the syndrome do not always correlate with compatible symptoms and signs. Soft tissue magnetic resonance imaging (MRI) signal abnormalities are present within the IFS in 9.1% of asymptomatic patients (edema only in 1.4% and fatty infiltration only in 7.7%) [117].

Arthroscopically, with the hip in adduction, external rotation, and extension, the lesser trochanter and ischial tuberosity are approximately 2.0 cm apart. This relationship allows the femur to

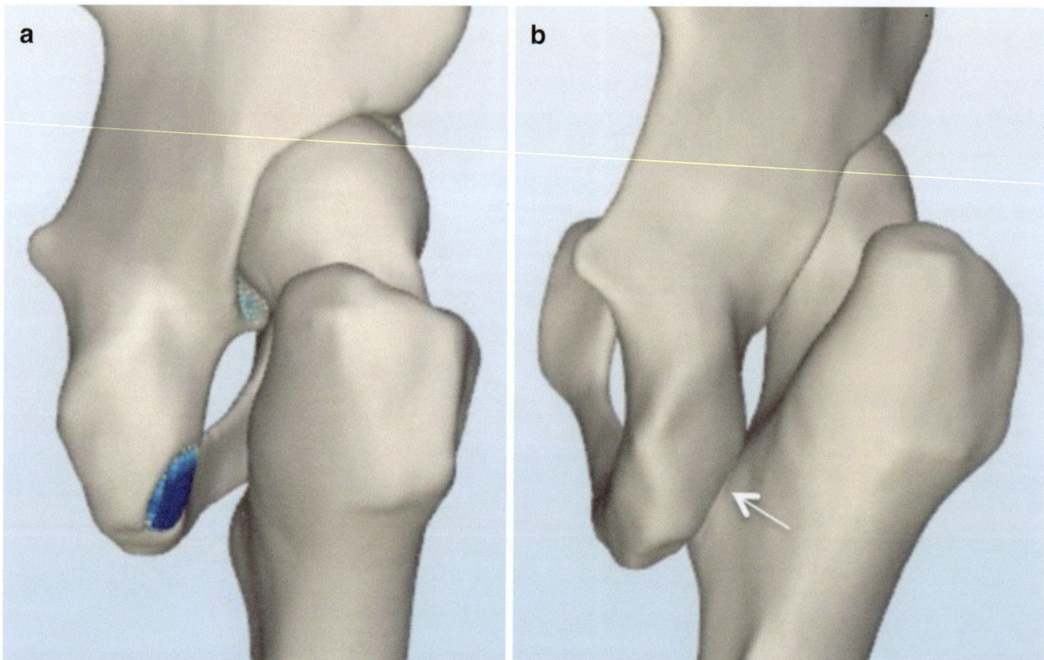

Fig. 5.83 3D CT images showing the positioning of the femur and the ischium before (**a**) and during (**b**) ischiofemoral impingement (arrow in **b**). The bluish area represents the area of maximum contact between both bone structures

rotate without contacting the ischial tuberosity or proximal hamstring tendons. Thus, any factor that alters this relationship can trigger IFI [118, 119].

Several studies have shown significant reductions of IFS and QFS with good to excellent intra- and interobserver reliability when comparing patients with QFM abnormalities and control individuals. Measures of the IFS of 13 ± 5/12.9 mm and QFS of 7 ± 3/6.71 mm have been identified in affected patients with the lower leg in internal and neutral rotation. These values in control subjects in internal rotation are significantly higher, corresponding to 23 ± 8 and 12 ± 4 mm, respectively [63, 64, 113] (Fig. 5.84).

Unfortunately, the resting position of the limb that is required for routine MRI does not reproduce the conditions leading to instability in daily life. Moreover, there is ≥10% width difference between the right and left IF spaces in approximately half of asymptomatic individuals [117]. These measurements depend on the degree of hip rotation, adduction, and extension during MRI. Therefore, the validity of these values remains unclear in these retrospective studies [64,

120]. Nevertheless, these studies are not invalid. Using a cutoff of ≤15 mm, a sensitivity of 76.9%, specificity of 81.0%, and overall accuracy of 78.3% have been reported. For QFS, a cutoff of ≤10.0 mm resulted in 78.7% sensitivity, 74.1% specificity, and 77.1% overall accuracy [2, 121].

Dynamic MRI utilizing a full range of rotation will help to confirm impingement, to evaluate the relationship between the QFM and adjacent structures, and to better assess associated findings, such as delineation of unnoticed partial tears of the anterior surface of the QFM. Currently, the sufficient time frame resolution with real-time demonstration of movements has been considered the main limitation of MRI [62, 122, 123].

Etiology and Predisposing Factors

In most cases it is possible to evaluate and discover by imaging the etiology of the impingement and to evaluate predisposing factors. Existing studies concerning the etiology of IFI

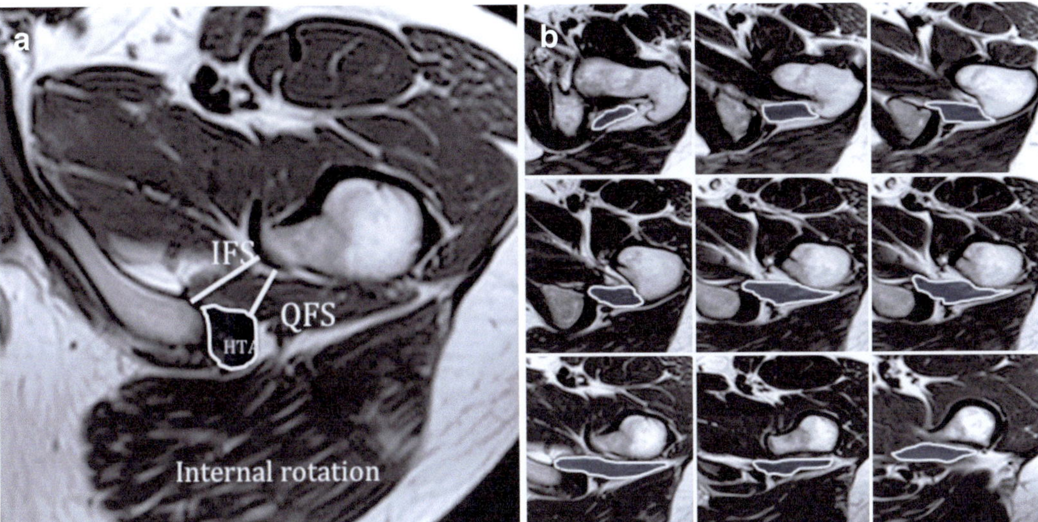

Fig. 5.84 Quantitative assessment of IFI. Axial T1-weighted MR image at the tip of the lesser trochanter (LT) in internal rotation (**a**) shows normal right IFS, QFS, and hamstring tendon area (HTA). IFS is defined as the gap between the ischium tuberosity and the iliopsoas tendon or the LT and QFS as the smallest gap between the superolat- eral surface of the hamstring tendons and the posteromedial surface of the iliopsoas tendon or the LT. HTA is measured by tracing the contours of the hamstring tendon where the QFS is measured. Highlighted muscle regions on sequen- tial axial T1-weighted images (**b**) are used to perform total quadratus femoris muscle volume (TQFMV) measurement

are not prospective and do not include sufficient sample sizes or standardized protocols, so a direct cause-and-effect relationship between IFI and particular described etiologies cannot be established. However, the analysis of individual patients has established potential etiologies and predisposing factors (Table 5.2). Imaging tests are essential to assess all of them [62, 124].

Coxa Valga

The neck-shaft angle or inclination angle (IA) is the deviation of the femoral neck from the femoral diaphysis. In adults, the IA ranges from 120° to 130°, and its value is greater in newborns (150°) and smaller in elderly popula- tions (120°) [125]. The IA differs with age, sex, stature, spinal deformities, and width of the pelvis, affecting the gait and increasing stress at the hip and knee joint. A higher preva- lence of extra-articular impingement has been found for coxa valga. Patients with IFI show increased femoral neck and ischial angles com- pared with controls, suggesting that increased IA may lead to the narrowing of the IFS [22, 126] (Fig. 5.85).

Table 5.2 Potential etiologies and predisposing factors of IFI according to the pathophysiological mechanisms

Primary or congenital (orthopedic disorders)
Coxa valga
Prominence of the lesser trochanter
Congenital posteromedial position of the femur
Larger cross section of the femur
Abnormal femoral antetorsion
Coxa breva
Variations of the pelvic bony anatomy
Secondary or acquired
Functional disorders
Hip instability
Pelvic and spinal instability
Abductor/adductor imbalance
Ischial tuberosity enthesopathies
Traumatic, overuse, and extreme hip motion
Iatrogenic causes
Tumors
Other etiologies

Other Proximal Femur Abnormalities

A congenital posteromedial position of the femur, larger cross section of the femur, prominence or hook-shaped lesser trochanter, abnormal femoral antetorsion, and coxa breva are congenital condi- tions that could lead to the syndrome since they

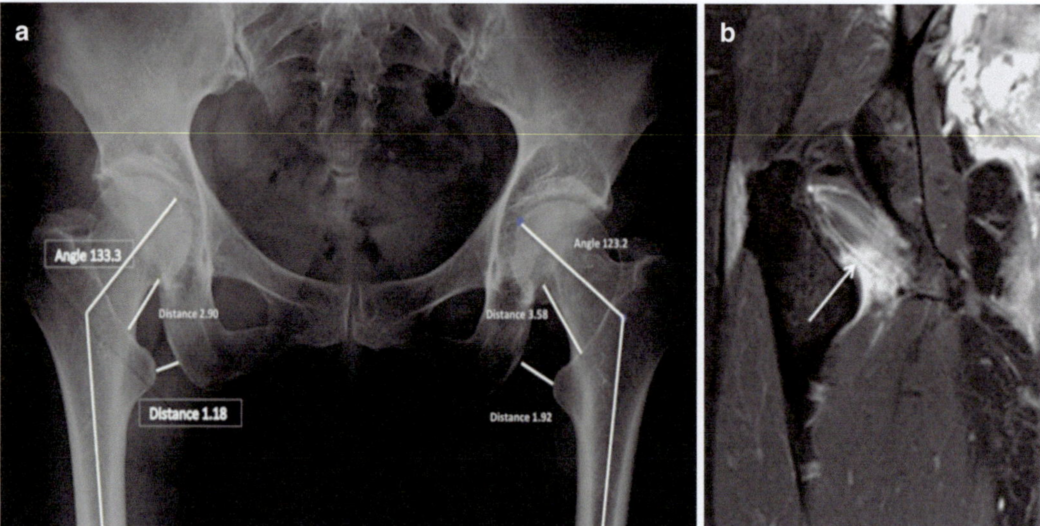

Fig. 5.85 IFI secondary to coxa valga and breva (short neck) in a 55-year-old woman. The PA simple pelvic radiograph shows a shortening of the femoral neck, an increased neck-shaft angle (inclination angle), and a decreased IF on the right side with respect to the contralateral side (**a**). Coronal PD fat-suppressed MR image shows QFM edema (arrow) secondary to the entrapment in the same patient (**b**)

determine an approach to the lesser trochanter of the femur [62] (Fig. 5.86).

In addition, coxa breva (short neck) decreases the abductor resting length and lever arm, increases joint reaction forces, and causes abductor fatigue and Trendelenburg gait contributing to the reduction of IFS [127].

Finally, higher antetorsion angles have been described in these patients compared to controls. The abnormal femoral antetorsion angle is measured on pure axial computed tomography (CT) or MRI images over the proximal and distal femur. This angle is normally anteverted to the bicondylar femoral plane at an angle of 35° to 50° at birth and gradually decreases by 1.5° per year and reaches an approximate value of 16° at 16 years of age and 10° in adults [62] (Fig. 5.86d).

Variations of the Pelvic Bony Anatomy: Female Pelvis

The incidence of IFI has been reported to be higher in women than men, and it has been hypothesized that this occurs because of the differing osseous configuration. In particular, the ischial tuberosities are prominent, more separated, and have a wider positioning in women. Prominence of the lesser trochanter and lower ischiopubic ramus with an angle closer to the coronal plane in the female pelvis may also explain why IFI is seen most commonly in women [126]. Projection of the ischial spines outward in the female pelvis may be another explanation. In patients with IFI, the ischial angle is higher than in the control population [62, 126] (Fig. 5.87). Furthermore, there is a significant association between the degree of degenerative change observed in the QFM and (1) an increased approximation of the QF attachments sites and (2) a narrower intertuberous diameter [128].

Functional Disorders Predisposing to or Causing IFI

Hip Instability

Hip dysplasia in adults causes chronic forces that exceed the level of tolerance causing bone deformation and articular soft tissue changes. The femoral head is displaced anteriorly and laterally, causing instability of the hip and the patient to adopt an exaggerated valgus position that contributes to IFS narrowing [129]. Some patients with IFI have a dysplastic-kind hip, but few correspond to true dysplasia and most correspond to minor dysplasia or instabilities. These forms can

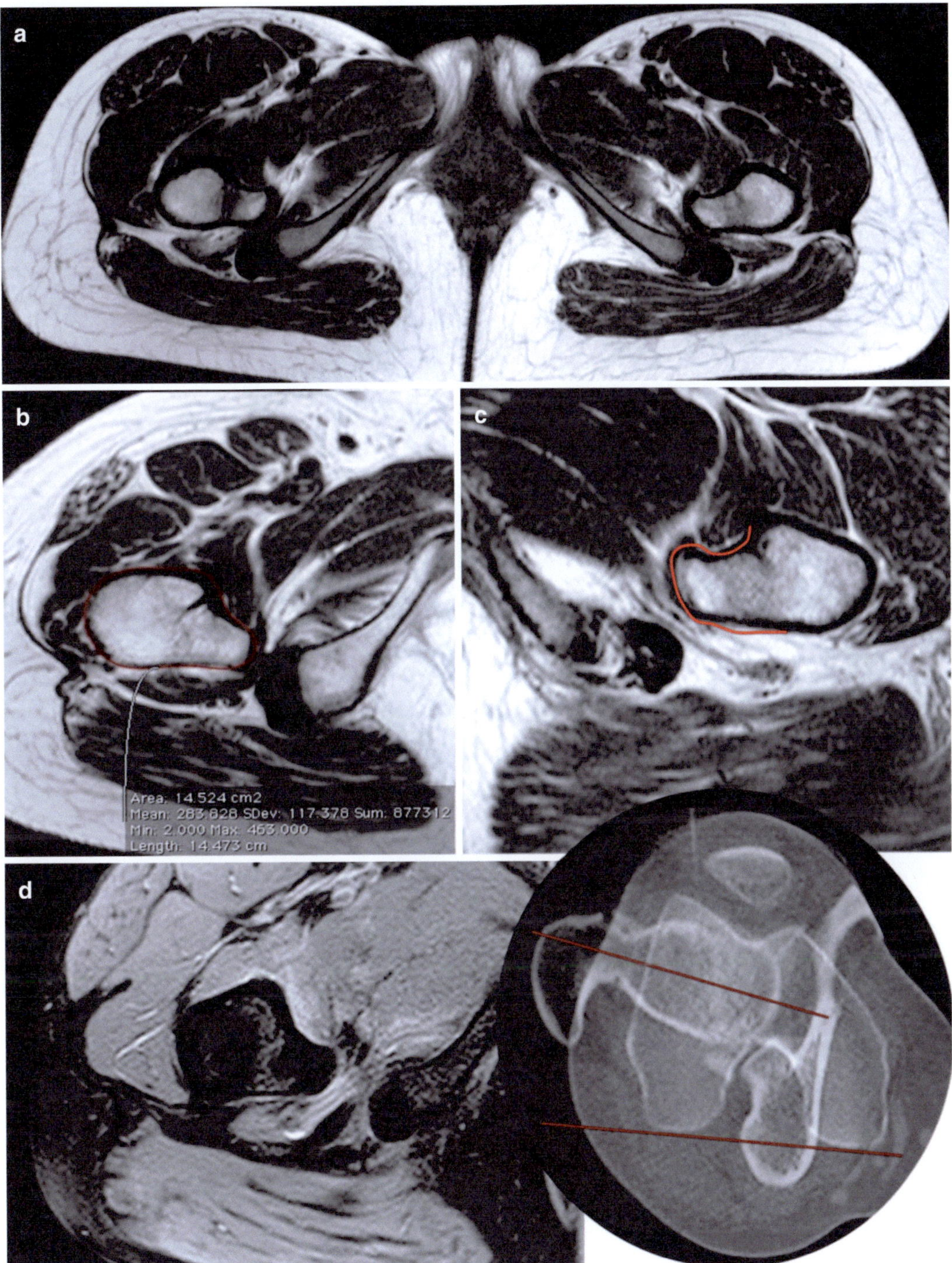

Fig. 5.86 IFI secondary to congenital posteromedial position of the femur (**a**), larger cross section of the femur at the level of the lesser trochanter (**b**), prominence and hook-shaped lesser trochanter (**c**), and abnormal femoral antetorsion (**d**)

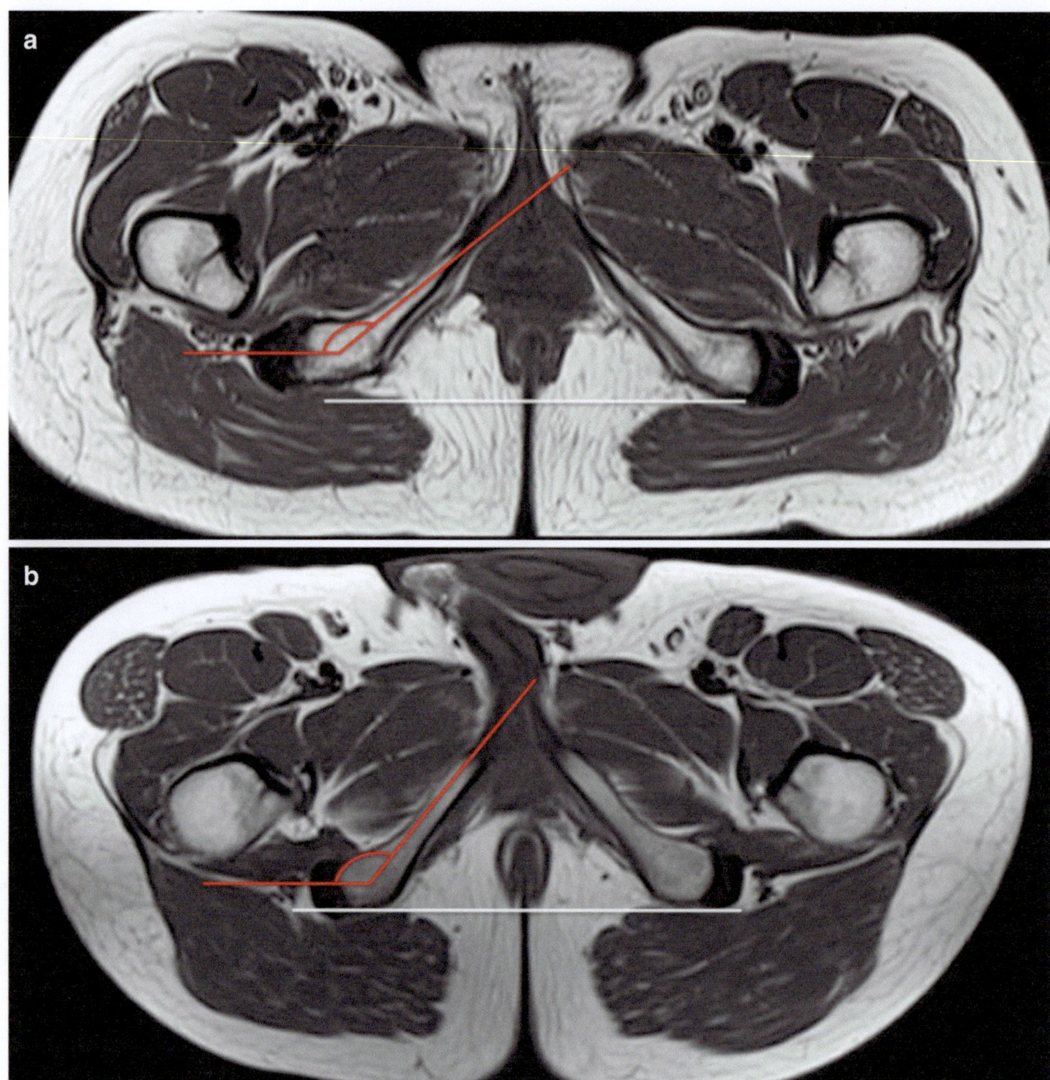

Fig. 5.87 Variations of the pelvic bony anatomy: female pelvis. Axial T1-weighted MR images of a woman (**a**) and a man (**b**) show an increased ischial angle (red angle) and a more separated ischial tuberosities (white line) in woman. Note that white lines in a and b are the same length

be classified according to the measurement of the anterior and posterior acetabular sector angles (AASA and PASA, respectively) as instability of the anterior column and posterior column (or both columns), leading to anterior or posterior instability [129, 130] (Fig. 5.88).

Pelvic and Spinal Instability
Abnormal pelvic tilt (PT) may promote the development of atypical impingement [131]. A close relationship has been described between the sagittal balance of the spine (SB), the PT, and ischiofemoral impingement. PT can increase or reduce the IFS. Moreover, PT increases (5.5–10.6%) when the effects of muscle damage on walking biomechanics at different speeds are studied [132].

Pelvic anteversion and retroversion movements are related to the position of the sacrum and ischium. When the pelvis is retroverted, the sacrum turns vertical, SI and lumbar lordosis

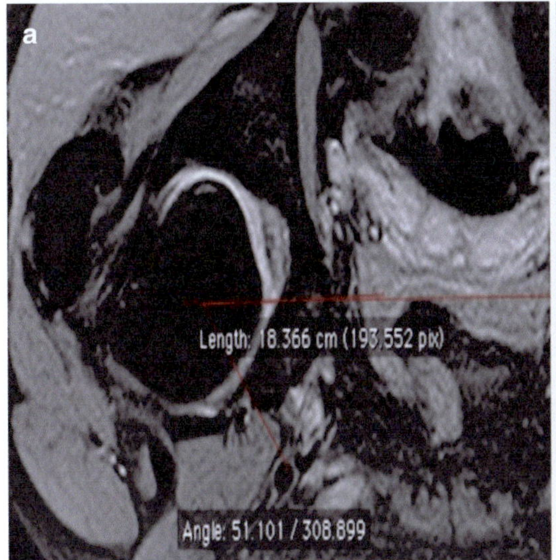
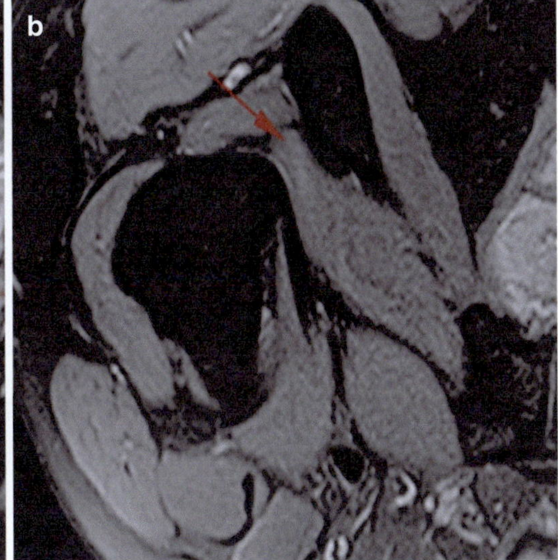

Fig. 5.88 IFI secondary to anterior acetabular coverage deficit and femoral dysplasia in a 45-year-old woman. Axial PD fat-suppressed MR images show a decreased AASA angle and impingement (arrow in a) and impingement of the quadratus femoris muscle (red arrow in b).

decrease, and the ischial tuberosities come close to the lesser trochanters (Fig. 5.89). In clinical practice, cervical lordosis, thoracic kyphosis and the lumbar lordosis angles, pelvic incidence angle, pelvis version angle, sagittal line at T9 angle, tibiofemoral angle, plumb line of C7, vertical line of the external auditory canal, and leg length discrepancy are the common measurements used to assess sagittal balance of the spine [133] (Fig. 5.90).

Abductor/Adductor Muscles Imbalance

Abnormal gait that results from abductor dysfunction and leads to subsequent pathology in the QFM has been hypothesized. Cases of abductor muscle pathology that develop IFI have been recently described [62]. The reason why some patients are prone to impingement following injury to the abductors is an unresolved question, but such damage has the potential to disturb the quadratus femoris space either directly, via an abnormal gait, or due to the secondary atrophy of abductors muscles (retroverted pelvic imbalance approximates the ischial tuberosity to the lesser trochanter). If prolonged adduction occurs as a result of abductor impairment, the ischiofemoral gap will be narrowed. A wide spectrum of conditions in the hip,

back, or any anatomical region could trigger IFI through this mechanism [62] (Figs. 5.91, 5.92, 5.93, and 5.94). This is by far, in my personal experience, the most common cause of IFI.

Of note, different rates of atrophy have been encountered in synergistic muscles after bed rest secondary to any body pathology. The QFM has a unique response among the hip external rotators to unload, showing a faster rate of atrophy and greater loss of muscle volume, and, expectedly, takes longer to recover. Research on other joints suggests that the local, rather than global, muscles are well suited to provide subtle joint stabilization. Indeed, QFM atrophy itself might reduce IFS. Moreover, muscle injury and inflammation have been documented in resting patients after any pathology and have been found to be associated with fluid changes, masking a lack of recovery of muscle volume in the initial recovery scans (which can be confused with edema on MRI). Future unloading studies could reduce this uncertainty by monitoring the recovery of musculature at frequent intervals and/or using muscle biopsies to understand the underlying histology to these signal changes [134].

Thus, any injury of the abductor or adductor muscles can thus trigger impingement. Gluteal

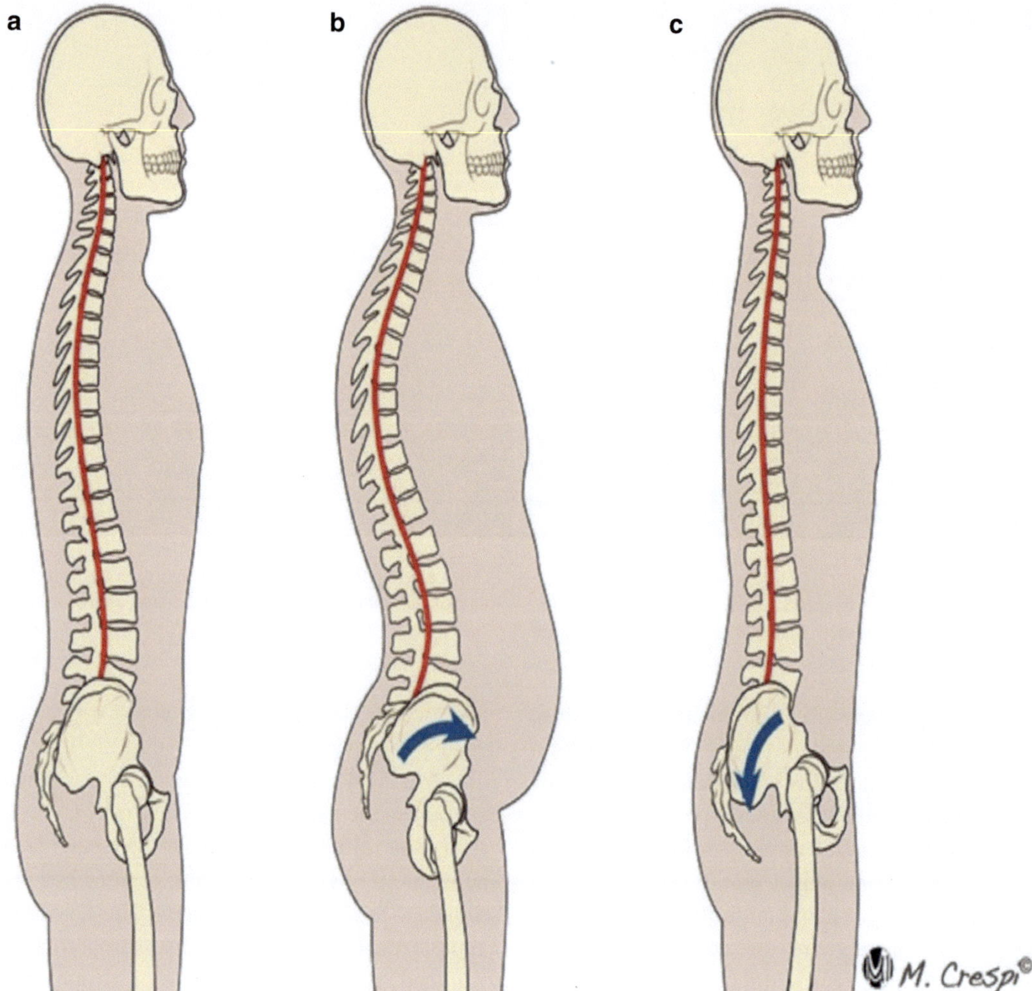

Fig. 5.89 Pelvic instability. Normal pelvic alignment is shown in the figure (**a**). Pelvic anteversion (**b**) and retroversion (**c**) movements are related to the position of the sacrum and ischium. When the pelvis is retroverted (**c**), the sacrum turns vertical, SI and lumbar lordosis decrease, and the ischial tuberosities come close to the lesser trochanters, causing the impingement. Reprinted with permission from Massimiliano Crespi

contractures require special attention because they have been related to IFI. Medial retraction of the muscle in advanced cases results in external rotation of the proximal femur that predisposes to IFI [5, 62, 66].

Ischial Tuberosity Enthesopathies

Hamstring disorders, as a cause of impingement, have been recently described. Tendinosis leads to swelling and widening of the proximal hamstring tendon insertion and results in narrowing of the QFS and thus impingement. Therefore, hamstring tendinosis might be the cause or the consequence of the dynamic changes described in IFI [22, 63, 115]. A wide spectrum of hamstring origin enthesopathies that are present in isolation or in combination may trigger IFI including partial/complete hamstring strain, tendon detachment, avulsion fractures, apophysitis, nonunited apophysis, proximal tendinopathy, calcifying tendinosis, and contusions. Imaging findings are specific to each type of injury [135] (Fig. 5.46).

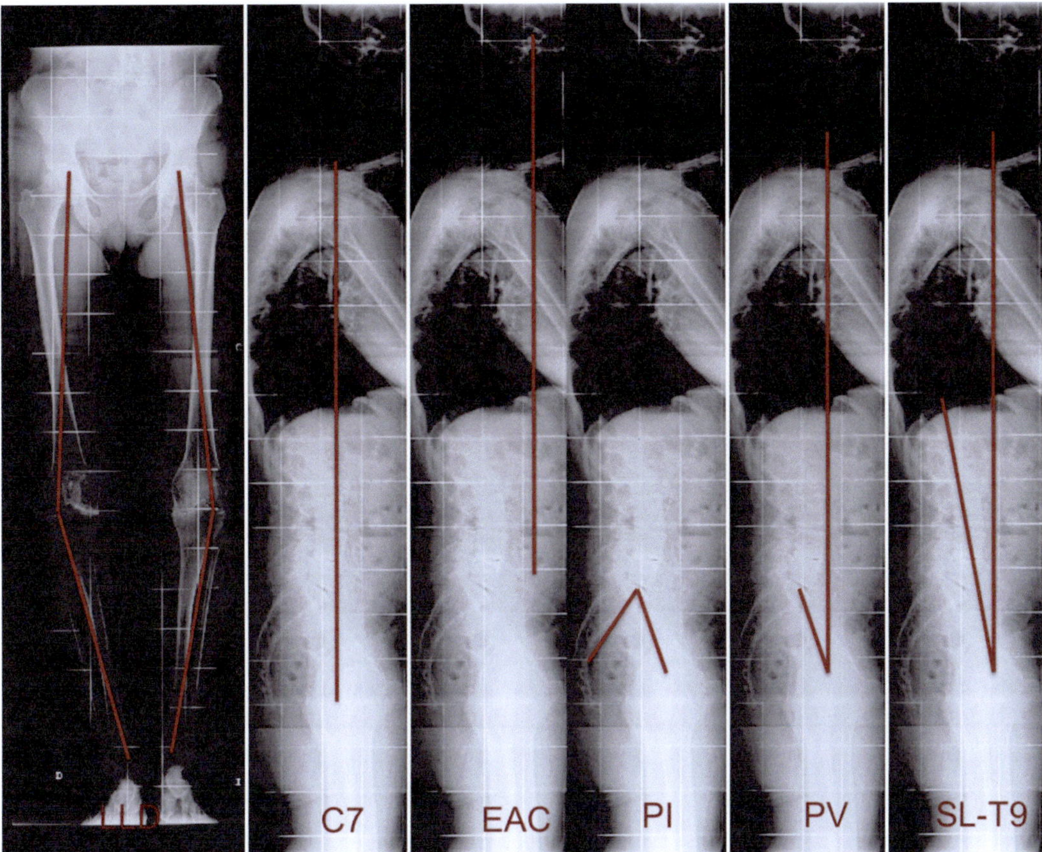

Fig. 5.90 Measurements used to assess sagittal balance of the spine. Images shows how to measure leg length discrepancy (LLD), plumb line of C7 (C7), vertical line of the external auditory canal (EAC), pelvic incidence angle (PI), pelvis version angle (PV), and sagittal line at T9 angle (SL-T9)

Injuries Related to Trauma, Overuse, or Extreme Movements of the Hip

A history of traumatic injury to the pelvis is likely relevant to IFI. Progressive narrowing of the IFS and quadratus femoris edema on MRI, over a long period, has been documented in patients who presented with posttraumatic hip pain and developed IFI. In particular, abnormal gait may have led to this IFS narrowing. IFI and other atypical forms of impingement may be associated with overuse or the extreme external rotation of the hip during extension in ballet, soccer players, martial arts, and other sports [62]. Intense, sudden positional QFS narrowing during intensive training can cause acute QFM damage and acute IFI (Fig. 5.95). Furthermore, intertro-chanteric fractures with involvement of the lesser trochanter and postfracture deformity may predispose to or cause IFI [62, 136].

Iatrogenic Causes

IFI was first described in patients after total hip joint replacement and after valgus-producing intertrochanteric osteotomies, but this is not a frequent cause. Although these and other iatrogenic causes are included in multiple articles, published cases are scarce [119].

Tumors

Osteochondroma (OC) is the most common bone tumor involved in IFI development. OC may be solitary or multiple, the latter being associated with hereditary multiple exostoses (HME) [137].

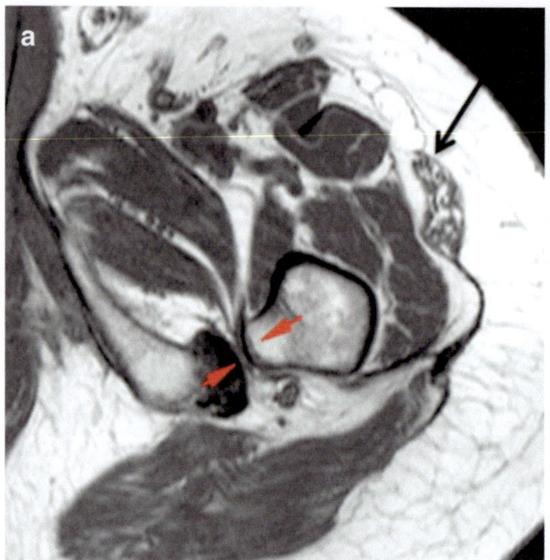
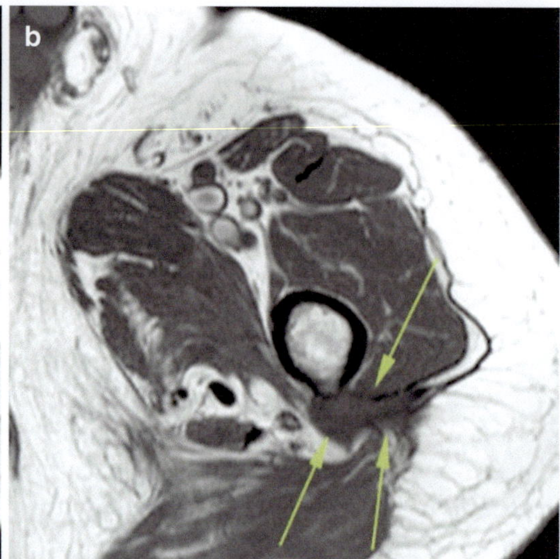

Fig. 5.91 IFI secondary to abductor/adductor muscles imbalance. Axial T1-weighted images show a 39-year-old man with left IFI (red arrows in image **a**) as a result of a degenerative tendinopathy and extensive partial tear of the distal insertion of the gluteus maximus muscle (green arrows in image **b**). Note the atrophy of the abductor muscles, especially affecting the tensor fascia latae muscle (black arrow in image **a**)

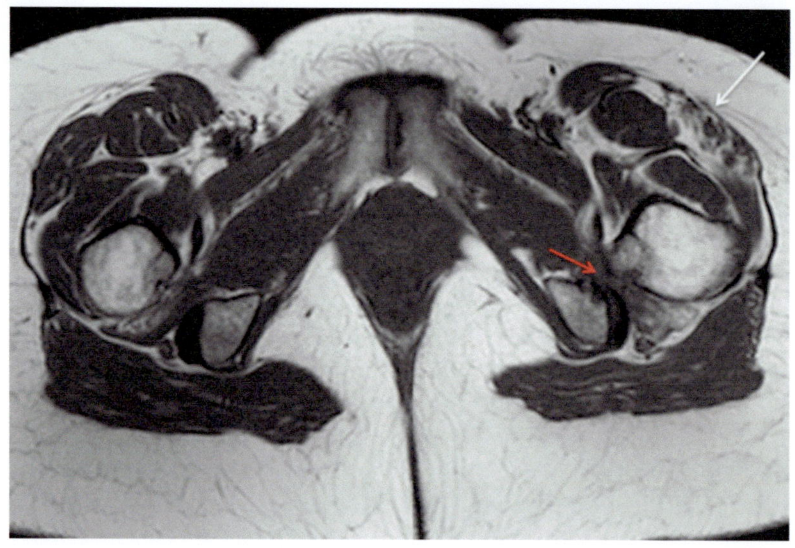

Fig. 5.92 IFI secondary to abductor/adductor muscles imbalance. Axial T1-weighted MR image shows a case of left IFI (red arrow) secondary to pelvic muscle imbalance as a result of a partial tear of the proximal insertion of the left tensor fascia lata muscle (white arrow)

Complications are more frequent with HME and include deformity, fracture, vascular compromise, neurologic sequelae, overlying bursa formation, and malignant transformation (seen in 1% of solitary OC and in 3–5% of patients with HME). Exostoses may narrow the IFS and cause impingement, even without malignant transformation (Fig. 5.96). Pain is improved by resection of the ischial or femur exostoses [138, 139].

Other Etiologies

Osteoarthritis leading to superior and medial migration of the femur has also been proposed as a possible mechanism for IFI in older women [119].

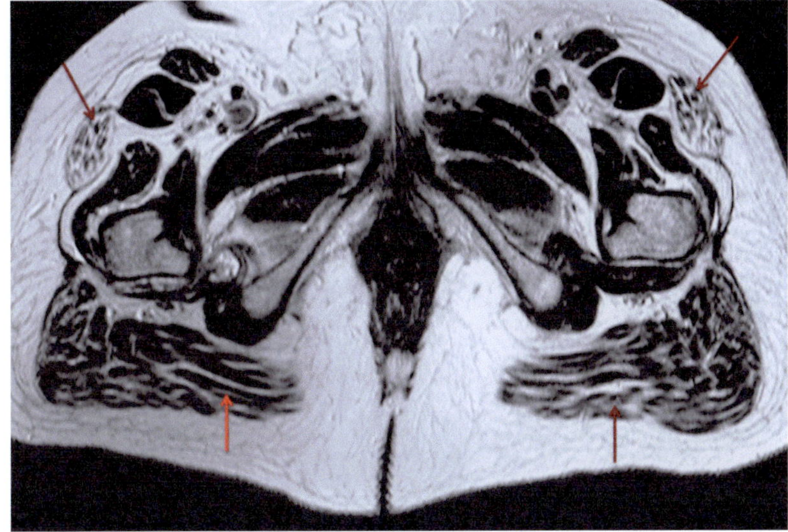

Fig. 5.93 IFI secondary to abductor/adductor muscle imbalance. Axial T1-weighted MR image shows a case of bilateral IFI that is more pronounced on the right side, secondary to bilateral and symmetrical atrophy of abductor muscles (red arrows) in a 45-year-old man after 2 months of bed rest due to a cerebrovascular accident

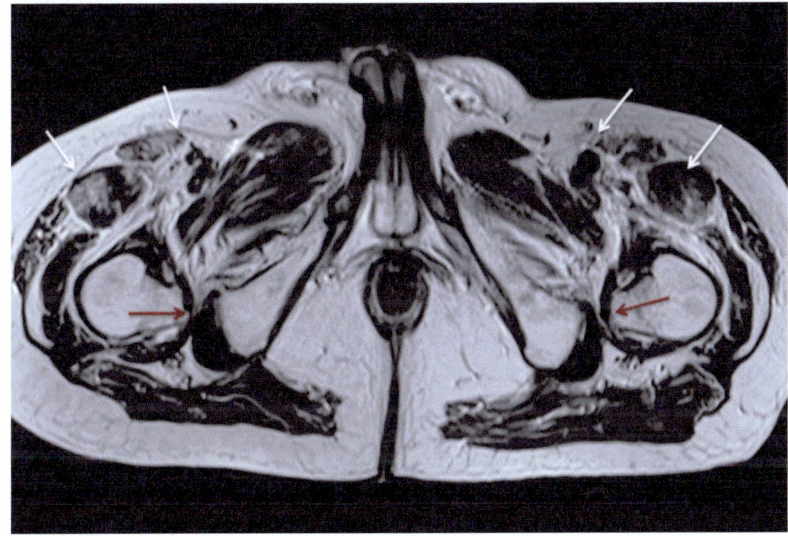

Fig. 5.94 IFI secondary to abductor/adductor muscle imbalance. Axial T1-weighted and PD fat-suppressed MR images show a case of bilateral IFI (red arrows) secondary to bilateral and symmetrical atrophy of the adductor and flexor muscle groups (white arrows) in a 62-year-old man diagnosed with an advanced autoimmune myopathy

Furthermore, although quadratus femoris wasting may simply be part of impingement, another possibility is that atrophy and edema-like signal alterations arise from denervation of the muscle, as the nerve runs in the area of space conflict. It is possible that any cause of QFM atrophy, such as injuries, burns, long-term corticosteroid therapies, immobilization, sciatic neuropathy, and spinal cord injury, may predispose an individual to IS narrowing because this muscle is a primary stabilizer of the hip joint. However, more functional studies need to be conducted to evaluate this hypothesis [62].

Imaging Findings

There are no specific radiographic findings for IFI. The IFS narrowing on radiographs is uncommon and has not been related to clinical findings

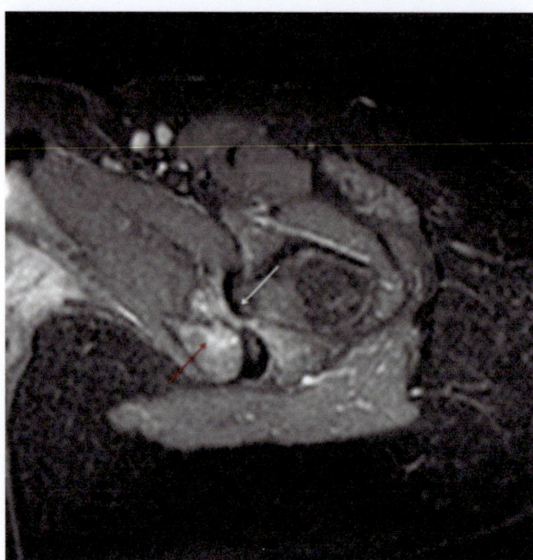

Fig. 5.95 Acute traumatic IFI: extreme external rotation in the extension position. Axial short tau recovery (STIR) MR image shows a cortical disruption of the anterior ischial tuberosity aspect (red arrow) secondary to sudden and intense osseous ischiofemoral impingement (white arrow) in a 29-year-old man during an international karate competition

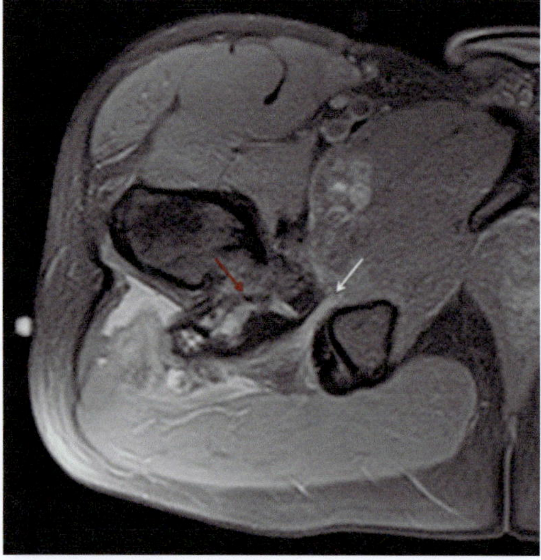

Fig. 5.96 Osteochondroma as a cause of IFI. Axial fat-suppressed PD-weighted MR image in a 32-year-old man shows an exostoses arising from the medial aspect of the femoral metaphysis (red arrow) with signs of osseous impingement (white arrow) and a full tear of the QFM. Exostoses bursata (adventitious bursa) is also seen. Osteochondroma removal resulted in complete resolution of symptoms

or other imaging tests. Although chronic osseous changes of the lesser trochanter and ischial tuberosity may be present, it is uncertain whether chronic contact between them represents the cause. However, hip and pelvic radiographs are useful to diagnose osseous abnormalities that may cause acquired IFI or to depict other causes of pain [64, 140].

Ultrasound (US) may show hyperemia within the IFS although normal results has been reported in patients found to have impingement changes on MRI [141, 142].

Currently, 3D/4D high-resolution multidetector CT scans provide interesting images simplifying the image interpretation to better evaluate the relationship between QFM and adjacent osseous structures through a full range of hip motion. Specific softwares have been developed to generate models for dynamization and preoperative templating of extra-articular impingement. As a result, insight can be gained as to whether an arthroscopic, open, or combined approach is necessary, where the specific location of mechanical conflict is occurring and how much must be resected to eliminate this mechanical conflict [143, 144] (Fig. 5.83).

MR imaging is the gold standard method to diagnose IFI. As Torriani and subsequently Tosun suggested, ischiofemoral narrowing can be evaluated by measuring the IFS, QFS, hamstring tendon area (HTA), and total QFM volume (TQFMV), with good to excellent intra-/interobserver reliability for all measures. The IFS, QFS, and TQFMV values of patient have found to be significantly lower than those of controls, whereas the HTA and IA measurements are significantly higher [22, 63] (Fig. 5.84).

Possible visible MRI abnormalities are listed below:

(a) *Quadratus femoris muscle*. The lesional spectrum description includes crowding of the fibers intramuscular edema at the maximal impingement point without disruption of the fibers [62] (Fig. 5.97), anterior myofascial disruption, and partial tear or full tear and muscle

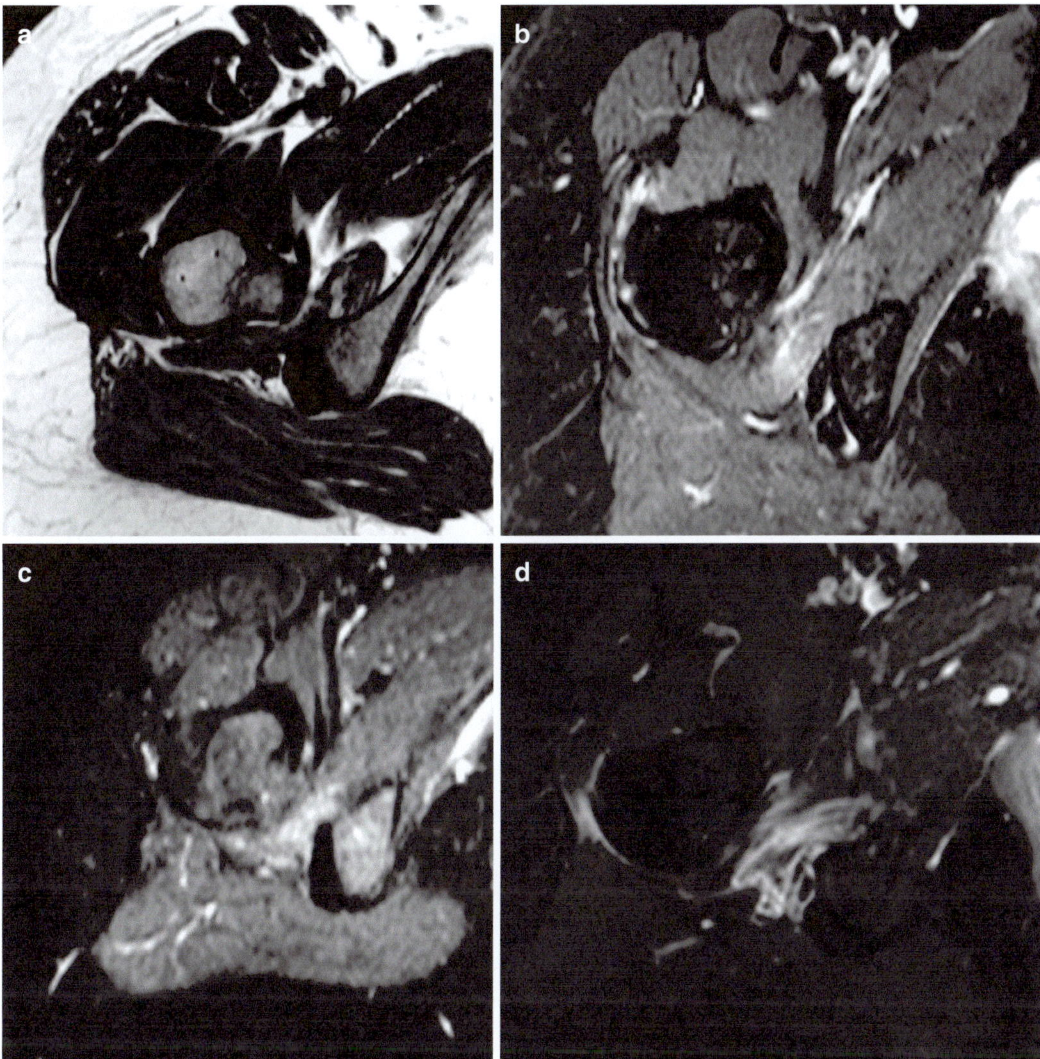

Fig. 5.97 Edema stages affecting QFM in patients with IFI. Crowding of the anterior surface of the QFM fibers as it passes between ischium/hamstring tendons and the posteromedial femur is the minor stage that can be seen on MRI (image **a**). The QFM edema may be considered mild or grade 1 if it consists of focal edema in the region where the narrowest IFS and QFS values are measured (image **b**), moderate or grade 2 if diffuse edema extends outside the narrowest point (image **c**), and severe or grade 3 if QFM edema extends to the surrounding soft tissues (image **d**)

wasting/fatty infiltration, which is best visualized on T1-weighted MRI images and usually occurs in patients with long-standing IFI (Figs. 5.98 and 5.99). Muscle atrophy may be graduated as grade 1 (tiny linear fat signal intensity between muscle fibers), grade 2 (thicker and linear-globular fat signal intensity occupying <50% of the QFM), and grade 3 (>50% of the muscle) [124].

(b) *Bones*. Bone marrow edema and subcortical changes are extremely rare unless a complete atrophy of QFM and a direct osseous impingement exists. If bone marrow edema is present in the lesser trochanter or ischial

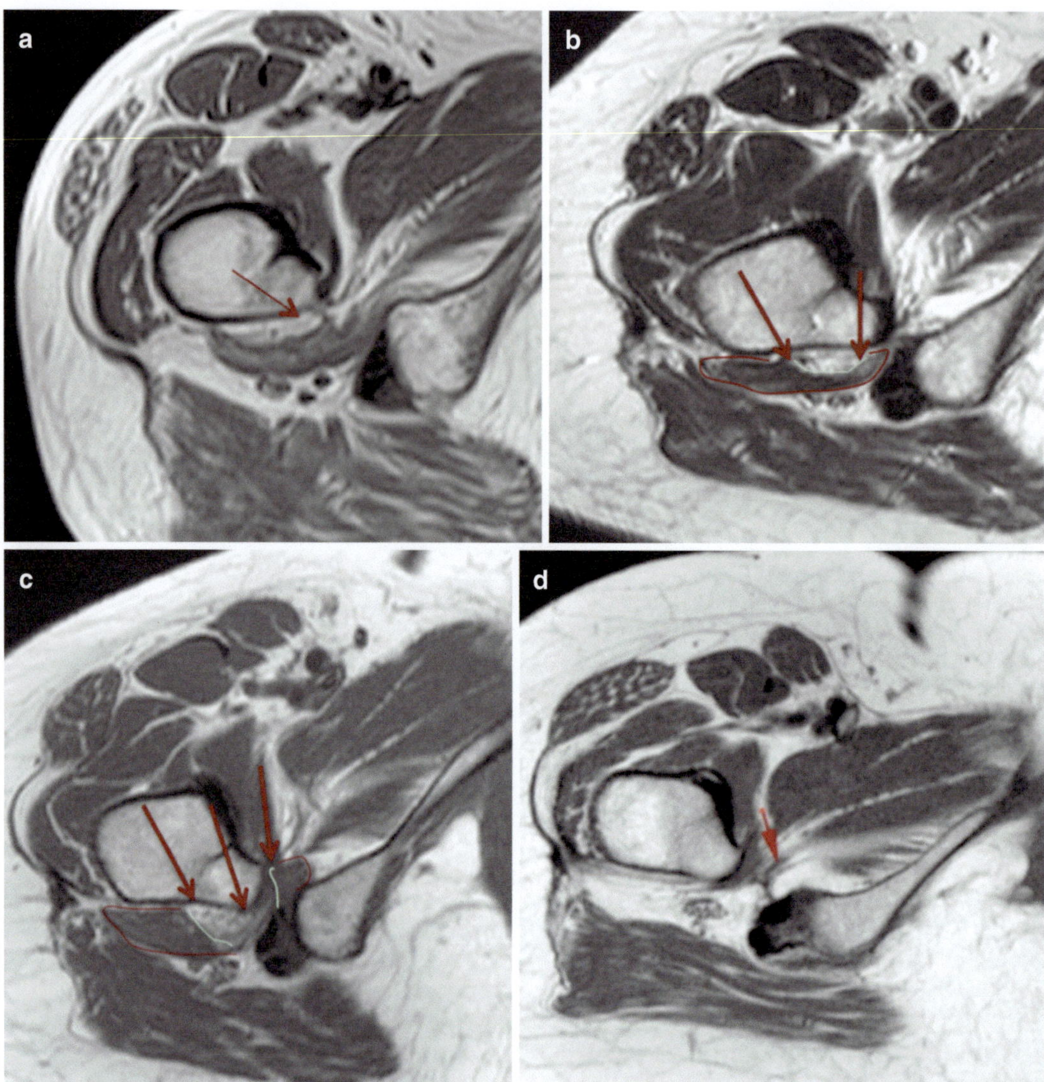

Fig. 5.98 Tear stages affecting QFM in patients with IFI are best evaluated on axial T1-weighted MRI images: anterior myofascial disruption (**a**), anterior partial tear (**b**), full-thickness partial tear (**c**), and complete atrophy (short arrow) (**d**). Red lines demarcate the normal limit of muscle fascia and green lines define tears. Long arrows mark the transition point between the normal fascia and the tear

tuberosity, it will likely be secondary to hamstring tendon abnormalities or spread by soft tissue edema [62, 136] (Fig. 5.100).

(c) *Tendons*. Cases of severe changes within the QFM are more likely to show edema surrounding the hamstring tendon attachments. However, adjacent inflammation, musculotendinous injury, unrelated enthesopathy, and overuse syndromes may also account for these findings [62]. The hamstring tendons of affected subjects may show edema, degenerative tendinopathy, partial tears, and, more rarely, full-thickness tears (Fig. 5.101). Although no tears are usually seen involving the iliopsoas tendon, edemas surrounding its insertion and tendinosis are not uncommon [143].

(d) *Bursae and adipose tissue*. Edema affecting the ischiofemoral fat is commonly seen in IFI. Bursa-like fluid collections (thickened

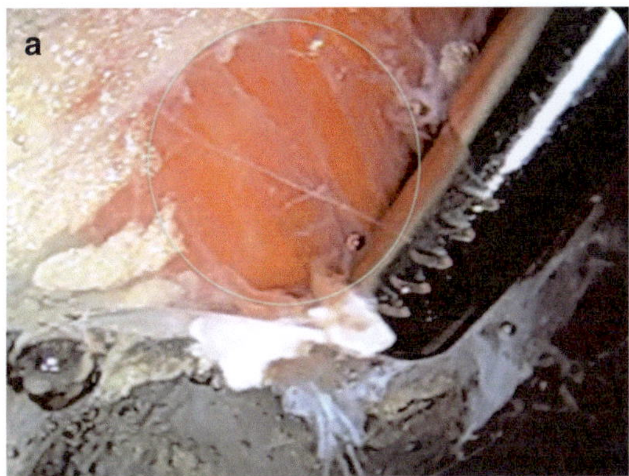
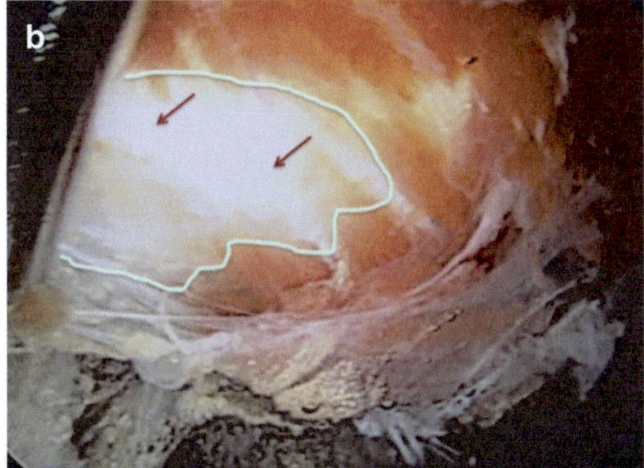
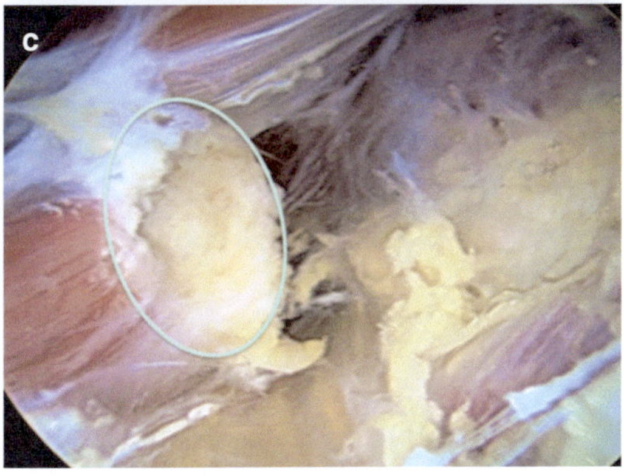

Fig. 5.99 Tear stages affecting QFM in patients with IFI. Endoscopic images show an anterior myofascial disruption (green lines define tears) (**a**), a full-thickness partial tear (**b**), and a complete tear (**c**)

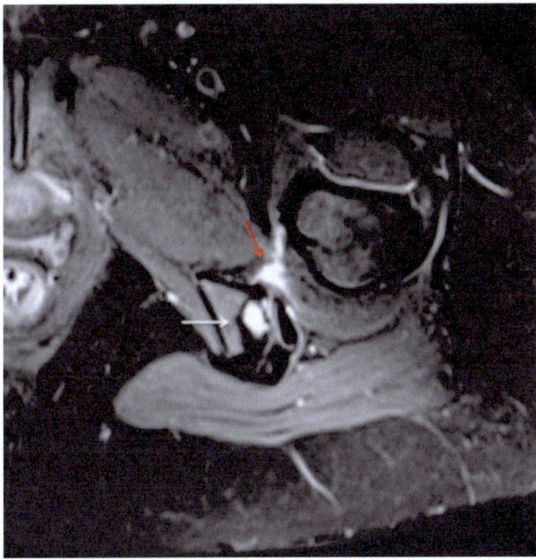

Fig. 5.100 Subcortical bone changes in a patient with an evolved IFI. Subcortical simple cysts affecting the ischial tuberosity (white arrow) are not common. Note the complete tear of the medial portion of the QFM (red arrow)

bursae that may be affected by IFI [62, 145–148] (Fig. 5.102).

(e) *Nerve*. The proximity of the sciatic nerve to an abnormal QFM may contribute to lower back pain [5]. With severe edema in the perisciatic fat, irritation of the adjacent sciatic nerve may cause acute deep gluteal syndrome (sciatic neuritis). Chronic inflammatory changes and adhesions causing scar tissue between the muscle and the sciatic nerve result in entrapment during hip motion, which causes chronic deep gluteal syndrome [5] (Figs. 5.44 and 5.45). In addition, any other nerve running along the deep gluteal space can be compressed, being especially relevant the compression of the quadratus femoris nerve. This nerve damage occurs at the level of its entry into the muscle, which is unique and coincides with the point of maximum impingement. Our current theory is that damage to this nerve can be a cause of early QFM atrophy. By failing to exercise its function as a stabilizer of the hip, impingement may progress resulting in the establishment of a vicious circle, which finishes with complete atrophy of the muscle [62].

bursal-type tissue) surrounding the lesser trochanter in the area of the impingement may be present due to friction between it and overlying soft tissues. This finding can mimic iliopsoas, obturator externus, or ischial bursitis. Obturator externus and ischiogluteal, gluteofemoral, and iliopsoas bursae are the hip

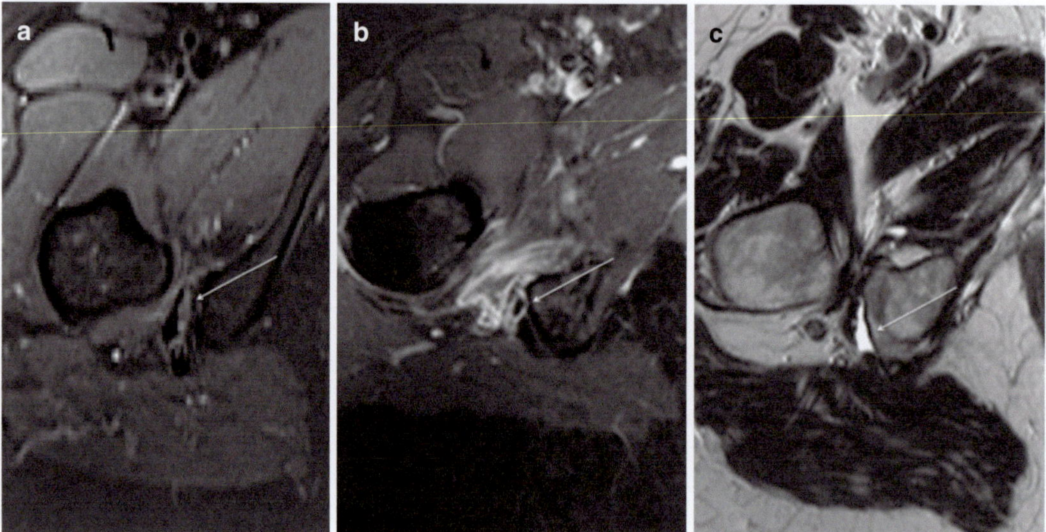

Fig. 5.101 Tendon injuries in the context of IFI. Axial PD fat-suppressed MRI images show peritendinous edema of the hamstring secondary to IFI without signs of tear (**a**) and extensive partial tear of the semimembranosus tendon (**b**). Axial T1-weighted MR image shows a complete tear of the conjoined tendon and semimembranosus tendon (**c**)

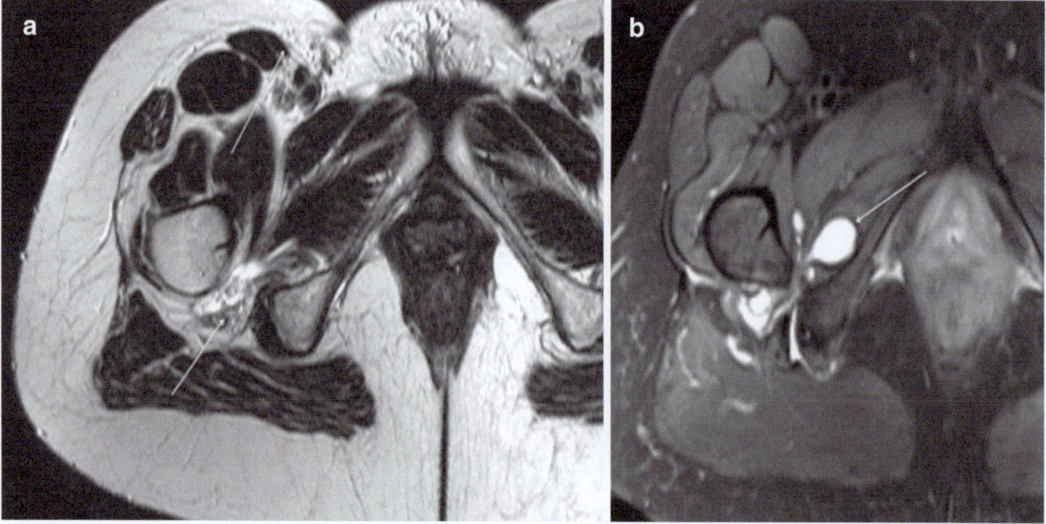

Fig. 5.102 Bursal abnormalities in patients with IFI. Axial T1-weighted MR image shows an inflammatory reaction of the ischiofemoral fat with a pseudobursa formation by accumulation and encapsulation of edema. Note the inflammatory and granulation tissue, blood remnants, and muscle tissue remnants within the bursa-like collection (white arrow) (**a**). Axial PD fat-suppressed MR image demonstrates a moderate obturator externus bursitis (arrow) (**b**), a distended ischiogluteal bursa (red arrows) (**c**), and a slight iliopsoas bursitis (arrows) (**d**)

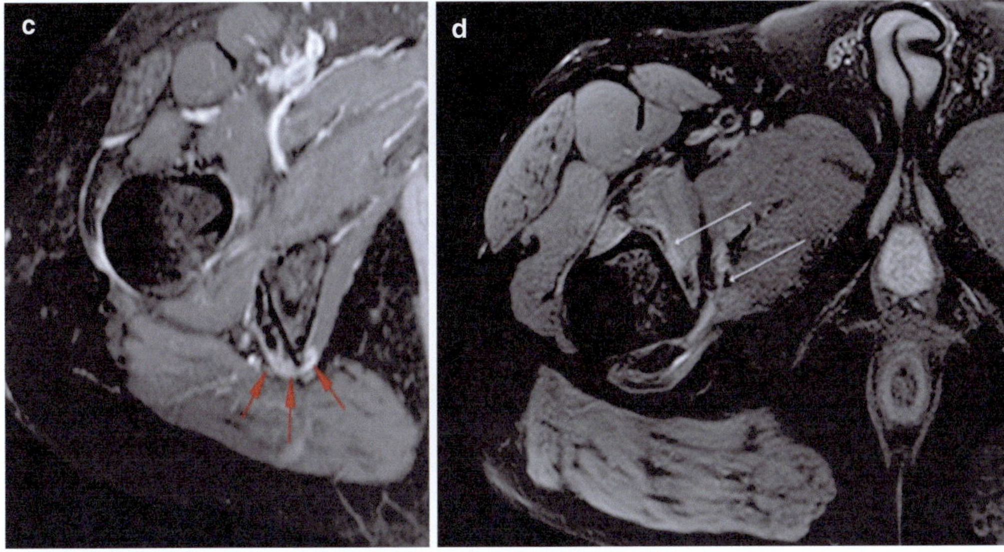

Fig. 5.102 (continued)

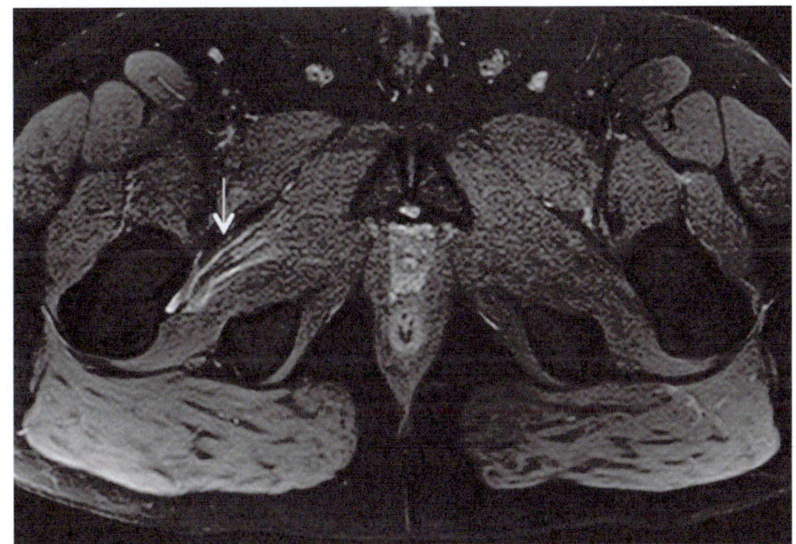

Fig. 5.103 DGS secondary to anterior myotendinous partial tear of the right obturator externus. Axial PD fat-suppressed MRI image shows a slight acute-subacute hemorrhage in the muscle thickness secondary to the injury in a 29-year-old patient with subgluteal syndrome. MRI did not show any other significant alteration

Differential Diagnosis

A wide range of conditions related to hip pain must be ruled out in the clinical and imaging differential diagnosis of IFI including deep gluteal syndrome [5], hamstring or iliopsoas injuries, femoroacetabular impingement (FAI), strain or tear of the QFM without narrowing of the IFS, bursitis without impingement, denervation patterns of the QFM, delayed-onset muscle soreness (DOMS), QFM tear, tendinosis, avulsion or agenesis, iliotibial band friction syndrome, and tendinosis or myotendinous tear of the obturator externus [149–152] (Figs. 5.103, 5.104, and 5.105).

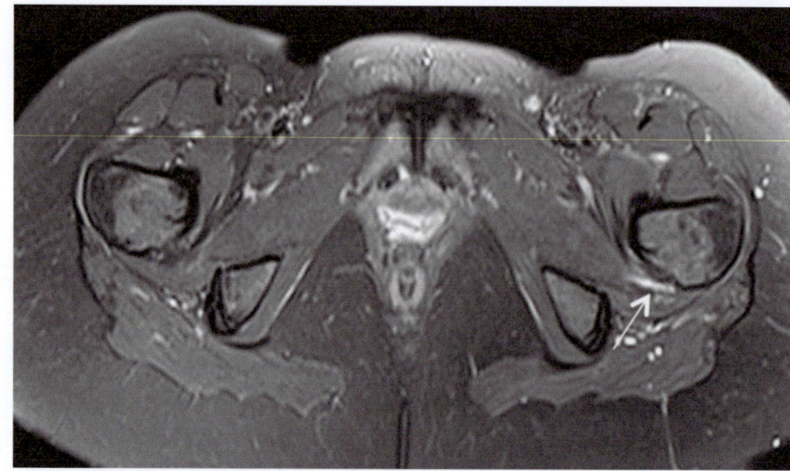

Fig. 5.104 DGS secondary to distal obturator externus tendinosis in a 46-year-old patient. Axial fat-suppressed PD-weighted MR image shows moderate thickening and hypersignal of obturator externus tendon at the level of the distal enthesis on the medial side of the left greater trochanter (arrow)

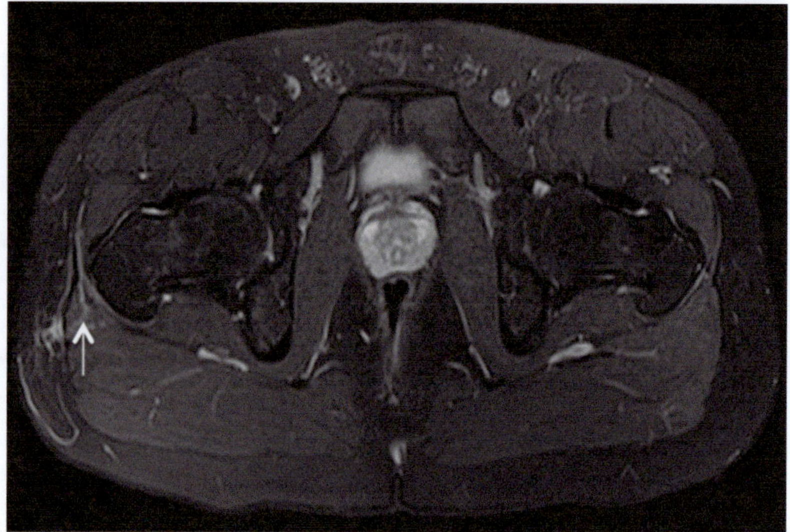

Fig. 5.105 DGS secondary to right iliotibial band friction syndrome. Axial fat-suppressed PD-weighted MR image shows moderate edema surrounding the iliotibial tract in the vicinity of the greater trochanter in a 24-year-old patient with no audible snapping

Imaging Assessment in Other Posterior Hip Pathologies

Proximal Hamstring Tendons Injuries

Injury to the hamstring muscle complex (HMC) is extremely common, especially in the athletic community, and an important cause of posterior thigh and buttock pain. Clinically it may at times be difficult to distinguish between hamstring origin pathologies [153]. Imaging allows to diagnose a wide spectrum of pathologic conditions that may affect the proximal region of this tendon group, including partial/complete hamstring strain (acute, recurrent, or chronic), tendon detachment, avulsion fractures (acute or chronic/nonunited), apophysitis, nonunited apophysis, proximal tendinopathy, calcifying tendinosis, and contusions. It also has a role in confirming the site of injury and characterizing its extent, providing some prognostic information, and helping plan treatment. MRI can have prognostic import as to time to return to sport. Some clinically diagnosed hamstring strains have no abnormal findings on MRI; these patients have a shorter time of recovery and returning to full activity than those with positive MRI findings. Generally, involvement of the proximal tendon(s) indicates a more prolonged recuperation period and return to sport than those without injury to the proximal tendon(s) [154].

Hamstring Avulsion Injuries MRI is the preferred imaging modality for demonstrating proximal hamstring avulsions, due to its superior contrast resolution and ability to easily demonstrate the full extent of injury. The axial plane is most useful in their evaluation given that they are seen in cross section in this plane. The extent of the tendon(s) retraction can easily be made on MRI, usually with the coronal sequence. The degree of tendon retraction measured by MRI is the main factor influencing the decision to perform surgery [155]. In some cases there may be a partial avulsion, usually involving the conjoint ST-BF component with an intact SMB component of the hamstring origin or vice versa. The other relatively common form of partial tear involves complete avulsion of the SMB origin and partial tear of the conjoint ST-BF component, sparing either the medial or lateral margin. With chronic avulsions, the retracted tendon edges will have no surrounding fluid collection. The tendon edges may be difficult to clearly define due to the formation of scar tissue within the tendon defect [153]. In the skeletally immature patient, acute apophyseal injuries may be less obvious on MRI than the typical acute hamstring tendon avulsion, particularly if there is no retraction (Figs. 5.106, 5.107, 5.108, 5.109, and 5.110).

Chronic Hamstring Origin Tendinosis and Tears Typical MRI findings in chronic hamstring origin tendinosis include tendon thickening and signal hyperintensity at the deep margin. Partial tears, when present, are generally seen at the deep margin. In general, the criterion for diagnosis of a tear is the presence of a fluid signal intensity cleft at the deep margin. Confident diagnosis of partial tear on ultrasound can be difficult in these cases. Edema, hemorrhage, and/or a hematoma is often prominent in the setting of high-grade partial and, particularly, full-thickness tears of the hamstring tendons; this is seen as amorphous and/or well-defined high signal on fluid-sensitive sequences in the soft tissues about the site of tear [156] (Fig. 5.111).

Acute Hamstring Muscle-Tendon Junction Injuries Isolated hamstring MTJ injuries most commonly involve the long head biceps femoris, followed by semimembranosus and lastly

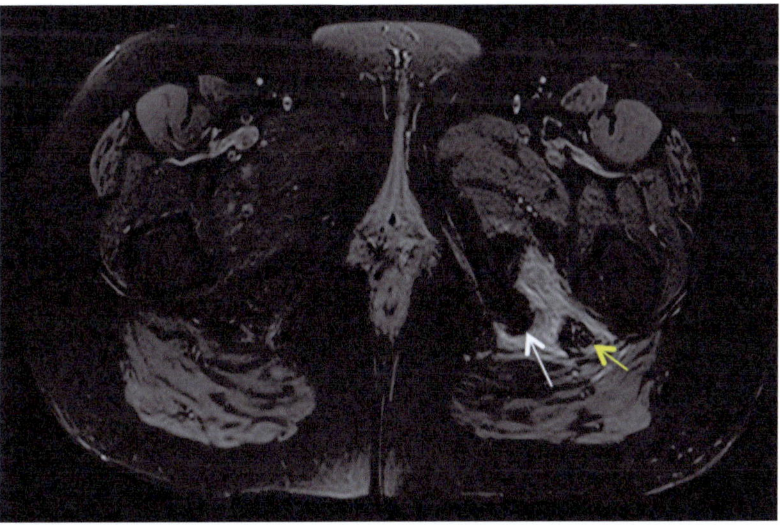

Fig. 5.106 DGS secondary to complete hamstring avulsion. Axial fat-suppressed PD-weighted MR image shows a complete avulsion of the hamstring origin involving both semimembranosus and conjoint semitendinosus-biceps femoris components (white arrow). Note moderate edema within the deep gluteal space and sciatic neuritis (yellow arrow) in this 24-year-old patient suffering from pain associated with acute sciatica

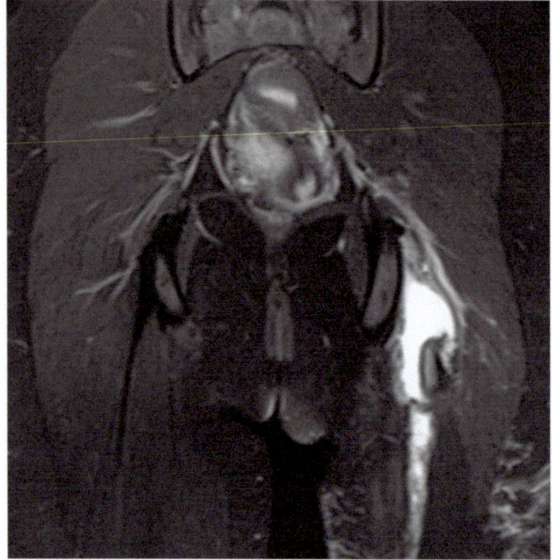

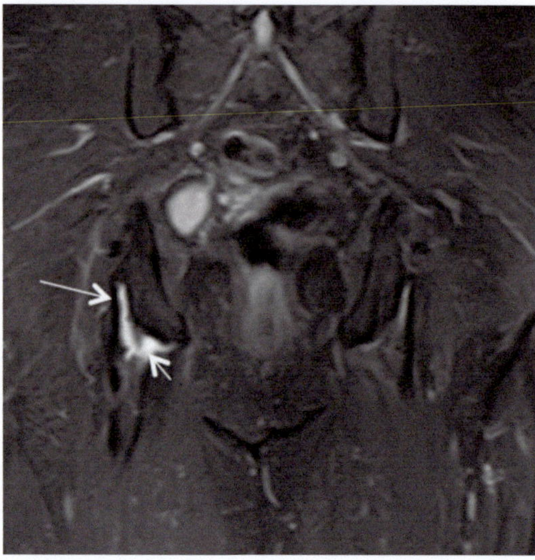

Fig. 5.107 DGS secondary to complete hamstring avulsion in the same patient showed in the previous figure. Coronal fat-suppressed PD-weighted MR image shows a complete avulsion of the hamstring origin involving both semimembranosus and conjoint semitendinosus-biceps femoris components with a significant retraction degree

Fig. 5.108 DGS secondary to partial hamstring avulsion. Coronal fat-suppressed PD-weighted MR image shows a partial avulsion of the hamstring origin involving the conjoint semitendinosus-biceps femoris component (short arrow) without significant retraction. Note how semimembranosus insertion remains intact (large arrow)

Fig. 5.109 DGS secondary to partial hamstring tear. Axial fat-suppressed PD-weighted MR image shows a partial tear of the hamstring origin involving the medial margin of both semimembranosus and conjoint semitendinosus-biceps femoris components (arrows)

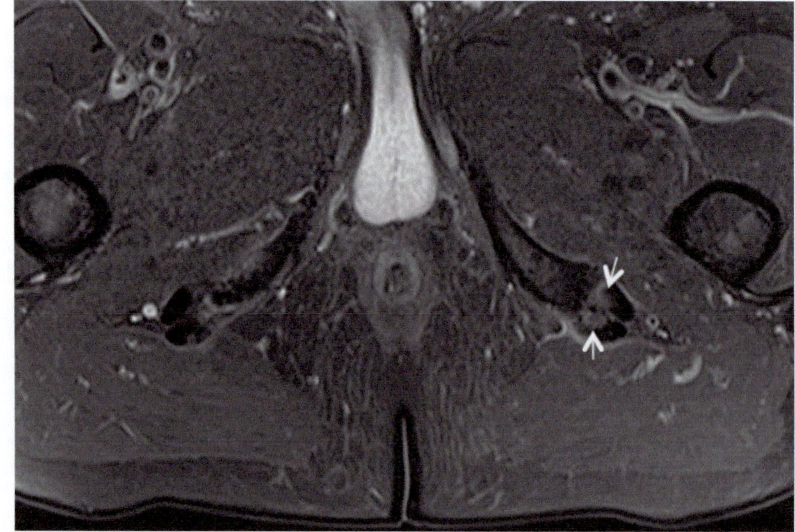

semitendinosus. Combined hamstring muscle strain injuries usually involve a combination of BF and ST, with BF predominant [157]. Muscle-tendon junction injury ranges from mild strain to partial-thickness tear to full-thickness disruption. Mild strain is seen as feathery fluid about the junction, having a comblike appearance of edema with thin elongated edema oriented craniocaudally along the central tendon with fine bands of edema radiating along the muscle-tendon junction fibrils at acute angles with the central tendon. Partial-thickness tears manifest with more significant edema/hemorrhage along and about the muscle-tendon junction with thinning and irregular contour of the tendon, sometimes with a focal hematoma. Disruption is seen as frank discontinuity of the tendon, usually with significant surrounding edema/hemorrhage and sometimes also a frank hematoma. In the subacute phase, there may be mild thickening and intermediate signal related to the adjacent tendon reflecting immature scarring of the tendon, which with remodeling will attenuate and become more markedly hypointense on all pulse sequences [158] (Fig. 5.112).

Calcifying Tendinosis of Hamstring Tendons Calcifying tendinosis results from the deposition of calcium hydroxyapatite crystals in muscular attachments. Historically, it is assumed that such depositions result from trauma, but no specific mechanism for their formation has been completely elucidated. More recently, genetic and metabolic factors have been postulated as other etiologies. CT and US allow proper visualization and localization of the calcium foci. US is valid for diagnosis affecting superficial tendons, such as the hamstrings, but not for calcifying tendonosis of the external rotators. MRI is useful to rule out other conditions but not to assess this condition [159]. Treatment of calcifying tendinosis varies with the clinical and radiologic phase of the calcification. Although the resorptive phase is usually self-limited, patient pain may be severe, and the need for relief may be urgent. US-guided needling, aspiration, and lavage are more likely to be successful in this phase. In the formative or resting phases, symptoms are milder and chronic [160] (Fig. 5.46).

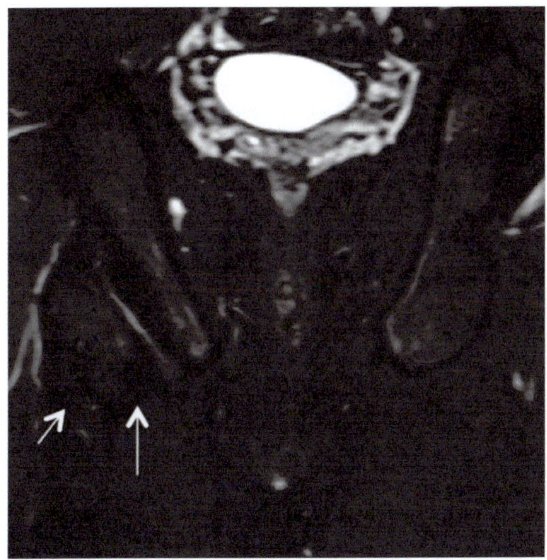

Fig. 5.110 DGS secondary to nonunited chronic apophysitis. Coronal fat-suppressed PD-weighted MR image shows a chronic nonunited fracture of the right ossification center of the ischial tuberosity (arrow). Note how both semimembranosus and conjoint semitendinosus-biceps femoris tendon-bone attachment remain intact (short arrow)

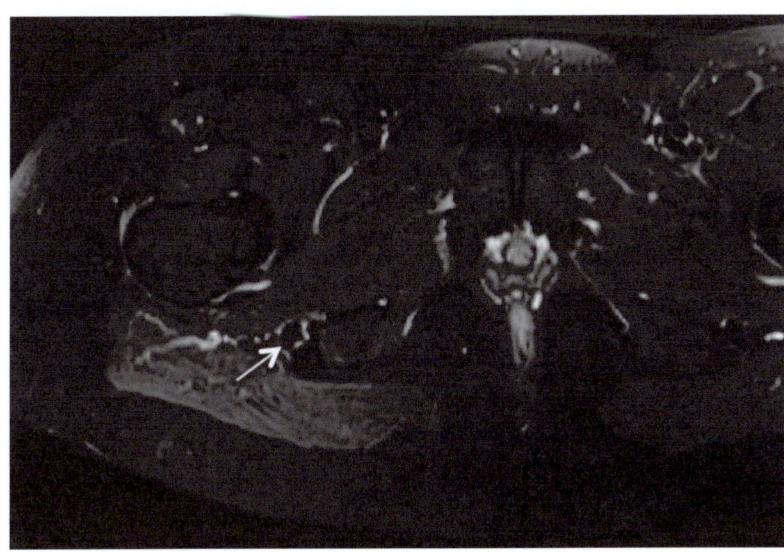

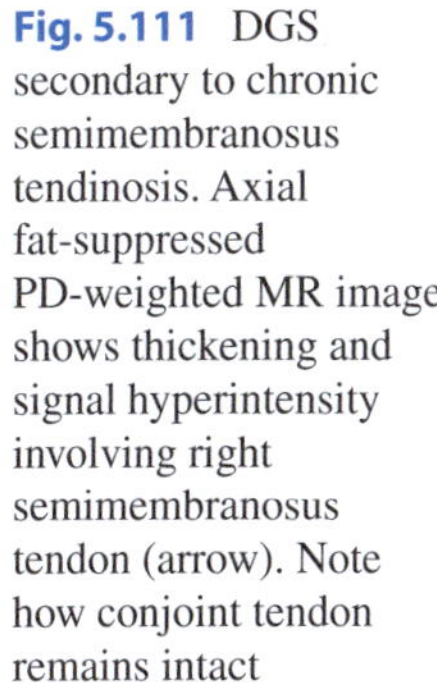

Fig. 5.111 DGS secondary to chronic semimembranosus tendinosis. Axial fat-suppressed PD-weighted MR image shows thickening and signal hyperintensity involving right semimembranosus tendon (arrow). Note how conjoint tendon remains intact

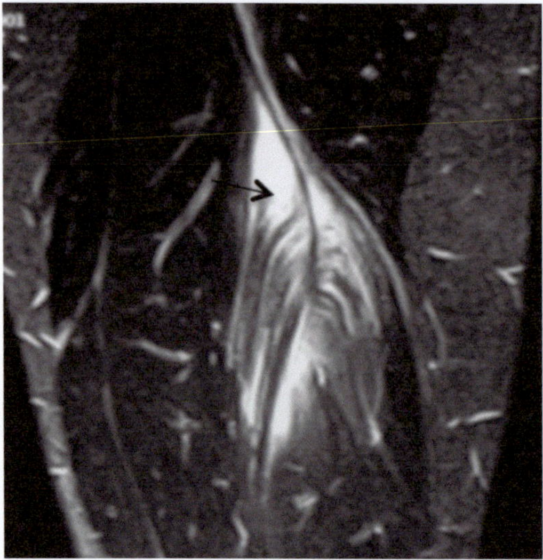

Fig. 5.112 Partial-thickness injury of the long head biceps femoris muscle-tendon junction. Note the disruption as a discontinuity of the muscle fibers, with significant surrounding edema/hemorrhage and a focal hematoma (arrow)

Bursae Conditions

Bursitis is a usual clinical entity that can cause severe disabling posterior hip pain and is often a result of inflammation secondary to excessive local friction, tendon pathologies, infection, arthritis, rheumatologic diseases, or direct trauma. Any pathology in the vicinity of a bursa may cause its distension and intra-bursal synovitis. We assume as standard that practically all bursitis are secondary. Bursitis can clinically be easily misdiagnosed as joint-, tendon-, or muscle-related pain and treatment of these conditions can be different. In general, it must be firstly treated the cause that brings this condition, such as tendinosis or a rheumatologic process. Treatment of each etiology is specific. The vast majority of bursitis has been reported to respond adequately to conservative management without surgical drainage. Thus, knowledge of the imaging features of bursitis can avoid unnecessary surgery. If there is no contraindication, ultrasound-guided evacuation and infiltration with corticosteroids are the treatment of choice for symptomatic control [62, 147, 148, 161–163].

Trochanteric or Subgluteus Maximus Bursa It covers the posterior facet of the GT and it is located beneath the gluteus maximus muscle and iliotibial tract. This bursa can be identified on axial MR images as an elongated structure paralleling the posterior facet and usually it does not extend over the anterior border of the lateral facet [161] (Fig. 5.12).

Piriformis Bursa This bursa, also named posterior subgluteus medius bursa, is situated posterior to the apex of the GT. The bursa lies on and follows the contour of the insertion of the piriformis tendon. Its superficial surface is in contact with, and often adhered to, the deep surface of the gluteus medius tendon [162] (Fig. 5.12).

Gluteofemoral Bursa This bursa is situated caudal to the GT and it lies beneath, and adhered to, the iliotibial band in the area where the tendinous fibers of gluteus maximus inserts. It is positioned over the posterior edge of the vastus lateralis, separating it from the iliotibial band [162] (Fig. 5.113).

Obturator Externus Bursa This bursa is thought to be formed by a protrusion of the posterior inferior hip synovium between the

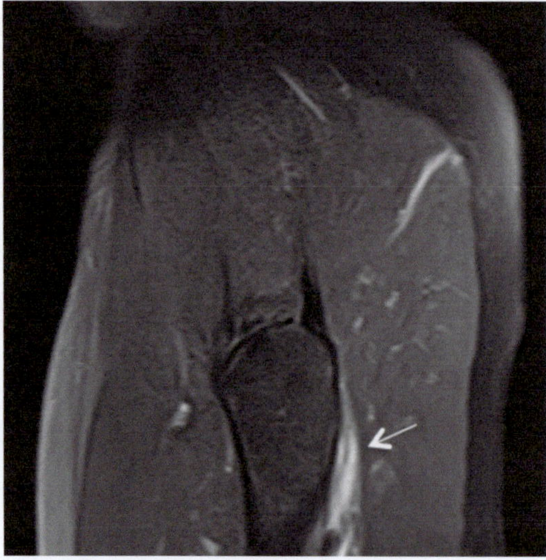

Fig. 5.113 Gluteofemoral bursitis. Sagittal fat-suppressed PD-weighted MR image demonstrates a moderate distension of gluteofemoral bursa in a 38-year-old patient with distal tendinosis of the gluteus maximus tendon

ischiofemoral ligament and the zona orbicularis. Bursitis usually occurs in patients with hip synovitis and chronically increased intra-articular pressure. When distended, this bursa displaces the obturator externus muscle inferiorly while extending medially toward the obturator foramen [148] (Figs. 5.12 and 5.102b).

Obturator Internus Bursa Normally, as in most hip bursae, the obturator internus bursa is in a collapsed state and is only distended when it is inflamed or infected. When present, it is a "boomerang"-shaped fluid distension between the obturator internus tendon and the posterior grooved surface of the ischium. Obturator internus bursa is usually secondary to dynamic compression of the sciatic nerve by the muscle belly, a piriformis-obturator scissor-like impingement, hypertrophied obturator internus bordering on the lesser sciatic notch or anatomical variant of the sciatic-obturator complex as we see previously [5] (Fig. 5.38).

Ischiogluteal Bursa It separates the gluteus maximus from the ischial tuberosity. Ischiogluteal bursitis is usually related to intermittent pressure upon the ischial tuberosity from prolonged sitting, hamstring tendinopathies, or ischiofemoral impingement [5, 62]. Tuberculosis, gout, rheumatoid arthritis, systemic lupus erythematous, ankylosing spondylitis, and Reiter's syndrome have also been reported to involve the ischiogluteal bursa. As the bursa lies in close contact to the sciatic and posterior femoral cutaneous nerve, ischiogluteal bursitis can mimic the symptoms of radiculopathy. It may have a very heterogeneous appearance on imaging studies, usually related to bleeding with blood-fluid levels, synovial proliferation, and internal septation [147] (Figs. 5.12 and 5.102c).

Pudendal Syndrome

Pudendal nerve entrapment neuropathies are rare entities in common practice. The clinical symptoms can be perineal or penile (clitoral-vulvar) pain (burning) or hypoesthesia, followed by erec-

tile dysfunction, as well as fecal incontinence, anal pain, or stress urinary incontinence. Isolated perineal pain and in the medial side of the posterior hip is frequently found in cyclists due to the entrapment of this nerve. Pudendal nerve entrapment is a recognized cause of chronic perineal pain, which is typically aggravated by sitting, relieved by standing, and absent when recumbent or sitting on a toilet seat [164].

The pudendal nerve arises from the sacral plexus. Subsequently, it passes around the ischial spine and reenters the pelvic cavity through the lesser sciatic foramen. It then courses under the levator ani muscle on top of the obturator internus muscle. Along its course in the ischiorectal fossa, the nerve gives off small inferior rectal branches and one or two perineal branches. It then pierces the superior urogenital fascia to penetrate the urogenital diaphragm. Up to that point, the bones of the pelvis protect the nerve [165]. Basically, the pudendal nerve is predisposed to entrapment at the level of the ischial spine and within Alcock's canal. At the ischial spine, the nerve can be compressed between the sacrotuberous and sacrospinous ligaments with a mechanism like a "lobster claw" with the nerve crushed while traversing the interligamentous space [166]. A shearing effect caused by the gluteus maximus on the sacrotuberous ligament seems to be possibly implicated in pudendal entrapment. More distally, at Alcock's canal, the pudendal nerve can be compressed by the anterior prolongation of the falciform process of the sacrotuberous ligament (lunate fascia), when this is focally thickened or tightly adherent to the underlying fascia of the obturator internus muscle [167]. No widely accepted confirmatory test is available for this neuropathy, although a neurophysiologic study may disclose the nerve damage. MR imaging can diagnose pudendal neuropathy if a space-occupying lesion is found along the nerve course or, in the absence of a mass, when focal nerve swelling and T2 hyperintensity are observed at Alcock's canal. One-to-one comparison with the contralateral nerve on axial planes may increase the confidence in the diagnosis. Proper diagnosis and treatment of pudendal nerve entrapment with CT-guided perineural injection offer a chance of long-term pain relief [168] (Figs. 5.114 and 5.115).

Pathology of the Distal Gluteus Maximus Tendon

There is not full agreement regarding the distal insertions of the gluteus maximus muscle. Tears affecting gluteus maximus are rare, underrecognized, and poorly described in the literature. Autopsy and imaging studies have shown gluteal tendon tears in up to 10% of individuals older than 60 years. The iliotibial band, fascia lata, lateral intermuscular septum, and linea aspera insertions may be involved [169] (Fig. 5.116).

Cases of calcifying tendinosis of the distal insertion of the gluteus maximus tendon have also been described. Plain radiography usually

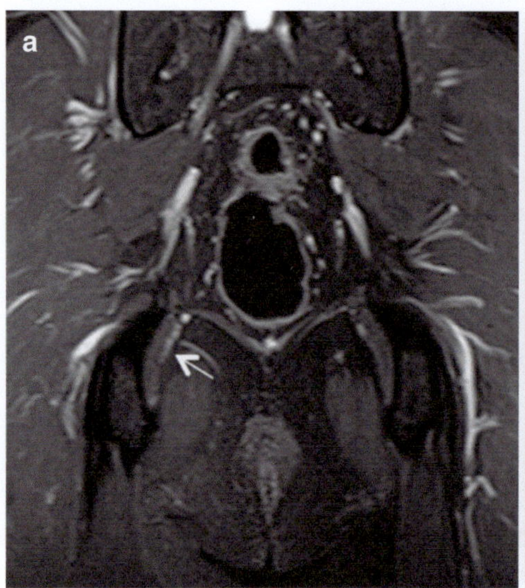
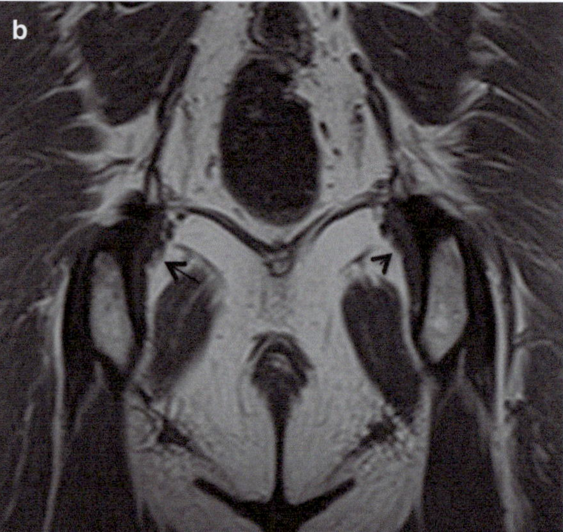

Fig. 5.114 Pudendal syndrome. Coronal PD-weighted (**b**) and fat-suppressed PD-weighted (**a**) MR image shows focal nerve swelling (black arrow) and T2 hyperintensity (white arrow) is observed at Alcock's canal in a 31-year-old cyclist. One-to-one comparison with the contralateral nerve (short black arrow) may increase the confidence in the diagnosis

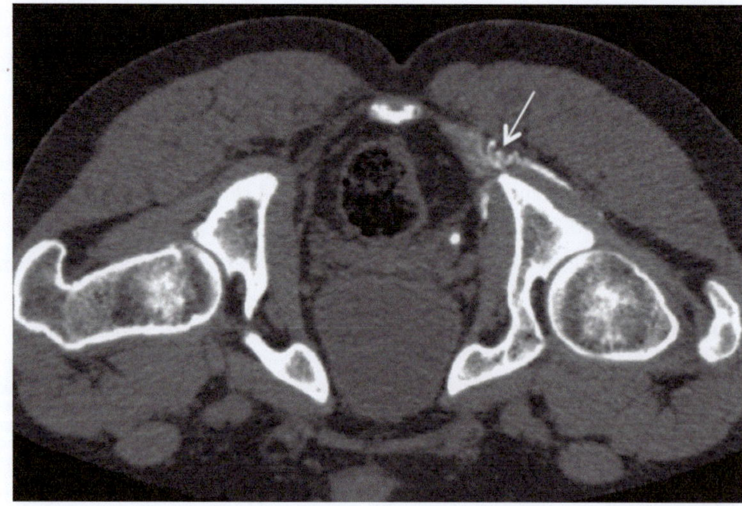

Fig. 5.115 Double injection of anesthetic and corticosteroid technique (pudendal infiltration test). Axial MDCT image shows the final result of CT-guided infiltration of the peripudendal space (arrow) at the level of the sacrotuberous-sacrospinous interligamentous space. The solution contains a small amount of iodinated contrast to assess the location of injection more accurately. Note how the solution runs along the perineural space and also reaches Alcock's canal

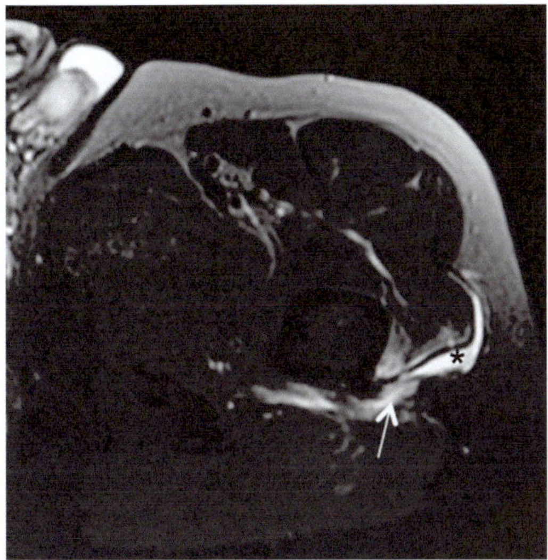

Fig. 5.116 DGS secondary to distal partial-thickness tear of the gluteus maximus tendon. Axial fat-suppressed PD-weighted MR image shows moderate thickening and signal hyperintensity of gluteus maximus tendon at the level of the distal enthesis on the gluteal tuberosity of the femur associated with peritendinous and perifascial bleeding. Note the partial discontinuity of the fibers of the distal tendon (arrow) and the hemorrhagic gluteofemoral bursa distension (asterisk)

shows amorphous calcific densities extending from the posterior border of the femur. Computed tomography can demonstrate cortical erosion associated with the calcified mass. The patients usually respond well to needle lavage and injection with local anesthesia and corticosteroids. Recognition of this entity makes biopsy unnecessary [170].

Posterior Wall Fractures of the Acetabulum

Most acetabular fractures involve the posterior wall. Although such fractures may appear to be simple on plain radiographs, many surgeons face difficulties when reducing the fragments. Most posterior wall fractures are comminuted or they are associated with an impaction injury of the articular surface into the underlying cancellous bone along the margin of the fracture line. Further, the soft tissues are frequently detached from fragments at the time of injury or during the surgery. In addition, after surgery it is difficult to

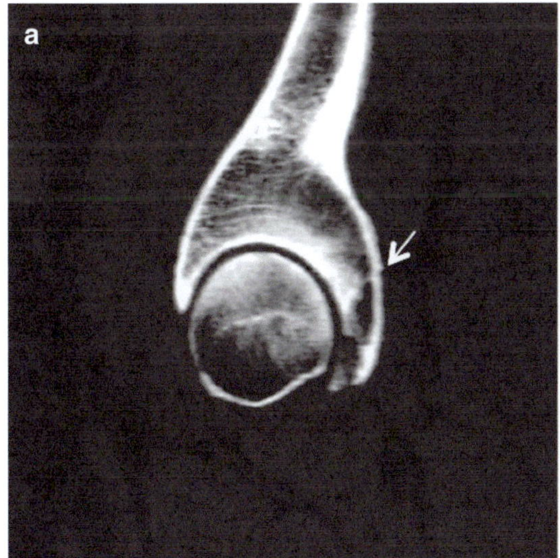

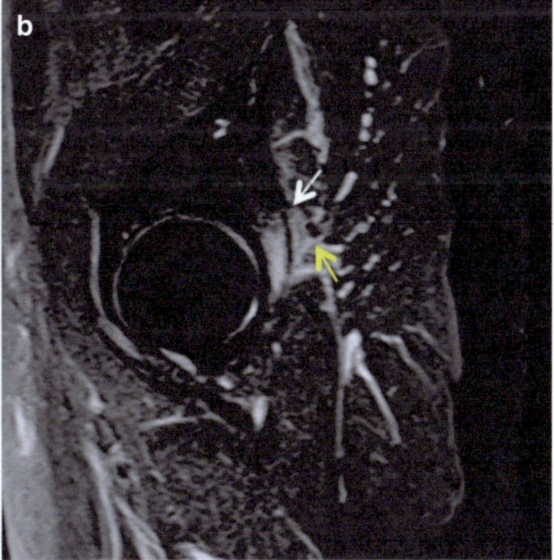

Fig. 5.117 DGS secondary to posterior wall fracture of the acetabulum. Sagittal-oblique MDCT reconstruction (**a**) and sagittal fat-suppressed PD-weighted MR image (**b**) shows a inconspicuously displaced fracture of the posterior wall of the acetabulum (white arrows) with reactive interfascial bleeding in piriformis-obturator internus space associated with moderate sciatica neuritis secondary to inflammatory changes in the vicinity of the fracture (yellow arrow)

know the exact quality of the reduction and the shape and congruity of the articular surface of the acetabulum due to its three-dimensionally complex shape and the interfering effect of metals on the radiologic images. Accurate evaluation of the resulting union and the likelihood of future osteoarthritis and posttraumatic arthritis are also hindered [171]. Therefore, radiologist should properly recognize and describe the fracture pattern, and surgeons should make every effort to obtain a stable congruous hip joint with complete union of the fragments during the primary surgery because a second operation is not feasible. CT has a key role in the diagnosis and monitoring of fracture healing and MRI in detecting associated injuries [5] (Fig. 5.117).

Summary

There is a broad spectrum of diseases affecting structures in the posterior hip. The deep gluteal space is the most extensive and significant anatomical space of this region and the seat of most of pathologies coursing with back hip pain. Many of the pathologic conditions that are located in this anatomical region are primary, but many have pathophysiological mechanisms in which are problems involved in other body areas.

The major complexity of the posterior hip anatomy requires high-quality MRI studies and the use of specific protocols. In recent years there has been a great development of imaging techniques and endoscopy that has allowed to understand the pathophysiological mechanisms underlying piriformis syndrome, which can currently be classified into six types, conditions of the external rotators of the hip, and nerve sciatic pathologies. It is especially important the discovery, classification, and development of endoscopic treatment of fibrovascular bands affecting the sciatic nerve mobility. It is also very important the knowledge of etiologies and predisposing factors of ischiofemoral impingement, many of them having a functional background.

There is great difficulty in formulating the diagnosis of posterior hip pathologies because clinical history and physical examination are imprecise and difficult to interpret. MR imaging is the diagnostic procedure of choice for assessing posterior disorders and therefore may substantially influence the management of these patients. In selected cases and for specific diseases, plane radiography, ultrasound, and MDCT can be useful for the diagnosis, although its use for the evaluation of the posterior hip has greatly reduced indications.

Counting on imaging techniques is essential when considering the most appropriate therapeutic approach in posterior hip pathology. Equally important are injection tests, with a dual diagnostic and also therapeutic purpose. Guiding infiltration tests by imaging allows carrying them out safely. Finally, MRI can play an important role in the timing of surgery.

References

1. Tibor LM, Sekiya JK. Differential diagnosis of pain around the hip joint. Arthroscopy. 2008;24(12):1407–21.
2. Martin HD, Shears SA, Johnson JC, Smathers AM, Palmer IJ. The endoscopic treatment of sciatic nerve entrapment/deep gluteal syndrome. Arthroscopy. 2011;27(2):172–81.
3. Martin HD, Palmer IJ, Hatem MA. Deep gluteal syndrome. In: Nho S, Leunig M, Kelly B, Bedi A, Larson C, editors. Hip arthroscopy and hip joint preservation surgery. New York: Springer; 2014. p. 1–17.
4. Guanche CA. Hip arthroscopy techniques: deep gluteal space access. In: Nho S, Leunig M, Kelly B, Bedi A, Larson C, editors. Hip arthroscopy and hip joint preservation surgery. New York: Springer; 2014. p. 1–12.
5. Hernando MF, Cerezal L, Pérez-Carro L, Abascal F, Canga A. Deep gluteal syndrome: anatomy, imaging, and management of sciatic nerve entrapments in the subgluteal space. Skelet Radiol. 2015;44(7):919–34.
6. Clohisy JC, Carlisle JC, Beaule PC, et al. A systematic approach to the plain radiographic evaluation of the young adult hip. J Bone Joint Surg Am. 2008;90:47–66.
7. Sartoris DJ, Resnick D. Plain film radiography: routine and specialized techniques and projections. In: Resnick D, Niwayana G, editors. Diagnosis of bone and joint disorders, vol. 1. 2nd ed. Philadelphia: Saunders; 1998. p. 38.
8. Miller TT. Abnormalities in and around the hip: MR imaging versus sonography. Magn Reson Imaging Clin N Am. 2005;13:799–809.

9. Joines MM, Motamedi K, Seeger LL, et al. Musculoskeletal interventional ultrasound. Semin Musculoskelet Radiol. 2007;11:192–8.
10. Klauser AS, Tagliafico A, Allen GM, Boutry N. Clinical indications for musculoskeletal ultrasound: a Delphi-based consensus paper of the European Society of Musculoskeletal Radiology. Eur Radiol. 2012;22(5):1140–8.
11. Martinoli C, Garello I, Marchetti A. Hip ultrasound. Eur J Radiol. 2012;81(12):3824–31.
12. Flohr TG, Schaller S, Stierstorfer K, et al. Multi-detector row CT systems and image-reconstruction techniques. Radiology. 2005;235:756.
13. Conway WF, Totty WG, McEnery KW. CT and MR imaging of the hip. Radiology. 1996;198:297–307.
14. Pritchard RS, Shah HR, Nelson CL, et al. MR and CT appearance of iliopsoas bursal distention secondary to diseased hips. J Comput Assist Tomogr. 1990;14:797–800.
15. Kneeland JB. MR imaging of sports injuries of the hip. Magn Reson Imaging Clin N Am. 1999;7:105–15.
16. Magee T. Comparison of 3 tesla MR versus 3 tesla MR arthrography of the hip for detection of acetabular labral tears in the same patient population. AJR Am J Roentgenol. 2010;194:A91–5.
17. Gary JL, Mulligan M, Banagan K. Magnetic resonance imaging for the evaluation of ligamentous injury in the pelvis: a prospective case-controlled study. J Orthop Trauma. 2014;28(1):41–7.
18. Bierry G, Simeone FJ, Borg-Stein JP, Clavert P, Palmer WE. Sacrotuberous ligament: relationship to normal, torn, and retracted hamstring tendons on MR images. Radiology. 2014;271(1):162–71.
19. Petchprapa CN, Rosenberg ZS, Sconfienza LM, Cavalcanti CF, Vieira RL, Zember JSMR. Imaging of entrapment neuropathies of the lower extremity part 1. The pelvis and hip. Radiographics. 2010;30(4):983–1000.
20. Solomon LB, Lee YC, Callary SA, Beck M, Howie DW. Anatomy of piriformis, obturator internus and obturator externus: implications for the posterior surgical approach to the hip. J Bone Joint Surg Br. 2010;92:1317–24.
21. Meknas K, Christensen A, Johansen O. The internal obturator muscle may cause sciatic pain. Pain. 2003;104:375–80.
22. Tosun O, Algin O, Yalcin N, Cay N, Ocakoglu G, Karaoglanoglu M. Ischiofemoral impingement: evaluation with new MRI parameters and assessment of their reliability. Skelet Radiol. 2012;41(5):575–87.
23. Kassarjian A, Tomas X, Cerezal L, Canga A, Llopis E. MRI of the quadratus femoris muscle: anatomic considerations and pathologic lesions. AJR Am J Roentgenol. 2011;197(1):170–4.
24. Aung HH, Sakamoto H, Akita K, Sato T. Anatomical study of the obturator internus, gemelli and quadratus femoris muscles with special reference to their innervation. Anat Rec. 2001;263(1):41–52.
25. Honma S, Jun Y, Horiguchi M. The human gemelli muscles and their nerve supplies. Kaibogaku Zasshi. 1998;73(4):329–35.
26. Wilson JT. Abnormal distribution of the nerve to the quadratus femoris in man, with remarks on its significance. J Anat Physiol. 1889;23(Pt 3):354–7.
27. Gudena R, Alzahrani A, Railton P, Powell J, Ganz R. The anatomy and function of the obturator externus. Hip Int. 2015;25(5):424–7.
28. Tatu L, Parratte B, Vuillier F, Diop M, Monnier G. Descriptive anatomy of the femoral portion of the iliopsoas muscle. Anatomical basis of anterior snapping of the hip. Surg Radiol Anat. 2001;23(6):371–4.
29. Obey MR, Broski SM, Spinner RJ, Collins MS, Krych AJ. Anatomy of the adductor magnus origin: implications for proximal hamstring injuries. Orthop J Sports Med. 2016;4(1). https://doi.org/10.1177/2325967115625055.
30. Miller SL, Gill J, Webb GR. The proximal origin of the hamstrings and surrounding anatomy encountered during repair. A cadaveric study. J Bone Joint Surg Am. 2007;89:44–8.
31. Martin HD, Palmer IJ, Hatem MA. Deep gluteal syndrome. Hip arthroscopy and hip joint preservation surgery. New York: Springer; 2014. p. 1–17.
32. Crock HV. Anatomy of the medial femoral circumflex artery and its surgical implications. J Bone Joint Surg Br. 2001;83(1):149–50.
33. Lazaro LE, Klinger CE, Sculco PK, Helfet DL, Lorich DG. The terminal branches of the medial femoral circumflex artery: the arterial supply of the femoral head. Bone Joint J. 2015;97-B(9):1204–13.
34. Dong Q, Jacobson JA, Jamadar DA, Gandikota G. Entrapment neuropathies in the upper and lower limbs: anatomy and MRI features. Radiol Res Pract. 2012;2012:230679.
35. Ergun T, Lakadamyali H. CT and MRI in the evaluation of extraspinal sciatica. Br J Radiol. 2010;83(993):791–803.
36. Enneking FK, Chan V, Greger J, Hadzić A, Lang SA. Lower-extremity peripheral nerve blockade: essentials of our current understanding. Reg Anesth Pain Med. 2005;30(1):4–35.
37. Moore KR, Tsuruda JS, Dailey AT. The value of MR neurography for evaluating extraspinal neuropathic leg pain: a pictorial essay. AJNR Am J Neuroradiol. 2001;22(4):786–94.
38. Bates D, Ruggieri P. Imaging modalities for evaluation of the spine. Radiol Clin N Am. 1991;29:675–87.
39. Coppieters MW, Alshami AM, Babri AS, Souvlis T, Kippers V, Hodges PW. Strain and excursion of the sciatic, tibial, and plantar nerves during a modified straight leg raising test. J Orthop Res. 2006;24(9):1883–9.
40. Kulcu DG, Naderi S. Differential diagnosis of intraspinal and extraspinal non-discogenic sciatica. J Clin Neurosci. 2008;15(11):1246–52.
41. Güvençer M, Akyer P, Iyem C, Tetik S, Naderi S. Anatomic considerations and the relationship

between the piriformis muscle and the sciatic nerve. Surg Radiol Anat. 2008;30(6):467–74.

42. Martin HD, Kivlan BR, Palmer IJ, Martin RL. Diagnostic accuracy of clinical tests for sciatic nerve entrapment in the gluteal region. Knee Surg Sports Traumatol Arthrosc. 2014;22(4):882–8.

43. Papadopoulos EC, Khan SN. Piriformis syndrome and low back pain: a new classification and review of the literature. Orthop Clin North Am. 2004;35(1):65–71.

44. Foster MR. Piriformis syndrome. Orthopedics. 2002;25(8):821–5.

45. Lewis AM, Layzer R, Engstrom JW, Barbaro NM, Chin CT. Magnetic resonance neurography in extraspinal sciatica. Arch Neurol. 2006;63(10):1469–72.

46. Boyajian-O'Neill LA, McClain RL, Coleman MK, Thomas PP. Diagnosis and management of piriformis syndrome: an osteopathic approach. J Am Osteopath Assoc. 2008;108:657–64.

47. Russell JM, Kransdorf MJ, Bancroft LW, Peterson JJ, Berquist TH, Bridges MD. Magnetic resonance imaging of the sacral plexus and piriformis muscles. Skelet Radiol. 2008;37(8):709–13.

48. Benzon HT, Katz JA, Benzon HA, Iqbal MS. Piriformis syndrome: anatomic considerations, a new injection technique, and a review of the literature. Anesthesiology. 2003;98(6):1442–8.

49. Fanucci E, Masala S, Sodani G. CT-guided injection of botulinic toxin for percutaneous therapy of piriformis muscle syndrome with preliminary MRI results about denervative process. Eur Radiol. 2001;11(12):2543–8.

50. Dezawa A, Kusano S, Miki H. Arthroscopic release of the piriformis muscle under local anesthesia for piriformis syndrome. Arthroscopy. 2003;19(5):554–7.

51. Masala S, Crusco S, Meschini A, Taglieri A, Calabria E, Simonetti G. Piriformis syndrome: long-term follow-up in patients treated with percutaneous injection of anesthetic and corticosteroid under CT guidance. Cardiovasc Intervent Radiol. 2012;35(2):375–82.

52. Beaton LE, Anson BJ. The relation of the sciatic nerve and its subdivisions to the piriformis muscle. Anat Rec. 1937;70:1–5.

53. Smoll NR. Variations of the piriformis and sciatic nerve with clinical consequence: a review. Clin Anat. 2010;23(1):8–17.

54. Natsis K, Totlis T, Konstantinidis GA. Anatomical variations between the sciatic nerve and the piriformis muscle: a contribution to surgical anatomy in piriformis syndrome. Surg Radiol Anat. 2014;36(3):273–80.

55. Güvençer M, Iyem C, Akyer P, Tetik S, Naderi S. Variations in the high division of the sciatic nerve and relationship between the sciatic nerve and the piriformis. Turk Neurosurg. 2009;19(2):139–44.

56. Windisch G, Braun EM, Anderhuber F. Piriformis muscle: clinical anatomy and consideration of the piriformis syndrome. Surg Radiol Anat. 2007;29(1):37–45.

57. Arora J, Mehta V, Kumar H, Suri RK, Rath G, Das S. A rare bimuscular conglomeration gluteopiriformis case report. Morphologie. 2010;94(305):40–3.

58. Diercks R, Bron C, Dorrestijn O. Guideline for diagnosis and treatment of subacromial pain syndrome: a multidisciplinary review by the Dutch Orthopaedic Association. Acta Orthop. 2014;85(3):314–22.

59. Filler AG, Gilmer-Hill H. Piriformis syndrome, obturator internus syndrome, pudendal nerve entrapment, and other pelvic entrapments. In: Winn HR, editor. Youmans neurological surgery. 6th ed. Philadelphia: Saunders; 2009. p. 2447–55.

60. Murata Y, Ogata S, Ikeda Y, Yamagata M. An unusual cause of sciatic pain as a result of the dynamic motion of the obturator internus muscle. Spine J. 2009;9(6):e16–8.

61. Meknas K, Kartus J, Letto JI, Christensen A, Johansen O. Surgical release of the internal obturator tendon for the treatment of retro-trochanteric pain syndrome: a prospective randomized study, with long-term follow-up. Knee Surg Sports Traumatol Arthrosc. 2009;17(10):1249–56.

62. Hernando MF, Cerezal L, Pérez-Carro L, Canga A, González RP. Evaluation and management of ischiofemoral impingement: a pathophysiologic, radiologic, and therapeutic approach to a complex diagnosis. Skelet Radiol. 2016;45(6):771–87.

63. Torriani M, Souto SC, Thomas BJ, Ouellette H, Bredella MA. Ischiofemoral impingement syndrome: an entity with hip pain and abnormalities of the quadratus femoris muscle. AJR Am J Roentgenol. 2009;193(1):186–90.

64. Taneja AK, Bredella MA, Torriani M. Ischiofemoral impingement. Magn Reson Imaging Clin N Am. 2013;21(1):65–73.

65. Bucknor MD, Steinbach LS, Saloner D, Chin CT. Magnetic resonance neurography evaluation of chronic extraspinal sciatica after remote proximal hamstring injury: a preliminary retrospective analysis. J Neurosurg. 2014;121(2):408–14.

66. Chen CK, Yeh L, Chang WN, Pan HB, Yang CF. MRI diagnosis of contracture of the gluteus maximus muscle. AJR Am J Roentgenol. 2006;187(2):W169–74.

67. Makhsous M, Lin F, Cichowski A, Cheng I. Use of MRI images to measure tissue thickness over the ischial tuberosity at different hip flexion. Clin Anat. 2011;24(5):638–45.

68. Delaney H, Bencardino J, Rosenberg ZS. Magnetic resonance neurography of the pelvis and lumbosacral plexus. Neuroimaging Clin N Am. 2014;24(1):127–50.

69. Fabeck L, Tolley M, Rooze M, Burny F. Theoretical study of the decrease in the femoral neck anteversion during growth. Cells Tissues Organs. 2002;171:269–75.

70. Issack PS, Helfet DL. Sciatic nerve injury associated with acetabular fractures. HSS J. 2009;5(1):12–8.

71. Daniilidis K, Stukenborg-Colsman CM, Ettinger M, Windhagen H. Huge sciatic neuroma presented

40 years after traumatic above knee amputation. Technol Health Care. 2013;21(3):261–4.

72. Wolf M, Bäumer P, Pedro M. Sciatic nerve injury related to hip replacement surgery: imaging detection by MR neurography despite susceptibility artifacts. PLoS One. 2014;9(2):e89154.

73. Von Roth P, Abdel MP, Wauer F. Significant muscle damage after multiple revision total hip replacements through the direct lateral approach. Bone Joint J. 2014;96-B(12):1618–22. https://doi.org/10.1302/0301-620X.96B12.34256.

74. Abitbol JJ, Gendron D, Laurin CA, Beaulieu MA. Gluteal nerve damage following total hip arthroplasty. A prospective analysis. J Arthroplast. 1990;5(4):319–22.

75. Wong M, Vijayanathan S, Kirkham B. Sacroiliitis presenting as sciatica. Rheumatology (Oxford). 2005;44(10):1323–4.

76. Crum-Cianflone NF. Bacterial, fungal, parasitic, and viral myositis. Clin Microbiol Rev. 2008;21:473–94.

77. Kraniotis P, Marangos M, Lekkou A. Brucellosis presenting as piriformis myositis: a case report. J Med Case Rep. 2011;5:125.

78. Chiedozi LC. Pyomyositis. Review of 205 cases in 112 patients. Am J Surg. 1979;137(2):255–9.

79. Dailey AT, Rondina MT, Townsend JJ. Sciatic nerve sarcoidosis: utility of magnetic resonance peripheral nerve imaging and treatment with radiation therapy. J Neurosurg. 2004;100(5):956–9.

80. Dalmau J. Carcinoma associated paraneoplastic peripheral neuropathy. J Neurol Neurosurg Psychiatry. 1999;67(1):4.

81. Bower EB, Smullens SN, Parke WW. Clinical aspects of persistent sciatic artery: report of two cases and review of the literature. Surgery. 1977;81(5):588–95.

82. Ishida K, Imamaki M, Ishida A. A ruptured aneurysm in persistent sciatic artery: a case report. J Vasc Surg. 2005;42(3):556–8.

83. Mousa A, Rapp Parker A, Emmett MK. Endovascular treatment of symptomatic persistent sciatic artery aneurysm: a case report and review of literature. Vasc Endovasc Surg. 2010;44(4):312–4.

84. Melikoglu MA, Kocabas H, Sezer I. Internal iliac artery pseudoaneurysm: an unusual cause of sciatica and lumbosacral plexopathy. Am J Phys Med Rehabil. 2008;87(8):681–3.

85. Kuma S, Mii S, Masaki I, Koike M, Nakahara I. Arteriovenous malformation arising on persistent sciatic vessels. Ann Vasc Surg. 2010;24(2):256.e1–3.

86. Berthelot JM, Pillet JC, Mitard D. Buttock claudication disclosing a thrombosis of the superior left gluteal artery: report of a case diagnosed by a selective arteriography of the iliac artery, and cured by per-cutaneous stenting. Joint Bone Spine. 2007;74(3):289–91.

87. Di Martino A, Papapietro N, Denaro V. Sciatic nerve compression by a gluteal vein varicosity. Spine J. 2014;14(8):1797.

88. Maniker A, Thurmond J, Padberg FT Jr, Blacksin M, Vingan R. Traumatic venous varix causing sciatic neuropathy: case report. Neurosurgery. 2004;55(5):1224.

89. Borghi C, Dell'Atti L. Pelvic congestion syndrome: the current state of the literature. Arch Gynecol Obstet. 2016;293(2):291–301.

90. Lemos N, Marques RM, Kamergorodsky G. Vascular entrapment of the sciatic plexus causing catamenial sciatica and urinary symptoms. Int Urogynecol J. 2016;27(2):317–9.

91. Al-Khodairy AT, Gerber BE, Praz G. Adenomyosis: an unusual cause of sciatic pain. Eur Spine J. 1995;4(5):317–9.

92. Al-Khodairy AW, Bovay P, Gobelet C. Sciatica in the female patient: anatomical considerations, aetiology and review of the literature. Eur Spine J. 2007;16(6):721–31.

93. Ghezzi L, Arighi A, Pietroboni AM. Sciatic endometriosis presenting as periodic (catamenial) sciatic radiculopathy. J Neurol. 2012;259(7):1470–1.

94. Kulowski J. Unusual causes of low back pain and sciatica during pregnancy. Am J Obstet Gynecol. 1962;84:627–30.

95. Roux A, Tréguier C, Bruneau B. Localized hypertrophic neuropathy of the sciatic nerve in children: MRI findings. Pediatr Radiol. 2012;42(8):952–8.

96. Johnson PC, Kline DG. Localized hypertrophic neuropathy: possible focal perineurial barrier defect. Acta Neuropathol. 1989;77(5):514–8.

97. Ma M, Guillerman RP. Paradoxic hypertrophy of the sciatic nerve. Pediatr Radiol. 2010;40(Suppl 1):S177.

98. Masuda N, Hayashi H, Tanabe H. Nerve root and sciatic trunk enlargement in Déjérine-Sottas disease: MRI appearances. Neuroradiology. 1992;35(1):36–7.

99. Torigian DA, Siegelman ES. CT findings of pelvic lipomatosis of nerve. AJR Am J Roentgenol. 2005;184(3 Suppl):S94–6.

100. Mahan MA, Howe BM, Amrami KK, Spinner RJ. Occult radiological effects of lipomatosis of the lumbosacral plexus. Skelet Radiol. 2014;43(7):963–8.

101. Murphey MD, Smith WS, Smith SE, Kransdorf MJ. Imaging of musculoskeletal neurogenic tumors: radiologic-pathologic correlation. Radiographics. 1999;19(5):1253–80.

102. Goddyn C, Passuti N, Leconte R, Redon H, Gouin F. Sciatic nerve compression related to ossification of the sacrospinous ligament secondary to pelvic balance abnormalities. Orthop Traumatol Surg Res. 2009;95(8):645–8.

103. Fathi I, Sakr M. Review of tumoral calcinosis: a rare clinico-pathological entity. World J Clin Cases. 2014;2(9):409–14.

104. Baek D, Lee SE, Kim WJ, Jeon S. Greater trochanteric pain syndrome due to tumoral calcinosis in a patient with chronic kidney disease. Pain Physician. 2014;17(6):E775–82.

105. Shaukat YM, Malik EF, Al Rashid M, Cannon SR. Large tumoral calcinosis in the gluteal region: a case report. Ortop Traumatol Rehabil. 2013;15(5):495–9.

106. Williams JB, Youngberg RA, Bui-Mansfield LT, Pitcher JD. MR imaging of skeletal muscle metastases. AJR Am J Roentgenol. 1997;168(2):555–7.

107. Ergun T. Bilateral sciatica secondary to mass lesions in the gluteal muscles. Intramuscular metastasis. J Clin Neurosci. 2008;15(12):1388–426.

108. Roncaroli F, Poppi M, Riccioni L, Frank F. Primary non-Hodgkin's lymphoma of the sciatic nerve followed by localization in the central nervous system: case report and review of the literature. Neurosurgery. 1997;40(3):618–21.

109. Stewart JD. The piriformis syndrome is overdiagnosed. Muscle Nerve. 2003;28(5):644–6.

110. Chhabra A, Andreisek G, Soldatos T. MR neurography: past, present, and future. AJR Am J Roentgenol. 2011;197(3):583–91.

111. Kasprian G, Amann G, Panotopoulos J. Peripheral nerve tractography in soft tissue tumors: a preliminary 3-tesla diffusion tensor magnetic resonance imaging study. Muscle Nerve. 2015;51(3):338–45.

112. Skorpil M, Karlsson M, Nordell A. Peripheral nerve diffusion tensor imaging. Magn Reson Imaging. 2004;22(5):743–5.

113. Wilson JJ, Furukawa M. Evaluation of the patient with hip pain. Am Fam Physician. 2014;89(1):27–34.

114. Sutter R, Pfirrmann CW. Atypical hip impingement. AJR Am J Roentgenol. 2013;201(3):437–42.

115. Ali AM, Teh J, Whitwell D, Ostlere S. Ischiofemoral impingement: a retrospective analysis of cases in a specialist orthopaedic centre over a four-year period. Hip Int. 2013;23(3):263–8.

116. López-Sánchez MC, Armesto Pérez V, Montero Furelos LÁ, Vázquez-Rodríguez TR, Calvo Arrojo G, Díaz Román TM. Ischiofemoral impingement: hip pain of infrequent cause. Reumatol Clin. 2013;9(3):186–7.

117. Maraş Özdemir Z, Aydıngöz Ü, Görmeli CA, Sağır Kahraman A. Ischiofemoral space on MRI in an asymptomatic population: normative width measurements and soft tissue signal variations. Eur Radiol. 2015;25(8):2246–53.

118. Sproul RC, Reynolds HM, Lotz JC, Ries MD. Relationship between femoral head size and distance to lesser trochanter. Clin Orthop Relat Res. 2007;461:122–4.

119. Johnson KA. Impingement of the lesser trochanter on the ischial ramus after total hip arthroplasty. Report of three cases. J Bone Joint Surg Am. 1977;59:268–9.

120. Finnoff JT, Bond JR, Collins MS, Sellon JL, Hollman JH, Wempe MK, Smith J. Variability of the ischiofemoral space relative to femur position: an ultrasound study. PM&R. 2015;7(9):930–7. https://doi.org/10.1016/j.pmrj.2015.03.010.

121. Hatem MA, Palmer IJ, Martin HD. Diagnosis and 2-year outcomes of endoscopic treatment for ischiofemoral impingement. Arthroscopy. 2015;31(2):239–46.

122. Tennant S, Kinmont C, Lamb G, Gedroyc W, Hunt DM. The use of dynamic interventional MRI in developmental dysplasia of the hip. J Bone Joint Surg Br. 1999;81(3):392–7.

123. Singer A, Clifford P, Tresley J, Jose J, Subhawong T. Ischiofemoral impingement and the utility of full-range-of-motion magnetic resonance imaging in its detection. Am J Orthop (Belle Mead NJ). 2014;43(12):548–51.

124. Kassarjian A. Signal abnormalities in the quadratus femoris muscle: tear or impingement? AJR Am J Roentgenol. 2008;190(6):W379. author reply W380-1.

125. Gujar S, Vikani S, Parmar J, Bondre KV. A correlation between femoral neck shaft angle to femoral neck length. Int J Biomed Adv Res. https://doi.org/10.7439/ijbar.v4i5.354. ISSN: 2229-3809 (Online).

126. Bredella MA, Azevedo DC, Oliveira AL, Simeone FJ, Chang CY, Stubbs AJ, Torriani M. Pelvic morphology in ischiofemoral impingement. Skelet Radiol. 2015;44(2):249–53.

127. Stevens PM, Coleman SS. Coxa breva: its pathogenesis and a rationale for its management. J Pediatr Orthop. 1985;5(5):515–21.

128. Sussman WI, Han E, Schuenke MD. Quantitative assessment of the ischiofemoral space and evidence of degenerative changes in the quadratus femoris muscle. Surg Radiol Anat. 2013;35:273–81.

129. Delaunay S, Dussault RG, Kaplan PA, Alford BA. Radiographic measurements of dysplastic adult hips. Skelet Radiol. 1997;26(2):75–81.

130. Tomás A, Domínguez R, Veras M, Roche S, Merino X, Pineda U. Ischiofemoral impingement: spectrum of findings. European Congress of Radiology, 2013/C-1005. Scientific exhibit. https://doi.org/10.1594/ecr2013/C-1005.

131. De Sa D, Alradwan H, Cargnelli S, Thawer Z, Simunovic N, Cadet E, Bonin N, Larson C, Ayeni OR. Extra-articular hip impingement: a systematic review examining operative treatment of psoas, subspine, ischiofemoral, and greater trochanteric/pelvic impingement. Arthroscopy. 2014;30(8):1026–41.

132. Tsatalas T, Giakas G, Spyropoulos G. The effects of muscle damage on walking biomechanics are speed-dependent. Eur J Appl Physiol. 2010;110(5):977–88.

133. Vital JM, García Suárez A, Sauri Barraza JC. Sagittal balance in spine disorders. Rev Ortop Traumatol. 2006;50:447–53.

134. Miokovic T, Armbrecht G, Felsenberg D, Belavy DL. Differential atrophy of the postero-lateral hip musculature during prolonged bedrest and the influence of exercise countermeasures. J Appl Physiol. 2011;110(4):926–34.

135. Hayat Z, Konan S, Pollock R. Ischiofemoral impingement resulting from a chronic avulsion injury of the hamstrings. BMJ Case Rep. 2014;25:bcr2014204017.

136. Singer AD, Subhawong TK, Jose J, Tresley J, Clifford PD. Ischiofemoral impingement syndrome: a meta-analysis. Skelet Radiol. 2015;44(6):831–7.

137. Viala P, Vanel D, Larbi A, Cyteval C, Laredo JD. Bilateral ischiofemoral impingement in a patient with hereditary multiple exostoses. Skelet Radiol. 2012;41(12):1637–40.

138. Mehta M, White LM, Knapp T, Kandel RA, Wunder JS, Bell RS. MR imaging of symptomatic osteochondromas with pathological correlation. Skelet Radiol. 1998;27(8):427–33.

139. Uri DS, Dalinka MK, Kneeland JB. Muscle impingement: MR imaging of a painful complication of osteochondromas. Skelet Radiol. 1996;25(7):689–92.

140. Patti JW, Ouellette H, Bredella MA, Torriani M. Impingement of lesser trochanter on ischium as a potential cause for hip pain. Skelet Radiol. 2008;37:939–41.

141. Backer MW, Lee KS, Blankenbaker DG, Kijowski R, Keene JS. Correlation of ultrasound-guided corticosteroid injection of the quadratus femoris with MRI findings of ischiofemoral impingement. AJR Am J Roentgenol. 2014;203(3):589–93.

142. Kim WJ, Shin HY, Koo GH, Park HG, Ha YC, Park YH. Ultrasound-guided Prolotherapy with Polydeoxyribonucleotide sodium in Ischiofemoral impingement syndrome. Pain Pract. 2014;14(7):649–55.

143. Blankenbaker DG, Tuite MJ. Non-femoroacetabular impingement. Semin Musculoskelet Radiol. 2013;17(3):279–85.

144. Monahan E, Shimada K. Verifying the effectiveness of a computer- aided navigation system for arthroscopic hip surgery. Westwood JD, Haluck RS, Hoffman HM, et al. medicine meets virtual reality 16–parallel, combinatorial, convergent: Nextmed by design. Stud Health Technol Informl. 2008;132:302–7.

145. Lee S, Kim I, Lee SM, Lee J. Ischiofemoral impingement syndrome. Ann Rehabil Med. 2013;37(1):143–6.

146. Ata AM, Yavuz H, Kaymak B, Ozcan HN, Ergen B, Özçakar L. Ischiofemoral impingement revisited: what physiatrists need to know in short. Am J Phys Med Rehabil. 2014;93(12):1104.

147. Cho KH, Lee SM, Lee YH, Suh KJ, Kim SM, Shin MJ, Jang HW. Non-infectious ischiogluteal bursitis: MRI findings. Korean J Radiol. 2004;5(4):280–6.

148. Robinson P, White LM, Agur A, Wunder J, Bell RS. Obturator externus bursa: anatomic origin and MR imaging features of pathologic involvement. Radiology. 2003;228(1):230–4.

149. Stibbe EP. Complete absence of the quadratus femoris. Anatomical notes. J Anat. 1929;64(Pt 1):97.

150. O'Brien SD, Bui-Mansfield LT. MRI of quadratus femoris muscle tear: another cause of hip pain. AJR Am J Roentgenol. 2007;189(5):1185–9.

151. Klinkert P Jr, Porte RJ, de Rooij TP, de Vries AC. Quadratus femoris tendinitis as a cause of groin pain. Br J Sports Med. 1997;31(4):348–9.

152. Lewis PB, Ruby D, Bush-Joseph CA. Muscle soreness and delayed-onset muscle soreness. Clin Sports Med. 2012;31(2):255–62.

153. Linklater JM, Hamilton B, Carmichael J, Orchard J, Wood DG. Hamstring injuries: anatomy, imaging, and intervention. Semin Musculoskelet Radiol. 2010;14(2):131–61.

154. Valle X, Tol JL, Hamilton B. Hamstring muscle injuries, a rehabilitation protocol purpose. Asian J Sports Med. 2015;6(4):e25411.

155. Heiderscheit BC, Sherry MA, Silder A. Hamstring strain injuries: recommendations for diagnosis, rehabilitation, and injury prevention. J Orthop Sports Phys Ther. 2010;40(2):67–81.

156. Hodgson RJ, O'Connor PJ, Grainger AJ. Tendon and ligament imaging. Br J Radiol. 2012;85(1016):1157–72.

157. Lempainen L, Sarimo J, Mattila K, Heikkilä J, Orava S, Puddu G. Distal tears of the hamstring muscles: review of the literature and our results of surgical treatment. Br J Sports Med. 2007;41(2):80–3. discussion 83.

158. Broadley P, Offiah AC. Hip and groin pain in the child athlete. Semin Musculoskelet Radiol. 2014;18(5):478–88.

159. Izadpanah K, Jaeger M, Maier D, Südkamp NP, Ogon P. Preoperative planning of calcium deposit removal in calcifying tendinitis of the rotator cuff – possible contribution of computed tomography, ultrasound and conventional X-ray. BMC Musculoskelet Disord. 2014;15:385.

160. Gosens T, Hofstee DJ. Calcifying tendinitis of the shoulder: advances in imaging and management. Curr Rheumatol Rep. 2009;11(2):129–34.

161. Pfirrmann CW, Chung CB, Theumann NH, Trudell DJ, Resnick D. Greater trochanter of the hip: attachment of the abductor mechanism and a complex of three bursae-MR imaging and MR bursography in cadavers and MR imaging in asymptomatic volunteers. Radiology. 2001;221:469–77.

162. Woodley SJ, Mercer SR, Nicholson HD. Morphology of the bursae associated with the greater trochanter of the femur. J Bone Joint Surg Am. 2008;90(2):284–94.

163. Swezey RL. Obturator internus bursitis: a common factor in low back pain. Orthopedics. 1993;16:783–5.

164. Hruby S, Ebmer J, Dellon AL, Aszmann OC. Anatomy of pudendal nerve at urogenital diaphragm – new critical site for nerve entrapment. Urology. 2005;66(5):949–52.

165. Martinoli C, Miguel-Perez M, Padua L. Imaging of neuropathies about the hip. Eur J Radiol. 2013;82(1):17–26.

166. Loukas M, Louis RG, Hallner B, et al. Anatomical and surgical considerations of the sacrotuberous ligament and its relevance in pudendal nerve entrapment syndrome. Surg Radiol Anat. 2006;28:163–9.

167. Filler AG. Diagnosis and treatment of pudendal nerve entrapment syndrome subtypes: imaging, injections and minimal access surgery. Neurosurg Focus. 2009;26:1–14.

168. Hough DM, Wittenberg KH, Pawlina W, et al. Chronic perineal pain caused by pudendal nerve entrapment: anatomy and CT-guided perineu-

ral injection technique. AJR Am J Roentgenol. 2003;181:561–7.
169. Stecco A, Gilliar W, Hill R, Fullerton B, Stecco C. The anatomical and functional relation between gluteus maximus and fascia lata. J Bodyw Mov Ther. 2013;17(4):512–7.
170. Thomason HC 3rd, Bos GD, Renner JB. Calcifying tendinitis of the gluteus maximus. Am J Orthop (Belle Mead NJ). 2001;30(10):757–8.
171. Kim HT, Ahn JM, Hur JO, Lee JS, Cheon SJ. Reconstruction of acetabular posterior wall fractures. Clin Orthop Surg. 2011;3(2):114–20.

Guided Injections of the Posterior Hip

6

Leon R. Toye

Introduction

After a detailed clinical examination has been performed, and proximal nerve root problems are ruled out, directed injections targeting sites of possible pain generation can be used to confirm clinical suspicions and potentially provide pain relief. Image guidance helps improve the accuracy and safety of these injections. In our practice, these procedures are performed by the musculoskeletal radiology department.

Pudendal Nerve Perineural Injections

Relevant Anatomy

The **pudendal nerve** is predominantly a sensory nerve arising from the sacral plexus (S2, S3, S4) ultimately terminating in three branches (inferior rectal, perineal, dorsal nerve of the penis/clitoris) [1] (Fig. 6.1a). The internal pudendal artery and a venous plexus accompany the nerve, creating a pudendal neurovascular bundle [2]. After taking origin from the sacral nerve roots, the pudendal nerve exits the pelvis through the

inferior aspect of the greater sciatic foramen, briefly entering the gluteal region while it wraps around the *ischial spine*, between the sacrotuberous (superficial) and sacrospinous (deep) ligaments [3] (Fig. 6.1b). The nerve then reenters the pelvis and enters the perineum through the lesser sciatic foramen, coursing through the ischioanal fossa, via the *pudendal canal*. The pudendal canal (also known as Alcock's canal) is a fascial tunnel along the medial margin of the obturator internus muscle, within the ischoanal fossa [1, 2] Fig. 6.1c).

Terminally, the nerve divides into three branches: The first **inferior rectal nerve** branch takes off within or just proximal to the pudendal canal, providing sensation to the skin around the anus. The second **perineal nerve** branch contains a deep motor portion and two sensory medial and lateral scrotal/labial branches. The third **dorsal nerve of the penis/clitoris** runs along skin of the penis/clitoris innervating the overlying skin [4].

The pudendal nerve is prone to entrapment at the pudendal (Alcock's) canal (due to compression at the falciform ligament or thickening at the obturator fascia) and at the ischial spine between the sacrospinous and sacrotuberous ligaments [3, 5]. The majority of compression is reported at the pudendal canal [4]. One author [6] describes four major types of pudendal nerve entrapment: type I (2.1%) exclusively at the level of the piriformis muscle, type II (4.8%) at the level of the ischial spine and sacrotuberous ligament, type III (79.9%) at the pudendal

L. R. Toye, MD
Radsource, Brentwood, TN, USA
e-mail: ltoye@radsource.us

© Springer International Publishing AG, part of Springer Nature 2019
H. D. Martin, J. Gómez-Hoyos (eds.), *Posterior Hip Disorders*,
https://doi.org/10.1007/978-3-319-78040-5_6

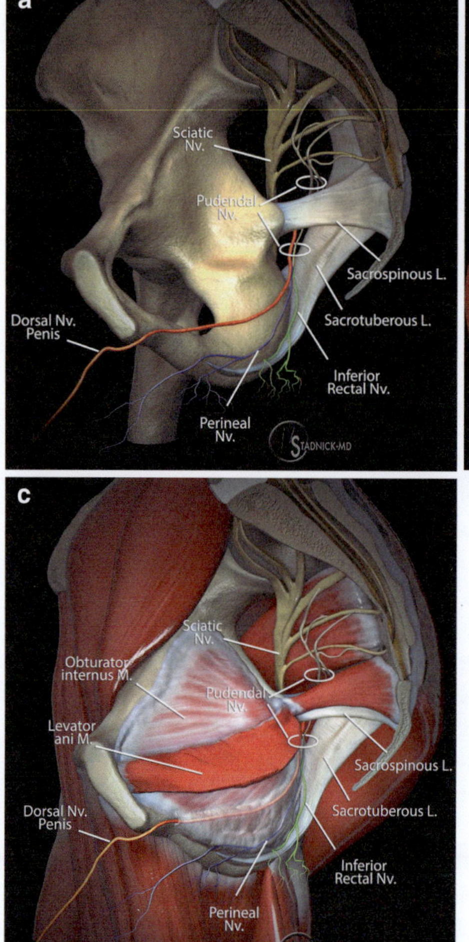

Fig. 6.1 (**a**) Pudendal nerve anatomy. The pudendal nerve arises from the S2, S3, S4 sacral plexus ultimately terminating in three branches: inferior rectal, perineal, dorsal nerve of the penis/clitoris. Courtesy of Dr. Michael Stadnick. (**b**) Pudendal nerve anatomy. The pudendal nerve exits the pelvis through the inferior aspect of the greater sciatic foramen, briefly entering the gluteal region, while it wraps around the *ischial spine*, between the sacro-tuberous (superficial) and sacrospinous (deep) ligaments. Courtesy of Dr. Michael Stadnick. (**c**) Pudendal nerve anatomy. The pudendal nerve reenters the pelvis and enters the perineum through the lesser sciatic foramen, coursing through the ischioanal fossa, via the *pudendal canal* (Alcock's canal), a fascial tunnel along the medial margin of the obturator internus muscle, within the ischoanal fossa. Courtesy of Dr. Michael Stadnick

(Alcock's) canal on the medial surface of the obturator internus muscle, and type IV (13%) involving distal branches of the pudendal nerve.

Injection Technique

Pudendal nerve blockade locations focus on the sites of typical pudendal nerve entrapment: near the ischial spine (between the sacrotuberous and sacrospinous ligaments) and within the pudendal canal. Some authors will first begin at the ischial spine (optionally repeating one or more times), with subsequent (optional or routine) injections at the pudendal canal [2, 4, 7]. One group of authors advocate performing all injections at the pudendal canal only, believing their pudendal canal injectate typically also backfills cranially into the space between the sacrotuberous and sacrospinous ligaments [3]. In our practice, we currently select the site of blockade based on clinical symptomatology. If the patient reports symptoms primarily related to the perianal region (suggesting a more proximal nerve entrapment involving the inferior rectal branch), we will perform blockade near the ischial spine. If the patient reports symptoms primarily related to the more distal perineal or penile/clitoral nerve branches, we will perform blockade at the pudendal canal/ obturator internus. Some authors advocate routinely performing repeat injections spaced 4 weeks apart [2], whereas others advocated performing repeat injections dictated by symptomatology [3, 4]. Injections may be done unilaterally or bilaterally, depending on symptoms. In our practice, unilateral injections are typically performed.

Imaging modalities used for peripudendal needle guidance include CT, ultrasound, fluoroscopy, and MRI. CT is our modality of choice based on reproducible accuracy and anatomic visualization.

Peripudendal Nerve Injection Near the Ischial Spine

Pudendal perineural injection near the level of the ischial spine targets the nerve more proximally. The patient is placed prone in the CT gantry, and localizer scout images are obtained (Fig. 6.2b). Radiopaque surface localizer markers are placed on the patient's skin, and planning 2.5 mm contiguous axial CT images are obtained from the level of the acetabular roof through the symphysis joint. Next, the patient's skin is marked at an entry point overlying the target near the ischial spine. The CT scanner is then placed into low-dose biopsy mode. A sterile field is then created, and local subcutaneous anesthesia is administered with 1% lidocaine. A 22-guage needle is then advanced under CT guidance immediately adjacent to the pudendal neurovascular bundle, just medial to the caudal portion of the ischial spine, to a small interligamentous space fat plane between the sacrotuberous (superficial) and sacrospinous (deep) ligaments (Fig. 6.2a and c). A small amount (e.g., 1 cc) of iodinated contrast (e.g., Isovue or Omnipaque) may be used to demonstrate perineural coating in the interligamentous space (Fig. 6.2c). Next, we typically inject a mixture of 40 mg (1 cc) methylprednisolone (Kenalog) and 2 cc of 0.25% bupivacaine.

Following the injection, we prefer to observe the patient for 30–45 min to monitor for complications and to assess the effects of the bupivacaine anesthetic. Commonly, patients will report perineal anesthesia postinjection. Potential complication risks include bleeding, infection,

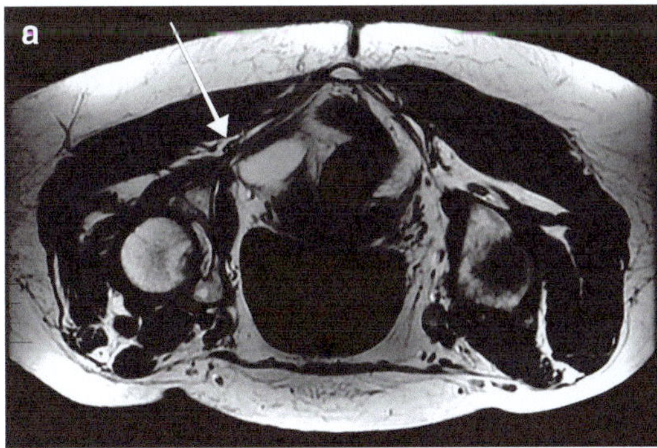

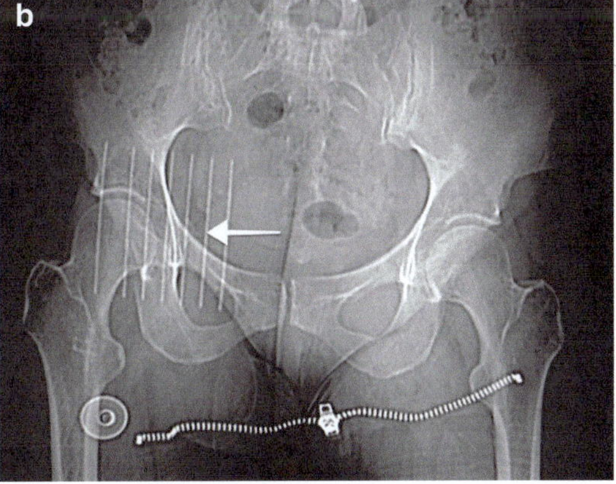

Fig. 6.2 (**a**) Pudendal perineural injection near the ischial spine. Axial T1-weighted MRI image at the level of the ischial tuberosity demonstrates the pudendal neurovascular bundle (arrow), just medial to the ischial spine, located between the sacrotuberous (superficial) and sacrospinous (deep) ligaments. (**b**) Pudendal perineural injection near the ischial spine. CT scout image is obtained, and localization surface markers are placed overlying the ischial spine (arrow). (**c**) Pudendal perineural injection near the ischial spine. Using axial CT guidance, a 22-gauge needle is placed just medial to the ischial spine. A small amount of contrast was injected, surrounding the pudendal neurovascular bundle

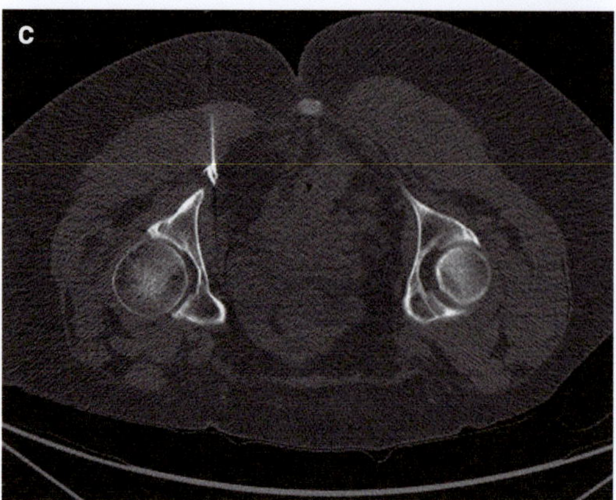

Fig. 6.2 (continued)

contrast allergy, vascular injury, and neurologic injury. Transient anesthesia of the sciatic nerve has also been reported, resulting in temporary leg weakness resolving in approximately 6 h [4].

Peripudendal Nerve Injection Pudendal Canal (Obturator Internus)

Pudendal perineural injection near the level of the pudendal (Alcock's) canal targets the nerve more distally. The patient is placed prone in the CT gantry, and localizer scout images are obtained (Fig. 6.3a). Radiopaque surface localizer markers are placed on the patient's skin, and planning 2.5 mm contiguous axial CT images are obtained from the level of the symphysis pubis. The CT scanner is then placed into low-dose biopsy mode. Next, the patient's skin is marked at an entry point overlying the target near the obturator internus muscle. A sterile field is then created, and local subcutaneous anesthesia is administered with 1% lidocaine. A 22G needle is then advanced transgluteally under CT guidance. The pudendal neurovascular bundle target is within the pudendal (Alcock's) canal, just medial/ superficial to the obturator internus muscle, lateral to the obturator fascia (Fig. 6.3b). A small amount (e.g., 1 cc) of iodinated contrast (e.g., Isovue or Omnipaque) may be used to demonstrate perineural coating in the pudendal canal.

Next, we typically inject a mixture of 40 mg (1 cc) methylprednisolone (Kenalog) and 2 cc of 0.25% bupivacaine.

As with injections near the ischial spine, we prefer to observe the patient for 30–45 min to monitor for complications and to assess the effects of the bupivacaine anesthetic. Potential complication risks again include bleeding, infection, contrast allergy, vascular injury, and neurologic injury. Transient anesthesia of the sciatic nerve is also possible.

Piriformis Injection

Relevant Anatomy

The piriformis muscle is a flat pyramidal-shaped muscle which originates from the anterior sacrum at the levels of S2–S4, the gluteal surface of the ilium near the iliac spine, and from the SI joint capsule [8]. The muscle exits the pelvis laterally through the greater sciatic foramen, inserting on the medial aspect of the femoral greater trochanter (Figs. 6.4a and b). Below the piriformis muscle courses the sciatic nerve, posterior femoral cutaneous nerve, and gluteal neurovascular bundle. The piriformis is innervated by branches of L5, S1, and S2. Several anatomic variations of the piriformis and sciatic nerve exist, whereby the sciatic nerve (or a divided branch) may course through or above the piriformis muscle [8].

The piriformis muscle may become inflamed, spasmodic, or stretched due to trauma, surgery, anatomic variations, and leg length discrepancy [8]. In this situation, inflammatory mediators such as prostaglandin, histamine, bradykinin, and serotonin may be released by the muscle causing inflammation of the adjacent sciatic nerve, resulting in buttock pain and sciatica [8].

Injection Technique

Injection of the piriformis muscle has been described with the assistance of fluoroscopy, CT, ultrasound, MRI, and nerve stimulation [8–13]. In our practice, we typically use fluoroscopy or CT.

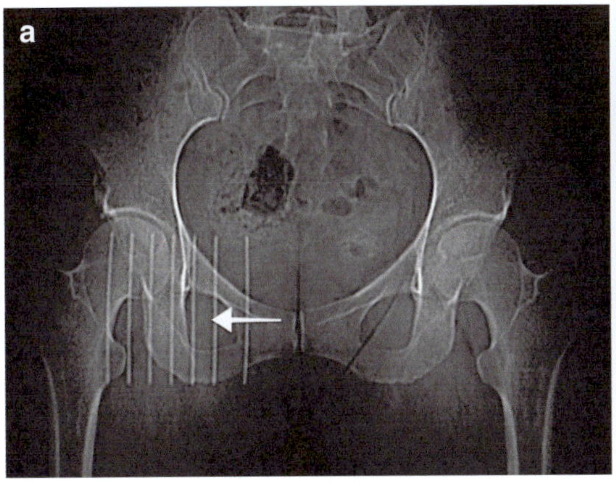
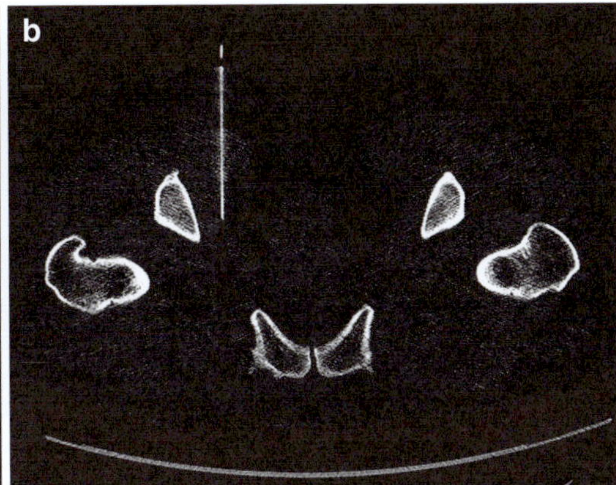

Fig. 6.3 (**a**) Pudendal perineural injection at the pudendal canal. CT scout image is obtained, and localization surface markers are placed near the level of the obturator foramen (arrow). (**b**) Pudendal perineural injection at the pudendal canal. Using axial CT guidance, a 22G needle is guided toward the pudendal (Alcock's) canal, along the superficial obturator internus muscle belly, medial to the ischial tuberosity

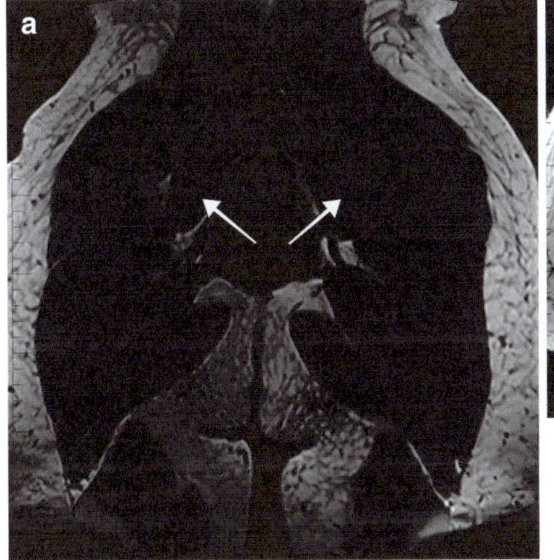
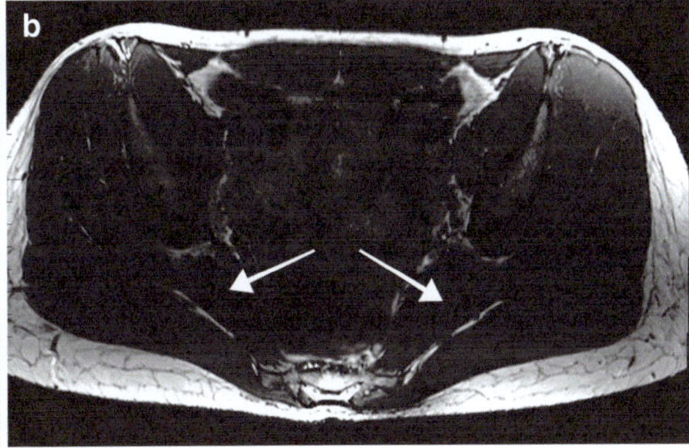

Fig. 6.4 Piriformis muscle on MRI. Coronal (**a**) and axial (**b**) T1-weighted MRI images demonstrate the piriformis muscles (arrows). The piriformis muscle originates (in part) from the anterior S2–S4 sacrum, exiting the pelvis laterally through the greater sciatic foramen, inserting on the medial aspect of the greater trochanter

Fluoroscopic Injection of the Piriformis

For fluoroscopic injection, the patient is placed in prone position on the fluoroscopy table, and scout imaging is performed focusing on the inferior aspect of the sacroiliac joint, of the symptomatic side (Fig. 6.5a).

Next, a skin surface entry point is determined, using fluoroscopy guidance, targeting a position, just lateral to the inferior aspect of the SI joint (Fig. 6.5b). A temporary mark is drawn on the patient's skin.

A sterile field is then created, and local subcutaneous anesthesia is administered with 1% lidocaine. A 22G needle (3.5″ or 5″ depending on patient size) is then advanced, using fluoroscopic guidance, targeting the posterior iliac cortical surface, just lateral to the inferior aspect of the SI joint (Fig. 6.5c). This area may be somewhat sensitive due to periosteal innervation, and patients usually appreciate advance notice before abutting the ilium.

After establishing the depth of the posterior ilium, the needle is slightly withdrawn and redirected caudally into the piriformis muscle (Fig. 6.5d). The target site within the piriformis muscle lies approximately 1 cm lateral, 1 cm inferior, and 1 cm deeper than the inferior SI joint [9]. Some practitioners opt for a more lateral (2 cm lateral to the inferior SI joint) placement of the needle tip within the muscle, striving to be closer in proximity to the sciatic nerve [8]. When the piriformis muscle is entered, sometimes a difference in resistance can be felt with the needle, perhaps related to muscle tension. It is important to monitor for any acute sciatica symptoms (e.g., electrical pain running down the back of the leg), as the goal is to land the needle within the muscle belly and not within the sciatic nerve. If sciatic symptoms are experienced, the needle is retracted back and repositioned into the muscle belly.

Once the needle tip has arrived at the target, aspiration is performed to ensure the needle is not intravascular. Confirmation of intramuscular placement is then obtained with a small amount (1–2 cc) of iodinated X-ray contrast (e.g., Isovue or Omnipaque). The contrast should flow away from the needle, along the muscle fascicles, diagonally along the orientation of the piriformis (Fig. 6.5e).

Next, we typically inject a mixture of 40 mg (1 cc) methylprednisolone (Kenalog) and 2 cc of 0.25% bupivacaine. If desired, postinjection imaging can be obtained to demonstrate the distribution pattern of the injectate (Fig. 6.5f).

CT-Guided Injection of the Piriformis

CT injection of the piriformis is relatively straightforward and similar to previously described techniques. Radiopaque surface localizer markers are placed on the patient's skin. Planning scout (Fig. 6.6a) and subsequent 2.5 mm contiguous axial CT images are obtained. The CT scanner is then placed into low-dose biopsy mode.

Next, the patient's skin is marked at an entry point overlying the target near the piriformis muscle. A sterile field is then created, and local subcutaneous anesthesia is administered with 1% lidocaine. A 22G needle is then advanced transgluteally under CT guidance into the posterior aspect of the piriformis muscle belly (Fig. 6.6b). The injectate is the same as in the fluoroscopic method, previously described.

Following the piriformis injection, we prefer to observe the patient for 30–45 min to monitor for complications and to assess the effects of the bupivacaine anesthetic. Potential complication risks include bleeding, infection, contrast allergy, vascular injury, and neurologic injury. Transient anesthesia of the sciatic nerve resulting in temporary leg weakness is also possible.

Sacroiliac Joint Injection

Relevant Anatomy

The sacroiliac (SI) joints are complex and contain both synovial and syndesmotic components. The upper portion of the SI joints is syndesmotic, containing fibrous ligaments; the inferior portion of the SI joints is synovial, containing a synovial capsule and articular cartilage. The inferiorly located synovial portion of the joint is therefore the target of typical SI joint injections. The SI joints often have a multiplanar orientation, irregular joint gap, facultative accessory auricular surfaces, osteophytes, and partial ankylosis which make blind and fluoroscopic-guided injections difficult [14].

Injection Technique

Injection of the SI joints has been described with the assistance of fluoroscopy, CT, ultrasound, and MRI [14–18]. In our practice, we typically use CT due to the direct cross-sectional visualization of the complex SI joint anatomy and availability of the modality. The patient is placed in prone position in the CT gantry, and scout images are obtained with surface markers placed along the dorsal skin surface near the level of the palpable posterior superior iliac spine (Fig. 6.7a).

Next, 3 mm axial CT images are obtained through the level of the SI joints to select an

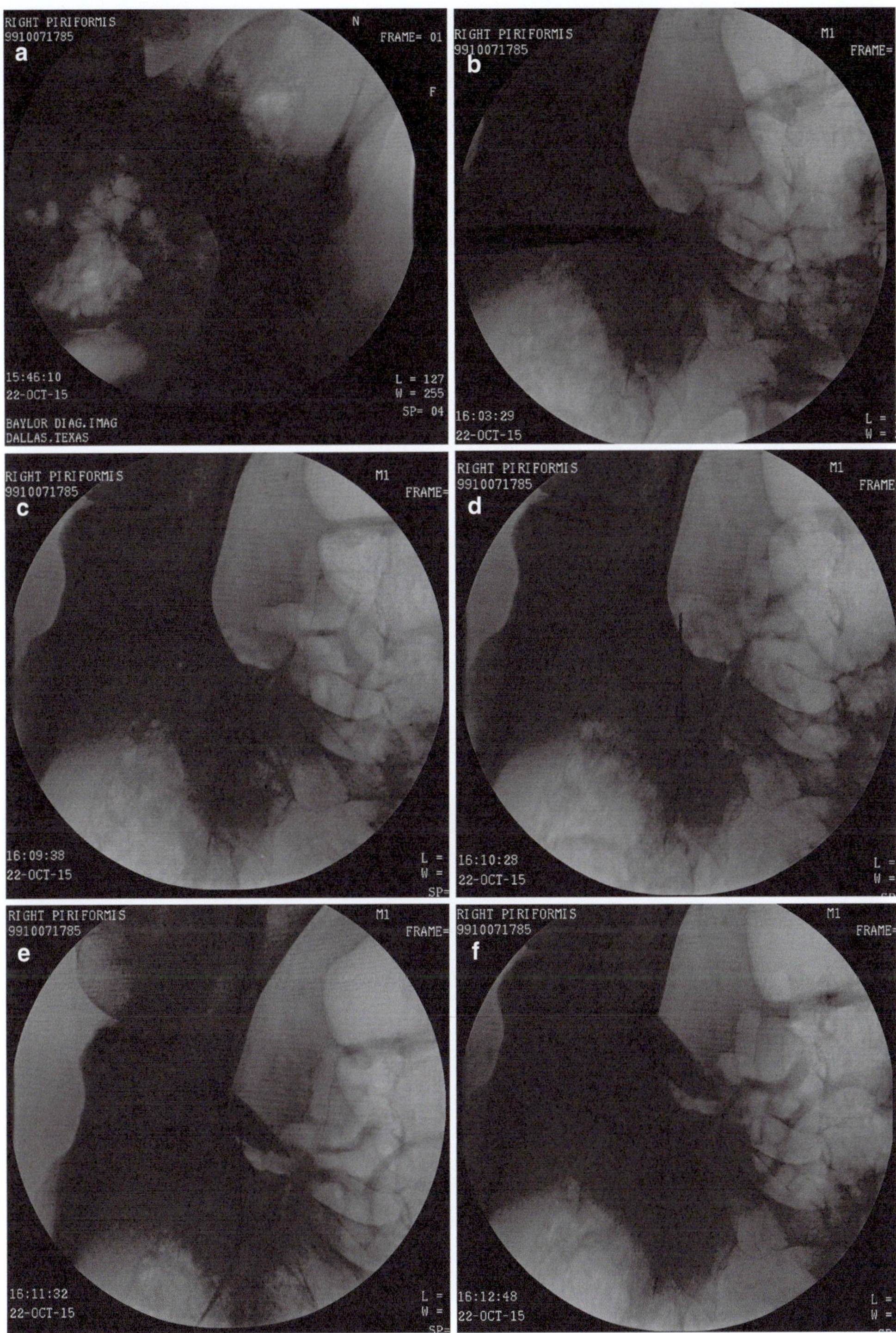

Fig. 6.5 (**a**) Fluoroscopic piriformis injection. Scout image targeting the inferior SI joint. (**b**) Fluoroscopic piriformis injection. Initial localization point, just lateral to the inferior SI joint. (**c**) Fluoroscopic piriformis injection. Initial advancement of 22G needle to the posterior ilium, just lateral to the SI joint. (**d**) Fluoroscopic piriformis injection. Redirection of 22G needle inferiorly into the piriformis muscle, approximately 1–2 cm lateral to the SI joint. (**e**) Fluoroscopic piriformis injection. Contrast injection demonstrating spread along the piriformis muscle. (**f**) Fluoroscopic piriformis injection. Imaging after the steroid/anesthetic mixture has been injected demonstrates expected dilution of the previously injected X-ray contrast

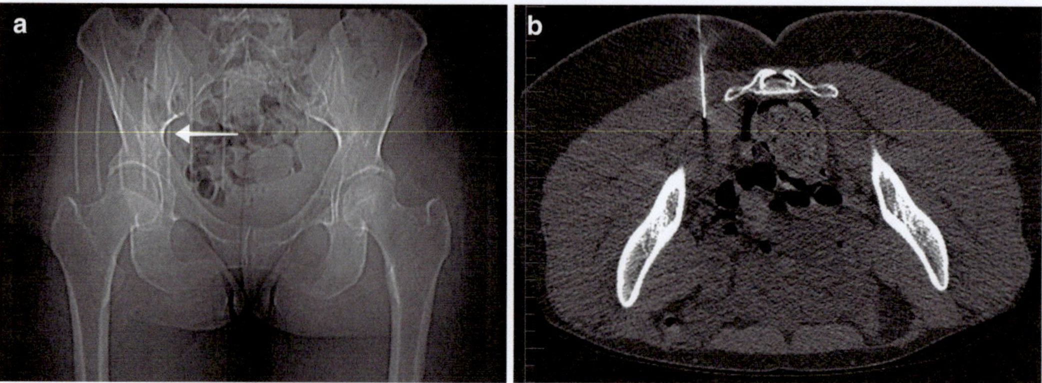

Fig. 6.6 (**a**) CT-guided piriformis injection. CT scout image is obtained, and localization surface markers are placed near the level of the greater sciatic notch (arrow). (**b**) CT-guided piriformis injection. Using axial CT guidance, a 22G needle is guided into the posterior aspect of the piriformis muscle belly

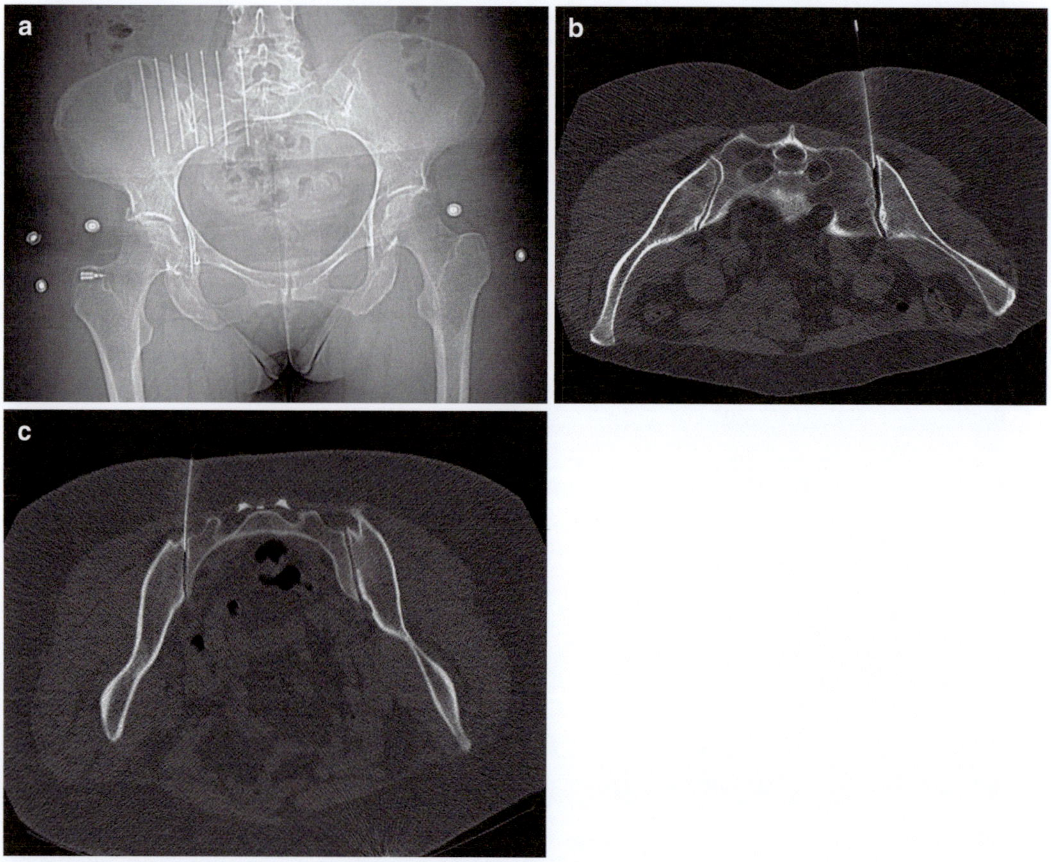

Fig. 6.7 (**a**) Sacroiliac joint injection. CT scout image is obtained, and localization surface markers are placed over the SI joint. (**b**) Sacroiliac joint injection. Using axial CT guidance, a 22G needle is guided into the SI joint. (**c**) Sacroiliac joint injection. Additional example

appropriate entry point, typically overlying the inferior third of the symptomatic SI joint, avoiding any abrupt joint curvature, ankyloses, or bridging osteophytes. After an entry point is selected, the patient's skin is marked with a temporary marker. The CT scanner is then placed into low-dose biopsy mode. A sterile field is then created, and local subcutaneous anesthesia is administered with 1% lidocaine. A 22G needle (3.5″ or 5″ depending on patient size) is then progressively advanced into the SI joint, obtaining periodic CT images (three contiguous slices at the level of the needle), after needle adjustments are performed. Contrast is typically not required with CT, as the needle can be directly visualized within the SI joint (Fig. 6.7b and c). The SI joint capacity is also fairly small, limiting the amount of fluid that can be routinely injected. Next, we typically inject a mixture of 40 mg (1 cc) methylprednisolone (Kenalog) and 1 cc of 0.25% bupivacaine. The SI joint often has significant resistance, and using a smaller-sized syringe (e.g., 3 cc) may decrease the required pressure for injection.

Following the injection, we prefer to observe the patient for 30–45 min to monitor for complications and to assess the effects of the bupivacaine anesthetic. Potential complication risks include bleeding, infection, and allergy. Transient lower extremity weakness or gait disturbance is also possible due to decreased pelvic girdle proprioception or anesthesia of the sciatic nerve.

Acknowledgment Special thanks to Michael Stadnick, MD (Radsource – Brentwood, Tennessee, USA) for creating the medical illustrations (Fig. 6.1a–c) for this chapter, used with permission.

References

1. Gajraj NM. Botulinum toxin a injection of the obturator internus muscle for chronic perineal pain. J Pain. 2005;6(5):333–7.
2. Hough DM, Wittenberg KH, Pawlina W, Maus TP, King BF, Vrtiska TJ, et al. Chronic perineal pain caused by pudendal nerve entrapment: anatomy and CT-guided perineural injection technique. Am J Roentgenol. 2003;181:561–7.
3. Mamlouk MD, van Sonnenberg E, Dehkharghani S. CT-guided nerve block for pudendal neuralgia: diagnostic and therapeutic implications. AJR Am J Roentgenol [Internet]. 2014;203(1):196–200. http://www.ncbi.nlm.nih.gov/pubmed/24951215.
4. Richard HM III, Marvel RP. CT guided pudendal nerve block. Open J Radiol. 2013;3(1):41–4.
5. Robert R, Prat-Pradal D, Labat JJ, Bensignor M, Raoul S, Rebai R, et al. Anatomic basis of chronic perineal pain: role of the pudendal nerve. Surg Radiol Anat [Internet]. 1998;20(2):93–8. http://www.ncbi.nlEm.nih.gov/pubmed/9658526.
6. Filler AG. Diagnosis and treatment of pudendal nerve entrapment syndrome subtypes: imaging, injections, and minimal access surgery. Neurosurg Focus [Internet]. 2009;26(2):E9. http://www.ncbi.nlm.nih.gov/pubmed/19323602.
7. Thoumas D, Leroi a M, Mauillon J, Muller JM, Benozio M, Denis P, et al. Pudendal neuralgia: CT-guided pudendal nerve block technique. Abdom Imaging. 1999;24:309–12.
8. Benzon HT, Katz JA, Benzon HA, Iqbal MS. Piriformis syndrome: anatomic considerations, a new injection technique, and a review of the literature. Anesthesiology [Internet]. 2003;98(6):1442–8. http://eutils.ncbi.nlm.nih.gov/entrez/eutils/elink.fcgi?dbfrom=pubmed&id=12766656&retmode=ref&cmd=prlinks\npapers2://publication/uuid/CD240315-78CD-4F56-96FC-D8D7E9A34BB8.
9. Faubel C. ThePainSource.com. Piriformis muscle injection with fluoroscopy [Internet]. 2013. p. 3–5. http://thepainsource.com/piriformis-muscle-injection-fluoroscopy/.
10. Chen CPC, Shen C-Y, Lew HL. Ultrasound-guided injection of the piriformis muscle. Am J Phys Med Rehabil [Internet]. 2011;90(10):871–2. http://journals.lww.com/ajpmr/Abstract/2011/10000/Ultrasound_Guided_Injection_of_the_Piriformis.12.aspx\npapers2://publication/doi/10.1097/PHM.0b013e31822de72c.
11. Smith J, Hurdle MF, Locketz AJ, Wisniewski SJ. Ultrasound-guided piriformis injection: technique description and verification. Arch Phys Med Rehabil. 2006;87:1664–7.
12. Ozisik P, Toru M, Denk C, Taskiran O, Gundogmus B. Ct-guided piriformis muscle injection for the treatment of piriformis syndrome. Turk Neurosurg [Internet]. 2013;3:471–7. http://www.turkishneurosurgery.org.tr/summary_en_doi.php3?doi=10.5137/1019-5149.JTN.8038-13.1.
13. Filler AG, Haynes J, Jordan SE, Prager J, Villablanca JP, Farahani K, et al. Sciatica of nondisc origin and piriformis syndrome: diagnosis by magnetic resonance neurography and interventional magnetic resonance imaging with outcome study of resulting treatment. J Neurosurg Spine. 2005;2(2):99–115.
14. Artner J, Cakir B, Reichel H, Lattig F. Radiation dose reduction in CT-guided sacroiliac joint injections to levels of pulsed fluoroscopy: a comparative study with technical considerations. J Pain Res. 2012;5:265–9.
15. Silbergleit R, Mehta B, Sanders WP, Talati SJ. Imaging-guided injection techniques with fluoroscopy and CT for spinal pain management. Radiographics. 2001;21(4):927–39. discussion 940–2.

16. Klauser A, De Zordo T, Feuchtner G, Sögner P, Schirmer M, Gruber J, et al. Feasibility of ultrasound-guided sacroiliac joint injection considering sonoanatomic landmarks at two different levels in cadavers and patients. Arthritis Rheum [Internet]. 2008;59(11):1618–24. https://doi.org/10.1002/art.24204.
17. D'Orazio F, Gregori LM, Gallucci M. Spine epidural and sacroiliac joints injections – when and how to perform. Eur J Radiol [Internet]. 2014;84(5):777–82. https://doi.org/10.1016/j.ejrad.2014.05.039.
18. Fritz J, Henes JC, Thomas C, Clasen S, Fenchel M, Claussen CD, et al. Diagnostic and interventional MRI of the sacroiliac joints using a 1.5-T open-bore magnet: a one-stop-shopping approach. AJR Am J Roentgenol [Internet]. 2008;191(6):1717–24. http://www.ncbi.nlm.nih.gov/pubmed/19020241.

Nucelio L. B. M. Lemos

Introduction

It is long known that a large portion of the lumbosacral plexus is located intra-abdominally, in the retroperitoneal space [1]. However, most of literature descriptions of lesions on this plexus refer to its extra-abdominal parts, whereas its intra-abdominal portions as well as the fact that these portions can be subject to entrapments are often neglected [2].

In 2007, Possover et al. [3] described the laparoscopic neuronavigation (LANN) technique, opening the doors to accessing the retroperitoneal portion of the lumbosacral plexus through a safe, minimally invasive, and objective way. Since then, multiple causes of intrapelvic nerve entrapments have been described, and a new field in medicine—the neuropelveology—was created.

In this chapter, we will review the laparoscopic anatomy of the intrapelvic nerve bundles and describe the symptoms and signs associated with intrapelvic neuropathies, as well as the diagnosis and treatment rationale of these conditions.

Laparoscopic Anatomy of the Intrapelvic Nerves

Iliohypogastric, Ilio-inguinal, and Genitofemoral Nerves

These nerves are sensitive branches of the lumbar plexus and enter the retroperitoneal space emerging on the lateral border of the psoas muscle and follow anteriorly and distally to leave the abdomen through the femoral and inguinal canals. Their fibrotic entrapment is related to post-herniorhaphy inguinodynia [4]. (Fig. 7.1).

Femoral Nerve

The femoral nerve is the largest motoric and sensitive nerve of the lumbar plexus. It enters the abdomen by the posterolateral aspect of the psoas muscle and leaves it through the femoral canal (Fig. 7.2) to innervate the quadriceps muscle and the skin covering the anterior thigh.

N. L. B. M. Lemos, MD, PhD
University of Toronto, Women's College Hospital and Mount Sinais Hospital, Department of Obstetrics and Gynecology, Toronto, ON, Canada
e-mail: nucelio.lemos@utoronto.ca

© Springer International Publishing AG, part of Springer Nature 2019
H. D. Martin, J. Gómez-Hoyos (eds.), *Posterior Hip Disorders*,
https://doi.org/10.1007/978-3-319-78040-5_7

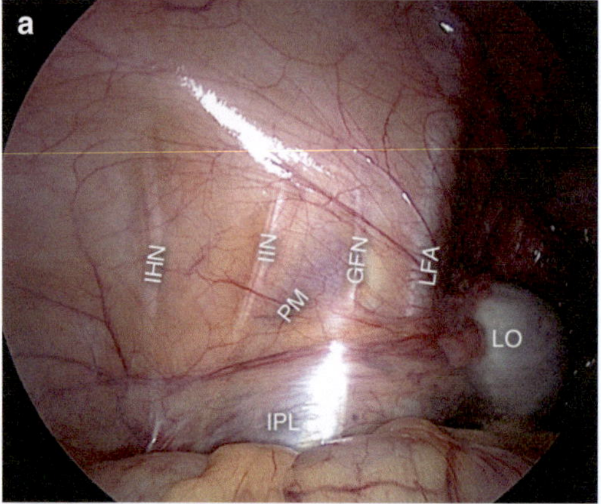

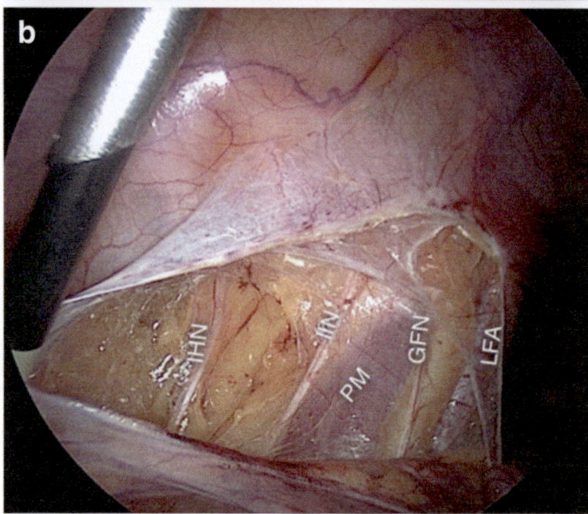

Fig. 7.1 Iliohypogastric (IHN), ilio-inguinalis (IIN), and genitofemoralis (GFN) nerves, with the overlying peritoneal intact (a) and exposed (b) (*PM* psoas muscle, *LO* left ovary, *IPL* infundibulopelvic ligament, *LFA* left femoral artery)

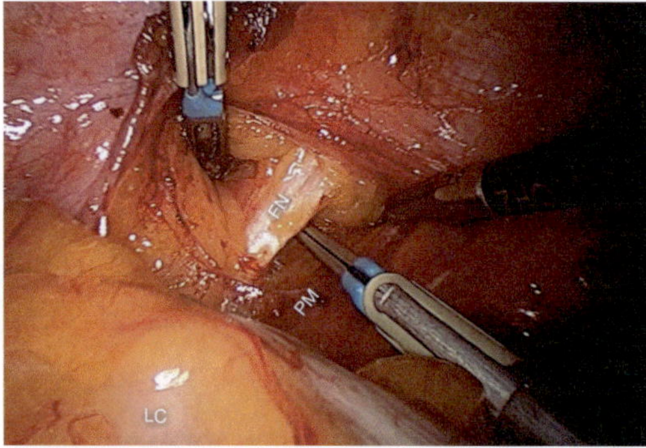

Fig. 7.2 The left femoral nerve (FN) entering the retroperitoneal space on the posterolateral aspect of the psoas muscle (PM). (*LC* left colon)

Nerves of the Obturator Space

The obturator nerve enters the obturator space at the level of the pelvic brim and leaves it through the obturator canal. It gives sensitive branches to the skin of the medial thigh and motoric branches to the hip adductors (Fig. 7.3a).

The lumbosacral trunk and the distal portions of the S1, S2, S3, and S4 nerve roots merge into the obturator space and form the sciatic and pudendal nerves (Fig. 7.3b).

The sciatic nerve is formed by the L4 and L5 fibers of the lumbosacral trunk and fibers from the

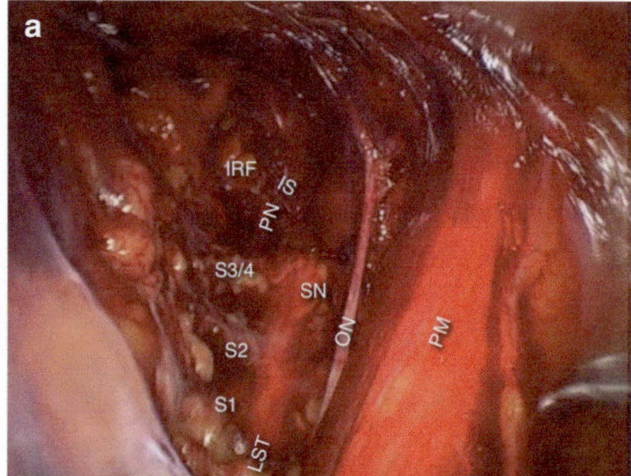

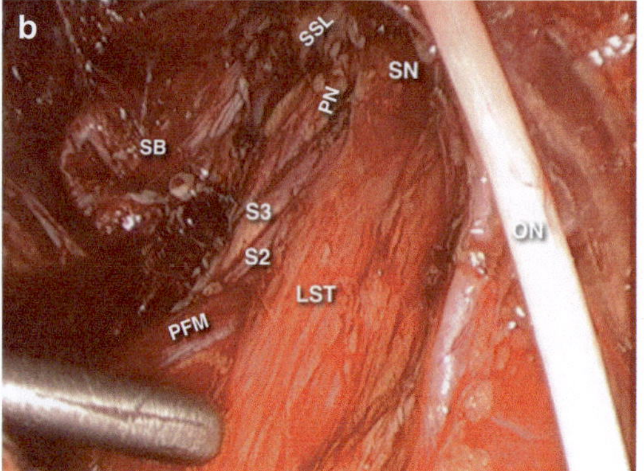

Fig. 7.3 Nerves of the obturator space (right side). Picture (**a**) is the final aspect of a laparoscopic approach to Alcock's canal syndrome, where the sacrospinous ligament has been transected to expose the pudendal nerve (PN). In picture (**b**), the sacrospinous ligament (SSL) is intact. In both pictures, the internal and external iliac vessels are retracted medially. (*ON* obturator nerve, *PM* psoas muscle, *SN* sciatic nerve, *LST* lumbosacral trunk, *PN* pudendal nerve, *IRF* ischiorectal fossa, *IS* ischial spine, *SB* sacral bone, *PFM* piriformis muscle)

S1, S2, and S3 nerve roots and leaves the pelvis through the sciatic notch. It gives out sensitive branches to the upper gluteal region, posterolateral thigh, leg ankle, and foot. It also controls the hip extensors, abductors and rotators, knee flexors, and all the muscles for the ankle and foot.

The pudendal nerve is formed by fibers of the second, third, and fourth nerve roots and leaves the pelvis through the pudendal (Alcock's) canal. It gives out sensitive branches to the lower gluteal region and the perineal skin. It also sends motoric branches to the perineal muscles and the anterior fibers of the levator ani muscles. Finally, there are direct motoric and sensitive nerves from the S3 and S4 nerve roots to the posterior fibers of the levator ani muscle [5–7].

Nerves of the Presacral and Pararectal Spaces

The superior hypogastric plexus is formed by fibers from para-aortic sympathetic trunk and gives rise to the hypogastric nerves. The hypogastric nerves run over the hypogastric fascia in an anterior and distal direction. After crossing about two thirds of the distance between the sacrum and the uterine cervix or the prostate, its fibers spread to join the pelvic splanchnic nerves (described below) to form the inferior hypogastric plexus (Fig. 7.4). The hypogastric nerves carry the sympathetic signals to the internal urethral and anal sphincters, rectum, and bladder, which cause detrusor relaxation and bladder contraction. They also carry proprioceptive and nociceptive afferent signals from the pelvic viscera [8].

The lateral limit of the presacral space is the hypogastric fascia, which is the formed by the medialmost fibers of the endopelvic fascia. The sacral nerve roots can be found juxta-laterally to this fascia (Fig. 7.5). They leave the sacral foramina and run anteriorly and distally, lying over the piriformis muscle and crossing the internal iliac vessels laterally to them, to merge and form the nerves of the sacral plexus [3]. Before crossing the internal iliac vessels,

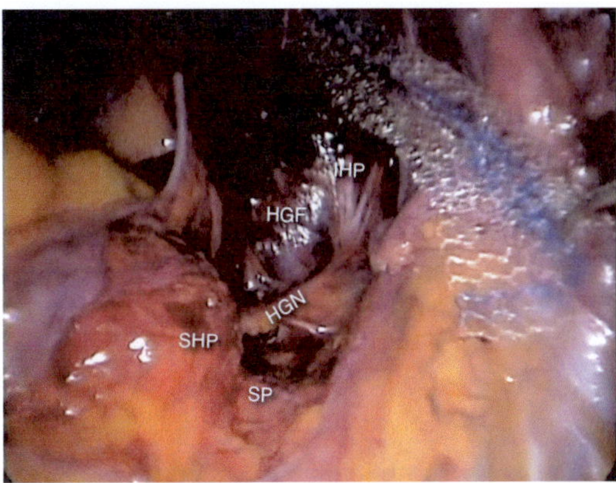

Fig. 7.4 The hypogastric nerve (HGN) emerges from the superior hypogastric plexus (SHP) at the level of the sacral promontory (SP) and runs anteriorly and distally, juxta-laterally to the hypogastric fascia (HGF), to merge with the pelvic splanchnic nerves to form the inferior hypogastric plexus (IHP)

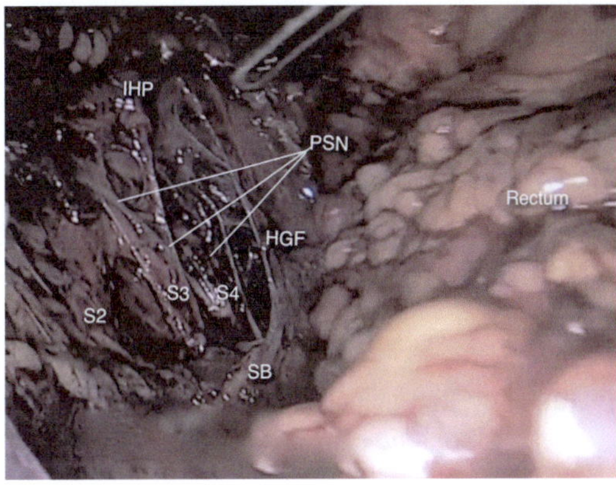

Fig. 7.5 The sacral nerve roots (S2–S4) can be found juxta-laterally to the hypogastric fascia (HGF) and give origin to the pelvic splanchnic nerves (PSN), which run anteriorly and distally to merge the hypogastric nerve and form the inferior hypogastric plexus (IHP)

they give out the thin parasympathetic branches called pelvic splanchnic nerves, which promote detrusor contraction and provide extrinsic parasympathetic innervation to the colon descendens, sigmoid, and rectum. They also carry nociceptive afferent signals from the pelvic viscera [8]. The pelvic splanchnic nerves join the hypogastric nerves to form the inferior hypogastric plexus in the pararectal fossae [3].

Intrapelvic Nerve Entrapment Syndrome

Definition and Symptoms

Nerve entrapment syndrome, or compression neuropathy, is a clinical condition caused by compression on a single nerve or nerve root. Its symptoms include pain, tingling, numbness, and muscle weakness on the affected nerve's dermatome [9]. Intrapelvic nerve entrapments are, therefore, entrapments of the intrapelvic portions of the nerves described in the previous sessions and will produce symptoms related to their dermatomes.

The above definition refers to the entrapment of somatic nerves. Autonomic nerve entrapment will produce visceral and vegetative symptoms, such as urinary frequency or urgency, dysuria, rectal pain, suprapubic and/or abdominal cramps, and chills. However, as described, above, the sacral nerve roots give origin to both somatic and parasympathetic nerves. Therefore, entrapments of these roots will produce pain on their somatic dermatomes, together with urinary and bowel dysfunction.

In a concise manner, the main symptoms of intrapelvic nerve entrapments are:

- Sciatica associated with urinary symptoms (urgency, frequency, dysuria) or without any clear orthopedic cause
- Gluteal pain associated with perineal, vaginal, or penile pain
- Dysuria and/or painful ejaculation
- Refractory urinary symptoms
- Refractory pelvic and perineal pain

It is important to emphasize that, due to the distance between both plexuses, intrapelvic nerve entrapments will usually cause unilateral symptoms.

Diagnostic Workup

Once the hypothesis of an intrapelvic entrapment is raised, it is mandatory to perform the topographic diagnosis, which is the determination of the exact point of entrapment. So far, careful neuropelveological evaluation, with detailed anamnesis and neurological examination, is the most reliable method for this.

To increase objectivity and accuracy of the diagnosis, we have been examining the use of high-definition pelvic MRI and sacral plexus tractography, which is a technique for functional MRI of peripheral nerves [10]. Asymmetries and structures that could entrap the plexus are identified at MRI and that specific portions are investigated on tractography for any gaps in neural activity (Fig. 7.6).

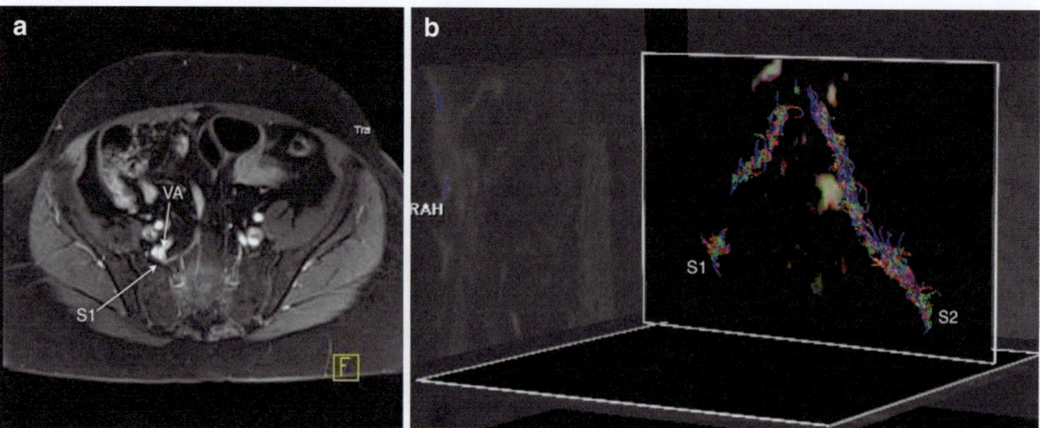

Fig. 7.6 (a) Contrasted MRI showing enlarged vessels (VA) in direct contact with S1 nerve root. (b) Tractography showing a signal gap in S1 (In collaboration with Dr. Suzan M. Goldman, MD, PhD and Homero Faria, PhD)

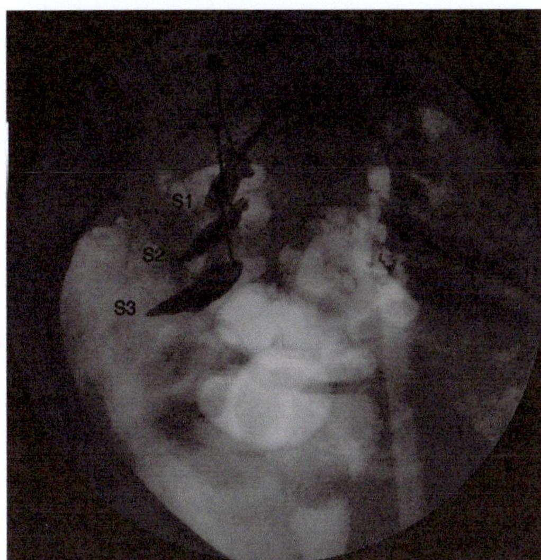

Fig. 7.7 Fluoroscopy-guided block of S1, S2, and S3 (Courtesy of Dr. Alexandra Raffaini)

The results so far are very promising, but the accuracy of this method still needs to be investigated. Therefore, for further assurance, the next step is a diagnostic block, guided by ultrasound or fluoroscopy and performed by an intervention pain therapist; the exact point where a signal gap was identified at the tractography is infiltrated with 0.5–1 mL of lidocaine 0.5%. If a 50% or greater reduction in pain (VAS) is observed, the test is considered positive (Fig. 7.7).

Etiology of Intrapelvic Entrapments

Endometriosis

The first report of intrapelvic nerve entrapment was made by Denton and Sherill [11], who described a case of cyclic sciatica due to endometriosis in 1955. After that, some other case reports and small series were published, until 2011, when Possover et al. [2] described the largest series so far, with 175 patients, all treated laparoscopically.

In endometriotic entrapments, the symptoms tend to be cyclic, worsening on the premenstrual and menstrual days and ameliorating or even disappearing on the post-menstrual period [2, 12, 13].

Treatment consists of preoperatively identifying the symptoms and determining the topographical localization of the lesions (by means, mainly, of anamnesis and neurological examination and, sometimes, by MRI) and laparoscopically exploring all suspect segments of the plexus, with radical removal of all endometriotic foci and fibrosis [2, 12, 13]. (Fig. 7.8).

The true incidence of endometriosis involving the sacral plexus is unknown, as this presentation of the disease is often neglected. In average, patients undergo four surgical procedures seeking to treat the pain before getting the right diagnosis [2]. Moreover, about 40% of women with endometriosis refer unilateral pain on the inferior limb [14], and, in 30% of patients with endometriosis, leg pain was demonstrated to be neuropathic, [15] which leads to the conclusion that endometriotic involvement of the lumbosacral plexus is probably underdiagnosed and much more frequent than reported.

Fibrosis

This is one of the most frequent causes of intrapelvic nerve entrapments and possibly the most well-known etiology, since Amarenco [16] described the pudendal neuralgia in cyclists, in whom the pain is a consequence of fibrotic entrapment due to continued trauma.

Despite the historical aspect, however, surgical manipulation seems to be the most frequent cause of fibrosis over the sacral plexus (Fig. 7.9). Among the surgeries with higher risks of inducing such kinds of entrapments are the pelvic reconstructive procedures [17].

Vascular Entrapment

Pelvic congestion syndrome is a well-known cause of cyclic pelvic pain. Patients commonly present with pelvic pain without evidence of inflammatory disease. The pain is worse during the premenstrual period and pregnancy and is exacerbated by fatigue and standing [18].

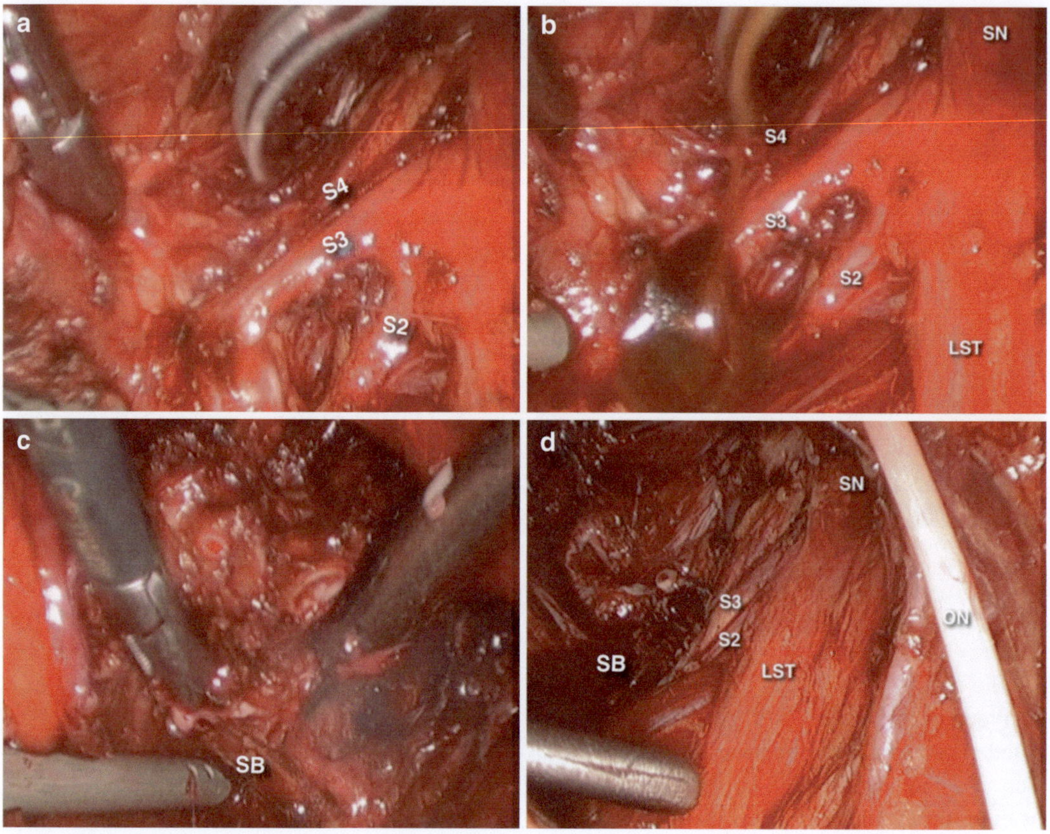

Fig. 7.8 (**a**) After partial detachment of the nodule, allowing for visualization of S2, S3, and S4 nerve roots, S3 was found to be dilated on its proximal part; (**b**) opening of the S3 nerve root sheath revealed an endometrioma inside the nerve; (**c**) the nodule was detached from the sacral bone (SB); (**d**) final aspect of the right pelvic sidewall; *ON* obturator nerve, *SN* sciatic nerve

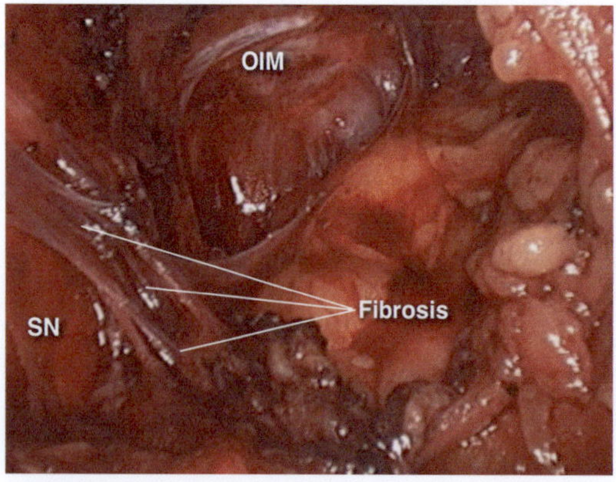

Fig. 7.9 Fibrotic entrapment of the left sciatic nerve

However, what is much less known is the fact that dilated or malformed branches of the internal or external iliac vessels can entrap the nerves of the sacral plexus against the pelvic sidewalls, producing symptoms such as sciatica or refractory urinary and anorectal dysfunction [2, 19] (Fig. 7.10).

Piriformis Syndrome

Numerous malformations of the piriformis muscle have been described in the deep gluteal space that can entrap branches of the sciatic nerve. The laparoscopic approach has revealed that the intrapelvic fibers of this muscle can also entrap the sacral nerve roots [20, 21]. Usually, these fibers originate from the sacral bone, laterally to the sacral foramina; some people present with some of the piriformis fibers originating medially to the sacral foramina and involving the sacral nerve roots (Fig. 7.11). Differentiating intrapelvic from extrapelvic piriformis syndrome can be very challenging. Bowel and urinary symptoms are a good indication that the entrapment is intrapelvic, but these are not always present.

Neoplasms

Tumors can also entrap the nerves or nerve roots. Tumors can be primary neural tumors, such as Schwannomas, or metastatic tumors entrapping the nerves, such as pelvic lymph nodes, in pelvic malignancies (Fig. 7.12).

Treatment of Intrapelvic Neuropathies

As a general rule, once a nerve entrapment has been diagnosed, decompression (usually surgical) is mandatory, since chronic ischemia can

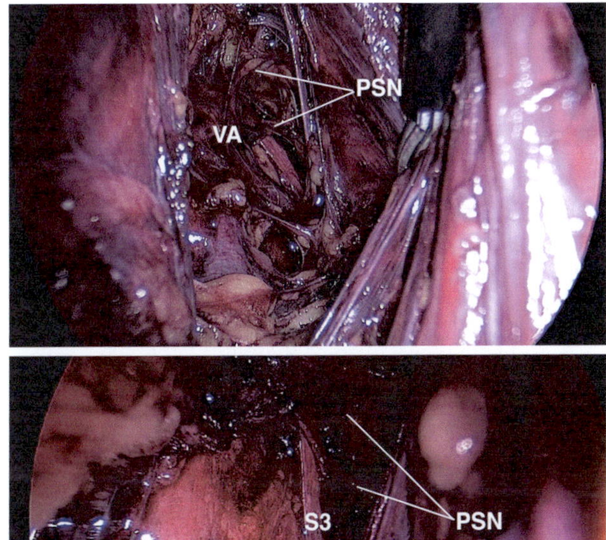

Fig. 7.10 Varicose tributary (VA) of the left internal iliac vein entrapping the S2 and S3 nerve roots against the left piriformis muscle (PM). PSN: perisplanchnic nerves

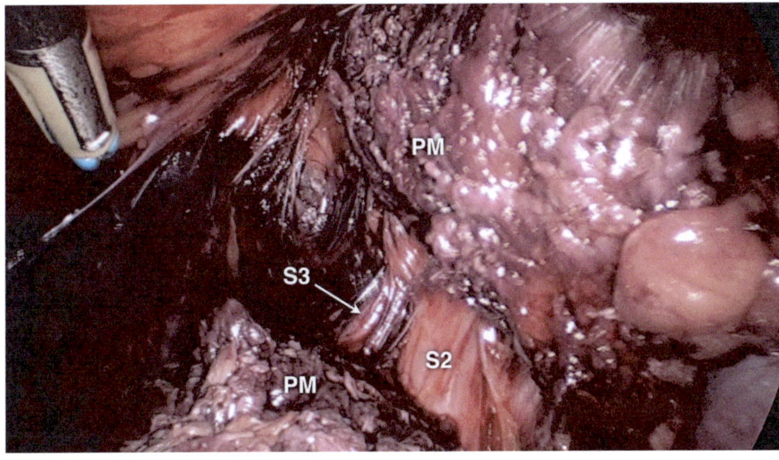

Fig. 7.11 Muscular entrapment of the right S2 and S3 nerve roots. Observe the transected piriformis muscle (PM) bundle originating from the sacral bone medially from the sacral nerve roots and, therefore, crushing the nerves every time the muscle contracts

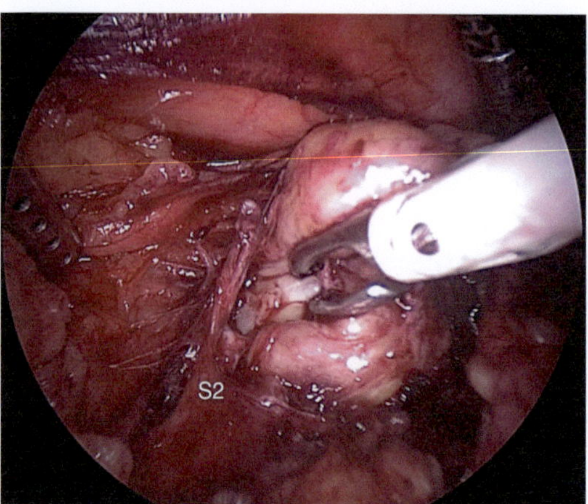

Fig. 7.12 Schwannoma in S2 (left)

lead to endoneurial degeneration [22]. Therefore, the longer the time between the beginning of symptoms and detrapment, the lower the chance of success.

Surgical decompression tends to solve the problem in about 30% of the patients; around 50% will experience 50% reduction in pain, and about 20% will not improve or, in some cases, experience worsening of their pain [23]. Approximately, 25% of patients will present post-decompression neuropathic pain, and 17% will present neuropathic strength loss, both of which tend to be transient; the former will last, in average, 5.5 months and the latter 2.5 months.

Patients who present transient post-decompression pain, persistent post-neuropathic pain or worsening of symptoms, should be treated like patients with primary neuropathic pain, as described in the following session.

Primary Neuropathic Pain, Nerve Transection, and Secondary Neuropathic Pain

All the previously described causes of intrapelvic neuropathies have extrinsic entrapment as the etiology of pain. Intrapelvic radiculopathies can also result from intrinsic dysfunctions of the nerves themselves.

Nerve transections can occur during surgery or trauma and can induce neuroma formation, resulting in phantom pain and anesthesia of the affected nerve dermatome. The pictorial example of this is the phantom pain secondary to amputations, where branches of the sciatic and femoral nerves are transected. In the same fashion, pudendal transection will induce perineal pain and perineal anesthesia, as well as unilateral atrophy of perineal muscles, frequently resulting in urinary and fecal incontinence.

In entrapment syndromes chronic ischemia induces cytoarchitectural changes to the neuron, which do not heal properly after the de-entrapment, resulting in neuropathic pain. The latter the de-entrapment is performed, the higher the risk of neuropathic pain [22].

Neuropathic pain can also result from metabolic disturbances of the neuron, infectious agents, chronic exposure to neurotoxic substances, or a myriad of other causes.

In such cases where there is no suspicion of entrapment as the primary cause of symptoms, extensive neurological investigation must be performed, preferably by a neurology with peripheral nerve pain as their main research interest, and symptoms must be clinically treated by a multiprofessional pain team composed by a pain physician (usually an anesthesiologist or neurologist), a physiotherapy team (pelvic and motor), and a mental healthcare team (psychologist and psychiatrist) and hip surgeon. The pain specialist will prescribe and adjust the pharmacological treatment and, in cases where poor response to medical treatment is observed, perform the intervention pain procedures (anesthetic blocks, pulsed radiofrequency, etc.).

In cases where medical and intervention pain treatment has failed or in cases where, although the topography of the lesion is determined, its etiology cannot be identified intraoperatively, the laparoscopic implantation of neuromodulation electrodes can be used to specifically modulate the affected nerve, producing very encouraging results when compared to the more commonly available epidural neuromodulation [4, 20, 21].

The laparoscopic implantation of neuroprosthesis—the LION procedure—was first reported

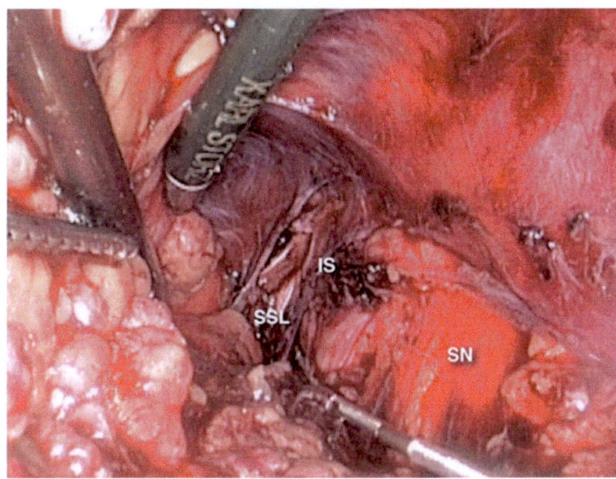

Fig. 7.13 LION electrode placed on right sciatic and pudendal nerves (*PM* psoas muscle, *IS* ischial spine, *SN* sciatic nerve, *SSL* sacrospinous ligament)

by Possover in 2009 as a rescue procedure in patients with local complications of a Brindley procedure [20, 21]. Due to its successful results and lesser invasiveness, it was then used as a primary procedure in spinal cord-injured patients, aiming to improve locomotion and bladder function [24]. Long-term data has shown improvement in voluntary motor function and sensitivity, suggesting positive effects on neuroplasticity [25] (Fig. 7.13).

Conclusion

Laparoscopy provides minimally invasive access with optimal visualization to virtually all abdominal portions of the lumbosacral plexus, which are also subject to entrapment neuropathies. Therefore, when facing sciatica, gluteal or perineal pain without any obvious spinal, or deep gluteal causes, the examiner should always remember that the entrapment could be in the intrapelvic portions, especially when urinary or anorectal symptoms are present.

The laparoscopic approach to the intrapelvic bundles of the lumbosacral nerves opened a myriad of possibilities to assess and treat this neglected portion of the plexus, by means of nerve decompression or selective neuromodulatio

Disclosures Nucelio Lemos received research grants from Medtronic Inc. and Laborie Inc. and travel and proctorship grants from Medtronic Inc. None of these grants are, however, directly related to the current publication.

References

1. Gray H. Anatomy of the human body. IX. Neurology. 6d. The lumbosacral plexus. London: Bounty; 1918.
2. Possover M, Schneider T, Henle KP. Laparoscopic therapy for endometriosis and vascular entrapment of sacral plexus. Fertil Steril. 2011;95(2):756–8.
3. Possover M, Chiantera V, Baekelandt J. Anatomy of the sacral roots and the pelvic splanchnic nerves in women using the LANN technique. Surg Laparosc Endosc Percutan Tech. 2007;17(6):508–10.
4. Possover M. Use of the LION procedure on the sensitive branches of the lumbar plexus for the treatment of intractable postherniorrhaphy neuropathic inguinodynia. Hernia. 2013;17(3):333–7. https://doi.org/10.1007/s10029-011-0894-x.
5. Grigorescu BA, Lazarou G, Olson TR, Downie SA, Powers K, Greston WM, Mikhail MS. Innervation of the levator ani muscles: description of the nerve branches to the pubococcygeus, iliococcygeus, and puborectalis muscles. Int Urogynecol J Pelvic Floor Dysfunct. 2008;19(1):107–16.
6. Barber MD, Bremer RE, Thor KB, Dolber PC, Kuehl TJ, Coates KW. Innervation of the female levator ani muscles. Am J Obstet Gynecol. 2002;187(1):64–71.
7. Wallner C, van Wissen J, Maas CP, Dabhoiwala NF, DeRuiter MC, Lamers WH. The contribution of the levator ani nerve and the pudendal nerve to the innervation of the levator ani muscles; a study in human fetuses. Eur Urol. 2008;54(5):1136–42.
8. DeGroat WC, Yoshimura N. Anatomy and physiology of the lower urinary tract. In: Handbook of clinical neurology 3rd series. Oxford: Elsevier; 2015.
9. Bouche P. Compression and entrapment neuropathies. Handb Clin Neurol. 2013;115:311–66. https://doi.org/10.1016/B978-0-444-52902-2.00019-9.
10. van der Jagt PK, Dik P, Froeling M, Kwee TC, Nievelstein RA, ten Haken B, Leemans A. Architectural configuration and microstructural properties of the sacral plexus: a diffusion tensor MRI and fiber tractography study. Neuroimage. 2012;62(3):1792–9. https://doi.org/10.1016/j.neuroimage.2012.06.001.
11. Denton RO, Sherrill JD. Sciatic syndrome due to endometriosis of sciatic nerve. South Med J. 1955;48(10):1027–31.
12. Lemos N, Kamergorodsky G, Ploger C, Castro R, Schor E, Girão M. Sacral nerve infiltrative endometriosis presenting as perimenstrual right-sided sciatica and bladder atonia: case report and description of surgical technique. J Minim Invasive Gynecol. 2012;19(3):396–400. https://doi.org/10.1016/j.jmig.2012.02.001.
13. Lemos N, D'Amico N, Marques R, Kamergorodsky G, Schor E, Girão MJ. Recognition and treatment of endometriosis involving the sacral nerve roots. Int Urogynecol J. 2016;27(1):147–50.
14. Missmer SA, Bove GM. A pilot study of the prevalence of leg pain among women with endometriosis. J Bodyw Mov Ther. 2011;15(3):304–8. https://doi.org/10.1016/j.jbmt.2011.02.001.

15. Pacchiarotti A, Milazzo GN, Biasiotta A, Truini A, Antonini G, Frati P, Gentile V, Caserta D, Moscarini M. Pain in the upper anterior-lateral part of the thigh in women affected by endometriosis: study of sensitive neuropathy. Fertil Steril. 2013;100(1):122–6. https://doi.org/10.1016/j.fertnstert.2013.02.045.

16. Amarenco G, Lanoe Y, Perrigot M, Goudal H. A new canal syndrome: compression of the pudendal nerve in Alcock's canal or perinal paralysis of cyclists. Presse Med. 1987;16(8):399.

17. Possover M, Lemos N. Risks, symptoms, and management of pelvic nerve damage secondary to surgery for pelvic organ prolapse: a report of 95 cases. Int Urogynecol J. 2011;22(12):1485–90. https://doi.org/10.1007/s00192-011-1539-4.

18. Ganeshan A, Upponi S, Hon LQ, Uthappa MC, Warakaulle DR, Uberoi R. Chronic pelvic pain due to pelvic congestion syndrome: the role of diagnostic and interventional radiology. Cardiovasc Intervent Radiol. 2007;30(6):1105–11.

19. Lemos N, Marques RM, Kamergorodsky G, Ploger C, Schor E, Girão M. Vascular entrapment of the sciatic plexus causing catamenial sciatica and urinary symptoms. In: 44th annual meeting of the International Continence Society (ICS), 2014, Rio de Janeiro. Neurourology and urodynamics, vol. 33. Hoboken: Wiley; 2014. p. 999–1000. https://doi.org/10.1016/j.jbmt.2011.02.001.

20. Possover M. Laparoscopic management of endopelvic etiologies of pudendal pain in 134 consecutive patients. J Urol. 2009;181(4):1732–6. https://doi.org/10.1016/j.juro.2008.11.096.

21. Possover M. The sacral LION procedure for recovery of bladder/rectum/sexual functions in paraplegic patients after explantation of a previous Finetech-Brindley controller. J Minim Invasive Gynecol. 2009;16(1):98–101.

22. Rempel D, Dahlin L, Lundborg G. Pathophysiology of nerve compression syndromes: response of peripheral nerves to loading. J Bone Joint Surg Am. 1999;81(11):1600–10.

23. Lemos N, et al. Intrapelvic nerve entrapments: a neglected cause of perineal pain and urinary symptoms. In: "Scientific Programme, 45th Annual Meeting of the International Continence Society (ICS), 6–9 October 2015, Montreal, Canada." Neurourology urodynamics, vol. 34(Suppl 3); 2015. p. S53–5. https://doi.org/10.1002/nau.22830.

24. Possover M, Schurch B, Henle K. New strategies of pelvic nerves stimulation for recovery of pelvic visceral functions and locomotion in paraplegics. Neurourol Urodyn. 2010;29:1433–8.

25. Possover M. Recovery of sensory and supraspinal control of leg movement in people with chronic paraplegia: a case series. Arch Phys Med Rehabil. 2014;95(4):610–4.

Deep Gluteal Syndrome

8

Hal D. Martin and Juan Gómez-Hoyos

Introduction

Posterior hip pain often represents a diagnostic challenge, and the examiner must be aware of the deep gluteal space abnormalities in order to obtain a correct diagnosis and treatment plan. The sources of symptoms can include conditions in one or more of the following hip layers: osseous, capsulolabral, musculotendinous, neurovascular, and kinematic chain.

Deep gluteal syndrome is characterized by non-discogenic, extra-pelvic sciatic nerve compression presenting with symptoms of pain and dysesthesias in the buttock area, hip or posterior thigh, and/or as radicular pain [1]. The nomenclature piriformis syndrome was widely utilized in the early years to characterize patients with deep gluteal pain, since the piriformis muscle was considered the only structure to compress the sciatic nerve in the deep gluteal space. However, the progress in diagnostic and surgical techniques has demonstrated a number of structures entrapping the sciatic nerve: fibrous bands containing blood vessels [2, 3], gluteal muscles [1], hamstring muscles [4, 5], the gemelli-obturator internus complex [6, 7], bone structures [8], vascular abnormalities [9, 10], ischiofemoral impingement, greater trochanteric impingement, and space-occupying lesions [11, 12]. Considering the variation of anatomical entrapment, the term "deep gluteal syndrome" [1] is preferred to describe the entrapment of the sciatic nerve in the deep gluteal space. The sciatic nerve can be also affected in locations above and below the deep gluteal space, as in intra-pelvic vascular and gynecologic abnormalities [13]. Furthermore, entrapments can occur in more than one place in the same nerve fiber or coexist with lumbosacral root compression. Considering the sciatic nerve can be entrapped by structures in each layer of the hip, a comprehensive physical examination with a thorough understanding of anatomy and biomechanics is critical in cases of deep gluteal pain.

H. D. Martin, DO
Medical and Research Director, Hip Preservation Center, Baylor University Medical Center, Dallas, TX, USA

J. Gómez-Hoyos, MD (✉)
International Consultant, Hip Preservation Center / Baylor Scott and White Research Institute, Baylor University Medical Center, Dallas, TX, USA

Department of Orthopaedic Surgery - Health Provider, Clínica Las Américas / Clínica del Campestre, Medellin, Antioquia, Colombia

Professor - School of Medicine - Sports Medicine Program, Universidad de Antioquia, Medellín, Antioquia, Colombia

Deep Gluteal Space Anatomy

A complete review of anatomy is comprehensively described in Chap. 1; however, a short review of the deep gluteal space and sciatic nerve anatomy will be given. The deep gluteal space is anterior to the gluteus maximus muscle and posterior to the acetabular column, hip joint capsule, and proximal femur. Other anatomical limits include the linea aspera (lateral), the sacrotuberous ligament and falciform fascia (medial), the inferior margin of the greater sciatic notch (superior), and the distal border of the ischial tuberosity (inferior) (Fig. 8.1). The sacrotuberous and sacrospinous ligaments create the greater and lesser sciatic foramen, which communicate the deep gluteal space with the true pelvis and ischioanal fossa. The sacrotuberous ligament is normally composed of two parts: a ligamentous band and a membranous falciform process [14]. Both sacrospinous and sacrotuberous ligaments are anatomically close to the pudendal nerve and may be involved in the entrapment of this nerve (Fig. 8.2).

The piriformis muscle occupies a central position in the buttock and is an important reference for identifying the neurovascular structures emerging above and below it (Fig. 8.3). This

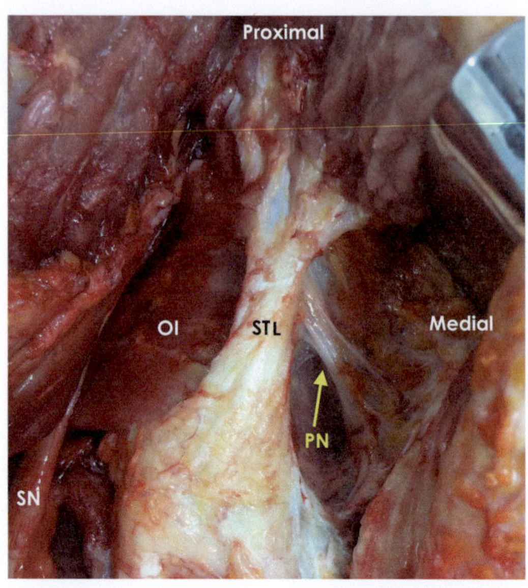

Fig. 8.2 Cadaveric dissection of the pudendal nerve (yellow arrow) running beneath the sacrotuberous ligament. *OI* obturator internus muscle, *STL* sacrotuberous ligament, *SN* sciatic nerve, *PN* pudendal nerve

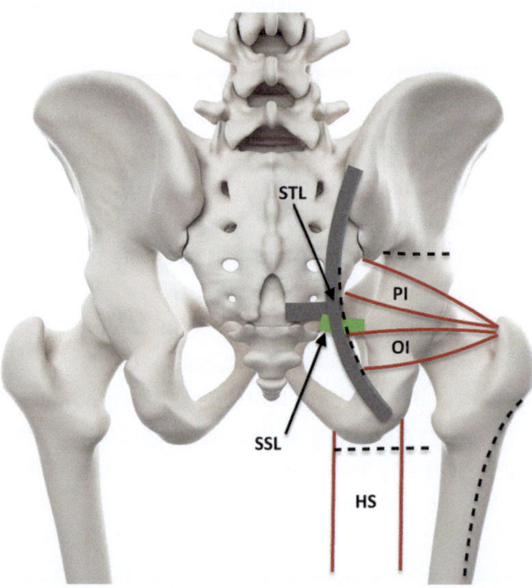

Fig. 8.1 Limits (dashed lines) of the deep gluteal space beneath the gluteus maximus muscle: lateral, linea aspera; medial, sacrotuberous ligament and falciform fascia; superior, inferior margin of the greater sciatic notch; and inferior; the distal border of the ischial tuberosity. *STL* sacrotuberous ligament, *SSL* sacrospinous ligament, *PI* piriformis muscle, *OI* obturator internus muscle, *HS* hamstring muscles

muscle arises from the ventrolateral surface of the sacrum, gluteal surface of the ileum, and sacroiliac joint capsule. The distal attachment of the piriformis is at the medial side of the upper border of the greater trochanter, often partially blended with the common tendon of obturator/gemelli complex [15–17]. Distal to the piriformis muscle is the cluster of short external rotators: the gemellus superior, obturator internus, gemellus inferior, and quadratus femoris muscle. At the ischium tuberosity, the long head of biceps femoris and semitendinosus have a common tendinous origin. The semimembranosus muscle also originates from the ischium, lateral and anteriorly to the long head of the biceps/semitendinosus muscles common origin [18] (Fig. 8.4).

Seven neural structures exit the pelvis through the greater sciatic notch: posterior femoral cutaneous nerve, superior gluteal nerve, inferior gluteal nerve, nerve to obturator internus, nerve to quadratus femoris muscle, pudendal nerve [19], and sciatic nerve (Fig. 8.3). Table 8.1 is a summary of the usual motor and sensory functions for each nerve. Accompanying the respective nerves are the

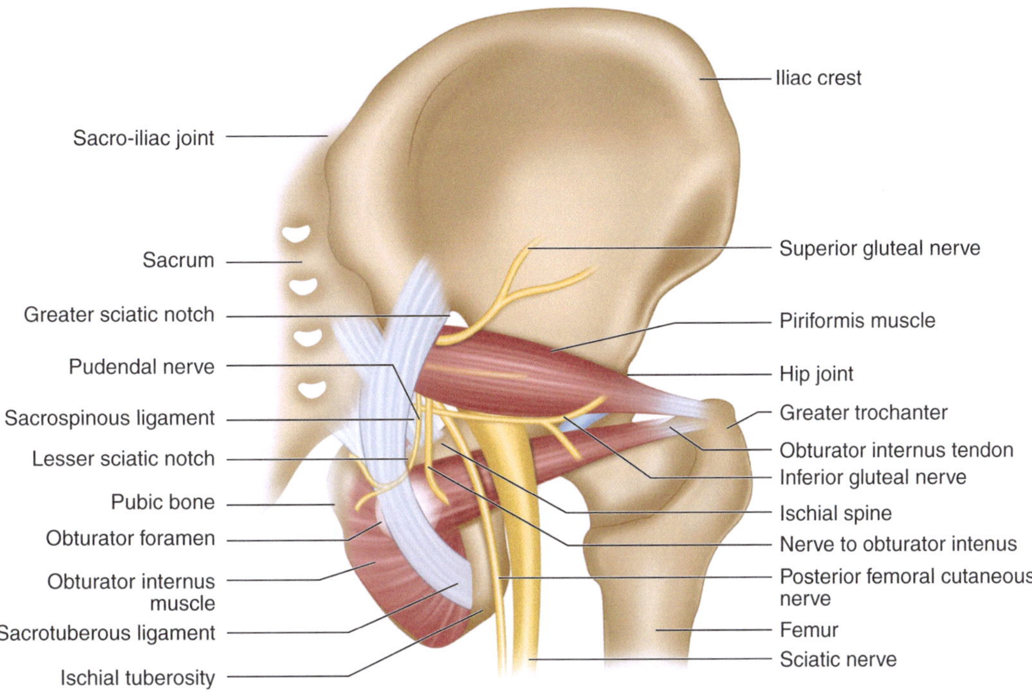

Fig. 8.3 Schematic illustrating the nerve anatomy of the deep gluteal space

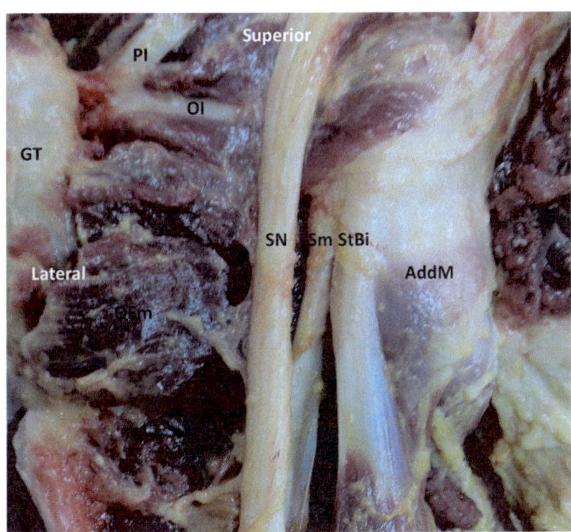

Fig. 8.4 Posterior view of a left hip. Origin of the hamstring muscles at ischial tuberosity. The semimembranosus muscle origin (Sm) is anterior and lateral to the conjoint origin of the semitendinosus and long head of the biceps femoris muscles (St/Bi). *GT* greater trochanter (posterior view), *PI* piriformis tendon, *OI* obturator internus tendon, *QFm* quadratus femoris muscle, *SN* sciatic nerve, *AddM* adductor magnus muscle origin

superior gluteal vessels, inferior gluteal vessels, and internal pudendal vessels.

The anatomic positions of the inferior gluteal artery (IGA) and medial circumflex femoral artery (MCFA) are relevant within the deep gluteal space. The IGA enters the deep gluteal space with the inferior gluteal nerve and supplies the gluteus maximus muscle. This artery also gives a superficial arterial branch that crosses the sciatic nerve laterally between the piriformis and superior gemellus muscles. Another branch of the IGA is the descending branch, which runs along the posterior femoral cutaneous nerve in a frequency of 72% according to a cadaveric study [21]. The MCFA follows the inferior border of the obturator externus and crosses over its tendon and under the external rotators and piriformis muscle [22]. The existence of an anastomosis between the inferior gluteal artery and the medial femoral circumflex artery is frequent [23] (Fig. 8.5).

Table 8.1 Summary of function of the nerves in the deep gluteal space

Nerve	Motor innervation	Sensory innervation
Posterior femoral cutaneous nerve		Gluteal region, perineum and posterior thigh, and popliteal fossa
Superior gluteal nerve	Gluteus medius, gluteus minimus, and tensor fascia lata	
Inferior gluteal nerve	Gluteus maximus	
Nerve to obturator internus	Superior gemellus and obturator internus	
Nerve to quadratus femoris	Inferior gemellus, and quadratus femoris	Hip capsule
Pudendal nerve	Perineal muscles, external urethral sphincter, and external anal sphincter	
Sciatic nerve	Semitendinosus, biceps femoris, semimembranosus, extensor portion of the adductor magnus and leg and foot musculature	Leg and foot, except for the saphenous nerve dermatome

Source: Moore [20] and Standring (Gray's Anatomy) [17]

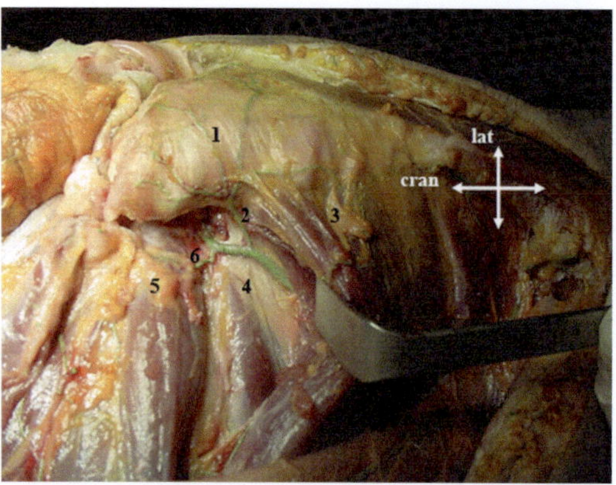

Fig. 8.5 Deep branch of the medial femoral circumflex artery. Posterior aspect of the right hip, demonstrating the anatomic position of the deep branch of the medial femoral circumflex artery. (1) greater trochanter, (2) trochanteric branch of the medial femoral circumflex artery, (3) quadratus femoris muscle, (4) obturator externus muscle, (5) obturator internus and gemellus muscles, and (6) anastomotic branch to the inferior gluteal artery. *Cran* cranial, *Lat* lateral (Reprint with permission from Kahlor et al. [22])

Sciatic Nerve Anatomy and Biomechanics

The sciatic nerve is formed by the L4-S3 ventral rami in the sacral plexus. Nerve fibers of the fibular and tibial components maintain a pattern of fiber separation in these branches and in the sciatic nerve. The sciatic nerve physically splits in tibial and fibular divisions at highly variable locations from the pelvis to the popliteal fossa, although this split is more frequent at the distal thigh [24]. Often, the split is oblique and may not be seen in a uniplanar MRI view [25]. Most sciatic neural fibers are destined to motor and sensory innervation distal to the knee. However, important branches arise from the nerve in the deep gluteal space and thigh. A summary of the sciatic nerve branches in the thigh is depicted in Fig. 8.6 according to Seidel et al. [26] and Sunderland and Hughes [25].

Neural tissue and non-neural tissue compose the sciatic nerve. The ratio neural/non-neural tissue changes from 2/1 at the level of piriformis muscle to 1/1 at the mid-femur, i.e., there is an increase in the non-neural tissue contribution as the sciatic nerve courses distally [27] (Fig. 8.7). The composition of the sciatic nerve also varies during the aging process, with increase in connective tissue and decrease of myelinated nerve fibers [28].

The nerve fibers of the sciatic nerve do not course between the tibial and fibular divisions [17]. However, fibers are often changing from one fascicle to another within each division [25]. Sunderland reported 6 mm as the maximum length of nerve trunk with a constant fascicular pattern, although an individual fascicle can maintain the same neural fibers for greater distances [25]. In general, most fascicles contain fibers for the majority, if not all, of the peripheral branches. Nevertheless, there is a tendency of grouping fibers for different muscles with similar function, for example, the fibers for the hamstring muscles are located anterior-medially in the proximal portion of the sciatic nerve. A progressive arrangement is found until the appearance of fascicles with nervous fibers exclusively destined to specific branches [25].

The sciatic nerve has a segmental arterial supply by branches of the inferior gluteal artery,

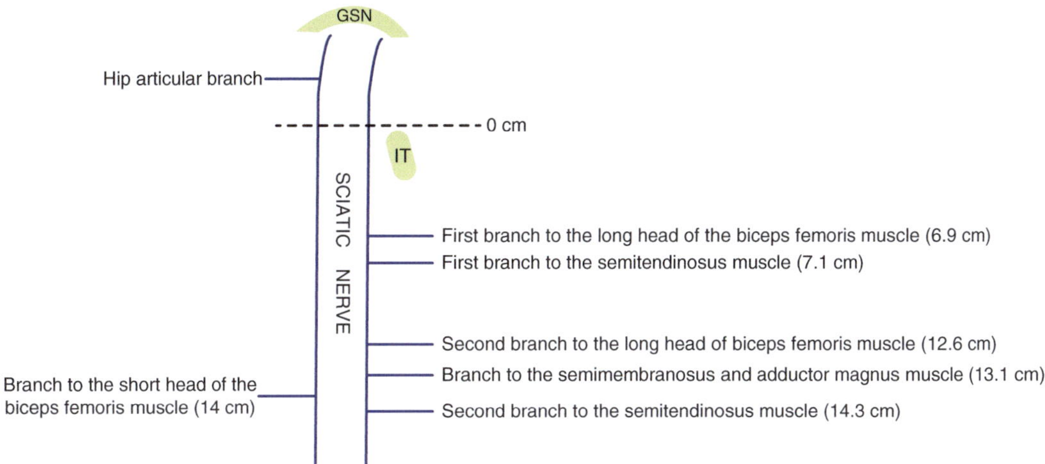

Fig. 8.6 Schematic showing the branches of the sciatic nerve before the physical separation in tibial and fibular nerves. The mean distance from the ischial tuberosity (IT) to the branch emergence is described between brackets. *GSN* greater sciatic notch, *IT* ischial tuberosity. Sunderland and Hughes [24] served as reference for the location of the BSH branch and Seidel et al. [26] for the other branches

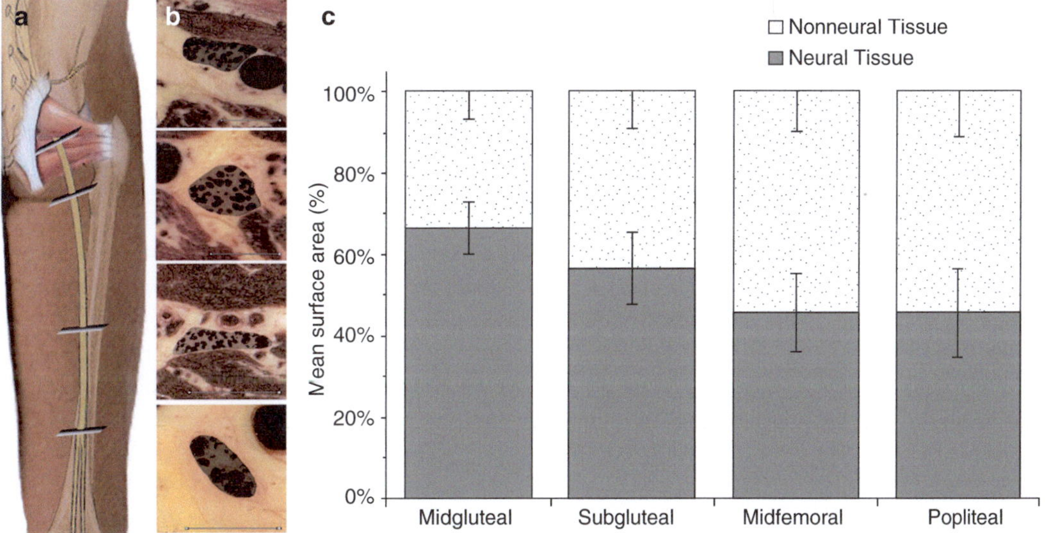

Fig. 8.7 Non-neural and neural tissue composition of the sciatic nerve at different locations. (**a**) Schematic diagram showing four locations of analysis: midgluteal, subgluteal, midfemoral, and popliteal sciatic nerve. (**b**) Transversal view of the sciatic nerve at the four locations, with details of the demarcated neural contents (right; black dots) and epineural areas (gray fields). (**c**) Relative values (percentages) of neural versus non-neural tissue inside the epineurium (means SDs). Reprint with permission from Moayeri [27]

medial circumflex femoral artery (MCFA), and perforating arteries of the thigh (usually the first and second) [29–31]. The venous drainage of the sciatic nerve is performed through the perforators to the femoral profunda system in the thigh and to the popliteal vein at the knee [32] (Fig. 8.8).

Nonfunctioning sciatic veins have been related to sciatic nerve symptoms [9].

The sacral plexus is anatomically close to the internal iliac vessels, their branches and tributaries. The superior gluteal vessels run either between the lumbosacral trunk (L4-L5 ventral

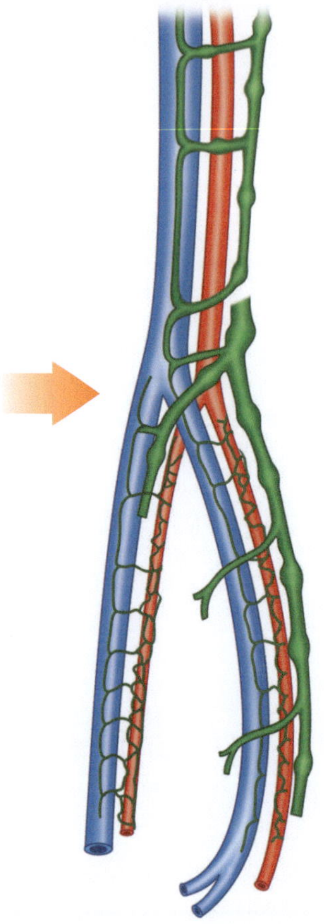

Fig. 8.8 Schematic diagram of the venous drainage of the sciatic nerves. Arrows designate the level of the knee. From proximal to distal, the dominant venous drainage of the sciatic nerve is via the perforators of the profunda system in the thigh and directly to the popliteal vein at the knee. In the leg, the tibial and peroneal nerves drain predominantly to the plexus around their accompanying arteries as well as to muscular veins. Reprinted with permission from Del Pinãl and Taylor [32]

rami) and first sacral ventral ramus or between the first and second sacral rami, whereas the inferior gluteal vessels lie between either the first and second or second and third sacral rami (Fig. 8.9a, b) [17, 33]. The ovaries are close to the sacral plexus, although on the left side, the sigmoid is usually between the ovary and sacral plexus. The intimate anatomic relation between the iliac vessels, ovaries, and sacral plexus is an important consideration in sciatica caused by sacral plexus vascular compression and endometriosis [34].

The sciatic nerve is the terminal branch of the sacral plexus and courses anterior to the piriformis muscle in the pelvis. Variation in the relationship between the sciatic nerve and the piriformis muscle is present in 16–17% of the subjects and can be a cause of sciatic nerve entrapment [35, 36]. After leaving the piriformis muscle, the sciatic nerve runs posteriorly to the obturator/gemelli complex and quadratus femoris muscle, located at an average of 1.2 ± 0.2 cm from the most lateral aspect of the ischial tuberosity and maintaining an intimate relationship with the hamstring origin [18] (Fig. 8.4). The sciatic nerve then enters the thigh posteriorly to the adductor magnus muscle and crosses anteriorly the long head of the biceps femoris. Next, the nerve runs between the semimembranosus and biceps before accessing the popliteal fossa.

Under normal conditions, the sciatic nerve is able to stretch and glide in order to accommodate moderate strain or compression associated with joint movement. During a straight leg raise with knee extension, the sciatic nerve experiences a proximal excursion of 28.0 mm [37] at 70–80° of hip flexion. Strain of the sciatic nerve increases 6.6% relative to the extended hip [37]. Fleming et al. measured the sciatic nerve strain throughout ten hip arthroplasty procedures [38]. The strain increased on average 26% during hip flexion with the knee in extension. This amount of strain is significant and may cause nerve dysfunction. An animal study reported the nerve conduction was completely blocked after stretching of 12% of the nerve length during 1 h [39]. At 6% strain, the authors found a decrease of 70% in amplitude of the action potential after 1 h [39]. The changes in femoral bone morphology may influence sciatic nerve kinematics during hip mobilization [2]. Therefore, it is always important to assess osseous parameters, including femoral and acetabular versions (Fig. 8.10a, b). Hip flexion, adduction, and internal rotation increases the distance between the greater trochanter and posterior superior iliac spine and the distance between the greater trochanter and ischial tuberosity. This hip position stretches the piriformis muscle and causes a narrowing

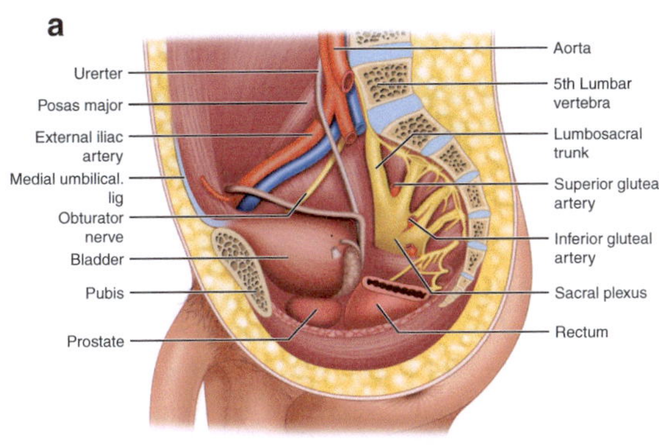

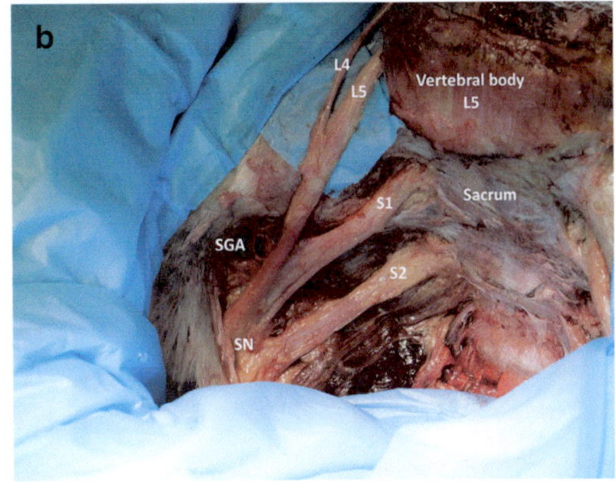

Fig. 8.9 (**a**) Superior and inferior gluteal arteries crossing the sacral plexus before accessing the deep gluteal space. (**b**) Cadaveric dissection of the intra-pelvic showing a close relationship between the superior gluteal artery (SGA) and nerve roots (L4, L5, S1, S2) forming the sciatic nerve (SN)

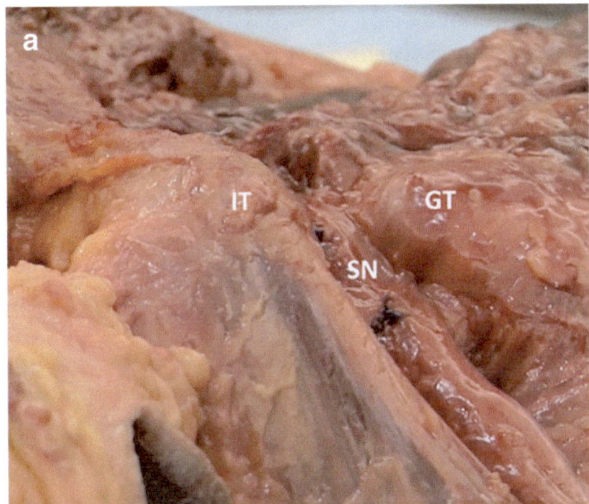

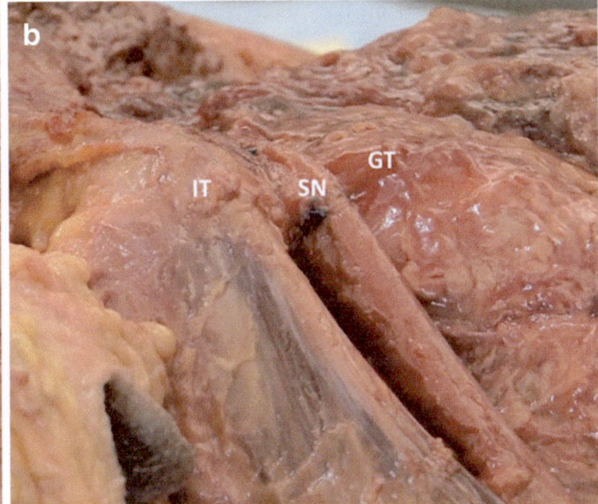

Fig. 8.10 Posterior view of the sciatic nerve (SN) excursion between the greater trochanter (GT) and ischial tuberosity (IT) in a cadaveric specimen, right hip. The sciatic nerve is forced posterior to the GT and ischium during increasing hip flexion and external rotation (**a**, **b**). This pattern of excursion of the sciatic nerve may change according to the bone morphology, adjacent soft tissue restriction, and knee position (flexion or extension)

of the space between the inferior border of the piriformis, the superior gemellus, and the sacrotuberous ligament [40].

Etiology

The piriformis muscle and tendon are the most common source of extra-pelvic sciatic nerve impingement. Yeoman first described the possibility of sciatic nerve entrapment by the piriformis muscle in 1928 [41]. The introduction of the term "piriformis syndrome" has been credited to Robinson, in 1947 [42]. The diagnostic resources have improved last decades, and a number of structures have been associated with sciatic nerve entrapment within the deep gluteal space: the piriformis muscle [2, 3, 11, 12, 43–49], fibrous bands containing blood vessels [2, 3, 43] (Fig. 8.11), gluteal muscles [1], gemelli-obturator internus complex [6, 7], hamstring muscles [4, 5], ischial

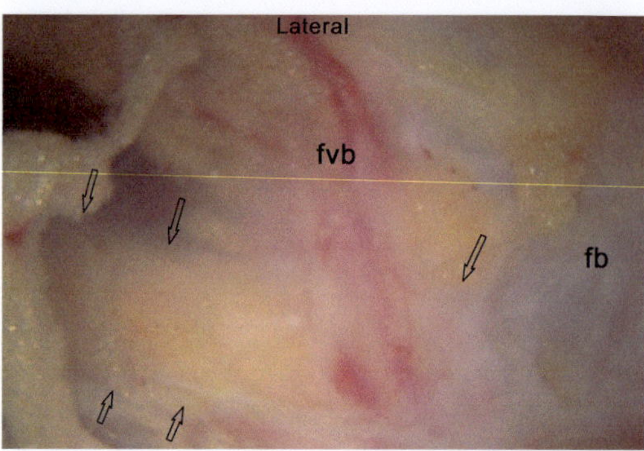

Fig. 8.11 Entrapment of the sciatic nerve by fibrovascular scar band, endoscopic visualization. The sciatic nerve is indicated by the open arrows and is anterior to a fibrovascular band (fvb) and another fibrous band (fb)

tuberosity [8, 50], and space-occupying lesions [11, 12]. Additionally, vascular abnormalities [10, 47], prolonged surgery in the seated position [51], acetabular reconstruction surgery [52], and total hip replacement [53] have been reported to cause compression of the sciatic nerve. Considering the variation of anatomical structures causing the entrapment, the term "deep gluteal syndrome" [1] seems to be a more accurate description of this non-discogenic sciatica.

The piriformis muscle is the most common source of sciatic nerve entrapment [2, 3, 11, 12, 43–49]. The risk of nerve compressive symptoms is increased by the existence of variation in the relationship between the piriformis muscle and the sciatic nerve. Six categories of piriformis-sciatic nerve variations have been reported [35] (Fig. 8.12). However, other sciatic nerve variants have been identified. For instance, the authors of this chapter incidentally found a bifid sciatic nerve that runs below the piriformis muscle in a male cadaver during a routine anatomic dissection (Fig. 8.13). The prevalence of anomalies was 16.9% in a meta-analysis of cadaveric studies [36] and 16.2% in a review of published surgical case series [36]. It is important to mention that the anomaly itself may not be the etiology of the DGS symptoms. Martin et al. [2] reported on 35 patients endoscopically treated for deep gluteal syndrome. Eighteen patients involved the pirifor-

mis muscle as etiology, including the sciatic nerve passing through the piriformis muscle or a portion of piriformis muscle/tendon passing through or anterior to the sciatic nerve [2]. A thick piriformis tendon hidden under the piriformis belly can also be identified causing sciatic nerve compression (Fig. 8.13). Hypertrophy of the piriformis muscle has also been associated with sciatic nerve compression [12, 46, 47, 56]. However, of 14 patients with posttraumatic piriformis syndrome, Benson and Schutzer found that only two had larger piriformis muscles on the symptomatic side and seven appeared smaller than the unaffected side [44].

Atypical fibrovascular scar bands and hypertrophy of the greater trochanteric bursae have been reported in many cases of sciatic nerve entrapment [2, 3] (Fig. 8.14). In 27 of the 35 patients previously described by Martin et al., the greater trochanteric bursa was found to be excessively thickened, and large fibrovascular scar bands were present in many patients [2]. The fibrovascular bands extended from the posterior border of the greater trochanter to the gluteus maximus onto the sciatic nerve and then proximally to the greater sciatic notch [2]. The obturator internus/gemelli complex is commonly overlooked in association with sciatica-like pain [6, 7, 15]. As the sciatic nerve passes under the belly of the piriformis and over the superior gemelli-obturator internus, a scissor effect between the two muscles can be the source of entrapment. In one case, Martin et al. found the obturator internus penetrating the sciatic nerve.

The sciatic nerve courses close to the hamstrings origin at the most lateral aspect of the ischium tuberosity (Fig. 8.4). Avulsions of the hamstring tendons or congenital fibrotic bands can affect the sciatic nerve causing symptoms of entrapment [4, 5, 57–59]. Other sources of sciatic nerve entrapment within the deep gluteal space include malunion of the ischium or healed avulsions, greater trochanter ischium impingement (Fig. 8.14), tumor, sciatic nerve venous varicosities [9] (Fig. 8.15), and gluteus maximus (from a prior iliotibial band release). Intra-

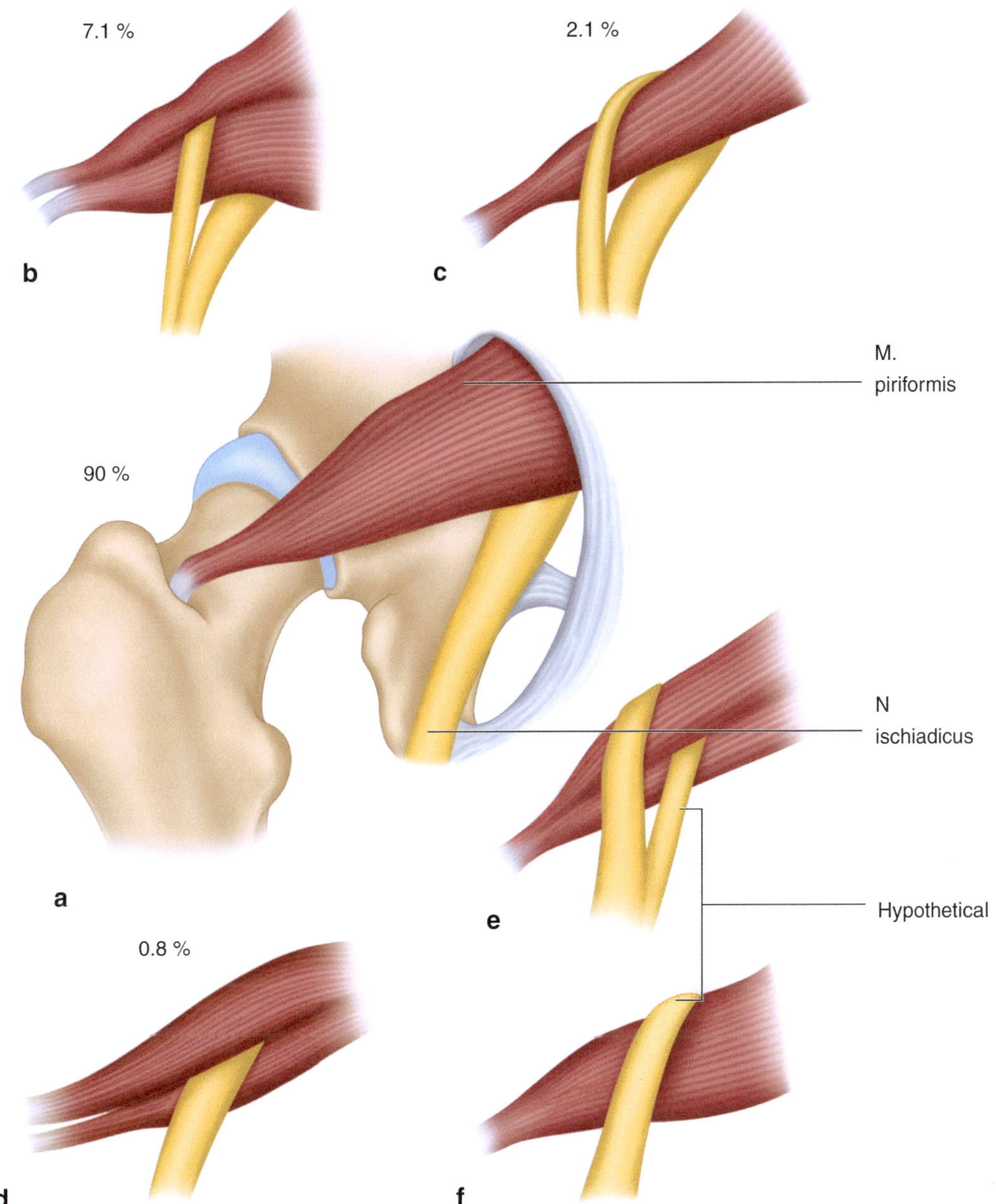

Fig. 8.12 Schematic of piriformis-sciatic nerve variants. Six types of arrangement of the sciatic nerve, or of its subdivisions in relation to the piriformis muscle, arranged in the order of frequency [35]. Gluteal (external) view. The percentage incidence in 240 examples is indicated. Figures (**e**) and (**f**) were hypothetical in 1938 [35]. (**a**) Nerve undivided passes out of greater sciatic foramen, below piriformis muscle, (**b**) divisions of nerve pass through and below heads of muscle, (**c**) divisions above and below undivided muscle, (**d**) nerve undivided between the heads of muscle, (**e**) divisions of nerve between and above heads, and (**f**) undivided nerve above undivided muscle [35]

Fig. 8.13 Posterior hip dissection in a 58 years-old male cadaver. Observe a bifid sciatic nerve (SN1 and SN2) running below the piriformis muscle (PM)

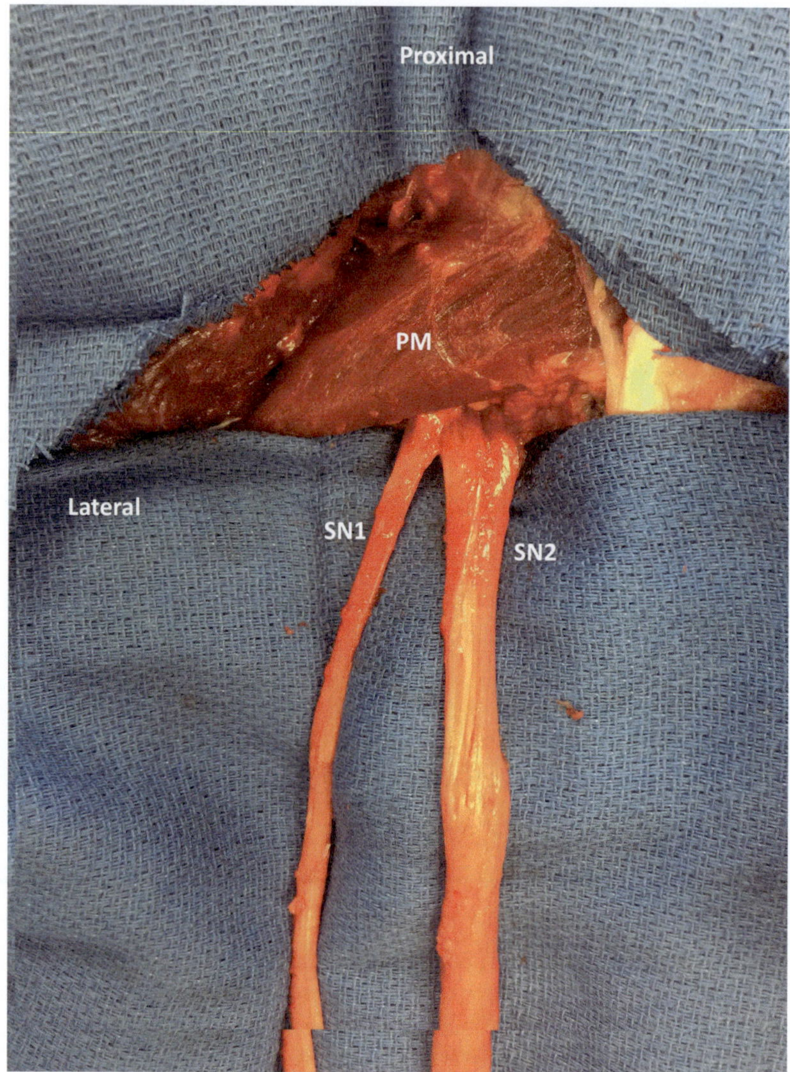

Fig. 8.14 Endoscopic view of sciatic nerve (SN) compression between the greater trochanter (GT) and ischial tuberosity. With hip flexion and external rotation, the sciatic nerve was not able to move due to the ischial outgrowth of the bone

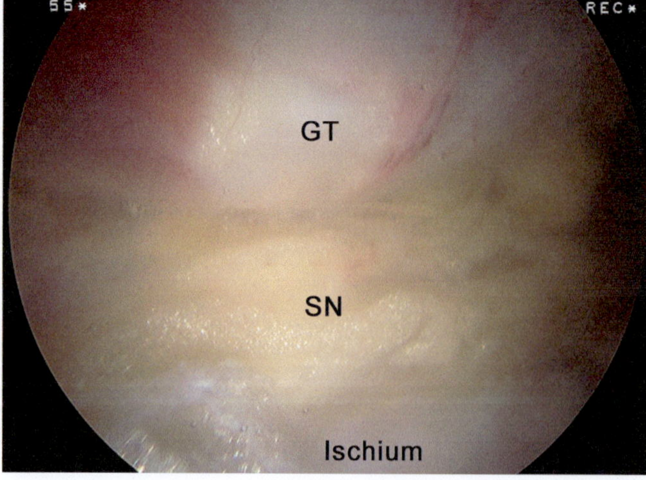

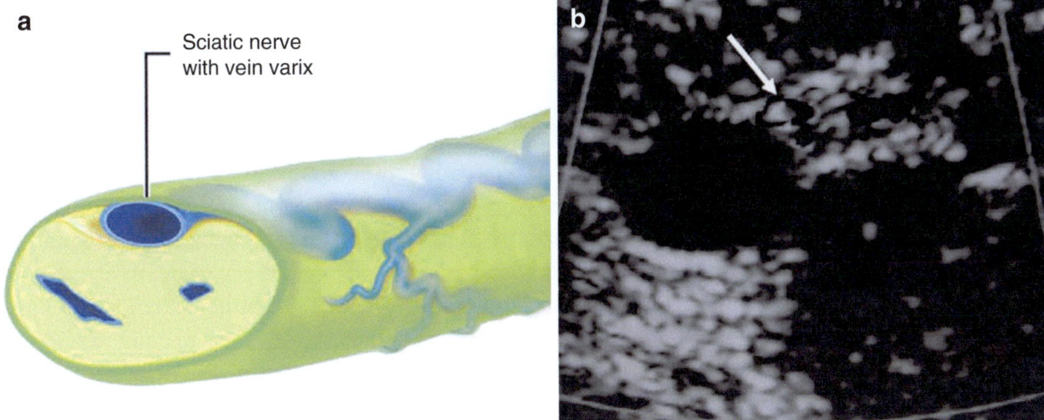

Fig. 8.15 Varicose veins around the sciatic nerve. (**a**) Schematic drawing of varicose veins within the perineurium and the sciatic nerve. (**b**) Sciatic nerve at the midthigh with varicose veins within the nerve (arrow) in a patient who presented with pain and swelling. A larger refluxing vein is also seen in adhesion with the nerve. Reprinted with permission from Labropoulos et al. [9]

Table 8.2 Entrapments of the sciatic nerve within the deep gluteal space in key publications

Piriformis muscle	Martin et al. [2], Guvencer et al. [40], Papadopoulos and Kahn [55], Adams [43], Beauchesne and Schutzer [11], Benson and Schutzer [44], Chen [12], Dezawa et al. [45], Filler et al. [46], Hughes et al. [47], Mayrand et al. [48], Sayson et al. [49], Vandertop and Bosma [3], McCrory and Bell [1]
Hamstring muscles	Martin et al. [2]; Puranen and Orava [4], Young et al. [5]
Gemelli-obturator internus complex	Martin et al. [2]; Meknas et al. [7, 15], Cox and Bakkum [6]
Fibrous bands containing blood vessels	Martin et al. [2]; Adams [43], Vandertop and Bosma [3]
Ischial tuberosity	Miller et al. [8], Patti et al. (2008), Torriani et al. (2009)
Sciatic varicosities and vascular abnormalities	Martin et al. [2], Papadopoulos and Kahn [55], Hughes et al. [47], Papadopoulos et al. [10], Labropoulos et al. [9]
Gluteal muscles	Martin et al. [2]; McCrory and Bell [1]
Acetabular reconstruction surgery	Issack et al. [52]
Prolonged surgery in the seated position	Brown et al. [51]
After total hip replacement	Uchio et al. [53]
Secondary to space-occupying lesions intra-pelvic	Beauchesne and Schutzer [11], Chen [12]
Gynecologic and vascular abnormalities	Possover [13], Possover et al. [34]

articular hip disorders may also be involved with sciatic nerve symptoms. Patients submitted to surgical treatment of femoroacetabular impingement often recovery hip mobility or can move the hip without having intra-articular pain. Considering that neural structures are sensitive to strain [39], increases in mobility can cause strain greater than habitual in the sciatic nerve, triggering the sciatic nerve entrapment symptoms in patients with variations in the piriformis-sciatic nerve relationship. This factor may be even more important in patients with capsular laxity and bone abnormal morphologies, as increased femoral version or retroversion.

The fibers of the sciatic nerve can be also entrapped in the lumbar spine, pelvis, and thigh. A discussion regarding intra-pelvic etiologies of sciatic nerve entrapment will be provided in the differential diagnoses section. Table 8.2 summarizes the etiologies of sciatic nerve entrapment reported in the main publications.

Clinical Presentation and Ancillary Testing

History and Physical Examination

A comprehensive physical examination, a detailed history, and standardized radiographic interpretation are paramount in evaluating hip pain [2, 60, 61]. When assessing posterior hip pain, the physical examination will allow for an assessment of osseous, capsular labral, musculotendinous, and neurovascular etiologies. Additionally, it is important to recognize the coexistence of many of these pathologies. The lumbar spine, abdominal, genitourinary problems are ruled out by history, physical examination, and ancillary testing. It is important to consider intra-pelvic causes of sciatic nerve entrapment, particularly in patients with previous gynecologic surgical procedures and menses-related pain [13, 34]. In all cases of suspected sciatic nerve entrapment, the spine must first be ruled out by MRI and history/physical examination.

Patients presenting with sciatic nerve entrapment often have a history of trauma and symptoms of sit pain (inability to sit for more than 30 min), radicular pain of the lower back or hip, and paresthesias of the affected leg [2, 44]. Patients may present with neurological symptoms of abnormal reflexes or motor weakness [55]. Some symptoms may mimic a hamstring tear or intra-articular hip pathology such as aching, burning sensation, or cramping in the buttock or posterior thigh. Symptoms of sit pain can also be caused by pudendal nerve entrapment, in which the pain is medial to the ischium and will be discussed later in this chapter. Upon palpation of the piriformis, Robinson described a tender sausage-shaped mass as a key feature of what he termed "piriformis syndrome" [42]. Physical examination

tests that have been used for the clinical diagnosis of sciatic nerve entrapment include passive stretching tests and active contraction tests. The space between the piriformis and obturator internus muscles narrows with flexion, adduction, and internal rotation [40].

The seated piriformis stretch test (Fig. 8.16a) is a flexion, adduction with internal rotation test performed with the patient in the seated position [60]. The examiner extends the knee (engaging the sciatic nerve) and passively moves the flexed hip into adduction with internal rotation while palpating 1 cm lateral to the ischium (middle finger) and proximally at the sciatic notch (index finger). A positive test is the recreation of the posterior pain at the level of the piriformis or external rotators. An active piriformis test (Fig. 8.16b) is performed by the patient pushing the heel down into the table, abducting and externally rotating the leg against resistance, while the examiner monitors the piriformis. In a recent published study, the combination of the seated piriformis stretch test with the piriformis active test presented a sensitivity of 91% and specificity of 80% for the endoscopic finding of sciatic nerve entrapment [62].

The palpation of the gluteal structures is fundamental for the diagnosis of gluteal and sit pain. Patient is seated with the pelvis square to the examination table, and the ischial tuberosity (IT) serves as the reference point for palpation (Fig. 8.17a–c). Pain superolateral to the IT at the sciatic notch is characteristic of deep gluteal syndrome [2]; pain lateral to the IT, ischial tunnel syndrome or ischiofemoral impingement is considered; pain at the IT, hamstring tendon pathologies are possible; and pain medial to the IT, pudendal nerve entrapment is considered. An active knee flexion test against resistance, with 30° versus 90° of knee flexion, can help evaluate the proximal hamstring tendons [5].

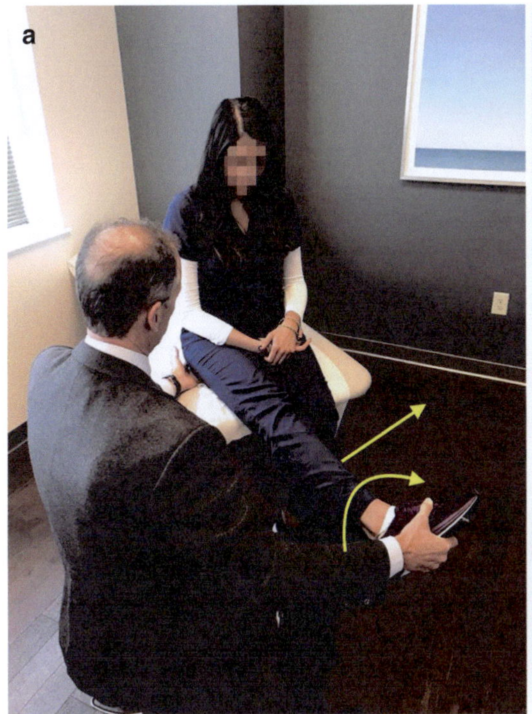

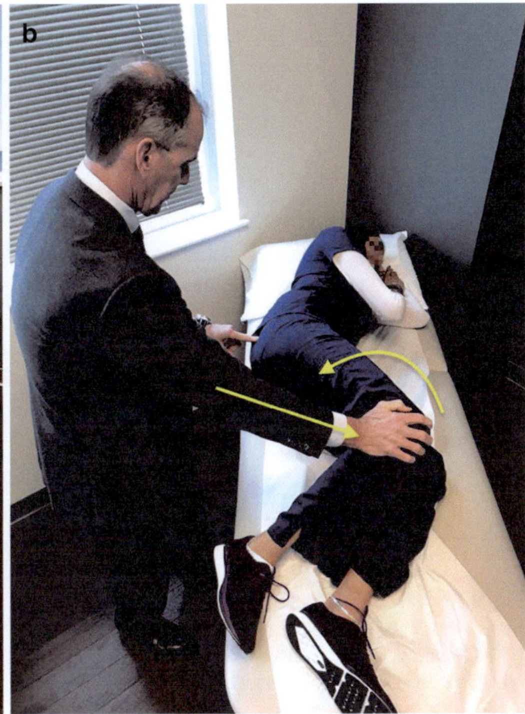

Fig. 8.16 (**a**) Seated piriformis stretch test. The patient is in the seated position with knee extension. The examiner passively moves the flexed hip into adduction with internal rotation while palpating 1 cm lateral to the ischium (middle finger) and proximally at the sciatic notch (index finger). (**b**) Active piriformis test. With the patient in the lateral position, the examiner palpates the piriformis. The patient drives the heel into the examining table thus initiating external hip rotation while actively abducting and externally rotating against resistance

Ischial tunnel syndrome or hamstring syndrome is described as pain in the lower buttock region that radiates down the posterior thigh to the popliteal fossa and is commonly associated with hamstring weakness [4]. This syndrome is related to sciatic nerve entrapment by scarring or a fibrotic band at the lateral insertion of the hamstring tendons to the ischial tuberosity [4, 5]. Patients experience pain with sitting, stretching, and with exercise, primarily running (sprinting and acceleration) [5, 63]. Palpable tenderness is located around the ischial tuberosity in the proximal hamstring region. Clinically, Young et al. reported that the straight leg raise test (Lasègue test) is slightly positive without neurological deficit. Marked weakness of the hamstring muscle at 30° knee flexion yet normal strength at 90° knee flexion is a suggestive finding in diagnosis [5].

Symptoms related to other nerves may be observed in cases of sciatic nerve entrapment, such as weakness of the gluteus medius and minimus muscles (superior gluteal nerve), weakness of the gluteus maximus (inferior gluteal nerve), perineal sensory loss (pudendal nerve) [64], or loss of posterior cutaneous sensation (posterior femoral cutaneous nerve) (Table 8.1) (Fig. 8.18).

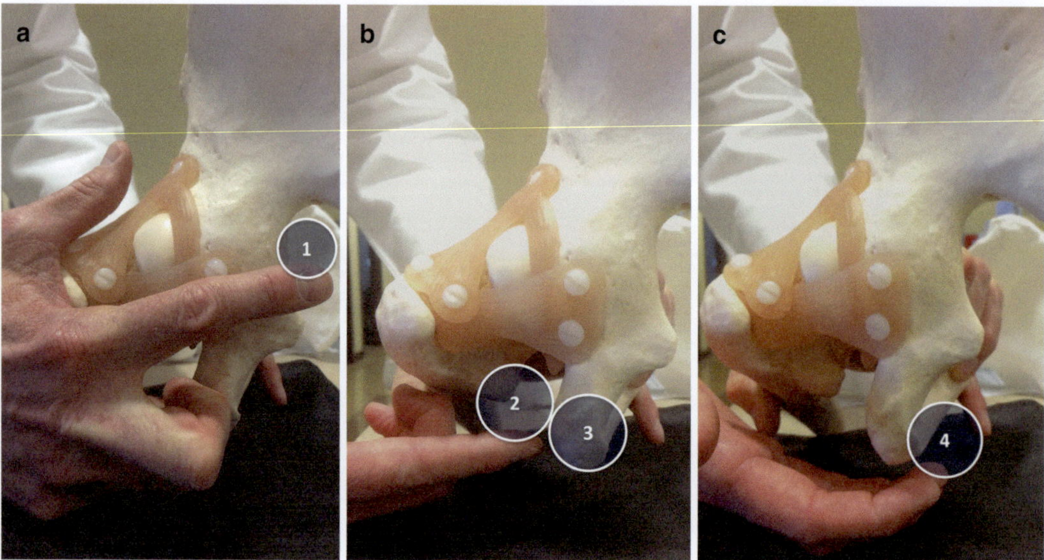

Fig. 8.17 Palpation of the deep gluteal space. The examiner palpates the gluteal area using the ischial tuberosity (IT) as reference: (1) superolateral at the piriformis muscle/sciatic nerve (index finger); (2) moving the index finger to palpate lateral to the IT, ischiofemoral impingement and ischial tunnel syndrome; (3) at the IT, hamstring origin tendinopathy and avulsion (middle finger); (4) medial at the obturator internus/pudendal nerve (ring finger)

Ancillary Testing

Guided injections are useful to support the diagnosis of DGS, mainly when the piriformis is involved. Computed tomography, fluoroscopy, ultrasonography, electroneuromyography, or magnetic resonance imaging is useful to obtain more precise injections [46]. The results and techniques for injections in deep gluteal space will be discussed in more detail in the treatment section. The association of physical examination and injection is also utilized to rule out intra-articular hip pathologies, nerve root compression at lumbar spine, and pudendal nerve entrapment.

Electromyography and nerve conduction studies may assist with the diagnosis of deep gluteal syndrome. Piriformis entrapment of the sciatic nerve is often indicated by H-reflex disturbances of the tibial and/or fibular nerves [65, 66]. It is important to compare side to side and perform a dynamic test with the knee in extension and hip in adduction with internal rotation. This position will tighten the piriformis muscle compressing the sciatic nerve sufficiently to disturb nerve conduction distally. Patients presenting with symptoms of sciatic nerve entrapment may fail to

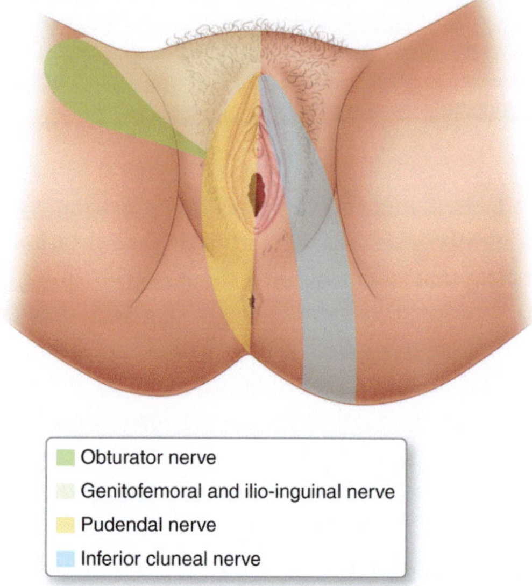

Fig. 8.18 Sensory zones of the perineum in female. The sensitive innervation territory is marked according to the nerve. The dotted area represents the obturator nerve territory. The vertical lines represent the genitofemoral and ilioinguinal nerves. The oblique lines represent the pudendal nerve. The crossed lines denote the inferior cluneal nerve innervation. Although the figure illustrates well-defined areas of innervation, it is important to remember that an overlap in dermatomes is frequent [64]

exhibit paraspinal denervation even when radiculopathy coexists [65]. Although electrodiagnostic assessment can be useful when associated with adequate physical examination and injection tests, obesity, edema, and age can impair the acquisition of sensory nerve action potentials in the lower limb, principally for the proximally located nerves [67]. Moreover, asymptomatic patients (usually elderly) often present neurogenic changes in electrodiagnostic studies [67]. These features may be problematic for the differential diagnosis between lumbosacral and peripheral entrapment [67].

Magnetic resonance imaging (MRI) is the most useful imaging method for evaluation of sciatic nerve entrapment. The sciatic nerve anatomy and potential sources of compression can be assessed through this imaging method, including anomalies of the piriformis muscle, scar from proximal hamstring avulsion, osseous compression, and intra-pelvic abnormalities (Fig. 8.19). The MRI is also helpful in detecting direct and indirect signs of nerve injury [68].

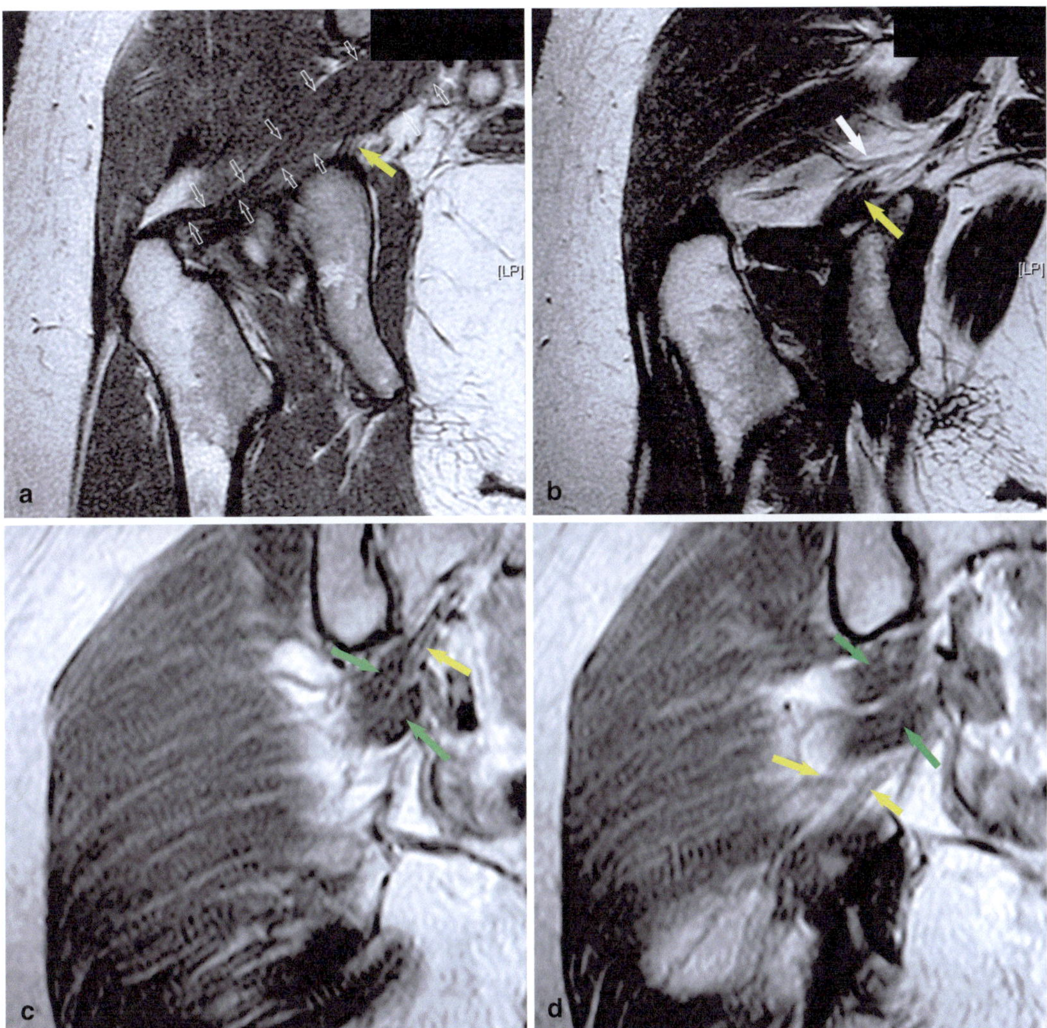

Fig. 8.19 Magnetic resonance images of deep gluteal space, coronal view of the right hip. (**a**) Normal relationship between the piriformis muscle (open arrows) and the sciatic nerve (yellow arrow). (**b**) More posterior cut of the same hip demonstrating the inferior gluteal artery (white arrow) leaving the sciatic notch close to the sciatic nerve (yellow arrow). (**c**) and (**d**) Variation of the sciatic nerve/piriformis relationship in a patient with deep gluteal syndrome. The superior division of the sciatic nerve (yellow arrow in **c**) is demonstrated crossing between the two piriformis muscle portions (green arrows)

Table 8.3 Main differential diagnosis of deep gluteal syndrome

Diagnosis	History	Physical examination	Ancillary tests
Pudendal nerve entrapment	Pain in the anatomical territory of the pudendal nerve, worsened by sitting, does not wake the patient at night Numbness	Tenderness at the medial ischium	Injection guided by imaging Intra-pelvic tests
Ischiofemoral impingement	Sciatic nerve complaints Lower back pain Limping	Long-stride walking reproduces the pain during terminal hip extension Tenderness at the lateral ischium Positive ischiofemoral impingement test	MRI showing decreased ischiofemoral and quadratus femoris space and quadratus femoris muscle edema
Greater trochanter ischial impingement	Sciatic nerve complaints Laxity? Limping	Tenderness at posterior aspect of the greater trochanter Pain in deep flexion, abduction, and external rotation	Injection guided by imaging
Ischial tunnel syndrome	Sciatic nerve complaints Limping Pain increased by flexion of the hip and extension of the knee	Tenderness at lateral ischium Positive hamstring active test	Injection guided by imaging MRI showing hamstring origin avulsion with edema around the sciatic nerve

Hyperintensity on fluid-sensitive images that is focal or similar to that of adjacent vessels is more likely to be significant [68]. However, hyperintensity in peripheral nerves may be seen in normal nerves due to the artifact known as magic angle effect [69]. Abnormalities in nerve size, fascicular pattern, or blurring of the perineural fat tissue are suggestive of neural injury, although those features are difficult to be noted in small diameter nerves [68]. The main indirect sign of nerve entrapment injury is the muscular denervation edema [70]. In addition to sciatic nerve compression assessment, the MRI is important to rule out spine issues, intra-articular hip pathology, and other differential diagnoses. Despite the usefulness of MRI in the diagnosis of deep gluteal pain, the potential false-positive and false-negative results reinforce the importance of a proficient physical examination. Ultrasonography is a valuable method to guide nerve blocks and has been increasingly utilized for nerve assessment, with the advantages of dynamic evaluation and Doppler assessment of the vascular nerve supply [9].

The differential diagnosis of sciatic nerve entrapment is established through the combination of physical examination, imaging studies, and piriformis injection test (Table 8.3).

Treatment

Nonoperative Treatment

The nonoperative treatment for deep gluteal syndrome begins addressing the suspected site of entrapment. Compression from a hypertrophied, contracted, or inflamed muscle (piriformis, quadratus femoris, obturator internus, superior/inferior gemellus) is initially treated with rest, anti-inflammatories, muscle relaxants, and physical therapy. The physical therapy program should include stretching maneuvers aimed at the external rotators. The piriformis stretch, or FAIR, involves placing the hip in flexion, adduction, and internal rotation (Fig. 8.20a). Patients with CAM impingement, anterior pincer impingement, or acetabular retroversion may not be able to stretch adequately into this position and should be evaluated and treated primarily for the intra-articular pathology, as most will resolve with appropriate surgical intervention. In a seated position, the patient brings the knee into the

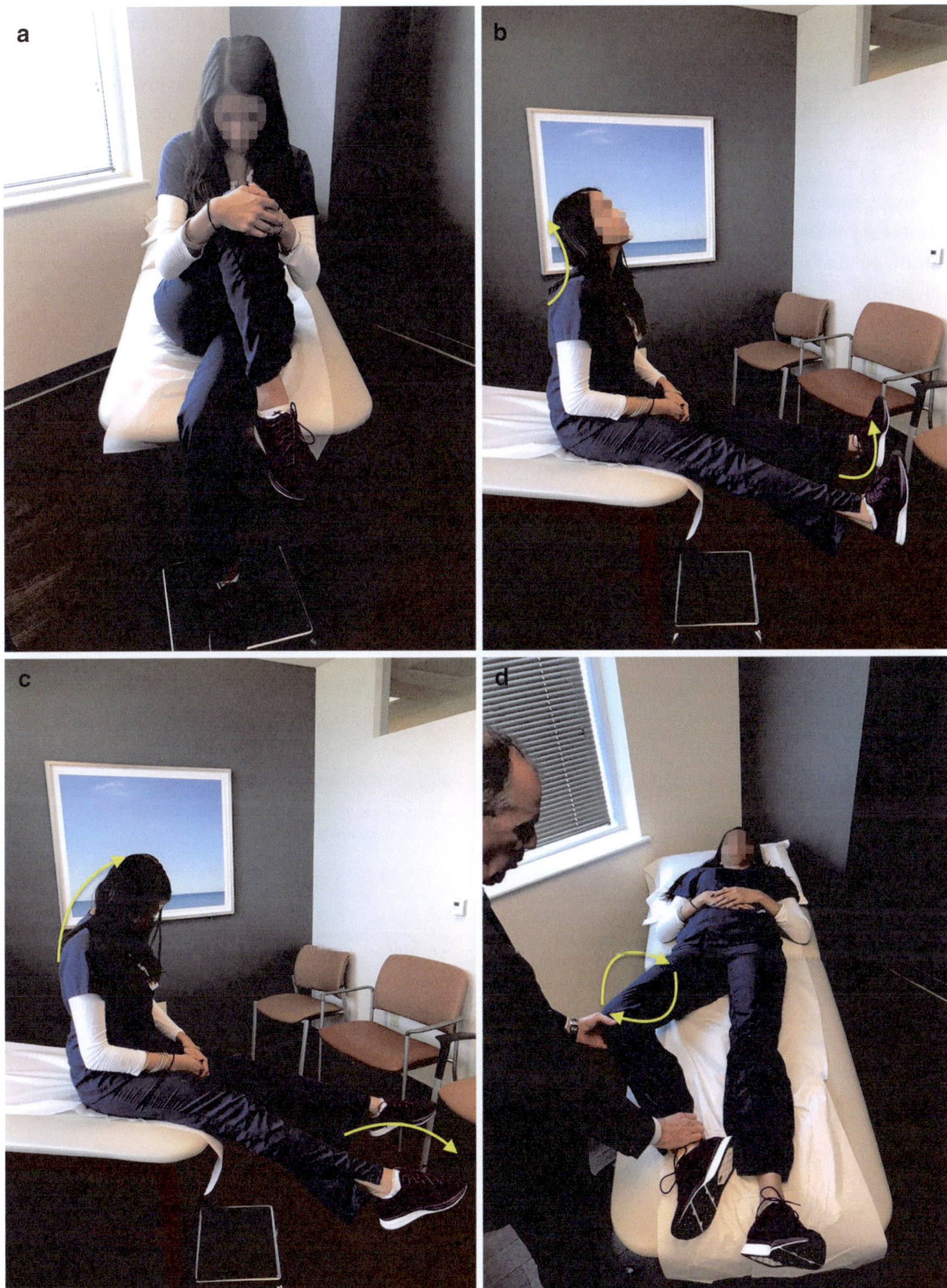

Fig. 8.20 Piriformis stretch, sciatic nerve glides, and hip circumduction. (**a**) The piriformis stretch is performed in a seated position. The patient brings the knee toward the opposite shoulder. (**b**) For the sciatic nerve glides, the patient first performs cervical extension and plantar flexion of the ankle, (**c**) followed by cervical flexion with ankle dorsiflexion. (**d**) Circumduction performed in supine position with gentle circular passive movements in the following sequence: abduction, external rotation, flexion, internal rotation, extension

chest and across midline and pulls the knee to the opposite shoulder during 20 s. Gradually progress the stretching by increasing duration and intensity until a maximal stretch is obtained. Sciatic nerve glides and hip circumduction exercises are useful to maintain the sciatic nerve excursion and should be gently performed (Fig. 8.20b–d). Additional physical therapy techniques that may be helpful include ultrasound and electrical stimulation. Patients with more intense or acute symptoms may not tolerate positions of hip flexion associated with knee extension. In this situation, a knee brace to avoid knee extension and maintain the sciatic nerve without tension may be helpful for some patients. The brace is adjusted according to the straight leg raise test, and gradual extension of the knee is performed toward full extension during 4–6 weeks.

Guided injections of anesthetic or corticosteroid into the piriformis muscle can provide pain relief in patients not responding to physical therapy. It is important to administer the injection to the correct site, and different techniques can be utilized for guidance, including fluoroscopy, CT, ultrasound, electromyography, and MRI. A trial of three injections has been recommended before opting for more aggressive therapy, taken on a case by case basis [46, 55, 71]. The literature has reported variable results for piriformis injection [46, 72, 73]. Pace and Nagle reported a double-injection technique of Kenalog and Xylocaine toward the piriformis muscle which relieved the pain in 41 out of 45 patients [73]. Filler et al. reported lasting pain relief in 37 out of 162 patients following 1 or 2 injections of Marcaine and Celestone [46]. The piriformis muscle may be also injected with botulinum toxin [54]. Another alternative is the perisciatic nerve injection of anesthetic and corticosteroid instead of the intra-piriformis muscle [74]. Most cases of deep gluteal syndrome/sciatic nerve entrapment will respond to nonoperative measures.

Operative Treatment

As a general guideline, only patients who have failed conservative measures are considered for operative treatment. The type of surgical procedure depends on the clinical and imaging diagnosis. The response to targeted injections is helpful to predict the treatment success.

Effective open and endoscopic techniques have been described for a number of posterior hip pathologies including sciatic nerve decompression (Fig. 8.13). Innovative surgical techniques as car-

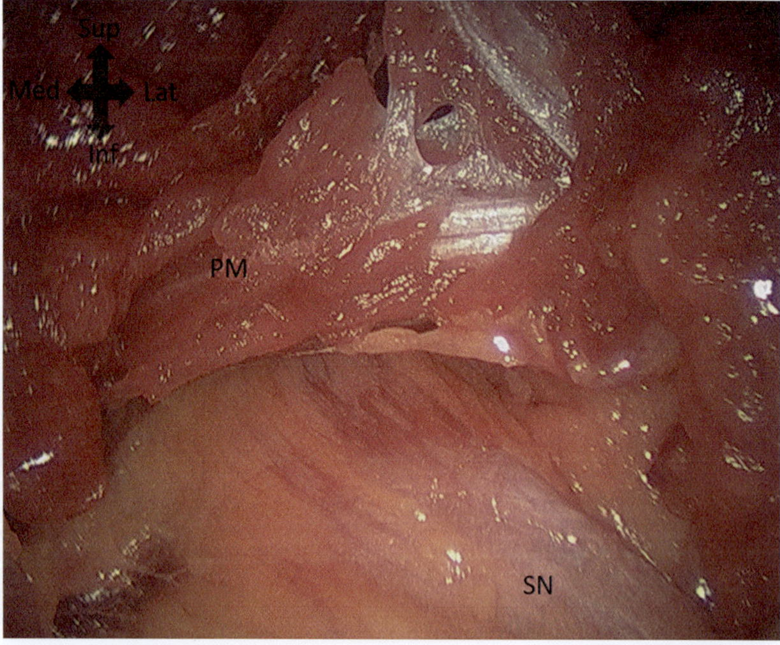

Fig. 8.21 Deep gluteal space exploration by using carbon dioxide (CO_2) gas as an insufflation medium. *PM* piriformis muscle, *SN* sciatic nerve

bon dioxide gas insufflation as a medium for deep gluteal endoscopy are being developed in order to simplify the technical aspects of the procedure while decreasing complications (Fig. 8.21).

A comprehensive and illustrative description of both open and endoscopic techniques for treating deep gluteal syndrome is presented in this book describing surgical approaches to the posterior hip.

References

1. McCrory P, Bell S. Nerve entrapment syndromes as a cause of pain in the hip, groin and buttock. Sports Med. 1999;27:261–74.
2. Martin HD, Shears SA, Johnson JC, Smathers AM, Palmer IJ. The endoscopic treatment of sciatic nerve entrapment/deep gluteal syndrome. Arthroscopy. 2011;27:172–81.
3. Vandertop WP, Bosma NJ. The piriformis syndrome. A case report. J Bone Joint Surg Am. 1991;73:1095–7.
4. Puranen J, Orava S. The hamstring syndrome. A new diagnosis of gluteal sciatic pain. Am J Sports Med. 1988;16:517–21.
5. Young IJ, van Riet RP, Bell SN. Surgical release for proximal hamstring syndrome. Am J Sports Med. 2008;36:2372–8.
6. Cox JM, Bakkum BW. Possible generators of retrotrochanteric gluteal and thigh pain: the gemelli-obturator internus complex. J Manip Physiol Ther. 2005;28:534–8.
7. Meknas K, Kartus J, Letto JI, Christensen A, Johansen O. Surgical release of the internal obturator tendon for the treatment of retro-trochanteric pain syndrome: a prospective randomized study, with long-term follow-up. Knee Surg Sports Traumatol Arthrosc. 2009;17:1249–56.
8. Miller A, Stedman GH, Beisaw NE, Gross PT. Sciatica caused by an avulsion fracture of the ischial tuberosity. A case report. J Bone Joint Surg Am. 1987;69:143–5.
9. Labropoulos N, Tassiopoulos AK, Gasparis AP, Phillips B, Pappas PJ. Veins along the course of the sciatic nerve. J Vasc Surg. 2009;49:690–6.
10. Papadopoulos SM, McGillicuddy JE, Albers JW. Unusual cause of 'piriformis muscle syndrome'. Arch Neurol. 1990;47:1144–6.
11. Beauchesne RP, Schutzer SF. Myositis ossificans of the piriformis muscle: an unusual cause of piriformis syndrome. A case report. J Bone Joint Surg Am. 1997;79:906–10.
12. Chen WS. Sciatica due to piriformis pyomyositis. Report of a case. J Bone Joint Surg Am. 1992;74:1546–8.
13. Possover M. Laparoscopic management of endopelvic etiologies of pudendal pain in 134 consecutive patients. J Urol. 2009;181:1732–6.
14. Loukas M, Louis RG Jr, Hallner B, Gupta AA, White D. Anatomical and surgical considerations of the sacrotuberous ligament and its relevance in pudendal nerve entrapment syndrome. Surg Radiol Anat. 2006;28:163–9.
15. Meknas K, Christensen A, Johansen O. The internal obturator muscle may cause sciatic pain. Pain. 2003;104:375–80.
16. Solomon LB, Lee YC, Callary SA, Beck M, Howie DW. Anatomy of piriformis, obturator internus and obturator externus: implications for the posterior surgical approach to the hip. J Bone Joint Surg Br. 2010;92:1317–24.
17. Standring S. Grays anatomy the anatomical basis of clinical practice. London: Elsevier; 2008.
18. Miller SL, Gill J, Webb GR. The proximal origin of the hamstrings and surrounding anatomy encountered during repair. A cadaveric study. J Bone Joint Surg Am. 2007;89:44–8.
19. Filler AG. Diagnosis and treatment of pudendal nerve entrapment syndrome subtypes: imaging, injections, and minimal access surgery. Neurosurg Focus. 2009;26:E9.
20. Moore K, Dalley A. Essential clinical anatomy. Philadelphia: Lippincott Williams and Wilkins; 1999.
21. Windhofer C, Brenner E, Moriggl B, Papp C. Relationship between the descending branch of the inferior gluteal artery and the posterior femoral cutaneous nerve applicable to flap surgery. Surg Radiol Anat. 2002;24:253–7.
22. Kalhor M, Beck M, Huff TW, Ganz R. Capsular and pericapsular contributions to acetabular and femoral head perfusion. J Bone Joint Surg Am. 2009;91:409–18.
23. Gautier E, Ganz K, Krugel N, Gill T, Ganz R. Anatomy of the medial femoral circumflex artery and its surgical implications. J Bone Joint Surg Br. 2000;82:679–83.
24. Sunderland S, Hughes ES. Metrical and non-metrical features of the muscular branches of the sciatic nerve and its medial and lateral popliteal divisions. J Comp Neurol. 1946;85:205–22.
25. Sunderland S, Ray LJ. The intraneural topography of the sciatic nerve and its popliteal divisions in man. Brain. 1948;71:242–73.
26. Seidel PM, Seidel GK, Gans BM, Dijkers M. Precise localization of the motor nerve branches to the hamstring muscles: an aid to the conduct of neurolytic procedures. Arch Phys Med Rehabil. 1996;77:1157–60.
27. Moayeri N, Groen GJ. Differences in quantitative architecture of sciatic nerve may explain differences in potential vulnerability to nerve injury, onset time, and minimum effective anesthetic volume. Anesthesiology. 2009;111:1128–34.
28. Sladjana UZ, Ivan JD, Bratislav SD. Microanatomical structure of the human sciatic nerve. Surg Radiol Anat. 2008;30:619–26.
29. Georgakis E, Soames R. Arterial supply to the sciatic nerve in the gluteal region. Clin Anat. 2008;21:62–5.

30. Karmanska W, Mikusek J, Karmanski A. Nutrient arteries of the human sciatic nerve. Folia Morphol (Warsz). 1993;52:209–15.

31. Ugrenovic SZ, Jovanovic ID, Vasovic LP, Stefanovic BD. Extraneural arterial blood vessels of human fetal sciatic nerve. Cells Tissues Organs. 2007;186:147–53.

32. Del Pinal F, Taylor GI. The venous drainage of nerves; anatomical study and clinical implications. Br J Plast Surg. 1990;43:511–20.

33. Testut L, Latarjet A. Traite d'anatomie humaine. Paris: G. Doin & Cie; 1949.

34. Possover M, Schneider T, Henle KP. Laparoscopic therapy for endometriosis and vascular entrapment of sacral plexus. Fertil Steril. 2011;95:756–8.

35. Beaton L, Anson B. The sciatic nerve and the piriformis muscle: their interrelation and possible cause of coccygodynia. J Bone Joint Surg Am. 1938;20:686–8.

36. Smoll NR. Variations of the piriformis and sciatic nerve with clinical consequence: a review. Clin Anat. 2010;23:8–17.

37. Coppieters MW, Alshami AM, Babri AS, Souvlis T, Kippers V, Hodges PW. Strain and excursion of the sciatic, tibial, and plantar nerves during a modified straight leg raising test. J Orthop Res. 2006;24:1883–9.

38. Fleming P, Lenehan B, O'Rourke S, McHugh P, Kaar K, McCabe JP. Strain on the human sciatic nerve in vivo during movement of the hip and knee. J Bone Joint Surg Br. 2003;85:363–5.

39. Wall EJ, Massie JB, Kwan MK, Rydevik BL, Myers RR, Garfin SR. Experimental stretch neuropathy. Changes in nerve conduction under tension. J Bone Joint Surg Br. 1992;74:126–9.

40. Guvencer M, Akyer P, Iyem C, Tetik S, Naderi S. Anatomic considerations and the relationship between the piriformis muscle and the sciatic nerve. Surg Radiol Anat. 2008;30:467–74.

41. Yeoman W. The relation of arthritis of the sacro-iliac joint to sciatica, with an analysis of 100 cases. Lancet. 1928;2:1119–22.

42. Robinson DR. Pyriformis syndrome in relation to sciatic pain. Am J Surg. 1947;73:355–8.

43. Adams JA. The pyriformis syndrome – report of four cases and review of the literature. S Afr J Surg. 1980;18:13–8.

44. Benson ER, Schutzer SF. Posttraumatic piriformis syndrome: diagnosis and results of operative treatment. J Bone Joint Surg Am. 1999;81:941–9.

45. Dezawa A, Kusano S, Miki H. Arthroscopic release of the piriformis muscle under local anesthesia for piriformis syndrome. Arthroscopy. 2003;19:554–7.

46. Filler AG, Haynes J, Jordan SE, Prager J, Villablanca JP, Farahani K, McBride DQ, Tsuruda JS, Morisoli B, Batzdorf U, Johnson JP. Sciatica of nondisc origin and piriformis syndrome: diagnosis by magnetic resonance neurography and interventional magnetic resonance imaging with outcome study of resulting treatment. J Neurosurg Spine. 2005;2:99–115.

47. Hughes SS, Goldstein MN, Hicks DG, Pellegrini VD Jr. Extrapelvic compression of the sciatic nerve. An unusual cause of pain about the hip: report of five cases. J Bone Joint Surg Am. 1992;74:1553–9.

48. Mayrand N, Fortin J, Descarreaux M, Normand MC. Diagnosis and management of posttraumatic piriformis syndrome: a case study. J Manip Physiol Ther. 2006;29:486–91.

49. Sayson SC, Ducey JP, Maybrey JB, Wesley RL, Vermilion D. Sciatic entrapment neuropathy associated with an anomalous piriformis muscle. Pain. 1994;59:149–52.

50. Bano A, Karantanas A, Pasku D, Datseris G, Tzanakakis G, Katonis P. Persistent sciatica induced by quadratus femoris muscle tear and treated by surgical decompression: a case report. J Med Case Rep. 2010;4:236.

51. Brown JA, Braun MA, Namey TC. Pyriformis syndrome in a 10-year-old boy as a complication of operation with the patient in the sitting position. Neurosurgery. 1988;23:117–9.

52. Issack PS, Kreshak J, Klinger CE, Toro JB, Buly RL, Helfet DL. Sciatic nerve release following fracture or reconstructive surgery of the acetabulum. Surgical technique. J Bone Joint Surg Am. 2008;90(Suppl 2 Pt 2):227–37.

53. Uchio Y, Nishikawa U, Ochi M, Shu N, Takata K. Bilateral piriformis syndrome after total hip arthroplasty. Arch Orthop Trauma Surg. 1998;117:177–9.

54. Porta M. A comparative trial of botulinum toxin type A and methylprednisolone for the treatment of myofascial pain syndrome and pain from chronic muscle spasm. Pain. 2000;85:101–5.

55. Papadopoulos EC, Khan SN. Piriformis syndrome and low back pain: a new classification and review of the literature. Orthop Clin North Am. 2004;35:65–71.

56. Filler AG. Piriformis and related entrapment syndromes: diagnosis & management. Neurosurg Clin N Am. 2008;19:609–622, vii.

57. Chakravarthy J, Ramisetty N, Pimpalnerkar A, Mohtadi N. Surgical repair of complete proximal hamstring tendon ruptures in water skiers and bull riders: a report of four cases and review of the literature. Br J Sports Med. 2005;39:569–72.

58. Orava S. Hamstring syndrome. Oper Tech Sports Med. 1997;5:143–9.

59. Wood DG, Packham I, Trikha SP, Linklater J. Avulsion of the proximal hamstring origin. J Bone Joint Surg Am. 2008;90:2365–74.

60. Martin H. Clinical examination and imaging of the hip. In: Byrd J, Guanche C, editors. AANA advanced arthroscopy: the hip. Philadelphia: Saunders; 2010.

61. Martin HD, Kelly BT, Leunig M, Philippon MJ, Clohisy JC, Martin RL, Sekiya JK, Pietrobon R, Mohtadi NG, Sampson TG, Safran MR. The pattern and technique in the clinical evaluation of the adult hip: the common physical examination tests of hip specialists. Arthroscopy. 2010;26:161–72.

62. Martin HD, Kivlan BR, Palmer IJ, Martin RL, Hatem M. Diagnostic accuray of clinical tests for sciatic nerve entrapent in the gluteal region. Knee Surg Sports Traumatol Arthrosc. 2013;22(4):882–8.

63. Migliorini S, Merlo M. The hamstring syndrome in endurance athletes. Br J Sports Med. 2011;45:363.

64. Labat JJ, Riant T, Robert R, Amarenco G, Lefaucheur JP, Rigaud J. Diagnostic criteria for pudendal neuralgia by pudendal nerve entrapment (Nantes criteria). Neurourol Urodyn. 2008;27:306–10.

65. Fishman LM, Wilkins AN. Piriformis syndrome: electrophysiology vs. anatomical assumption. In: Fishman LM, Wilkins AN, editors. Functional electromyography. New York: Springer; 2011.

66. Jawish RM, Assoum HA, Khamis CF. Anatomical, clinical and electrical observations in piriformis syndrome. J Orthop Surg Res. 2010;5:3.

67. Katirji B. Electrodiagnostic approach to the patient with suspected mononeuropathy of the lower extremity. Neurol Clin. 2002;20:479–501, vii.

68. Petchprapa CN, Rosenberg ZS, Sconfienza LM, Cavalcanti CF, Vieira RL, Zember JS. MR imaging of entrapment neuropathies of the lower extremity. Part 1. The pelvis and hip. Radiographics. 2010;30:983–1000.

69. Chappell KE, Robson MD, Stonebridge-Foster A, Glover A, Allsop JM, Williams AD, Herlihy AH, Moss J, Gishen P, Bydder GM. Magic angle effects in MR neurography. AJNR Am J Neuroradiol. 2004;25:431–40.

70. Kim SJ, Hong SH, Jun WS, Choi JY, Myung JS, Jacobson JA, Lee JW, Choi JA, Kang HS. MR imaging mapping of skeletal muscle denervation in entrapment and compressive neuropathies. Radiographics. 2011;31:319–32.

71. Barton PM. Piriformis syndrome: a rational approach to management. Pain. 1991;47:345–52.

72. Benzon HT, Katz JA, Benzon HA, Iqbal MS. Piriformis syndrome: anatomic considerations, a new injection technique, and a review of the literature. Anesthesiology. 2003;98:1442–8.

73. Pace JB, Nagle D. Piriform syndrome. West J Med. 1976;124:435–9.

74. Hanania M, Kitain E. Perisciatic injection of steroid for the treatment of sciatica due to piriformis syndrome. Reg Anesth Pain Med. 1998;23:223–8.

Pudendal Nerve Neuralgia/Entrapment

Sung-Jung Yoon, Juan Gómez-Hoyos,
William Henry Márquez-Arabia,
and Hal D. Martin

Introduction

Chronic pelvic pain situations such as pudendal pain, chronic proctalgia, coccygodynia, vulvodynia, and pudendal neuralgia (PN) occur in 7–24% of the population and are associated with impaired quality of life and high health-care costs [1].

Pain in the distribution of the pudendal nerve is frequently due to identifiable organic problems; however a number of cases occur under circumstances in which no organic cause can be found. Pudendal nerve neuralgia due to entrapment at the Alcock's canal is commonly overlooked by physicians, thus delaying access to etiological treatment. The abnormal hip biomechanics affects the entire pelvis and kinematic chain, therefore putting the pudendal nerve under strain during hip movements. The most common patient's profile is a patient who had seen multiple doctors, with no clear evidence of organic problem, normal urogynecological and colorectal evaluations, and failed multiple pharmacologic treatments.

The cause of the pudendal neuralgia is not always clear, but it is believed that neuronal insult caused by stretching or compression is the primary etiology. Pudendal neuralgia is said to be a diagnosis of exclusion and requires a high index of suspicion. Although there are no pathognomonic signs and symptoms, clinical diagnostic criteria are helpful. Clinical neurophysiology tests have quite low diagnostic efficacy and must therefore be considered to be complementary investigations. Optional treatments include behavioral modifications, physical therapy, analgesics, pudendal nerve block, and surgical nerve decompression [2].

Neurologic pathology in the pelvic region can produce extreme pain, which greatly affects quality of life by limiting the ability to sit, void/defecate, and engage in sexual intercourse. This review provides an overview of the main causes

S.-J. Yoon, MD, PhD
Chonbuk National University Hospital, Department of Orthopedic Surgery, Jeonju, South Korea

J. Gómez-Hoyos, MD (✉)
International Consultant, Hip Preservation Center / Baylor Scott and White Research Institute, Baylor University Medical Center, Dallas, TX, USA

Department of Orthopaedic Surgery - Health Provider, Clínica Las Américas / Clínica del Campestre, Medellin, Antioquia, Colombia

Professor - School of Medicine - Sports Medicine Program, Universidad de Antioquia, Medellín, Antioquia, Colombia

W. H. Márquez-Arabia, MD
Clínica Las Americas, Orthopedic Surgery, Medellin, Antioquia, Colombia

Sports Medicine Program, School of Medicine, Medellin, Antioquia, Colombia

H. D. Martin, DO
Medical and Research Director, Hip Preservation Center, Baylor University Medical Center, Dallas, TX, USA

© Springer International Publishing AG, part of Springer Nature 2019
H. D. Martin, J. Gómez-Hoyos (eds.), *Posterior Hip Disorders*,
https://doi.org/10.1007/978-3-319-78040-5_9

of neurogenic pelvic pain, along with information on diagnosis and treatment options [3].

Anatomy

The pudendal nerve arises from sacral nerves 2, 3, and 4 and passes in close association with the sciatic nerve between the piriformis and coccygeus muscles. The nerve crosses the ischial spine as it first leaves and then reenters the pelvis through the greater and lesser sciatic foramina, respectively. At the area of the ischial spine, it is superficial to the sacrospinous ligament and deep to the sacrotuberous ligament, an area of possible compression or fixation. The nerve then accompanies the internal pudendal vessels along the lateral wall of the ischioanal fossa in a tunnel formed by a splitting of the obturator fascia (Alcock's canal). This tunnel is another area of possible compression adhesion [4, 5].

The pudendal nerve sensory distribution course is generally via the three terminal branches: inferior rectal, perineal, and dorsal nerve of the penis/clitoris. The inferior rectal supplies the integument around the anus and communicates with the perineal branch of the posterior femoral cutaneous nerve and its terminal branch, the posterior scrotal (labia majora) nerve. The perineal branch has a deep motor portion and two superficial sensory branches, the medial and lateral posterior scrotal (labial) nerves. The dorsal nerve of the penis/clitoris runs along the dorsum of the penis/clitoris, supplying the overlying skin. Pudendal neuralgia may present with pain in the distribution of some or all of these branches [6].

The pudendal nerve can become entrapped in several locations from the greater sciatic notch to the lesser sciatic notch and even distally to the obturator internus/levator ani fascia. The anatomy of the pudendal nerve can have significant individual variation. In 87 of 100 cadaveric hips, the sacrotuberous ligament has been found to be composed of the two parts: a ligamentous band and a membranous falciform process [7]. The attach-

ment of the falciform process to the ischial ramus showed two variations. Most commonly, the falciform process continued toward and along the ischial ramus to the obturator fascia. The second type coursed along the ischial ramus, fused with the obturator fascia, and continued to the ischioanal fossa. The medial border of the falciform process descended to fuse with the lateral anococcygeal ligament. Superior to the sacrotuberous ligament is the sacrospinous ligament. A very rare anomaly of the pudendal nerve was discovered in a cadaver involving the pudendal nerve and vessels coursing posterior to the sacrotuberous ligament [7]. Pudendal nerve relationship with the sacrospinous ligament is varied and could be prone to entrapment [8] (Figs. 9.1 and 9.2).

Epidemiology and Etiology

About 4% of all cases of chronic pelvic pain are caused by pudendal neuralgia. This condition is most commonly seen in women, but it also affects men. Pudendal neuralgia has an average age at onset of 50–70 years [3]. A pudendal nerve disorder can occur due to extrinsic or intrinsic causes, most of them being a mechanical insult such as iatrogenic injury during pelvic surgery, stretching of the nerve during vaginal childbirth, compression from prolonged sitting, and prolonged positions of stretching, which have been documented in orthopedic surgical cases involving traction [9–13]. Chemoradiation, tumors, and endometriosis have also been documented as causes of nerve compression [14]. Anatomic variation of the falciform process of the sacrotuberous ligament may also predispose the nerve to stretching in some individuals [7]. Intrinsic causes are much less common than entrapment, but there have been documented cases caused by autoimmune or inflammatory illness.

Four main types of pudendal nerve entrapment are based upon the location of entrapment, which is very important for injections: Type I, at the exit of the greater sciatic notch accompanied by piriformis muscle spasm; Type II, at the ischial

Fig. 9.1 (a and b) Cadaveric dissection of the pudendal nerve running beneath the sacrotuberous ligament

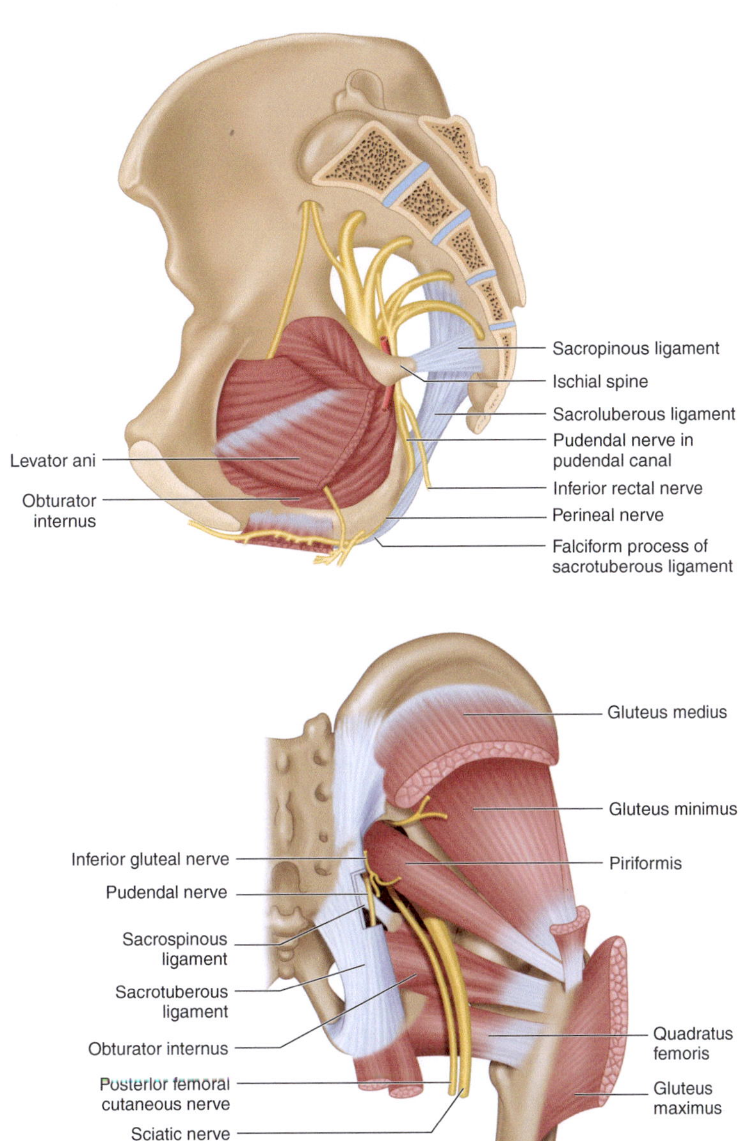

spine, sacrotuberous ligament, and lesser sciatic notch entrance; Type III, at the entrance of the Alcock's canal associated with obturator internus muscle spasm; and Type IV, tidal entrapment of terminal branches [15].

In many cases, the nerve is not truly entrapped at these sites along its winding course but rather under traction due to biomechanical factors, such as pelvic floor muscle spasm or the presence of a pelvic obliquity. It has been hypothesized that repetitive flexion of the hip, such as in sports or strength training, may cause hypertrophy of the muscles of the pelvic floor as well as elongation and posterior remodeling of the ischial spine causing stretch of the nerve over the sacrospinous ligament [10].

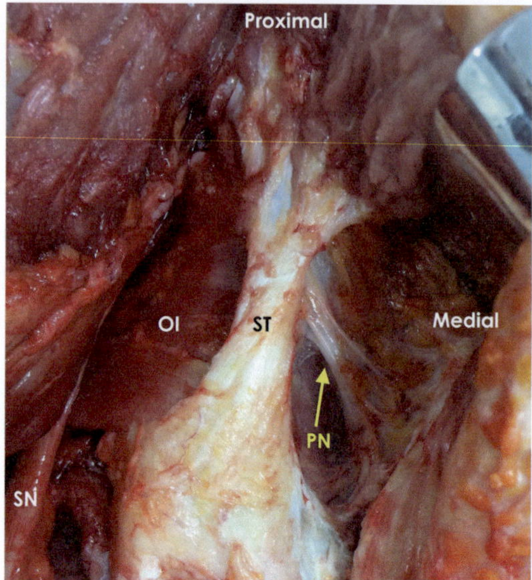

Fig. 9.2 Anatomy of the pudendal nerve (PN). Posterior view of the nerve and its relationship with other important structures such as sacrotuberous (ST) ligament, sciatic nerve (SN), and obturator internus (OI) muscle

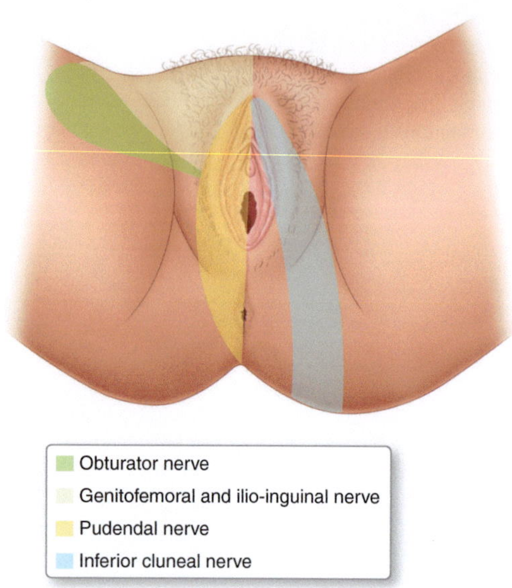

Fig. 9.3 The innervation of the perineum

Diagnosis

History and physical examination are the most relevant components leading to diagnosis. Problems that can present with similar clinical findings such as painful bladder syndrome, vulvodynia, piriformis syndrome, cauda equine syndrome, and neuralgias of other close nerves must be excluded [16] (Fig. 9.3).

Detailed history should report the pain characteristics including onset, type, duration, aggravating and alleviating factors, and frequency. Examination should include any inspection for any peri-genital lesions and a complete hip physical exam focusing on the posterior aspect of the hip and the peri-ischial area [17].

Palpation on the ischial spine or pudendal nerve that produces paresthesias or pain is referred to as Tinel's sign. Some patients start favoring one side of their pelvis while sitting, which can be discretely observed during history and physical examination [18].

In 2008, Labat el al. validated the Nantes criteria with five essential diagnostic criteria: (1) pain in the anatomical territory of the pudendal nerve, (2) worsened by sitting (although no pain when sitting on a toilet seat), (3) the pain does not wake the patient at night, (4) pain with no objective sensory impairment, and (5) pain is relieved by diagnostic pudendal nerve block [19]. Also defined in the report are complementary diagnostic criteria, exclusion criteria, and associated signs not excluding the diagnosis (Table 9.1). Neurophysiologic testing techniques have been used to aid in diagnosis [20]. The physical examination is useful for preliminarily sorting patients into four categories: Type I, sciatic notch tenderness only; Type II, mid-ischial tenderness; Type IIIa, obturator internus muscle tenderness only; Type IIIb, obturator and piriformis muscle tenderness; and Type IV, no palpable tenderness. MR neurography or MRI can then be helpful to identify abnormalities in nerve or adjacent muscles/vessels [15]. Positive MRI findings will lead to injection sites according to category: Type I, piriform injection; Type II, blocking the pudendal nerve at the ischial spine; Type IIIa, obturator internus injection; Type IIIb, piriformis and obturator internus injection; and Type IV, blocking the pudendal nerve in the area of the Alcock's canal [15]. If there is no relief and no specific aggravation, evaluate immune/rheumatological issues and end-organ causes, which if negative, consider a ganglion block. A

Table 9.1 Diagnostic criteria for pudendal neuralgia by pudendal nerve entrapment (Nantes criteria)

Essential criteria for the diagnosis of pudendal neuralgia
- Pain in the territory of the pudendal nerve: from the anus to the penis or clitoris
- Pain is predominantly experienced while sitting
- Pain does not wake the patient at night
- Pain with no objective sensory impairment
- Pain relieved by diagnostic pudendal nerve block

Complementary diagnostic criteria
- Burning, shooting, stabbing pain, numbness
- Allodynia or hyperpathia
- Rectal or vaginal foreign body sensation (sympathalgia)
- Worsening of pain during the day
- Predominantly unilateral pain
- Pain triggered by defecation
- Presence of exquisite tenderness on palpation of the ischial spine
- Clinical neurophysiology findings in men or nulliparous women

Exclusion criteria
- Exclusively coccygeal, gluteal, pubic, or hypogastric pain
- Pruritus
- Exclusive paroxysmal pain
- Imaging abnormalities able to account for the pain

Associated signs no excluding the diagnosis
- Buttock pain on sitting
- Referred sciatic pain
- Pain referred to the medial aspect of the thigh
- Suprapubic pain
- Urinary frequency and/or pain on a full bladder
- Pain occurring after ejaculation
- Dyspareunia and/or pain after sexual intercourse
- Erectile dysfunction
- Normal clinical neurophysiology

Labat J-J, Riant T, Robert R, Amarenco G, Lefaucheur J-P, Rigaud J. Diagnostic criteria for pudendal neuralgia by pudendal nerve entrapment (Nantes criteria). Neurourol. Urodyn. 2008;27:306–10.

repeat injection may be required if necessary for diagnosis and treatment. Details about imaging-guided injections are developed in Chap. 6 of this book.

Ancillary Tests

Imaging studies are not helpful for diagnosing pudendal nerve entrapment. However, radiographs, CT scan, and MRI may assist in ruling out other causes of pain and/or in determining a potential cause of entrapment.

Electromyography and other neurophysiology aids may help as complementary measures [21]. However they lack specificity. Those tests could result in a lot of false-positive reports. Thus, a normal test does not rule out pudendal neuralgia as only motor fibers are being tested, while an abnormal test indicates that the pudendal nerve is affected, but it is not specific for this diagnosis.

Ultrasound-guided pudendal nerve injection is the useful method for confirming and differentiating this pathology from other pelvic-related sources of pain. A patient is placed in see chapter pelvic floor therapy a prone position. Place a convex probe on the gluteal region to visualize the transverse view of the ilium. Move the probe in a cephalad-caudal direction until the ischial spine can be seen in position when the probe places transversely between sacrum and ischial spine levels. The ischial spine appears as a flatten hyperechoic line. The sacrospinous ligament (SSL) and the sacrotuberous ligament (STL) are also visualized at this position. The pudendal nerve resides between the SSL and STL. Insert a 100 mm spinal needle in a medial-to-lateral direction, and advance it until the needle tip penetrates the STL. When the needle tip penetrates the STL, a click can be felt. After negative aspiration test for the blood can be checked, injection of 5 mL of local anesthetics with corticosteroid is performed. The spreading of local anesthetics can be confirmed between the STL and the SSL using ultrasound. This ultrasound-guided infiltration test allowed precision in performing the procedure and in making a differential diagnosis.

Treatment

A number of therapeutic options have been reported depending on the cause of pudendal neuropathy. The most effective strategies can be broken in three parts: (1) conservative measures, (2) pudendal nerve block, and (3) surgical decompression.

Physical therapy interventions, such as pelvic floor therapy, have been considered the first option of treatment by most of authors. A detailed description of this strategy is presented in Chap. 22.

Other strategies include electrical stimulation and biofeedback. In some cases botulinum toxin has been utilized with variable results. A randomized controlled trial investigating whether botulinum toxin is more effective than placebo found objective reduction of pelvic floor spasm as compared with placebo. This intervention may be useful in women with pelvic floor muscle spasm and chronic pelvic pain who do not respond to conservative physical therapy [22].

Pudendal nerve block could be performed through transgluteal, transrectal, or transvaginal approach. The ischial bone is used as an important landmark for identifying the injection spot. Imaging-guided approaches have been reported in several studies. CT-guided injection, as described in Chap. 6, improves the accuracy of locating the pudendal nerve [23, 24].

Multiple injection protocols for treating pudendal nerve neuralgia have been proposed. Those protocols vary in terms of utilized medications, number of injections, and timing. Most of the authors use a combination of a local anesthetic and steroid. Patients may benefit from repetitive nerve blocks, and conservatives measures should be individualized [2, 25].

Surgical pudendal nerve decompression is offered to patients who have failed conservative measures. Open, endoscopic and laparoscopic techniques have shown good results in case series [15, 26]. Filler reported on 200 patients with pudendal nerve entrapment, and 12% achieved long-standing relief (over 1 year) with injection alone. One hundred and eighty-five operations were performed (some patients bilateral). The application of targeted minimal access surgical techniques has led to sustained good to excellent outcomes (50–100% improvement in the pain score or functional score) in 87% of patients. Many of these patients obtained most of their improvement within 4 weeks of surgery, and some continued to experience progressive improvements up to 12 months after surgery [15]. Other authors have reported successful outcomes in a range between 57% and 81% [27, 28].

Robert et al. published the results of a prospective, randomized controlled trial that compared transgluteal decompression with nonsurgical treatment and repetitive pudendal blocks. A total of 32 patients were included in this study (16 in each group). After 1 year of treatment, 71.4% of the surgery group compared with 13.3% of the nonsurgery group showed improvement [29].

According to the literature, after surgical decompression, approximately 40% of patients are pain-free, 30% have some improvement in pain, and 30% neither show improvement nor worsening [16].

References

1. Possover M, Forman A. Voiding dysfunction associated with pudendal nerve entrapment. Curr Bladder Dysfunct Rep. 2012;7:281–5.
2. Stav K, Dwyer PL, Roberts L. Pudendal neuralgia: fact or fiction? Obstet Gynecol Surv. 2009;64(3):190–9.
3. Elkins N, Hunt J, Scott KM. Neurogenic pelvic pain. Phys Med Rehabil Clin N Am. 2017;28(3):551–69.
4. Robert R, Prat-Pradal D, Labat JJ, Bensignor M, Raoul S, Rebai R, Leborgne J. Anatomic basis of chronic perineal pain: role of the pudendal nerve. Surg Radiol Anat. 1998;20(2):93–8.
5. Thor KB, Donatucci C. Central nervous system control of the lower urinary tract: new pharmacological

approaches to stress urinary incontinence in women. J Urol. 2004;172(1):27–33.

6. Benson JT, Griffis K. Pudendal neuralgia, a severe pain syndrome. Am J Obstet Gynecol. 2005;192(5):1663–8.

7. Loukas M, Louis RG, Hallner B, Gupta AA, White D. Anatomical and surgical considerations of the sacrotuberous ligament and its relevance in pudendal nerve entrapment syndrome. Surg Radiol Anat. 2006;28:163–9.

8. Mahakkanukrauh P, Surin P, Vaidhayakarn P. Anatomical study of the pudendal nerve adjacent to the sacrospinous ligament. Clin Anat. 2005;18:200–5.

9. Bohrer JC, Walters MD, Park A, et al. Pelvic nerve injury following gynecologic surgery: a prospective cohort study. Am J Obstet Gynecol. 2009;201:531.e1–7.

10. Antolak SJ, Hough DM, Pawlina W, et al. Anatomical basis of chronic pelvic pain syndrome: the ischial spine and pudendal nerve entrapment. Med Hypotheses. 2002;59:349–53.

11. Alevizon SJ, Finan MA. Sacrospinous colpopexy: management of postoperative pudendal nerve entrapment. Obstet Gynecol. 1996;88:713–5.

12. Pailhe R, Chiron P, Reina N, et al. Pudendal nerve neuralgia after hip arthroscopy: retrospective study and literature review. Orthop Traumatol Surg Res. 2013;99:785–90.

13. Leibovitch I, Mor Y. The vicious cycling: bicycling related urogenital disorders. Eur Urol. 2005;47:277–86.

14. Elahi F, Callahan D, Greenlee J, et al. Pudendal entrapment neuropathy: a rare complication of pelvic radiation therapy. Pain Physician. 2013;16:E793–7.

15. Filler AG. Diagnosis and treatment of pudendal nerve entrapment syndrome subtypes: imaging, injections, and minimal access surgery. Neurosurg Focus. 2009;26:E9.

16. Khoder W, Hale D. Pudendal neuralgia. Obstet Gynecol Clin N Am. 2014;41(3):443–52.

17. Martin HD, Reddy M, Gómez-Hoyos J. Deep gluteal syndrome. J Hip Preserv Surg. 2015;2(2):99–107.

18. Amarenco G, Lanoe Y, Ghnassia RT, Goudal H, Perrigot M. Alcock's canal syndrome and perineal neuralgia. Rev Neurol (Paris). 1988;144(8–9):523–6.

19. Labat J-J, Riant T, Robert R, Amarenco G, Lefaucheur J-P, Rigaud J. Diagnostic criteria for pudendal neuralgia by pudendal nerve entrapment (Nantes criteria). Neurourol Urodyn. 2008;27:306–10.

20. Popeney C, Ansell V, Renney K. Pudendal entrapment as an etiology of chronic perineal pain: diagnosis and treatment. Neurourol Urodyn. 2007;26:820–7.

21. Olsen AL, Ross M, Stansfield RB, Kreiter C. Pelvic floor nerve conduction studies: establishing clinically relevant normative data. Am J Obstet Gynecol. 2003;189(4):1114–9.

22. Abbott JA, Jarvis SK, Lyons SD, Thomson A, Vancaille TG. Botulinum toxin type A for chronic pain and pelvic floor spasm in women: a randomized controlled trial. Obstet Gynecol. 2006;108(4):915–23.

23. McDonald JS, Spigos DG. Computed tomography-guided pudendal block for treatment of pelvic pain due to pudendal neuropathy. Obstet Gynecol. 2000;95(2):306–9.

24. Calvillo O, Skaribas IM, Rockett C. Computed tomography-guided pudendal nerve block. A new diagnostic approach to long-term anoperineal pain: a report of two cases. Reg Anesth Pain Med. 2000;25(4):420–3.

25. Hibner M, Desai N, Robertson LJ, Nour M. Pudendal neuralgia. J Minim Invasive Gynecol. 2010;17(2):148–53.

26. Shafik A. Endoscopic pudendal canal decompression for the treatment of fecal incontinence due to pudendal canal syndrome. J Laparoendosc Adv Surg Tech A. 1997;7:227–34.

27. Shafik A. Pudendal canal syndrome as a cause of vulvodynia and its treatment by pudendal nerve decompression. Eur J Obstet Gynecol Reprod Biol. 1998;80(2):215–20.

28. Beco J, Climov D, Bex M. Pudendal nerve decompression in perineology: a case series. BMC Surg. 2004;4:15.

29. Robert R, Labat JJ, Bensignor M, Glemain P, Deschamps C, Raoul S, Hamel O. Decompression and transposition of the pudendal nerve in pudendal neuralgia: a randomized controlled trial and long-term evaluation. Eur Urol. 2005;47(3):403–8.

Hamstring Origin Avulsions and Ischial Tunnel Syndrome

Carlos A. Guanche

Introduction

With the refinement of hip pathologies has come a better understanding of the management of several areas previously treated rarely and with much trepidation [1, 2]. The development of endoscopic techniques to understand the posterior aspect of the hip has been a process in evolution, which continues today. Hamstring injuries are common in athletic populations and can affect all levels of athletes [3–7]. There is a continuum of hamstring injuries that can range from musculotendinous strains to avulsion injuries [3, 4]. By definition, a strain is a partial or complete disruption of the musculotendinous unit [4]. A complete tear or avulsion, in contrast, is a discontinuity of the tendon bone unit. Most hamstring strains do not require surgical intervention and resolve with a variety of modalities and rest [3–7].

With the exception of the short head of the biceps femoris, the hamstring complex originates from the ischial tuberosity and inserts distally below the knee on the proximal tibia. The tibial branch of the sciatic nerve innervates the semitendinosus, semimembranosus, and the long head of biceps femoris, while the short head of the biceps femoris is innervated by the peroneal branch of the sciatic nerve [5].

The proximal hamstring complex has a strong bony attachment on the ischial tuberosity. The footprint on the ischium is comprised of the semitendinosus and the long head of biceps femoris beginning as a common proximal tendon and footprint, while there is a distinct semimembranosus footprint [8]. The semimembranosus footprint is lateral (and anterior) to the crescent-shaped footprint of the common insertion of the semitendinosus and long head of the biceps femoris.

The history of an acute injury usually involves a traumatic event with forced hip flexion and knee in extension, as is classically observed in waterskiing [9, 10]. However, the injury can result from a wide variety of sporting activities that involve rapid acceleration and deceleration [11, 12].

Proximal hamstring injuries can be categorized as complete tendinous avulsions, partial tendinous avulsions, apophyseal avulsions, and degenerative (tendinosis) avulsions [11]. Degenerative tears of the hamstring origin are more insidious in onset and are commonly seen in overuse situations. The mechanism of injury is presumably repetitive irritation of the medial aspect of the hamstring tendon (typically along the lateral aspect of the tuberosity, where the bursa resides) ultimately causing an attritional tear of the tendon.

C. A. Guanche, MD
Southern California Orthopedic Institute,
Los Angeles, CA, USA
e-mail: cguanche@scoi.com

© Springer International Publishing AG, part of Springer Nature 2019
H. D. Martin, J. Gómez-Hoyos (eds.), *Posterior Hip Disorders*,
https://doi.org/10.1007/978-3-319-78040-5_10

Commonly, athletes with proximal hamstring tendon tears describe a popping or tearing sensation with associated acute pain and bruising over the posterior hip [13, 14]. Occasionally, patients who present with either acute or chronic tears may complain of pins and needles sensation in the sciatic nerve distribution, much like sciatica [14, 15]. This may be due to the acute compression of a hematoma in the proximity of the sciatic nerve or chronic scarring and tethering of the tendon to the nerve. Similarly, symptoms of ischial bursitis include buttock pain or hip pain and localized tenderness overlying the ischial tuberosity. Additional symptoms of chronic ischial bursitis may also include tingling into the buttock that spreads down the leg [14].

One aspect that briefly deserves mention is the need for advanced imaging in many of the cases of partial tears. To begin with, standard radiographs of the pelvis and a lateral of the affected hip are performed to rule out any apophyseal avulsions, particularly to the ischial tuberosity in younger patients. In others, the ischiofemoral distance may be markedly decreased, and this needs to be taken into consideration in posterior hip pain (Fig. 10.1). Most commonly, MRI is utilized to assess the proximal hamstring insertion on the ischial tuberosity, where several types of injuries may be seen. A complete rupture of all three tendons is common and easily identified on MRI.

Partial hamstring origin tears, however, are more difficult to evaluate. This is particularly the case in two tendon tears, which commonly have an associated musculotendinous junction injury to the third tendon [7]. Partial insertional tears without any significant retraction can be seen on MRI as a sickle sign. These are typically partial avulsions (Fig. 10.2). Often, the sciatic nerve is also involved in the imaging assessment and should be thoroughly evaluated. In some situations, actual entrapment of the nerve can be visualized in a variety of ways (Fig. 10.3).

Nonoperative treatment of proximal hamstring injuries is most commonly recommended in the

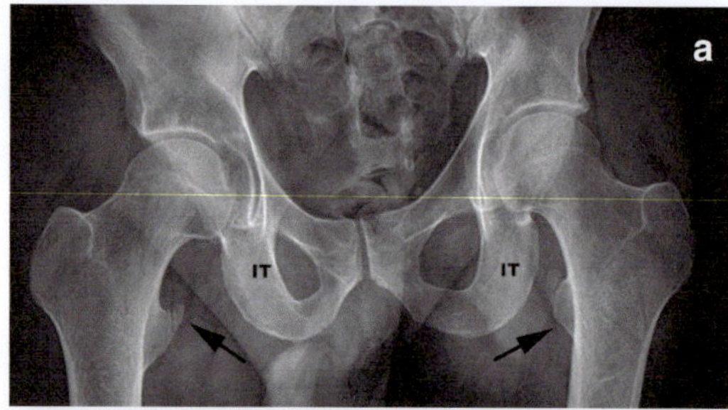
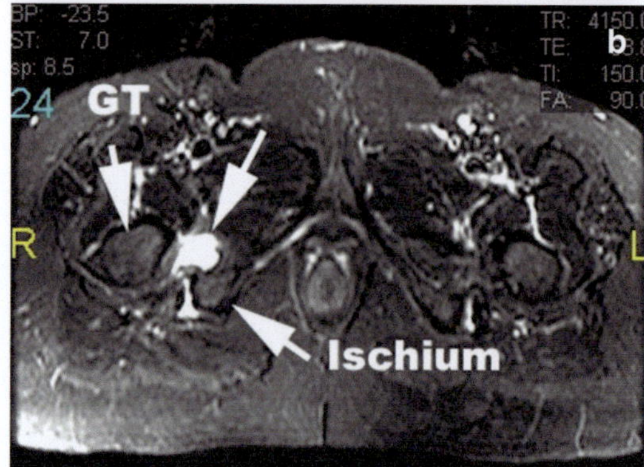

Fig. 10.1 Ischiofemoral impingement. (**a**) AP pelvis showing bilateral ischiofemoral impingement, with the ischiofemoral space being markedly narrower than the right. The arrows show the lesser trochanters. (*IT* ischial tuberosity) (**b**) T2-weighted axial MRI showing a narrowed ischiofemoral space with fluid along the ischium and a tear of the hamstring. (*GT* greater trochanter; top arrow, fluid in between quadratus space; lower arrow, ischial tuberosity)

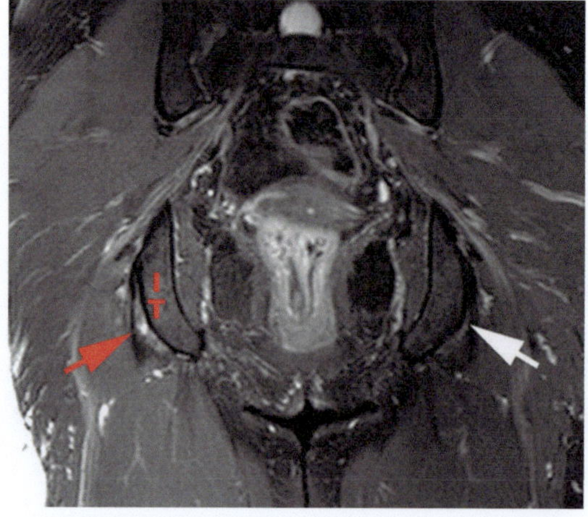

Fig. 10.2 Coronal MRI (T2 weighted) of a partial insertional tear with a sickle sign, indicating fluid in the ischial bursa (red arrow). *IT* ischial tuberosity. Note the right side (red arrow) showing the sickle sign and the normal left side (white arrow)

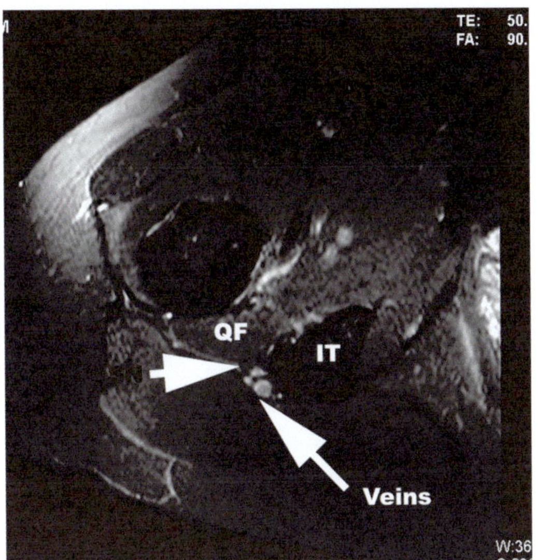

Fig. 10.3 Sciatic nerve with perineural venous dilatation. This is an axial MRI image, T1 weighted, showing the proximity of the dilated veins (vein) to the sciatic nerve (SN). (*IT* ischial tuberosity, *QF* quadratus femoris)

setting of low-grade partial tears and insertional tendinosis. Initial treatment consists of active rest, oral nonsteroidal anti-inflammatory medications, and a physical therapy program [16]. If the patient is unable to progress, an ultrasound-guided corticosteroid injection may be used and has been shown to provide initial relief in up to 50% of patients at 1 month [17]. Failure of nonoperative treatment of partial tears may benefit from surgical debridement and repair, similar to other commonly seen partial tendon tears (patella, quadriceps, and biceps) [18].

There are several series and descriptions of open surgical techniques that are available in the literature [12–14, 19–21]. To date, there has been no report of endoscopic management of these injuries. It is expected that the benefits of this endoscopic approach, without elevating the gluteus maximus and with the use of endoscopic magnification to protect the sciatic nerve, will improve the management of these injuries and reduce the morbidities associated with the open approach, thus allowing for further improvement in the management of these pathologies.

Surgical Technique

The technique positions the patient in the prone position after induction of anesthesia, with all prominences and neurovascular structures protected. The posterior aspect of the hip is then sterilized assuring that the leg and thigh are free so that the leg and hip can be repositioned (Fig. 10.4).

Two portals are then created, 2 cm medial and lateral to the palpable ischial tuberosity (Fig. 10.5). The lateral portal is established first, using blunt dissection with a switching stick, as

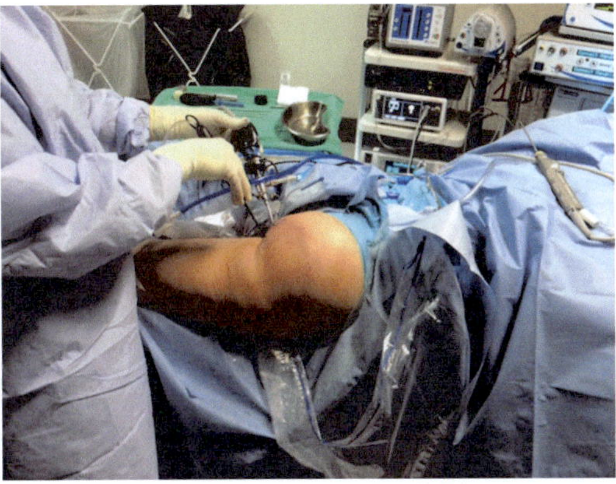

Fig. 10.4 Positioning of the patient in the prone position with the leg draped free. This is a right hip, positioned prone. Note the arthroscopic equipment is on the opposite side. The table is tilted about 20° toward the surgeon to make the access more comfortable

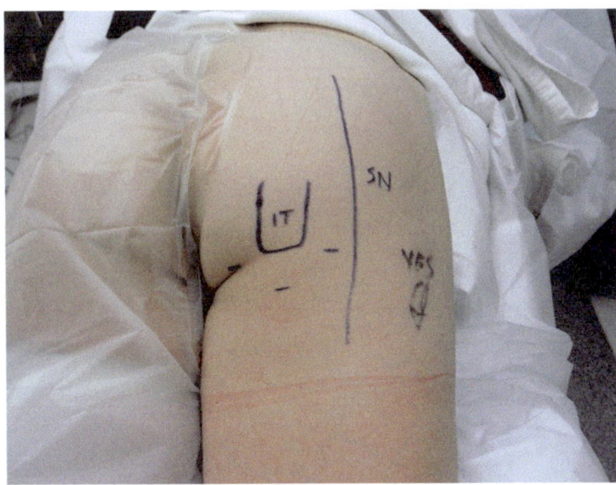

Fig. 10.5 Portals for endoscopic approach with the arthroscope in the medial portal. The shaver is in the distal portal

the gluteus maximus muscle is penetrated and the submuscular plane is developed. The prominence of the ischial tuberosity is identified, and the medial and lateral borders are located. The medial portal is then established, taking care to palpate the medial aspect of the ischium. A 30° arthroscope is then inserted in the lateral portal, and an electrocautery device is placed in the medial portal. Any remaining fibrous attachments between the ischium and the gluteus muscle are then released, staying along the central and medial portions of the ischium to avoid any damage to the sciatic nerve. The tip of the ischium and the medial aspect are delineated; the lateral aspect is then exposed with the use of a switching stick as a soft tissue dissector. With the lateral aspect identified, the dissection continues anteriorly and laterally toward the known area of the sciatic nerve (Fig. 10.6). A very careful and methodical release of any soft tissue

bands is then undertaken in a proximal to distal direction in order to mobilize the nerve and protect it throughout the exposure and ultimate repair of the hamstring tendon. In patients where the predominant problem is sciatic nerve symptomatology and impingement along the hamstring tunnel, this is an important part of the procedure. In many cases, bands of scar tissue are evident along the nerve course (Fig. 10.6). In some situations, there is a local vascular dilatation that must be addressed. This most commonly takes the form of venous distension. An important observation that can be made endoscopically is the status of the nerve's blood supply. Specifically, if the pump pressure is decreased to a minimum for a few seconds, the pulsatile flow of the perineural vessels can be observed. In situations where a nerve entrapment exists, the vessels are seen to be constricted with either poor flow or, in some cases, an area of post-stenotic dilation that is obvious below the site of compression.

With the nerve identified and protected, the tip of the ischium is identified. The tendinous origin is then inspected to identify any obvious tearing (Fig. 10.7). In acute tears, the area is obvious, and the tendon is often retracted distally. In these cases, there is occasionally a large hematoma that requires evacuation. It is especially important to protect the sciatic nerve during this portion of the procedure, as it may be obscured by the hematoma.

Once the area of pathology is identified (in incomplete tears), an endoscopic knife can be employed to longitudinally split the tendon along its fibers (Fig. 10.8). This area can be identified through palpation, as there is typically softening over the detachment, making the tissue ballottable against the ischium. The hamstring is then undermined, and the partial tearing and lateral ischial wall are debrided with an oscillating shaver. The devitalized tissue is removed, and a bleeding corticocancellous bed is fashioned in preparation for tendon repair. The more distal and inferior ischium and the ischial bursa can also be resected and cleared of inflamed tissues as the lateral ischial tissue is mobilized. By

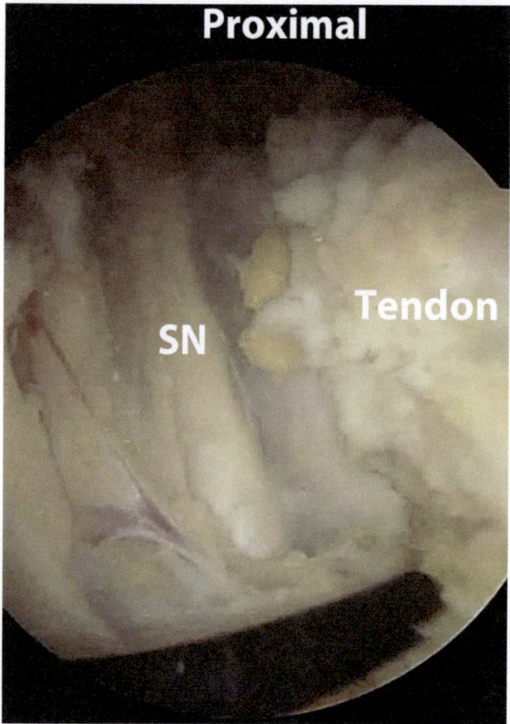

Fig. 10.6 Normal arthroscopic anatomy exposure in a left hip, viewed from the lateral portal. Sciatic nerve and lateral ischium. Note the tool entering from the medial portal

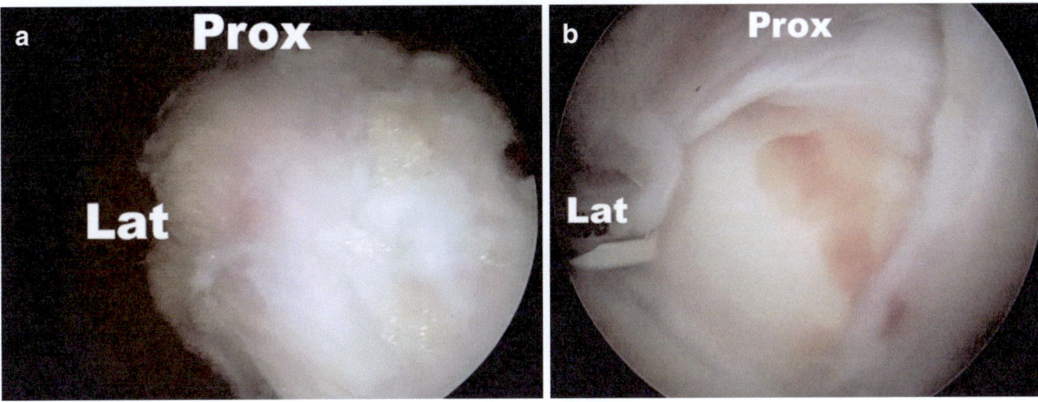

Fig. 10.7 The distal end of the ischium cleared of soft tissue. View is from the lateral portal and shows all of the soft tissue cleared from the hamstring sheath in a left hip. (**a**) Ischial prominence as seen prior to incising the hamstring sheath. (**b**) Exposed ischium following incision of the sheath

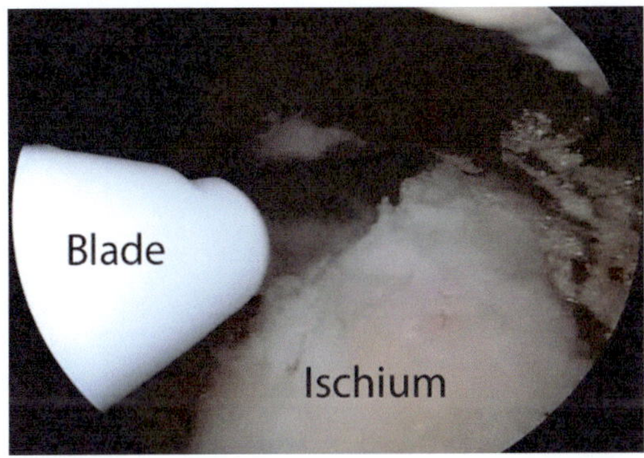

Fig. 10.8 Incision of tendon to explore area of tearing and ischial bursa

retracting the anterior tissues, the bursa can be entered and debrided (Fig. 10.9).

An inferior portal is then created approximately 4 cm distal to the tip of the ischium and equidistant from the medial and lateral portals (Fig. 10.5). This portal is employed for insertion of suture anchors, as well as suture management. Any variety of suture passing devices can then be used for the repair. The principles are essentially the same as those employed in arthroscopic rotator cuff repair. Once all of the sutures are passed through the tissue of the avulsed hamstring, the sutures are tied and a solid repair of the tendon is completed. In general, one suture anchor is used per centimeter of detachment (Fig. 10.10).

Postoperatively, the patient is fitted with a hinged knee brace that is fixed at 90° of flexion for 4 weeks to maintain the patient non-weight-bearing. The brace will also serve to restrict excursion of the hamstring tendons and protect the repair. At 4 weeks, the knee is gradually extended by about 30° per week, in order to allow full weight bearing by 6–8 weeks while maintaining the use of crutches. Physical therapy is instituted at this point, with the initial phase focused on hip and knee range of motion. Hamstring strengthening is begun at 10–12 weeks, predicated on full range of motion and a painless gait pattern. Full, unrestricted activity is allowed at approximately 4 months.

Summary

Historically, the surgical approach to hamstring repairs has not received much attention, as this is not a common area for surgical treatment that is encountered throughout orthopedic training. Those patients with partial tears and chronic bursitis are an even smaller percentage of hamstring problems, with few clinical studies available [22]. More importantly, patients with chronic sciatic nerve irritation have also been either not treated at all and simply placed in pain management algorithms or more possibly thought

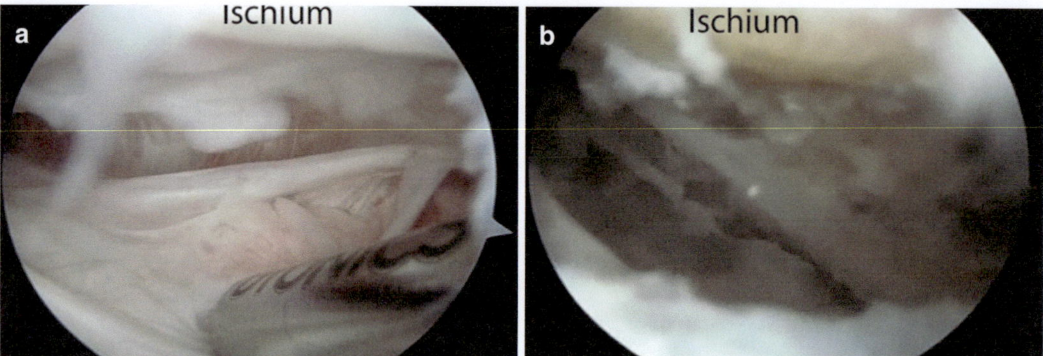

Fig. 10.9 Debridement and exposure of lateral and inferior ischium, including the ischial bursa. (**a**) Lateral ischium debridement and preparation. Note the tool is serving to retract the detached tissue. (**b**) Final debridement of bursa. Note the exposed bony surface at the top of the image and the lack of villonodular tissue

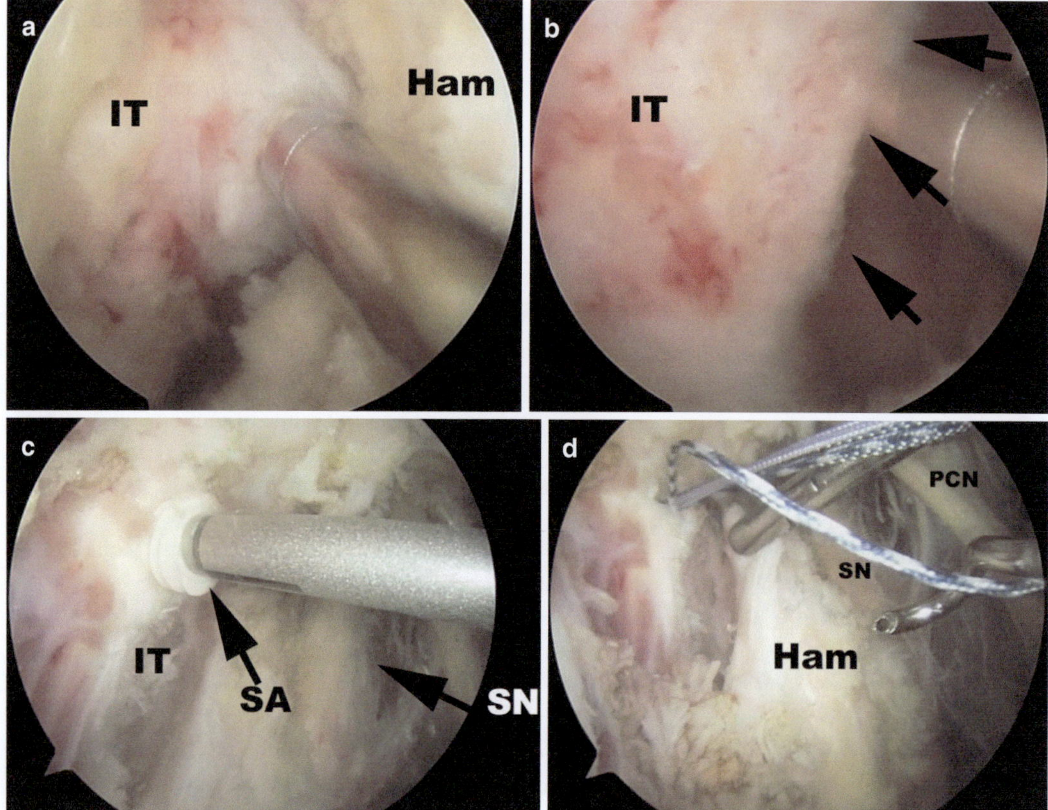

Fig. 10.10 Repair of tendinous avulsion in a right hip, visualized from the medial portal and working from lateral. (**a**) Initial exposure of frayed tissue (*IT* ischial tuberosity, *Ham* detached hamstring origin). (**b**) Prepared surface with edge of ischium (arrows) exposed. (**c**) Suture anchor (SA) in place. Note the proximity of the sciatic nerve to the repair (black arrow). (*IT* ischial tuberosity) (**d**) Repairing of the tendon with a suture passive device and a grasper holding the tendon. Note the proximity of the sciatic nerve (SN) and the posterior cutaneous nerve (PCN) to the repair. (*Ham* hamstring tendon). (**e**) Final tendon repair, prior to cutting the sutures (*SN* sciatic nerve, *PCN* posterior cutaneous nerve, *Ham* hamstring tendon)

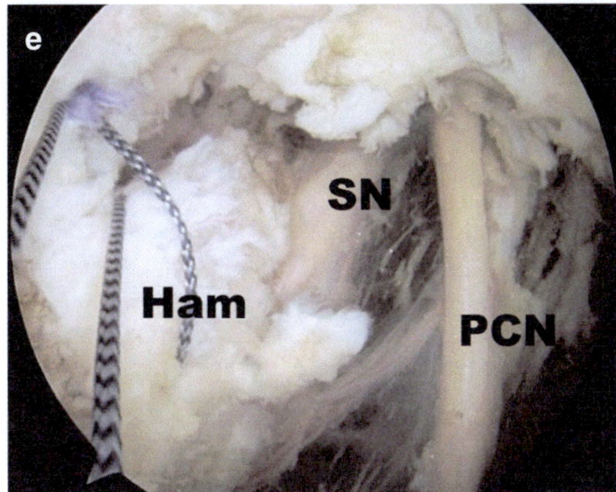

Fig. 10.10   (continued)

to be malingerers. With the advent of hip arthroscopy, the further development of physical examination and surgical techniques has allowed us to explore the use of the arthroscope in many previously unchartered areas. The treatment of these pathologies is one such area.

One important aspect in the treatment of proximal hamstring ruptures is early recognition and early treatment. Patients with acute repairs have had better outcomes in the literature when compared to chronic repair [13, 14]. Delayed complications of nonoperative treatment of proximal hamstring ruptures have been described, and these include knee flexion and hip extension weakness, difficulty sitting, and hamstring deformity [23]. The author has employed this technique successfully on several acute ruptures as well as chronic partial tears.

Surgical repair of proximal hamstring ruptures also has its inherent risks. With open methods, superficial as well as deep wound infections can occur similar to other surgeries; however the location of the incision can potentially increase this risk due to the proximity of the incision to the perineum. With the endoscopic techniques, this possibility should be substantially lessened. Additionally the three main nervous structures at risk to iatrogenic injury are the posterior femoral cutaneous, inferior gluteal nerve, and sciatic nerves [18, 24]. The sciatic nerve is in close proximity to the ischial tuberosity as it runs along the

lateral aspect. With the endoscopic technique, the need for retraction is essentially nonexistent since the nerve is identified and visualized during the repair, but no retraction is necessary.

A concern unique to the endoscopic approach is fluid extravasation into the pelvis as a result of the fluid used in the distension of the potential space around the hamstring tendon. Every effort should be made to regularly check the abdomen for any evidence of abdominal distension. Likewise, any unusual blood pressure decreases that may be due to fluid compression from retroperitoneal extravasation need to be kept in mind. In general, an attempt should be made to maintain the fluid inflow pressures as low as it is feasible for good visualization, and an attempt should be made to keep track of fluid volumes and assure that extravasation is avoided.

Through the judicious application of this technique, many of the chronic hamstring injuries and some of the acute injuries previously addressed through a more invasive, open method can be effectively addressed. With this improved technique, it is hoped that a further understanding of hamstring injuries and their sequelae can be further developed.

References

1. Martin HD, Shears SA, Johnson JC, et al. The endoscopic treatment of sciatic nerve entrapment/deep gluteal syndrome. Arthroscopy. 2011;27:172–81.
2. Byrd JWT, Polkowski G, Jones KS. Endoscopic management of the snapping iliopsoas tendon. Arthroscopy. 2009;25(6):e18.
3. Brown T. Thigh. In: Drez DD, JC DL, Miller MD, editors. Orthopaedic Sports medicine. Principles and practice, vol. 2. Philadelphia: Saunders; 2003. p. 1481–523.
4. Clanton TO, Coupe KJ. Hamstring strains in athletes: diagnosis and treatment. J Am Acad Orthop Surg. 1998;6:237–48.
5. Garrett WE Jr. Muscle strain injuries. Am J Sports Med. 1996;24(6 Suppl):S2–8.
6. Garrett WE Jr, Rich FR, Nikolaou PK, et al. Computed tomography of hamstring muscle strains. Med Sci Sports Exerc. 1989;2:506–14.
7. Elliott MC, et al. Hamstring muscle strains in professional football players: a 10-year review. Am J Sports Med. 2011;39:843–50.
8. Miller SL, Gill J, Webb GR. The proximal origin of the hamstrings and surrounding anatomy encountered

during repair. A cadaveric study. J Bone Joint Surg. 2007;89A:44–8.

9. Blasier RB, Morawa LG. Complete rupture of the hamstring origin from a water skiing injury. Am J Sports Med. 1990;18:435–7.

10. Orava S, Kujala UM. Rupture of the ischial origin of the hamstring muscles. Am J Sports Med. 1995;23(6):702–5.

11. Klingele KE, Sallay PI. Surgical repair of complete proximal hamstring tendon rupture. Am J Sports Med. 2002;30(5):742–7.

12. Mica L, Schwaller A, Stoupis C, et al. Avulsion of the hamstring muscle group: a follow-up of 6 adult non-athletes with early operative treatment: a brief report. World J Surg. 2009;33(8):1605–10.

13. Sallay PI, Friedman RL, Coogan PG, et al. Subjective and functional outcomes following surgical repair of complete ruptures of the proximal hamstring complex. Orthopedics. 2008;31(11):1092–6.

14. Sarimo J, Lempainen L, Mattila K, et al. Complete proximal hamstring avulsions: a series of 41 patients with operative treatment. Am J Sports Med. 2008;36(6):1110–5.

15. Konan S, Haddad F. Successful return to high level sports following early surgical repair of complete tears of the proximal hamstring tendons. Int Orthop. 2010;34(1):119–23.

16. Mendiguchia J, Brughelli M. A return-to-sport algorithm for acute hamstring injuries. Phys Ther Sport. 2011;12(1):2–14.

17. Zissen MH, Wallace G, Steven KJ, et al. High hamstring tendinopathy: MRI and ultrasound imaging and therapeutic efficacy of percutaneous corticosteroid injection. Am J Roentgenol. 2010;195(4):993–8.

18. Lempainen L, Sarimo J, Mattila K, et al. Proximal hamstring tendinopathy: results of surgical management and histopathologic findings. Am J Sports Med. 2009;37(4):727–34.

19. Chakravarthy J, Ramisetty N, Pimpalnerkar A, et al. Surgical repair of complete proximal hamstring tendon ruptures in water skiers and bull riders: a report of four cases and review of the literature. Br J Sports Med. 2005;39(8):569–72.

20. Cross MJ, Vandersluis R, Wood D, et al. Surgical repair of chronic complete hamstring tendon rupture in the adult patient. Am J Sports Med. 1998;26(6):785–8.

21. Cohen S, Bradley J. Acute proximal hamstring rupture. J Am Acad Orthop Surg. 2007;15(6):350–5.

22. Harris JD, Griesser MJ, Best TM, et al. Treatment of proximal hamstring ruptures – a systematic review. Int J Sports Med. 2011;32(7):490–5.

23. Puranen J, Orava S. The hamstring syndrome. A new diagnosis of gluteal sciatic pain. Am J Sports Med. 1988;16(5):517–21.

24. Lempainen L, Sarimo J, Heikkila J, et al. Surgical treatment of partial tears of the proximal origin of the hamstring muscles. Br J Sports Med. 2006;40(8):688–91.

Obturator Nerve Entrapment

11

Elan Jack Golan and Srino Bharam

Anatomy

The obturator nerve originates from the confluence of the ventral rami of L2, L3, and L4 as they exit the lumbar plexus. The rami of L3 is most commonly the largest of the three rami with L2 usually representing the smallest of the three nerve roots. Once joined, the nerve runs through the fibers of the psoas major muscles, emerging at its medial border to extend distally just superior and superficial to the common iliac artery and just lateral to the internal iliac bifurcation and ureter. The nerve then continues along the lateral border of the pelvis as it extends with the obturator vessels toward the obturator foramen. The nerve next passes through the obturator canal as it passes from the pelvis to the hip, through a channel created by the surrounding membrane.

Classically, the obturator nerve was thought to divide into its terminal anterior and posterior branches while traversing the obturator canal; however, the variability in the origin of these two terminal branches has been extensively documented [1–9]. Cadaveric studies have demonstrated that the classic bifurcation within the obturator canal does indeed occur in about 50 percent of individuals, with cases of aberrant bifurcation either proximally in the pelvis or distally in the thigh, with each variation occurring roughly 25% of the time [1]. During their decent into the pelvis, the two branches of the nerve are briefly separated by fibers of the obturator externus muscle. Eventually the anterior and posterior divisions come to lie on either side of the adductor brevis muscle.

When viewed from superficial to deep, the anterior division of the obturator can be found just deep to the adductor longus muscle belly, lying superficial to the adductor brevis. Conversely, the posterior branch of the obturator nerve passes just deep to the adductor brevis deep to its muscle belly and superficial to the adductor magnus. In this way, starting anteriorly and moving from deep to superficial, one will encounter in sequence the adductor longus, the anterior branch of the obturator nerve, the adductor brevis, the posterior branch of the obturator nerve, and finally the adductor magnus (Fig. 11.1).

Anterior Branch of the Obturator Nerve

The anterior branch of the obturator nerve takes a variable course as it descends through the

E. J. Golan, MD
Maimonides Medical Center, Department of
Orthopaedic Surgery, Brooklyn, NY, USA

S. Bharam, MD (✉)
Orthopaedic Surgery, Mount Sinai School of
Medicine, Lenox Hill Hospital, New York, NY, USA

© Springer International Publishing AG, part of Springer Nature 2019
H. D. Martin, J. Gómez-Hoyos (eds.), *Posterior Hip Disorders*,
https://doi.org/10.1007/978-3-319-78040-5_11

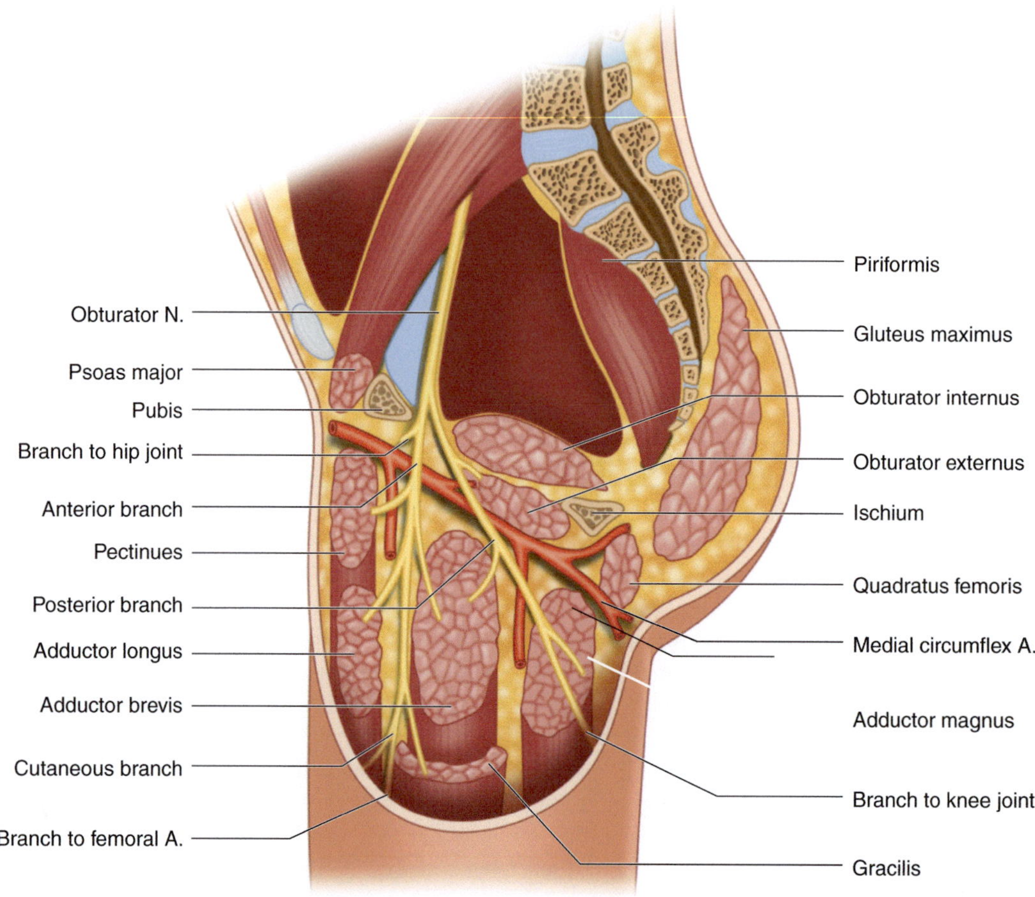

Fig. 11.1 Anatomy of the obturator nerve

obturator foramen, making its way distal to its terminal bifurcation in the thigh. The anterior branch of the obturator nerve contributes an articular branch to the hip joint at or adjacent to its origin in the obturator canal. The nerve provides muscular innervation to adductor longus and brevis as well as the gracilis and rarely to the pectineus muscle. Classical anatomic texts (*Gray's Anatomy*) describe the nerve as passing superficial to the superior border of the obturator externus along with the obturator vein.

A more recent cadaveric study demonstrated only half of all examined obturator nerves to follow this course [4]. Much additional variability has also been described in the nerve's course, including a segment of the nerve branching more distally through the externus muscle mass to later rejoining the main nerve bundle, as well as both anterior and posterior branches of the nerve emerging much more proximally in the thigh. Accessory obturator nerves have also been described, with variable reports of occurrence ranging between 8% and 30% of the population [2, 10, 11].

While the exact number of variations in nerve's course through the obturator foramen remains unclear, the nerve's highly variable anatomy [1] along with the presence of multiple adjacent structures including the inguinal ligament and pubic body [12] places the anterior branch of the obturator nerve at an increased susceptibility for compression.

Several studies investigating potential compression of the anterior division of the obturator nerve between the adductor brevis and the overlying adductor longus and pectineus have described a distinct fascial layer, located between these two muscle layers [4, 8, 12–15]. It is believed that this fascial interval represents the main site of compression in obturator neuropathy. This thin but distinct layer of fascia contains several components including fat, connective tissue adjacent to the surrounding vascular structures, and a well-vascularized intramuscular layer.

Authors have noted a correlation between a more vascular medial intramuscular septum and decreased separation between the adductor brevis and the overlying adductor longus and pectineus. Indeed, in cases of a particularly thickened intramuscular septum, these three muscles have been encountered as on confluent mass, with seemingly no separation between fascial plains.

The anterior branch of the obturator nerve terminates in numerous small branches, with three consistently noted main bundles. The first lies most superiorly, passing lateral to the superior border of the adjacent adductor longus. The second bundle passes medially to provide supply to the adductor longus and brevis. The third and final bundle occupies the most medial course, supplying the gracilis muscle while descending to join the subsartorial plexus. Additional terminating branches of the nerve also form cutaneous branches that descend into the adductor canal, ultimately providing sensation to the skin and fascial of the distal, medial thigh.

The anterior bundle of the obturator nerve also demonstrates several close relationships with the surrounding vasculature. At obturator foramen the nerve runs closely with obturator vein. Soon after, a branch of the medial femoral circumflex artery (MFCA) is found adjacent to the nerve at the interval between the pectineus and adductor

longus. Finally, two to three vascular bundles cross the artery from medial to lateral as it descends toward the subsartorial plexus. It is believed the vascular pedicle of the MFCA, which contributes to the pectineus along with the adductor longus and brevis, may represent the main culprit in the thickening of the fascial layer that results in nerve entrapment. The MFCA vascular pedicle surrounds the nerve as it runs along the triangularly shaped adductor brevis muscle, resulting in local tissue thickening, which likely increases the risk of compression.

Other Etiologies of Obturator Compression

Current literature is filled with case reports of external causes of obturator nerve compression. A comprehensive review of all such causes of secondary compression is beyond the scope of the chapter. Briefly, aside from the fascial compression that is the focus of the current chapter, obturator pathology can result from multiple organ system disorders, with some of the most commonly reported additional causes including malignant compression, [16] iatrogenic or postsurgical changes following gynecologic [17] or orthopedic procedures, [18] inflammatory [19] or infectious changes, and pelvic fracture [20].

Clinical Presentation

The clinical evaluation of hip pain, especially in the high-level athlete, represents one of the most complex diagnostic dilemmas known to orthopedic practice. The complex anatomy and myriad of structures enclosed in such a small area provide a troubling number of potential pain generators that must be systematically considered and eliminated in order to reach a final diagnosis. This diagnostic process often represents a challenge for even the most experienced clinicians. The differential for hip pain in the athlete is quite expansive, including tendonitis, bursitis, osteitis, hernia, conjoined tendon pathology, stress fracture, and enthesopathy among other potential etiologies of pain. A multipronged approach, including a focused physical exam and advanced imaging, in addition to a detailed and accurate history in a cooperative patient, is of utmost importance in arriving at an ultimate diagnosis [4, 21–26].

Current literature descriptions of obturator neuropathy are almost exclusively described in males. In the largest described series of obturator nerve compression, 28/29 examined patients were men [13]. It is unknown if this difference is due to an anatomic discrepancy between genders that predisposes males to such compressive neuropathies or if this finding is the result of a discrepancy in participation rates between genders in sports that require repeated rapid lateral movements such as rugby and Australian rules football. Similar trends of male predominant injury patterns have been demonstrated in other groin-related injuries such as sportsman's hernias or adductor longus injury [23–25, 27–29].

Though there is no physical exam finding that serves as pathognomonic for entrapment of the obturator nerve, several physical exam findings of patients ultimately found to have obturator neuropathy as diagnosed with focused EMG have been described.

It is important to note that many patients suffering from obturator entrapment may function normally at rest, with symptoms only manifesting following a period of exercise [13]. Patients will frequently present with a history of insidious onset of vague anterior, medial, and/or posterior thigh pain that is difficult to localize. This pain can often be diffuse, encompassing the entire area adjacent to the adductor longus's origin on the pubic tubercle, with some patients describing a concomitant referred pain along the ipsilateral ASIS.

In a review of 29 patients diagnosed with obturator neuropathy, Bradshaw et al. described a triad of the most important physical exam findings, namely, adductor muscle weakness, adductor spasm, and paresthesias over the medial aspect of the thigh. Of these, the most reliable

physical exam finding for obturator entrapment is weakness and spasm of the adductor muscles with accompanying paresthesias of the medial thigh following a period of exercise [15, 30, 31]. Athletes may report such symptoms following an attempt to perform a jump from a position of ipsilateral, single leg stance, with patients complaining of medial thigh and adductor weakness soon after [22, 32]. Such weakness is almost always incomplete secondary to the dual innervation of the adductor longus (femoral n) and adductor magnus (sciatic nerve) musculature, respectively [33, 34].

Ipsilateral loss of the hip's adductor reflex is also suggestive, but not diagnostic, of entrapment neuropathy. As this reflex is naturally absent in many individuals, both extremities must be tested, with an absence of the reflex in the effected extremity while simultaneously present in the contralateral extremity, diagnostic of obturator pathology [31]. Finally, in rare cases of long-standing entrapment neuropathy, clinicians may appreciate a noticeable weakness in the adduction of the effected extremity. This finding manifests as a circumducting, wide-based gait, with the affected hip held in a position of abduction and external rotation [8, 30, 35].

Several physical exam tests have also been described in the context of suspected adductor neuropathy. Patients will often experience pain with a *pectineal muscle stretch*, a maneuver eliciting pain with passive external rotation and abduction of the effected hip or resisted hip internal rotation [13]. Forced hip abduction may also elicit the *Howship-Romberg's sign*, in which medial knee pain is induced with progressive hip abduction, extension, and internal rotation [36, 37].

Diagnostic Imaging

While imaging is a critical part of correctly diagnosing obturator entrapment neuropathy, it is crucial to maintain a working differential at all times throughout the examination process. In this way, clinicians will not blindly rely on advanced imaging to arrive at a diagnosis but rather will incorporate such tests as a method of confirming and excluding other potential etiologies of groin pain that were part of their initial differential.

As with any orthopedic injury, routine evaluation begins with appropriate plain-film radiography. Especially in the setting of a questionable history of trauma, an AP view of the pelvis along with dedicated imaging of the affected hip should be obtained to rule out bony processes such as occult fracture as a possible etiology of symptoms.

In the setting of true isolated obturator neuropathy, plain films will be nondiagnostic. In setting of appropriate history and physical exam, EMG represents an inexpensive logical next step in diagnostic testing. In one series of athletes treated for obturator entrapment neuropathy, chronic denervation of the adductor longus and adductor brevis on EMG was reported as the most significant diagnostic finding in patients ultimately diagnosed with compressive obturator neuropathy, with all 29 diagnosed patients in the series demonstrating EMG evidence of such denervation [13]. These findings are commonly manifested as fibrillation potentials or high-amplitude complex motor unit potentials of a long duration [8]. Further, following surgical release of obturator compression, repeat EMGs of this patient cohort at 6 weeks and 12 months of follow-up demonstrated resolution of such changes, [13] further supporting the use of EMG for both initial diagnosis and tracking progression following treatment of obturator neuropathy.

Post-compression changes on diagnostic ultrasound have also been described in the setting of obturator entrapment neuropathy. Assessment will often reveal localized edema proximal to the site of compression along with atrophy and regressive changes in the distal musculature supplied by the anterior division of the nerve [5]. While not always visible, a recent study reported that the anterior division of the obturator nerve is detectable by ultrasound in 85% of patients surveyed. The divisions of the obturator are notably flat on ultrasound evaluation, with median anterior-posterior and medial to lateral dimension ratios of 0.32 and 0.18, respectively, representing the flattest peripheral nerves described in ultrasound evaluation of the

lower extremity [14]. A recent correlative cadaveric study defined a hyperechoic triangular area bordered by the pubic ramus along with the femoral artery and vein that predictably allowed for localization of the obturator nerve's anterior division [38].

Following EMG and/or ultrasound evaluation, individuals are routinely sent for MRI should the diagnosis remain in question. By obtaining an MRI, clinicians are able to screen for other causes of athletic pain such as fracture, [39] tendinous avulsion, [40–43] or intrapelvic masses [16, 44]. Upon MRI evaluation, the anterior branch of the obturator nerve is quickly found traversing the fat between the adductor longus and brevis. In the coronal plane, MRI will enhance the nerve as a thin, hypo-echoic cord within abundant epineural fat. The nerve is easily followed as it descends vertically to travel posteromedial to the psoas muscle. At the obturator canal, axial imaging is the preferred method of nerve localization. It is often difficult to clearly visualize the distal branching of the obturator anterior division. This is especially true in the setting of a younger, muscular patient, due to the relative lack of intramuscular fat adjacent to the epineurium [45].

Often no specific MRI findings are present on evaluation of the anterior division of the sciatic nerve as it emerges both from the obturator foramen and more distally in the thigh. MRI may reveal atrophy of the muscles supplied by the nerve, suggestive of longer-standing compressive pathology [22, 32]. Such changes are best visualized with the assistance of fluid-sensitive sequences [45].

It is important to differentiate between obturator denervation and more commonly found straining of the adjacent musculature. This distinction is best drawn by the more focal concentration of signal localized around muscle origins in the setting of muscular strain, along with relative sparing of the obturator externus [45]. More diffuse denervation changes can also be appreciated in the obturator nerve in the setting of osteitis pubis, especially following surgical procedures performed in the lithotomy position [46].

Bone scan will often demonstrate a mild increase in uptake at the level of the pubic ramus, coinciding with the origin of the adductor longus or brevis. It is unclear if this finding is representative of obturator compression itself or concomitant strain and irritation to the surrounding musculature [22].

Other Tests for Detection of Obturator Neuropathy: Nerve Block

An obturator nerve block can also be attempted as both a diagnostic and therapeutic approach to the patient exhibiting signs of compressive obturator neuropathy. Obturator nerve block is commonly used as a postoperative supplement to femoral nerve block in the setting of lower extremity procedures such as total knee arthroplasty [47, 48]. The reported success of obturator nerve blockade varies widely in the literature, with current success rates varying widely depending on technique employed [49, 50]. Clinically, accurate placement of a nerve block is presumed with resultant paresthesias in the anterior branch of the obturator nerve sensory division along the distal medial thigh [13].

Probably the most compelling argument for incorporation of a nerve block as part of patient assessment is the ability to predict resolution of symptoms following surgical release. The results of such localized anesthesia are especially important in the setting of a patient with a secondary, coexisting etiology of pain such as a hernia or adductor strain. Indeed, incomplete resolution of symptoms following a well-performed obturator nerve block should serve a clue that further evaluation is needed to rule out a coexisting source of pain. Further, while no long-term studies of their efficacy exist in the context of obturator-related pathology, similar "pubic cleft" injections have been demonstrated to result in favorable outcomes in the setting of other causes of chronic pain [25].

Surgical Treatment

In the acute setting, initial management of such injuries includes rest and activity modification along with a course of oral anti-inflammatory medications. In addition to formal physical therapy, secondary modalities such as massage, stretching, and myofascial manipulation are also encouraged in the setting of acute injury. Sorenson et al. reported favorable outcomes with such conservative treatment of patients presenting soon after the acute onset of obturator neuropathic symptoms [15]. However, as with more common compressive neuropathies in other parts of the body, literature suggests that conservative treatment has a limited role once a definitive diagnosis of obturator entrapment has been established [4, 8, 13, 22].

Ultimately, when confronted with a patient with electrodiagnostic evidence of decreased nerve conduction velocity, the role of the treating physician is to relieve the compression to allow for the best chance of recovery. Surgery is considered in those with prolonged, non-relenting symptoms along with either demonstrated EMG changes or positive response to obturator nerve block [4, 8, 13, 22].

To perform a release, an oblique incision 3 cm in length is centered over the lateral border of the adductor longus approximately 1 cm distal to the pubic tubercle [13]. The saphenous vein is identified and protected with the fascia overlying the adductor longus opened. Blunt dissection is then employed to develop the space between the adductor longus and pectineus and the deep adductor brevis muscle mass. The thick fascial layer lying in this interval is carefully opened and the anterior division of the nerve identified. Careful in-line dissection is then employed to trace the nerve proximally to its position in the obturator foramen with cautery used to coagulate any traversing vessels encountered during dissection. If any branches of the MFCA are encountered, it is crucial to divide these branches with proximal dissection as it has been hypothesized that these structures play a vital role in maintaining the thick fascial layer implicated in obturator entrapment [4, 8]. Once identified within the obturator foramen, blunt dissection is used to remove an excess fat that may contribute to compression of the anterior branch of the obturator nerve prior to its descent inferiorly toward its terminal branches.

Harvey describes three main sites of potential bleeding when performing a decompression of the anterior branch of the nerve, all secondary to the close relationship of the nerve to surrounding vasculature as it courses inferiorly in the lower extremity [4]. The first and most problematic site is due to the aforementioned branches of the MFCA at the level between the adductor longus and pectineus. It is here that these branches undergo their final bifurcations prior to forming the terminal supply to the surrounding musculature. Bleeding in this area is best avoided by ensuring dissection remains deep to the pectineus muscle, with the MFCA maintaining a course that is superficial and transverse to this muscle mass. The second potential site of bleeding is encountered with more distal dissection of the fascial layer enclosing the obturator nerve. This area often proves less problematic as vascular anatomy here can be quite variable. However, dissection should be advanced cautiously with immediate coagulation of any traversing vessels to avoid unnecessary bleeding. Lastly, the final site of bleeding is localized to the level of the obturator foramen where numerous anastomotic connections exist between the MFCA and the obturator vasculature. In addition to numerous venous tributaries, the obturator artery can also be encountered in this area within the obturator canal. However, as this tends to be a deeper structure, the area remains relatively safe for removable of any obstructing fat with careful, blunt dissection.

Outcomes

Measured outcomes of surgical neurolysis of the anterior branch of the obturator nerve are relatively rare in current literature. Fortunately, the largest reported outcome study of 29 patients reported excellent results in all patients following the surgical technique described above [13]. In this series, patients were divided into three groups based on presentation. Group I was composed of 24 patients who demonstrated symptoms of compressive obturator neuropathy with no known history of prior trauma or surgical intervention. These patients had uniformly good results following surgical neurolysis. Group II met the same initial criteria as Group I but were found to have concomitant direct inguinal hernia at the

time of surgical evaluation. In addition to neurolysis, these patients were also treated with concurrent hernia repair. Finally Group III consisted of three patients with a history of previous groin surgery (adductor tenotomy, symphyseal curettage, and femoral nerve exploration) prior to development of obturator-related symptoms. In all three cases, vast amounts of scar tissue were encountered with successful resolution of symptoms reported for all three patients following surgical neurolysis.

References

1. Anagnostopoulou S, Kostopanagiotou G, Paraskeuopoulos T, Chantzi C, Lolis E, Saranteas T. Anatomic variations of the obturator nerve in the inguinal region: implications in conventional and ultrasound regional anesthesia techniques. Reg Anesth Pain Med. 2009;34(1):33–9.
2. Anloague PA, Huijbregts P. Anatomical variations of the lumbar plexus: a descriptive anatomy study with proposed clinical implications. J Man Manip Ther. 2009;17(4):e107–14.
3. Gerlach U, Lierse W. Functional construction of the superficial and deep fascia system of the lower limb in man. Cells Tissues Organs. 1990;139(1):11–25.
4. Harvey G, Bell S. Obturator neuropathy. An anatomic perspective. Clin Orthop Relat Res. 1999;363:203–11.
5. Kowalska B, Sudol-Szopinska I. Ultrasound assessment of selected peripheral nerves pathologies. Part II: entrapment neuropathies of the lower limb. J Ultrasonography. 2012;12(51):463–71.
6. Quain J, Sharpey-Schäfer EA, Symington J, Godlee RJ, Thane GD. Quain's elements of anatomy. London: Longmans, Green; 1894.
7. Sinnatamby CS. Last's anatomy: regional and applied. Amsterdam: Elsevier Health Sciences; 2011.
8. Tipton JS. Obturator neuropathy. Curr Rev Musculoskelet Med. 2008;1(3–4):234–7.
9. Warwick R, Williams PL. Gray's anatomy. Edinburgh: Longman; 1973.
10. Akkaya T, Comert A, Kendir S, Acar HI, Gumus H, Tekdemir I, et al. Detailed anatomy of accessory obturator nerve blockade. Minerva Anestesiol. 2008;74(4):119–22.
11. Katritsis E, Anagnostopoulou S, Papadopoulos N. Anatomical observations on the accessory obturator nerve (based on 1000 specimens). Anat Anz. 1980;148(5):440–5.
12. Jo SY, Chang JC, Bae HG, Oh JS, Heo J, Hwang JC. A morphometric study of the obturator nerve around the obturator foramen. J Korean Neurosurg Soc. 2016;59(3):282–6.
13. Bradshaw C, McCrory P, Bell S, Brukner P. Obturator nerve entrapment. A cause of groin pain in athletes. Am J Sports Med. 1997;25(3):402–8.

14. Soong J, Schafhalter-Zoppoth I, Gray AT. Sonographic imaging of the obturator nerve for regional block. Reg Anesth Pain Med. 2007;32(2):146–51.

15. Sorenson EJ, Chen JJ, Daube JR. Obturator neuropathy: causes and outcome. Muscle Nerve. 2002;25(4):605–7.

16. Sureka J, Panwar S, Mullapudi I. Intraneural ganglion cysts of obturator nerve causing obturator neuropathy. Acta Neurol Belg. 2012;112(2):229–30.

17. Van Ba OL, Wagner L, de Tayrac R. Obturator neuropathy: an adverse outcome of a trans-obturator vaginal mesh to repair pelvic organ prolapse. Int Urogynecol J. 2014;25(1):145–6.

18. Ghijselings S, Bruyninckx F, Delport H, Corten K. Inflammatory neuropathy of the lumbosacral plexus following periacetabular osteotomy. Case Rep Orthop. 2016;2016:3632654.

19. Stuplich M, Hottinger AF, Stoupis C, Sturzenegger M. Combined femoral and obturator neuropathy caused by synovial cyst of the hip. Muscle Nerve. 2005;32(4):552–4.

20. Lehmann W, Hoffmann M, Fensky F, Nuchtern J, Grossterlinden L, Aghayev E, et al. What is the frequency of nerve injuries associated with acetabular fractures? Clin Orthop Relat Res. 2014;472(11):3395–403.

21. Ashby EC. Chronic obscure groin pain is commonly caused by enthesopathy: 'tennis elbow' of the groin. Br J Surg. 1994;81(11):1632–4.

22. Brukner P, Bradshaw C, McCrory P. Obturator neuropathy: a cause of exercise-related groin pain. Phys Sportsmed. 1999;27(5):62–73.

23. Harmon KG. Evaluation of groin pain in athletes. Curr Sports Med Rep. 2007;6(6):354–61.

24. LeBlanc KE, LeBlanc KA. Groin pain in athletes. Hernia. 2003;7(2):68–71.

25. Schilders E, Talbot JC, Robinson P, Dimitrakopoulou A, Gibbon WW, Bismil Q. Adductor-related groin pain in recreational athletes: role of the adductor enthesis, magnetic resonance imaging, and entheseal pubic cleft injections. J Bone Joint Surg Am. 2009;91(10):2455–60.

26. Suarez JC, Ely EE, Mutnal AB, Figueroa NM, Klika AK, Patel PD, et al. Comprehensive approach to the evaluation of groin pain. J Am Acad Orthop Surg. 2013;21(9):558–70.

27. Dimitrakopoulou A, Schilders E. Current concepts of inguinal-related and adductor-related groin pain. Hip Int. 2016;26(Suppl 1):2–7.

28. Schilders E, Dimitrakopoulou A, Cooke M, Bismil Q, Cooke C. Effectiveness of a selective partial adductor release for chronic adductor-related groin pain in professional athletes. Am J Sports Med. 2013;41(3):603–7.

29. Robinson P, Barron DA, Parsons W, Grainger AJ, Schilders EM, O'Connor PJ. Adductor-related groin pain in athletes: correlation of MR imaging with clinical findings. Skelet Radiol. 2004;33(8):451–7.

30. Dawson D, Hallett M, Wilbourn A. Miscellaneous uncommon syndromes of the lower extremity. In:

31. Entrapment neuropathies. 3rd ed. Philadelphia: Lippincott-Raven; 1988. p. 369–79.

31. Stewart JD. Peripheral nerve fascicles: anatomy and clinical relevance. Muscle Nerve. 2003;28(5):525–41.

32. Bradshaw C, McCrory P. Obturator nerve entrapment. Clin J Sport Med. 1997;7(3):217–9.

33. Gottschalk F. Transfemoral amputation: biomechanics and surgery. Clin Orthop Relat Res. 1999;361:15–22.

34. Vasilev SA. Obturator nerve injury: a review of management options. Gynecol Oncol. 1994;53(2):152–5.

35. Mumenthaler M, Schliack H. Lesions of individual nerves of the lower limb plexus and the lower extremity. In: Peripheral nerve lesions diagnosis and therapy. New York: Thieme Medical; 1991. p. 297–343.

36. Pecina MM, Markiewitz AD, Krmpotic-Nemanic J. Tunnel syndromes. Boca Raton: CRC; 2001.

37. Saurenmann P, Brand S. Obturator neuralgia (Howship-Romberg phenomenon). Schweiz Med Wochenschr. 1984;114(42):1462–4.

38. Akkaya T, Ozturk E, Comert A, Ates Y, Gumus H, Ozturk H, et al. Ultrasound-guided obturator nerve block: a sonoanatomic study of a new methodologic approach. Anesth Analg. 2009;108(3):1037–41.

39. Pavlov H, Nelson TL, Warren RF, Torg JS, Burstein AH. Stress fractures of the pubic ramus. A report of twelve cases. J Bone Joint Surg Am. 1982;64(7):1020–5.

40. Freire M, Winalski CS, Miniaci A, Sundaram M. Radiologic case study. Avulsion of the right adductor longus from the symphysis pubis. Orthopedics. 2012;35(2):85, 158–60.

41. Dimitrakopoulou A, Schilders EM, Talbot JC, Bismil Q. Acute avulsion of the fibrocartilage origin of the adductor longus in professional soccer players: a report of two cases. Clin J Sport Med. 2008;18(2):167–9.

42. Vogt S, Ansah P, Imhoff AB. Complete osseous avulsion of the adductor longus muscle: acute repair with three fiberwire suture anchors. Arch Orthop Trauma Surg. 2007;127(8):613–5.

43. Tehranzadeh J, Kurth LA, Elyaderani MK, Bowers KD. Combined pelvic stress fracture and avulsion of the adductor longus in a middle-distance runner: a case report. Am J Sports Med. 1982;10(2):108–11.

44. Redwine DB, Sharpe DR. Endometriosis of the obturator nerve. A case report. J Reprod Med. 1990;35(4):434–5.

45. Martinoli C, Miguel-Perez M, Padua L, Gandolfo N, Zicca A, Tagliafico A. Imaging of neuropathies about the hip. Eur J Radiol. 2013;82(1):17–26.

46. Litwiller JP, Wells RE Jr, Halliwill JR, Carmichael SW, Warner MA. Effect of lithotomy positions on strain of the obturator and lateral femoral cutaneous nerves. Clin Anat. 2004;17(1):45–9.

47. Macalou D, Trueck S, Meuret P, Heck M, Vial F, Ouologuem S, et al. Postoperative analgesia after total knee replacement: the effect of an obturator nerve block added to the femoral 3-in-1 nerve block. Anesth Analg. 2004;99(1):251–4.

48. McNamee D, Parks L, Milligan K. Post-operative analgesia following total knee replacement: an evalu-

ation of the addition of an obturator nerve block to combined femoral and sciatic nerve block. Acta Anaesthesiol Scand. 2002;46(1):95–9.

49. Jo YY, Choi E, Kil HK. Comparison of the success rate of inguinal approach with classical pubic approach for obturator nerve block in patients undergoing TURB. Korean J Anesthesiol. 2011;61(2):143–7.

50. Wassef M. Interadductor approach to obturator nerve blockade for spastic conditions of adductor thigh muscles. Reg Anesth Pain Med. 1993;18(1):13–7.

Ischiofemoral Impingement

12

Juan Gómez-Hoyos and Hal D. Martin

Introduction

The development of posterior hip pain in a non-arthritic hip is related to the structural anatomy and kinematics of the entire biomechanical axis. The impact of different phases of gait on dynamically changing different bony spaces around the hip joint should be harmonious in normal conditions. When anatomy and kinematics are distorted, impingement and/or instability could be generated depending upon the specifics of the problem. Ischiofemoral impingement (IFI) likely represents one of the most common and unfortunately overlooked causes of posterior hip pain.

A rubbing mechanism between the ischium and the lesser trochanter could lead to the development of quadratus femoris edema, hamstring origin tendonitis/tears, sciatic nerve entrapment, and disabling symptoms.

IFI is a recently described condition, and little demographic data of this problem is currently available. A recent meta-analysis by Singer et al. [1] reported 166 cases of IFI from four studies. Female patients were predominant (142), and the mean age was 50.8 years (SD ±12.7). Reports of IFI in pediatric population have been also published [2–5].

Patients with suspected IFI require a comprehensive history, clinical evaluation, and radiologic assessment. The best therapeutic options range between physical therapy and surgical procedures depending on the cause of the impingement and response to conservative measures.

Anatomy

The quadratus femoris muscle is a flat and quadrilateral muscle, situated along the posterior aspect of the hip joint. It originates on the anterior border of the ischial tuberosity and inserts on the posteromedial aspect of the proximal femur. The quadratus femoris muscle is bordered by the obturator externus muscle anteriorly, sciatic nerve posteriorly, inferior gemellus superiorly, and adductor magnus inferiorly. As defined by Torriani et al. [6], the ischiofemoral space (IFS) is the smallest distance between the lateral cortex of the ischial tuberosity and the medial cortex of the lesser trochanter, and the quadratus femoris

J. Gómez-Hoyos, MD (✉)
International Consultant, Hip Preservation
Center / Baylor Scott and White Research Institute,
Baylor University Medical Center, Dallas, TX, USA

Department of Orthopaedic Surgery - Health
Provider, Clínica Las Américas / Clínica del
Campestre, Medellin, Antioquia, Colombia

Professor - School of Medicine - Sports Medicine
Program, Universidad de Antioquia,
Medellín, Antioquia, Colombia

H. D. Martin, DO
Medical and Research Director, Hip Preservation
Center, Baylor University Medical Center,
Dallas, TX, USA

© Springer International Publishing AG, part of Springer Nature 2019
H. D. Martin, J. Gómez-Hoyos (eds.), *Posterior Hip Disorders*,
https://doi.org/10.1007/978-3-319-78040-5_12

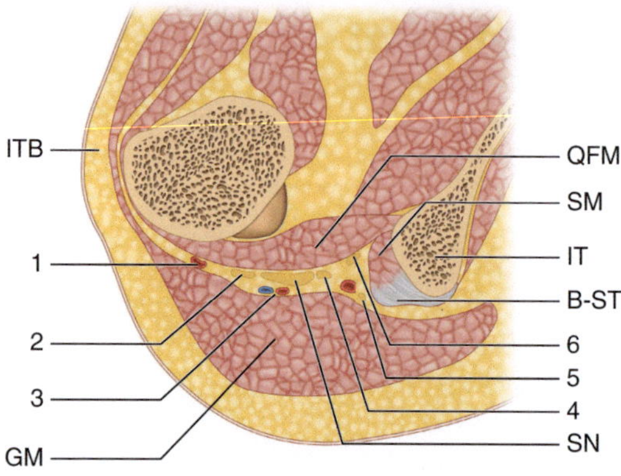

Fig. 12.1 Cranial view of an axial section at the level of the ischiofemoral space and surrounding structures. *ITB* iliotibial band, *QFM* quadratus femoris muscle, *SM* semimembranosus, *B-ST* conjoined tendon (biceps femoris and semitendinosus), *IT* ischial tuberosity, *GM* gluteus maximus, *SN* sciatic nerve, *APCFA* ascending posterior circumflex femoral artery, *PFCN* posterior femoral cutaneous nerve, *IGA-N* inferior gluteal artery and nerve

space (QFS) is the smallest space of passage of the quadratus femoris muscle delimited by the superolateral surface of the hamstring tendons and the posteromedial surface of the iliopsoas tendon or lesser trochanter (Fig. 12.1).

Within the ischiofemoral space, the sciatic nerve shares the same spatial location with the lesser trochanter, which is separated from the sciatic nerve by the quadratus femoris muscle [7]. The proximal insertion of the semimembranosus muscles at the lateral aspect of the ischium also shares the same anatomic spatial location within the ischiofemoral space (Fig. 12.2) [8].

Another anatomic structure worth mentioning is the distal insertion of the iliopsoas tendon on the lesser trochanter, which can be detached when decompressing ischiofemoral impingement by lesser trochanterplasty [9].

More anatomic details of the deep gluteal space are presented in Chap. 1.

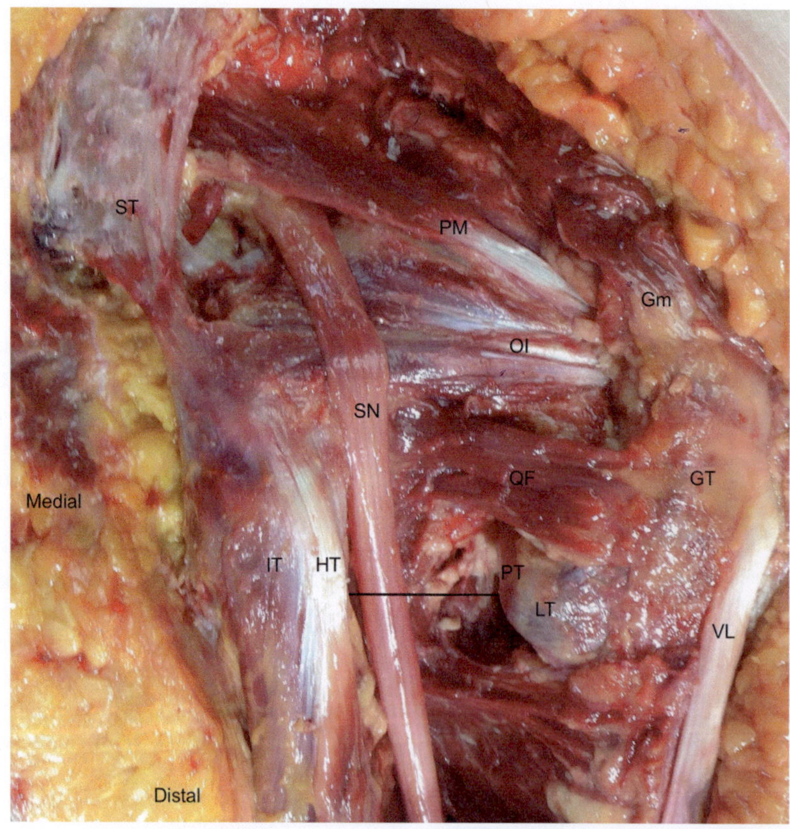

Fig. 12.2 Posterior view to the deep gluteal space in a 65-year-old male cadaver. The femur is in neutral position showing the normal ischiofemoral space (solid line). *ST* sacrotuberous ligament, *PM* piriformis muscle, *Gm* gluteus medius, *OI* obturator internus muscle, *SN* sciatic nerve, *QF* quadratus femoris muscle (partially resected in order to show the lesser trochanter), *GT* greater trochanter, *PT* psoas tendon insertion, *LT* lesser trochanter, *IT* ischial tuberosity, *HT* hamstring tendon, *VL* vastus lateralis

Definition

IFI was first described by Johnson in 1977 [10]. He stated that a pain that persists in a hip after an otherwise successful hip replacement might be due to a "pinching" of soft tissues between bone prominences. He described three cases of patients who had painful impingement between the lesser trochanter and the ischium and who were relieved of their pain by excision of the lesser trochanter (Fig. 12.3). After the first description, IFI has been reported in a number of patients with no previous history of surgery [11].

In his first description, Johnson proposed that the lesser trochanter and the ischium are within two centimeters of each other in normal conditions when the hip is in slight adduction, external rotation, and extension [10]. However, normal ischiofemoral space values (IFS) remain controversial.

Torriani et al. reported the first study about the definition of normal ischiofemoral space. They measured the IFS and quadratus femoris space (QFS) on magnetic resonance images (MRI) of 12 hips in nine patients with hip pain and abnormal MRI signal intensity of the quadratus femoris muscle. Data were compared with 11 hips in ten control subjects. A significantly narrower IFS and QFS in patients with quadratus femoris edema when compared with control subjects were found (13 ± 5 vs. 23 ± 8 and 7 ± 3 vs. 12 ± 4, respectively). Additionally, ROC cutoff values to detect affected subjects were reported as ≤17 mm for IFS and ≤ 8 mm for QFS [6]. Torriani's cutoff values are now commonly used in order to determine whether a patient has abnormal IFS or QFS. However, the ischiofemoral space (IFS) should be understood dynamically and related to gait. A normal gait pattern would allow the proximal femur moving from flexion to extension without any conflict with the lateral part of the ischium. An impingement could occur if normal gait patterns are disturbed from different causes. Abnormal frontal plane drift of the pelvis, increased leg adduction, and/or increased external rotation during gait will narrow IFS.

Although MRI has been traditionally used to evaluate IFS and QFS dimensions, a recent study used diagnostic ultrasound to measure the dimensions of the IFS during varying degrees of femoral abduction-adduction and internal-external rotation [12]. The results of the study suggested that femoral positions significantly affect IFS dimensions, with the narrowest dimension occurring during femoral adduction and external rotation and the widest occurring with the femoral abduction and internal rotation.

Apart from measuring IFS and QFS and identifying quadratus femoris edema, new criteria based on measurements of these spaces have

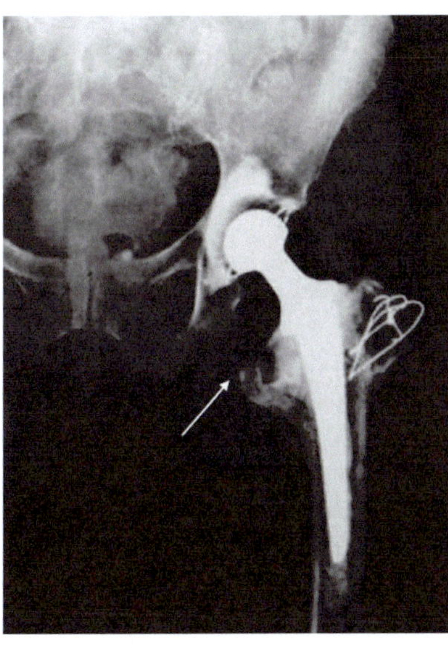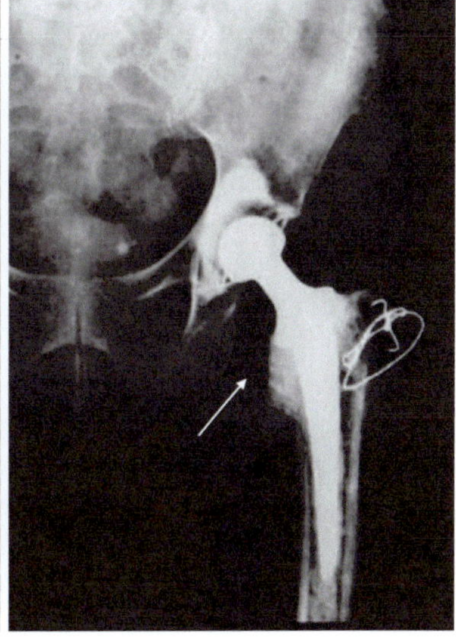

Fig. 12.3 Original case published in 1977 by Kenneth Johnson. *Left.* Radiograph made after total hip arthroplasty showing enlarged lesser trochanter (white arrow). *Right.* Radiograph made after a lesser trochanterplasty (white arrow)

recently been suggested. However, because these measurements are position-dependent, full-range-of-motion imaging techniques are supposed to increase the diagnostic yield. By evaluating through a range of motion using MRI, Springer et al. [13] detected a case of impingement involving the ischial tuberosity and greater trochanter. They propose that range-of-motion MRI can improve diagnostic accuracy of extra-articular hip impingement.

Further studies are warranted to expand and improve the definition of ischiofemoral impingement, as the measurement of the described spaces could be affected by a number of factors such as race, age, sex, and height of the patient.

Etiology

The combination of static and dynamic factors impacts the complex mechanics of the hip joint. Abnormalities in hip morphology can reduce range of motion. Structural issues around the proximal femur or ischium and their influence on native hip range of motion have been poorly studied. A recent study about the effect of angular deformities of the proximal femur on impingement-free hip range of motion used a three-dimensional model to simulate incremental deformation of the proximal femur. They found that when increasing neck-shaft angles ($\geq 135°$) and femoral torsion ($\geq 25°$), ischiofemoral impingement occurred [14].

In native hips, IFI has been discussed as a result of marked coxa valga deformities [15]. These suggestions are supported by specific MRI findings in severe coxa valga deformities, with a close relationship between the lesser trochanter and the ischial tuberosity together with a typical signal alteration within the quadratus femoris muscle [6]. Furthermore, other authors have suggested excessive femoral antetorsion and other changes in pelvic anatomy in patients with IFI [16]. Gómez-Hoyos et al. [17] assessed the femoral neck version (FNV) and the lesser trochanter version (LTV) in 11 patients with confirmed diagnosis of IFI. No difference was found in mean LTV between groups ($-23.6°$ vs. $-24.2°$;

$P = 0.8$; 95% CI, -7.5 to 6.4); however, the mean FNV ($21.7°$ vs. $14.1°$; $P = 0.02$; 95% CI, -14.2 to -1.1) was higher in symptomatic than in asymptomatic patients, with statistical significance.

Oliveira et al. [18] recently found no narrowing of the IFS after total hip replacement in 250 cases; however a femoral component abnormally anteverted could help explain iatrogenic IFI after a hip prosthesis.

Apart from anatomic abnormalities, space-occupying lesions could also produce IFI symptoms. Spencer-Gardner et al. [19] reported ten cases of ischiofemoral impingement related to ischial tuberosity nonunion/malunion. All cases underwent surgery and showed functional improvement during a 2-year follow-up. Other similar cases have been reported in young athletes [20].

Similarly, bone or soft tissue tumors could narrow the IFS and generate symptoms. Secondary IFI due to a solitary or bilateral bone exostosis is a rare cause; however this diagnosis is probably one of the most common musculoskeletal tumors linked to narrowing of the ischiofemoral space. In 20–45% of the patients, IFI is bilateral or occurs in young people, supporting the hypothesis of predisposing congenital narrowing of the IFS [4, 21, 22].

Yoong et al. [23] performed an MRI case-control study to assess whether there is a significant difference in the ischiofemoral impingement space in patients with multiple hereditary exostosis (MHE) affecting the proximal femur compared to normal subjects. After analyzing 42 hips, they found a significant difference in the minimum ischiofemoral space in individuals with multiple hereditary exostosis (mean, 10.7 mm, ranging from 0 to 21 mm), compared to a control group (mean, 18.1 mm, ranging from 10.5 to 26.5 mm). Features suggestive of IFI were seen in 62% of hips in the MHE group as compared with 0% in the control group.

Soft tissue problems associated with IFI have also been reported. Papoutsi et al. [24] described an unusual case of ischiofemoral impingement caused by an intermuscular lipoma. Surgical resection of the tumor and histology confirmed the lipomatosus nature of the tumor with subsequent resolution of the symptoms.

Table 12.1 Potential etiologies and predisposing factors of ischiofemoral impingement [26]

1. *Primary or congenital (orthopedic disorders)*:
1.1. Coxa valga
1.2. Prominence of the lesser trochanter
1.3. Congenital posteromedial position of the femur
1.4. Larger cross section of the femur
1.5. Abnormal femoral anteversion
1.6. Coxa breva
1.7. Variations of the pelvic bony anatomy
2. *Secondary or acquired*:
2.1. Functional disorders
(a) Hip instability
(b) Pelvic and spinal instability
(c) Abductor/adductor imbalance
2.2. Ischial tuberosity enthesopathies
2.3. Traumatic, overuse, and extreme hip motion
2.4. Iatrogenic causes
2.5. Tumors
2.6. (genu valgum, leg discrepancy, pronated foot)

The ischiofemoral space should be understood as a gait-related dynamic area with several contributing factors. As an example, one of the patients reported by Ali et al. [25] had an abnormal gait as the underlying cause of ischiofemoral narrowing. The gait abnormality in this 48-year-old woman resulted from abductor dysfunction, thereby putting the quadratus femoris at risk of impingement because of the resultant adduction during gait.

A list of potential etiologies and predisposing factors of ischiofemoral impingement is presented in Table 12.1.

History and Clinical Findings

The clinical presentation of IFI can vary, but the most common symptom is posterior hip pain lateral to the ischium deep into the gluteal space. Likewise, these patients may refer a snapping phenomenon and/or a variety of sciatic-like symptoms that spread down the leg, because of the proximity of the quadratus femoris muscle with pressure and irritation effect on the sciatic nerve (Fig. 12.2) [26].

Patients with sciatic nerve entrapment often have a history of trauma and symptoms of sit pain (inability to sit for >30 min), radicular pain of the lower back or hip, and paresthesias of the affected leg [27]. The coexistence of IFI and sciatic nerve problems should be considered.

Impingement between the lesser trochanter and ischium can be easily unnoticed regarding the complex anatomy of the deep gluteal space and the general similarities in clinical presentation for other causes of posterior hip pain. In a case series, Hatem et al. [28] documented that patients with IFI had 29.2 months (range, 16.6–59.3) of duration of symptoms on average.

Because of the pathologic narrowing of the ischiofemoral space, an abnormal stress between the lateral part of the ischium and the posteromedial part of the lesser trochanter leads to inflammation and posterior hip pain that can be reproduced on physical examination.

The original description of IFI proposed that the pain could be reproduced by having the hip in extension, adduction, and external rotation; however, no validated clinical tests were available until 2016, when Gómez-Hoyos et al. [29] reported the accuracy of two clinical tests for ischiofemoral impingement in patients with posterior hip pain and endoscopically confirmed diagnosis.

The IFI test is performed with the patient in a lateral position (Fig. 12.4). The examiner passively takes the patient's hip into extension. The IFI test is intended to provoke impingement in extension with a neutral or adducted hip (re-creating the posterior pain lateral to the ischium) and relieves the impingement pain in extension with an abducted hip. This test has a sensitivity of 0.82, specificity of 0.85, positive predictive value of 0.88, negative predictive value of 0.79, positive likelihood ratio of 5.35, negative likelihood ratio of 0.21, and diagnostic odds ratio of 25.6.

The long-stride walking (LSW) test is expected to provoke impingement between the lesser trochanter and ischium in terminal hip extension when the patient walks (Fig. 12.5). The findings of this test are considered positive if the posterior pain is reproducible lateral to the ischium during extension with long strides, whereas pain is alleviated when walking with short strides or abducted gait. This test had a sensitivity of 0.94, specificity of 0.85, positive predictive value of 0.89, negative

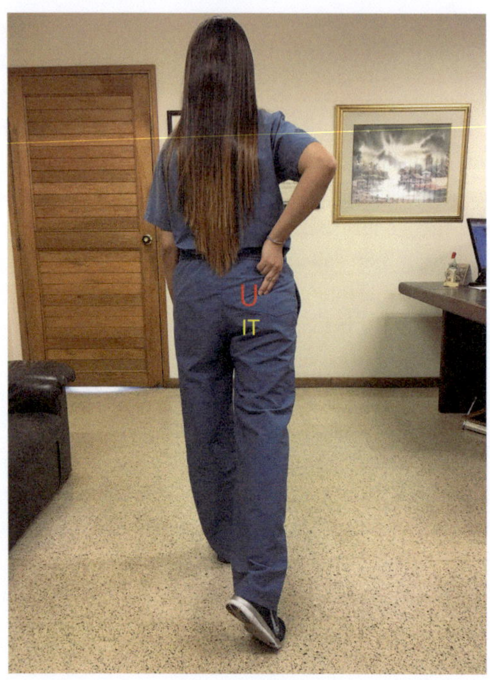

Fig. 12.4 The IFI test is performed with the patient in the contralateral decubitus position and taking the affected hip into passive extension. The findings of this test are considered positive when the symptoms are reproduced in adduction or the neutral position, whereas extension with abduction does not reproduce the symptoms. *IT* ischial tuberosity

predictive value of 0.92, positive likelihood ratio of 6.12, negative likelihood ratio of 0.07, and diagnostic odds ratio of 88.8.

In patients with other associated problems such as hamstring syndrome and/or sciatic nerve entrapment, other symptoms can be added.

The differential diagnosis of posterior hip pain can be localized to proximal or distal regions. Those producing distal sciatic nerve impingement have different complaints from those who exhibit pain with walking or sitting. An example of pain exacerbated by sitting can include driving; when the hip is in 30° flexion, the hamstrings (semimembranosus) show a different force vector angle in comparison with 90° activation. Activities holding the hip in 30° hip flexion can reproduce SN complaints when the hamstrings are activated. Conversely, patients with IFI are more comfortable sitting; however walking during terminal hip extension when the space between ischium and the lesser trochanter is diminished exacerbates the pain [7, 30]. This diminished space is the location of the SN. If the normal biomechanics of this space is disrupted, the SN has the dynamic potential to be impinged.

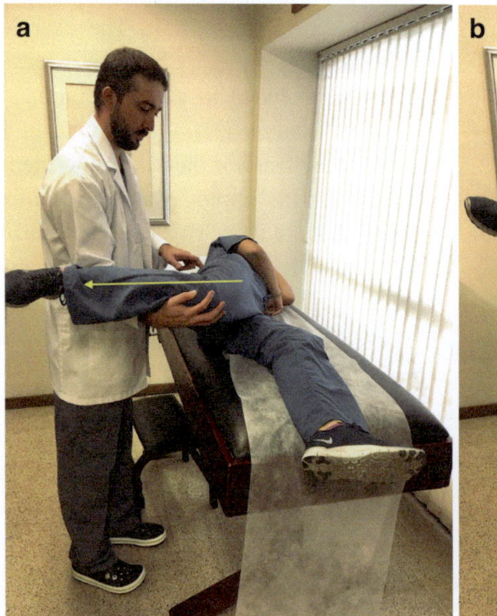

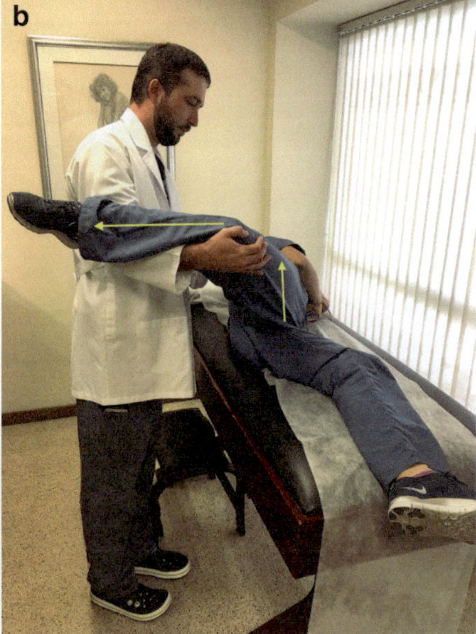

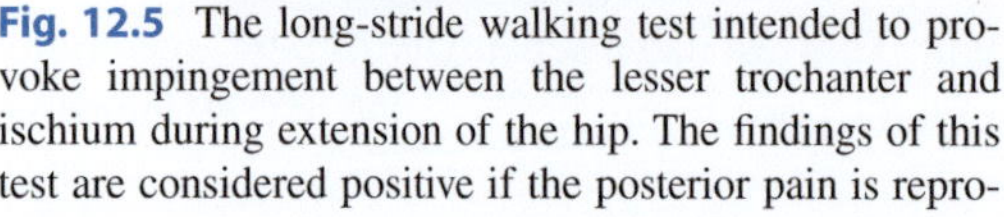

Fig. 12.5 The long-stride walking test intended to provoke impingement between the lesser trochanter and ischium during extension of the hip. The findings of this test are considered positive if the posterior pain is reproducible and the patient grabs the affected hip lateral to the ischium during extension (**a**) while pain is alleviated when walking with short strides (**b**)

The influence of limited hip range of motion on spine mobility and function has been shown as one of the causes of chronic low back pain. Patients with IFI may present associated symptoms of low back pain due to the limited hip extension. This clinical observation was confirmed by Gómez-Hoyos et al. [31] in a cadaveric study. Limiting hip extension by decreasing the ischiofemoral space resulted in significant increased facet joint pressure of the lumbar spine (L3–L4 and L4–L5). A complete physical examination of the hip must comprise a lumbar spine evaluation; in the same way, cases of low back pain should also include a hip evaluation.

Imaging Diagnosis

The standard imaging studies include the standing anterior-posterior pelvis, false profile, and lateral images. There are no specific radiographic findings for IFI. The IFS narrowing on anterior-posterior pelvic radiographs could lead to error, as the lesser trochanter is posterior to the ischial tunnel. Although false profile images are suggested to be useful for determining a narrow ischiofemoral space (Fig. 12.6), hip and pelvic radiographs are mainly utilized for diagnosing osseous abnormalities that may cause acquired IFI such as multiple exostosis, lesser trochanter malunion, and/or idiopathic narrowing of the ischiofemoral space (Fig. 12.7) [26].

Ultrasound has been traditionally used for identifying the presence of quadratus femoris edema within the IFS in patients with suspected IFI. However, in a recent study Finnoff et al. [12] used ultrasound to assess changes in IFS dimensions with femoral internal and external rotation and with adduction and abduction. Femoral position significantly changed the IFS dimensions. The widest IFS dimension occurred with femoral abduction and internal rotation (mean 51.8 mm; range 49.2–54.5 mm), and the narrowest with hip adduction and external rotation (mean 30.8, range 25.5–36.0 mm). Although this study provides valuable information regarding the relationship between hip position and IFS dimensions, the authors did not provide evidence that ultrasound could accurately measure the IFS. One year later, Finnoff et al. [32] published a new study aiming to determine whether ultrasound could accurately measure the IFS dimensions when compared with the gold standard imaging modality of MRI (Fig. 12.8). They found the IFS measurements obtained with ultrasound to be similar and not statistically different to those obtained with MRI (29.5 mm, SD 4.99 vs. 28.25 mm SD 5.91).

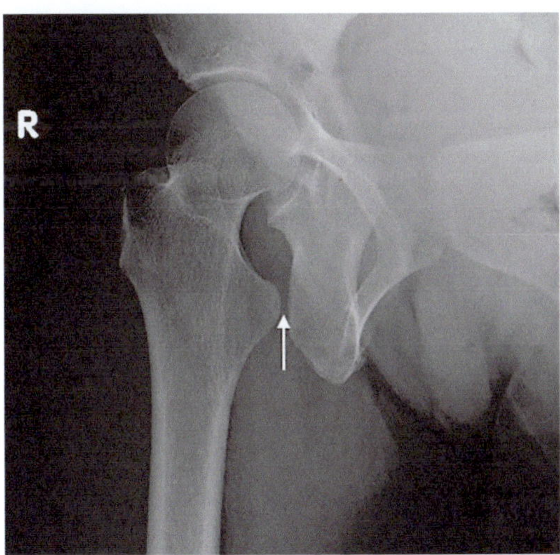

Fig. 12.6 False profile hip radiograph in a 56-year-old female with symptomatic ischiofemoral impingement. Observe the narrowing of the ischiofemoral space (white arrow). This case was confirmed by performing an MRI. Radiographs have not been validated for measuring the ischiofemoral space

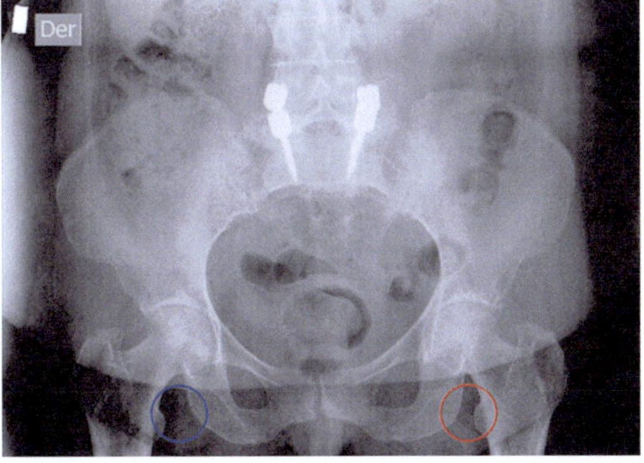

Fig. 12.7 Anteroposterior radiograph of the pelvis in a 63-year-old female. A diminished ischiofemoral space is seen on the left hip (red circle) as compared with the right side (blue circle)

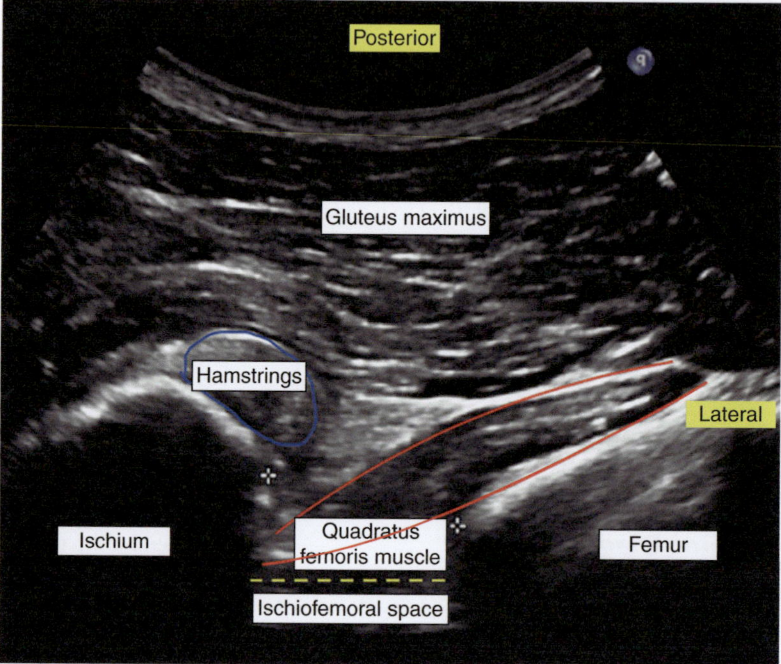

Fig. 12.8 Ultrasound image of the ischiofemoral space. A curved transducer was placed over the posterior part of the hip in a healthy volunteer. Observe the close relationship between the quadratus femoris muscle and the ischiofemoral space

In spite of new evidence showing ultrasound techniques being useful for measuring IFS, MRI remains as the gold standard for imaging assessment of patients with suspected IFI.

Before we assess the ischiofemoral space on MRI, all intra-articular and intrapelvic sources of posterior hip pain should be ruled out.

The patient positioning is important for IFI assessment when using MRI. The feet are secured in a neutral walking position, which will most closely simulate a dynamic assessment of the ischiofemoral space. If the feet are not secured in this functional position, a false impression of decreased ischiofemoral space could occur. The assessment of the semimembranosus and its orientation to the lateral ischium is best visualized on T2 axial or T2 coronal MRI. This view allows for the detection of a partial tear or undersurface tears of the semimembranosus [33].

Width measurements of two spaces at the ischiofemoral region were both initially described by Torriani et al. [6] as the smallest distance between the lateral cortex of the ischial tuberosity and medial cortex of the lesser trochanter (IFS), and the smallest space for passage of the quadratus femoris muscle delimited by the superolateral surface of the hamstring tendons and the

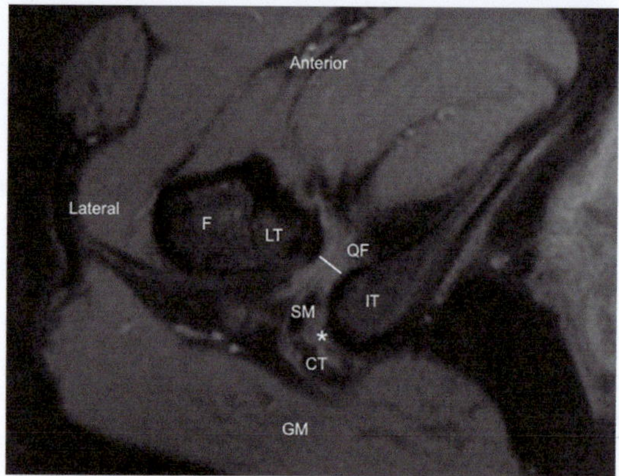

Fig. 12.9 T2 MRI of the right hip with narrow ischiofemoral space (solid white line) in a 54-year-old female. IFS is defined as the smallest distance between the lateral cortex of the ischial tuberosity and medial cortex of the lesser trochanter (8 mm in this case). Observe an associated hamstring origin tendon avulsion (asterisk). *F* femur, *LT* lesser trochanter, *QF* quadratus femoris muscle (with edema), *IT* ischial tuberosity, *SM* semimembranosus, *CT* conjoined tendon, *GM* gluteus maximus

posteromedial surface of the iliopsoas tendon or lesser trochanter (QFS), Fig. 12.9.

To date, Torriani et al. [6] cutoff values (IFS ≤ 17 mm and QFS ≤ 8 mm) for helping to diagnose ischiofemoral impingement are widely utilized. Nonetheless, several authors are still try-ing to find a reliable way to measure IF spaces in order to be more accurate in differentiating normal from abnormal.

Ozdemir et al. [34] performed a study in order to make normative width measurements of the IFS in an asymptomatic population and to record the soft tissue MRI signal variations within the IFS in order to determine whether such variations are associated with IFS dimensions. They included 418 1.5T hip MRI from 209 asymptomatic volunteers. They found a mean IFS width of 2.56 ± 0.75 cm (right, 2.60 ± 0.75 cm; left, 2.53 ± 0.75 cm). Soft tissue MRI signal abnormalities were present within the IFS in 19 (9.1%) of 209 volunteers. Soft tissue abnormalities within the IF space included edema (3/209, 1.4%) of the QF and/or surrounding soft tissue and fatty infiltration (16/209, 7.7%) of the QF.

Although the previous study reported that not all patients with QF edema have ischiofemoral impingement, MRI images which show QF edema and atrophy should prompt the health provider to check for IFS narrowing [35]. Narrowing of the ischiofemoral and QF spaces can compress the quadratus femoris muscle causing edema and atrophy. On the other hand, QFM edema and fatty infiltration can cause narrowing of these spaces.

Apart from QF edema, other associated MRI abnormalities such as bone marrow edema, hamstring tendonitis, ischial bursitis, and sciatic nerve irritation can also be identified [26].

IFI is a dynamic problem not based on imaging assessment. Diagnosis should be made correlating imaging to physical examination assessing all anatomical and functional layers.

Nonoperative Treatment

Conservative treatment is often advisable for IFI and typically consists of activity modification (such as teaching the patient to restrict the length of the stride), anti-inflammatory medication, abductor strengthening, core strengthening, and hip-motion exercises. The physical therapy program should be individualized on the basis of factors such as athletic demands, restriction in range of motion, and objective weakness in muscle strength. The intervention strategy for those with IFI is directed to rebalance the muscle-articular functioning of the hip/pelvis and spine through soft tissue mobilization, stretching and strengthening exercises, and aerobic conditioning. A patient with ischiofemoral impingement due to abductor weakness should get complete relief after a personalized physical therapy program directed to recover abductor strength and gait balance. Cases that involve hyperpronation, orthotics can be utilized.

Imaging-guided injections are used as a diagnosis tool and treatment alternative (see Chap. 6). For those with suspected IFI, the utilization of injections can help to differentiate the source of pain from other diagnosis, when correctly administered at the structure under investigation, producing relief of pain [7, 36].

Ultrasound-guided corticosteroid injection of the quadratus femoris has shown promising results as an effective treatment of IFI syndrome. Backer et al. [37] reported mild to good relief in 100% of a case series. However, location of pain may no longer be in the IFS, but be transfered proximally.

Case reports have been published about ultrasound-guided botulin toxin and polydeoxyribonucleotide sodium injection within the ischiofemoral space [38, 39]. Caution is advised when using these therapies as no enough evidence supports their utilization.

Operative Treatment

In the event that a patient does not achieve pain relief with conservative treatment, surgical intervention is considered. The surgical treatment chosen will depend on both the clinical diagnosis and imaging evaluation and to the patients' response to targeted injections during the conservative treatment stage. The goal of surgery is to reestablish a normal distance, wich may not require a complete resection of the lesser trochanter.

Decompression of the ischiofemoral space can be achieved by performing a lesser trochanterplasty [40, 41], an ischioplasty [42], or both when necessary.

The surgical treatment options can involve open and/or endoscopic techniques to restore the normal anatomy [28, 43]. Posterior approach to perform lesser trochanterplasty is safer to avoid medial circumflex artery. See Chap. 1.

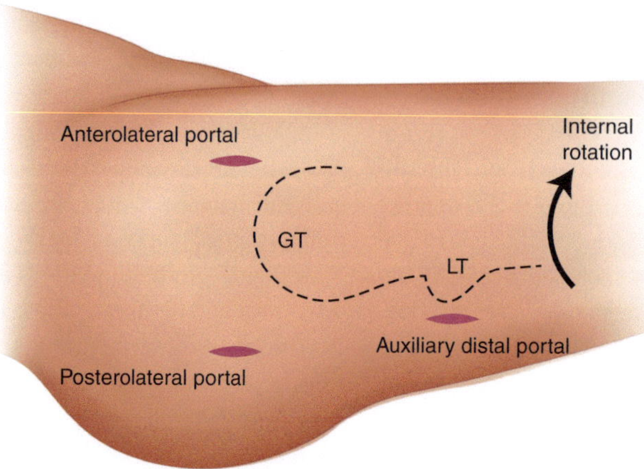

Fig. 12.10 Portal placement for endoscopic treatment of IFI. Three portals are used: anterolateral, posterolateral, and auxiliary distal at level of lesser trochanter (LT). *GT* greater trochanter

The full endoscopic procedure is performed similar to Hatem et al. [28]. The patient is placed supine on a traction table with 20° contralateral tilt. Three portals are used: anterolateral, posterolateral, and auxiliary distal at level of lesser trochanter, as seen in Fig. 12.10. Traction is used for a maximum of 15 min, while the intra-articular space was arthroscopically examined, with the remainder of the procedure performed without traction. A 70° high-definition arthroscope is used in the anterolateral portal, while the posterolateral and auxiliary distal portal are primarily used for a probe, arthroscopic burr, curved retractors, or arthroscope. Resection of the quadratus femoris is necessary to provide a window to access the lesser trochanter between the medial circumflex femoral artery and first perforating femoral artery. Lesser trochanterplasty of the posterior one-third (Leaving distal piece of QF to avoid vascular damage) is then performed to obtain a functionally normal ischiofemoral space. Dynamic hip movements of adduction-extension and internal-external rotation are used to verify the lesser trochanter decompression (Fig. 12.11) [28].

Regardless of the resection technique, to reduce the size of the lesser trochanter and/or the lateral aspect of the ischium could detach the iliopsoas and/or hamstring tendons, respectively. Gómez-Hoyos et al. [9] performed a cadaveric study in order to describe the exact location of the iliopsoas tendon insertion on the lesser trochanter clarify the implications of the lesser trochanterplasty. They found that a partial or total lesser trochanterplasty for increasing the ischiofemoral space without detaching partially or entirely the iliopsoas insertion is improbable.

The cases presenting with hamstrings avulsions in conjunction with IFI can be addressed with a combination of ischioplasty and hamstrings repair or with lesser trochanterplasty. The goal is to recreate the standard IFS so as to achieve normal terminal hip extension and to avoid any kinematic lumbar consequences. Identifying and decompressing the SN, which is often concomitantly involved, is critical to achieving optimal results [33].

An alternative approach is a mini-open surgical technique, which is assisted by dry endoscopy and neuromonitoring. The neuromonitoring reduces risk of intraoperative nerve damage [44–46]. The mini-open transgluteal approach is performed with the patient in a prone position. The ischial tuberosity and ischiofemoral space are identified under fluoroscopy, and an 8 cm transverse line is drawn. Ischiofemoral space, quadratus femoris muscle, and hamstrings are accessed through the gluteus maximus two-thirds proximal and one-third distal to the muscle (Fig. 12.12) [43].

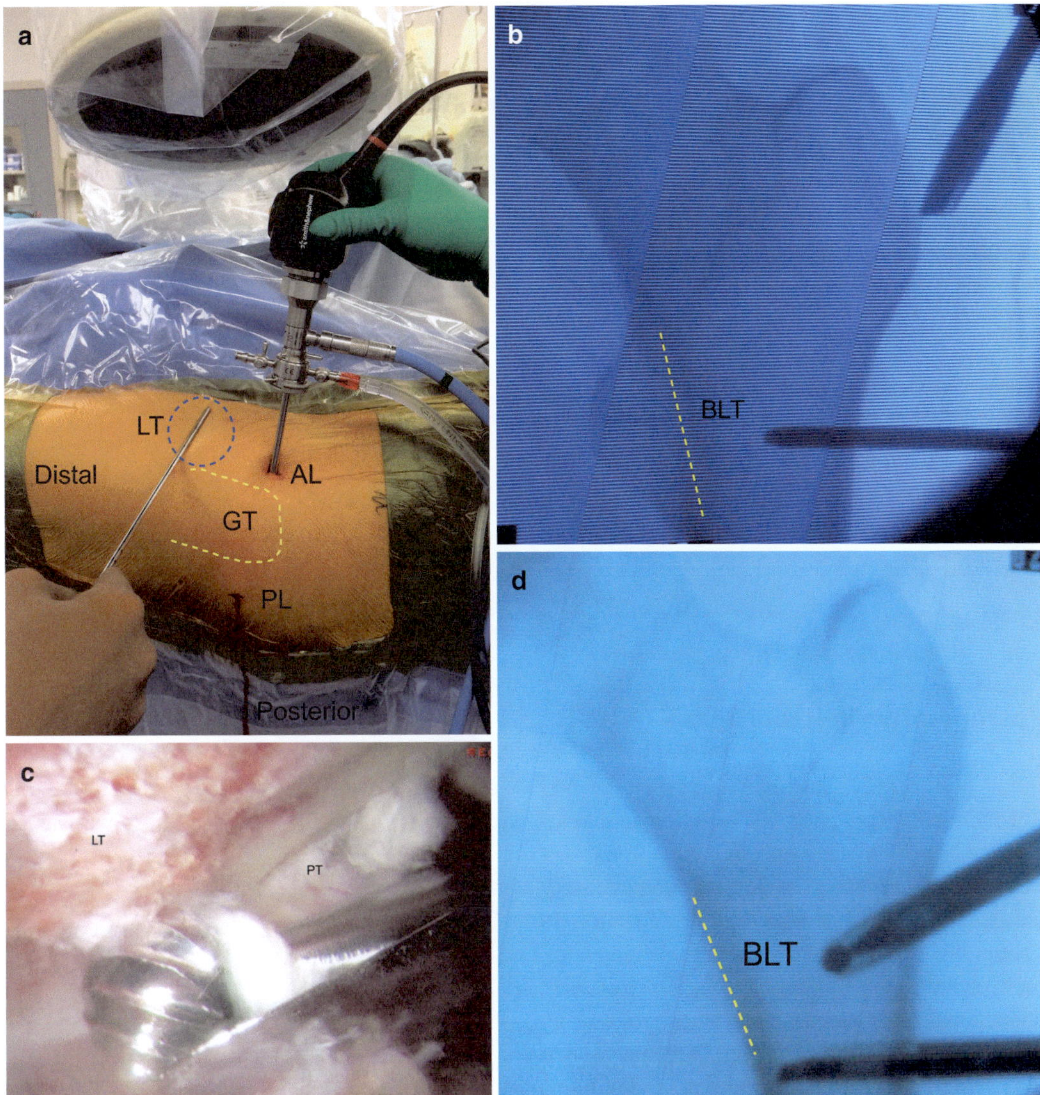

Fig. 12.11 Endoscopic lesser trochanterplasty. Patient in supine on a traction table. (**a**) The anterolateral (AL) portal was used for access to obtain visualization with a 70° high-definition arthroscope. The posterolateral (PL) portal and auxiliary distal portal are used for the introduction of a probe, arthroscopic burr, curved retractors, or the arthroscope. (**b**) Fluoroscopic image of the probe for determining the lesser trochanter location. (**c**) Endoscopic view of the lesser trochanterplasty by using an endoscopic burr through the posterolateral portal. (**d**) Fluoroscopic view of the final aspect of the femur after resecting the lesser trochanter. *GT* greater trochanter, *LT* lesser trochanter, *BLT* base of the lesser trochanter

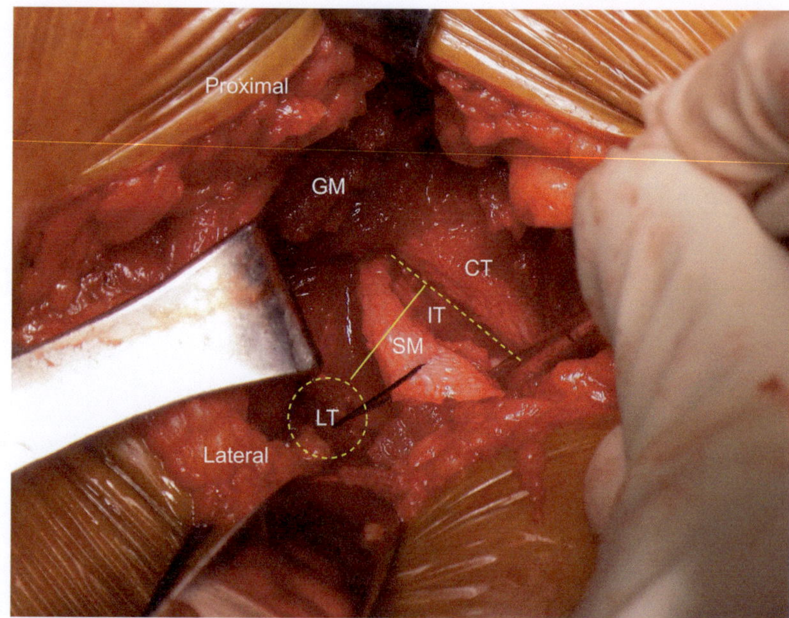

Fig. 12.12 Patient in prone position, left side, posterior approach. Ischiofemoral space (solid yellow line) decompression by performing ischioplasty through an open approach in a patient with concomitant hamstring origin avulsion. *GM* gluteus maximus, *LT* lesser trochanter (dashed yellow circle), *SM* semimembranosus tendon, *IT* ischial tuberosity (dashed yellow line), *CT* conjoined tendon

Postoperative Rehabilitation

Initial postoperative instructions during the first 4 weeks include crutches and partial weight bearing and neutral hip flexors stretching. Important milestones for an adequate postoperative recovery are lumbopelvic alignment and stabilization to control hip extension and abductor strengthening; then, avoiding lower pelvic drop or excessive adduction of the lower limb during weight bearing [33]. No active lifting of the leg is recommended in order to protect for the remaining tendon insertion. Please see neural mobilization in Physical Therapy Chapter and Appendix of this book.

References

1. Singer AD, Subhawong TK, Jose J, Tresley J, Clifford PD. Ischiofemoral impingement syndrome: a meta-analysis. Skelet Radiol. 2015;44(6):831–7.
2. Tosun Ö, Çay N, Bozkurt M, Arslan H. Ischiofemoral impingement in an 11-year-old girl. Diagn Interv Radiol. 2012;18(6):571–3.
3. Stenhouse G, Kaiser S, Kelley SP, Stimec J. Ischiofemoral impingement in children: imaging with clinical correlation. AJR Am J Roentgenol. 2016;206(2):426–30.
4. Duque Orozco MD, Abousamra O, Rogers KJ, Thacker MM. Magnetic resonance imaging in symptomatic children with hereditary multiple exostoses of the hip. J Pediatr Orthop. 2018;38(2):116–21.
5. Aydıngöz Ü, Özdemir Z, Güneş A, Ergen FB. MRI of lower extremity impingement and friction syndromes in children. Diagn Interv Radiol. 2016;22(6):566–73.
6. Torriani M, Souto SCL, Thomas BJ, Ouellette H, Bredella MA. Ischiofemoral impingement syndrome: an entity with hip pain and abnormalities of the quadratus femoris muscle. AJR Am J Roentgenol. 2009;193(1):186–90.
7. Martin HD, Reddy M, Gomez-Hoyos J. Deep gluteal syndrome. J Hip Preserv Surg. 2015;2(2):99–107.
8. Miller SL, Webb GR. The proximal origin of the hamstrings and surrounding anatomy encountered during repair. Surgical technique. J Bone Joint Surg Am. 2008;90(Suppl 2):108–16.
9. Gómez-Hoyos J, Schröder R, Palmer IJ, Reddy M, Khoury A, Martin HD. Iliopsoas tendon insertion footprint with surgical implications in lesser trochanterplasty for treating ischiofemoral impingement: an anatomic study. J Hip Preserv Surg. 2015;2(4):385–91.
10. Johnson KA. Impingement of the lesser trochanter on the ischial ramus after total hip arthroplasty. Report of three cases. J Bone Joint Surg Am. 1977;59:268–9.
11. Patti J, Ouellette H, Bredella M, Torriani M. Impingement of the lesser trochanter on ischium as a potential cause of hip pain. Skelet Radiol. 2008;37:939–41.
12. Finnoff J, Bond JR, Collins MS, Sellon JL, Hollman JH, Wempe MK, Smith J. Variability of the ischiofemoral space relative to femur position: an ultrasound study. PM&R. 2015;7:930–7.

13. Singer A, Clifford P, Tresley J, Jose J, Subhawong T. Ischiofemoral impingement and the utility of full-range-of-motion magnetic resonance imaging in its detection. Am J Orthop (Belle Mead NJ). 2014;43(12):548–51.

14. Vallon F, Reymond A, Fürnstahl P, Zingg P, Kamath A, Snedeker J. Effect of angular deformities of the proximal femur on impingement-free hip range of motion in a three-dimensional rigid body model. Hip Int. 2015;25(6):574–80.

15. Bedi A, Dolan M, Leunig M, Kelly BT. Static and dynamic mechanical causes of hip pain. Arthroscopy. 2011;27(2):235–51.

16. Bredella MA, Azevedo DC, Oliveira AL, Simeone FJ, Chang CY, Stubbs AJ, Torriani M. Pelvic morphology in ischiofemoral impingement. Skelet Radiol. 2015;44(2):249–53.

17. Gómez-Hoyos J, Schröder R, Reddy M, Palmer IJ, Martin HD. Femoral neck anteversion and lesser trochanteric retroversion in patients with ischiofemoral impingement: a case-control magnetic resonance imaging study. Arthroscopy. 2016;32(1):13–8.

18. Oliveira AL, Azevedo DC, Eajazi A, Palmer WE, Kwon YM, Bredella MA, Torriani M. Assessment of total hip arthroplasty as a predisposing factor for ischiofemoral impingement. Skelet Radiol. 2015;44(12):1755–60.

19. Spencer-Gardner L, Bedi A, Stuart MJ, Larson CM, Kelly BT, Krych AJ. Ischiofemoral impingement and hamstring dysfunction as a potential pain generator after ischial tuberosity apophyseal fracture non-union/malunion. Knee Surg Sports Traumatol Arthrosc. 2015;25(1):55–61.

20. Hayat Z, Konan S, Pollock R. Ischiofemoral impingement resulting from a chronic avulsion injury of the hamstrings. BMJ Case Rep. 2014;25:2014.

21. Schatteman J, Vanhoenacker FM, Somville J, Verstraete KL. Ischiofemoral impingement due to a solitary exostosis. JBR-BTR. 2015;98(1):39–42.

22. Viala P, Vanel D, Larbi A, Cyteval C, Laredo JD. Bilateral ischiofemoral impingement in a patient with hereditary multiple exostoses. Skelet Radiol. 2012;41:1637–40.

23. Yoong P, Mansour R, Teh JL. Multiple hereditary exostoses and ischiofemoral impingement: a case-control study. Skelet Radiol. 2014;43(9):1225–30.

24. Papoutsi D, Daniels J, Mistry A, Chandraseker C. Ischiofemoral impingement due to a lipoma of the ischiofemoral space. BMJ Case Rep. 2016;8:2016.

25. Ali AM, Whitwell D, Ostlere SJ. Ischiofemoral impingement: a retrospective analysis of cases in a specialist orthopaedic centre over a four-year period. Hip Int. 2013;23:263–8.

26. Hernando MF, Cerezal L, Pérez-Carro L, Abascal F, Canga A. Deep gluteal syndrome: anatomy, imaging, and management of sciatic nerve entrapments in the subgluteal space. Skelet Radiol. 2015;44(7):919–34.

27. Young IJ, van Riet RP, Bell SN. Surgical release for proximal hamstring syndrome. Am J Sports Med. 2008;36(12):2372–8.

28. Hatem MA, Palmer IJ, Martin HD. Diagnosis and 2-year outcomes of endoscopic treatment for ischiofemoral impingement. Arthroscopy. 2015;31(2):239–46.

29. Gómez-Hoyos J, Martin RL, Schröder R, Palmer IJ, Martin HD. Accuracy of 2 clinical tests for ischiofemoral impingement in patients with posterior hip pain and endoscopically confirmed diagnosis. Arthroscopy. 2016;32(7):1279–84.

30. Schroder R, Reddy M, Hatem M, et al. A MRI study of the lesser trochanteric version and its relationship to proximal femoral osseus anatomy. J Hip Preserv Surg. 2015;2(4):1–7.

31. Gómez-Hoyos J, Khoury A, Schroder R, et al. The hip-spine effect: A cadaveric study of ischiofemoral impingement in hip extension effecting loads in lumbar facet joints. Arthroscopy. 2017;33(1):101–7.

32. Finnoff JT, Johnson AC, Hollman JH. Can ultrasound accurately assess ischiofemoral space dimensions? A validation study. PM&R. 2017;9(4):392–7.

33. Martin HD, Khoury A, Schröder R, Palmer IJ. Ischiofemoral impingement and hamstring syndrome as causes of posterior hip pain: where do we go next? Clin Sports Med. 2016;35(3):469–86.

34. Özdemir Z, Aydıngöz Ü, Görmeli CA, Sağır Kahraman A. Ischiofemoral space on MRI in an asymptomatic population: normative width measurements and soft tissue signal variations. Eur Radiol. 2015;25(8):2246–53.

35. Tosun O, Algin O, Yalcin N, Cay N, Ocakoglu G, Karaoglanoglu M. Ischiofemoral impingement: evaluation with new MRI parameters and assessment of their reliability. Skelet Radiol. 2012;41(5):575–87.

36. Michel F, Decavel P, Toussirot E, et al. Piriformis muscle syndrome: diagnostic criteria and treatment of a monocentric series of 250 patients. Ann Phys Rehabil Med. 2013;56(5):371–83.

37. Backer MW, Lee KS, Blankenbaker DG, Kijowski R, Keene JS. Correlation of ultrasound-guided corticosteroid injection of the quadratus femoris with MRI findings of ischiofemoral impingement. AJR Am J Roentgenol. 2014;203(3):589–93.

38. Kim WJ, Shin HY, Koo GH, Park HG, Ha YC, Park YH. Ultrasound-guided prolotherapy with polydeoxyribonucleotide sodium in ischiofemoral impingement syndrome. Pain Pract. 2014;14(7):649–55.

39. Jenkins K, Chen YT. Poster 111 ultrasonographic finding of ischiofemoral impingement syndrome and novel treatment with botulinum toxin: a case report. PM&R. 2016;8(9S):S198.

40. Howse EA, Mannava S, Tamam C, Martin HD, Bredella MA, Stubbs AJ. Ischiofemoral space decompression through posterolateral approach: cutting block technique. Arthrosc Tech. 2014;3(6):e661–5.

41. Jo S, O'Donnell JM. Endoscopic lesser trochanter resection for treatment of ischiofemoral impingement. J Hip Preserv Surg. 2015;2(2):184–9.

42. Truong WH, Murnaghan L, Hopyan SKS. Ischioplasty for femoroischial impingement. JBJS Case Connect. 2012;2(3):e51.

43. Gómez-Hoyos J, Reddy M, Martin HD. Dry endoscopic-assisted mini-open approach with neuromonitoring for chronic hamstring avulsions and ischial tunnel syndrome. Arthrosc Tech. 2015;4(3):e193–9.

44. Porat M, Orozco F, Goyal N, et al. Neurophysiologic monitoring can predict iatrogenic injury during acetabular and pelvic fracture fixation. HSS J. 2013;9(3):218–22.

45. Calder HB, Mast J, Johnstone C. Intraoperative evoked potential monitoring in acetabular surgery. Clin Orthop Relat Res. 1994;305:160–7.

46. Baumgaertner MR, Wegner D, Booke J. SSEP monitoring during pelvic and acetabular fracture surgery. J Orthop Trauma. 1994;8:127–33.

Greater Trochanteric-Ischial Impingement

Jeremy A. Ross, Jennifer Marland, and Hugh S. West Jr.

Introduction

Extra-spinal compression of the sciatic nerve about the hip has been previously described in various conditions including piriformis syndrome, deep gluteal syndrome (DGS), and ischiofemoral impingement syndrome (IFI) [1]. A potential new source for extra-spinal sciatic nerve impingement has been described between the posterior aspect of the greater trochanter and the ischium and may be termed greater trochanteric-ischial impingement syndrome (GTII) (Fig. 13.1). While there is no clinical data to date regarding this entity, anatomic analysis implicates this as a potential site for sciatic nerve impingement and posterior hip/buttock pain.

Anatomy and Biomechanics

The sciatic nerve is comprised of nerve roots from the L4-S3 spinal levels which combine to form a large multifunction nerve. After passing beneath or around the piriformis muscle belly,

the sciatic nerve exits the greater sciatic foramen to enter the deep gluteal space and travel distally in the posterior compartment of the thigh. As it passes the ischium, it is intimately associated with the hamstring tendons and quadratus femoris muscle. Potential sites of extra-spinal sciatic nerve compression include the piriformis muscle, deep gluteal space, and ischiofemoral space (IFS) which have been discussed in previous chapters. A new potential site for extra-spinal sciatic nerve compression exists between the posterior aspect of the greater trochanter and the lateral aspect of the ischium, described as greater trochanteric-ischial impingement (GTII). Compression of the sciatic nerve at this site could lead to posterior hip pain and symptoms of sciatic nerve entrapment similar to the clinical syndromes previously described. This is a distinct clinical entity from greater trochanteric-pelvic impingement (GTPI) which involves impingement between the medial aspect of the greater trochanter and the ilium leading to lateral hip pain with no symptoms of nerve compression [2].

While no clinical data exists to date on GTII, a recently published cadaveric study by Kivlan et al. has shed light on the anatomic basis for impingement of the sciatic nerve at this site [3]. Impingement may occur when the hip is flexed, abducted, and externally rotated (Fig. 13.2). This study examined 25 hips from 14 embalmed cadavers to determine the presence of impingement in different hip positions. The hip was brought from 90° of flexion,

J. A. Ross, MD
UMass Memorial Health Care, Orthopaedics and Physical Rehabilitation, Worcester, MA, USA

J. Marland, DPT · H. S. West Jr., MD (✉)
Intermountain Healthcare, Department of Orthopedics, Murray, UT, USA
e-mail: Jenny.Marland@imail.org;
Hugh.West@imail.org

© Springer International Publishing AG, part of Springer Nature 2019
H. D. Martin, J. Gómez-Hoyos (eds.), *Posterior Hip Disorders*,
https://doi.org/10.1007/978-3-319-78040-5_13

60° of external rotation, and either 30° or 0° of abduction into extension to determine the flexion angle at which contact between the greater trochanter and ischium occurred (Fig. 13.3).

The data demonstrated contact between 20° and 60° of flexion with the hip abducted 30° and contact between 52° and 70° of flexion with the hip in neutral abduction. Thus, there is greater potential for contact between the posterior aspect of the greater trochanter and the ischium with increased hip abduction as the hip is brought from flexion to extension. The study also examined the

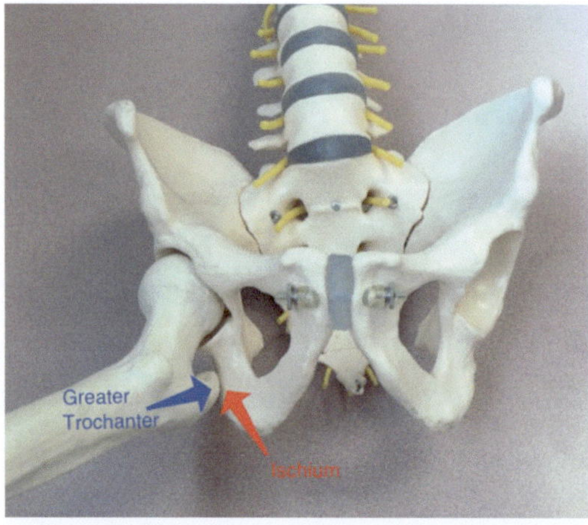

Fig. 13.1 GTII

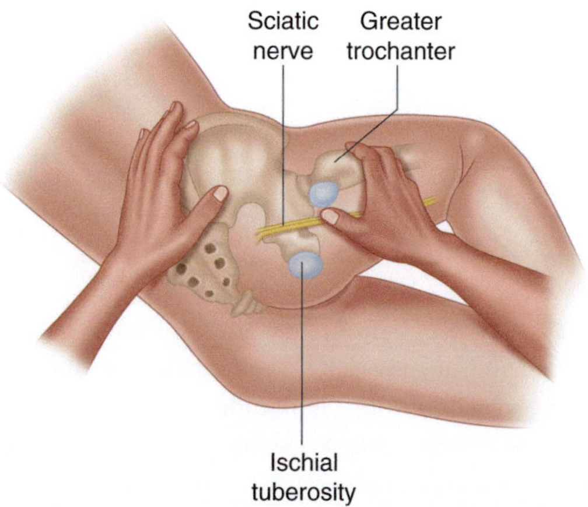

Fig. 13.2 Greater trochanteric ischial

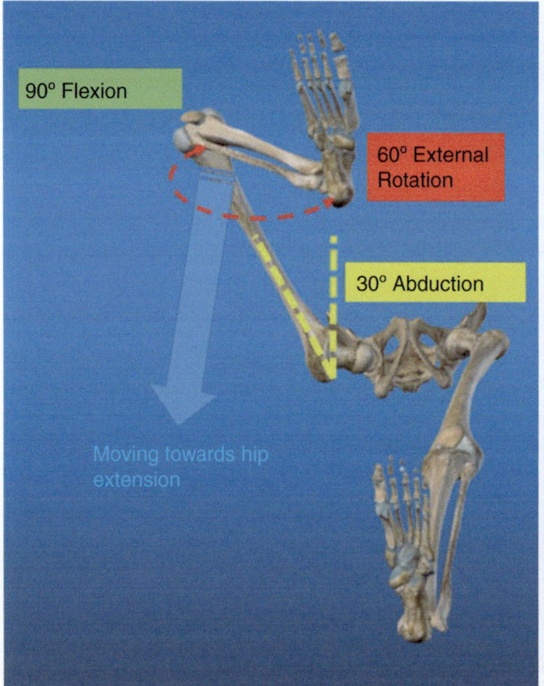

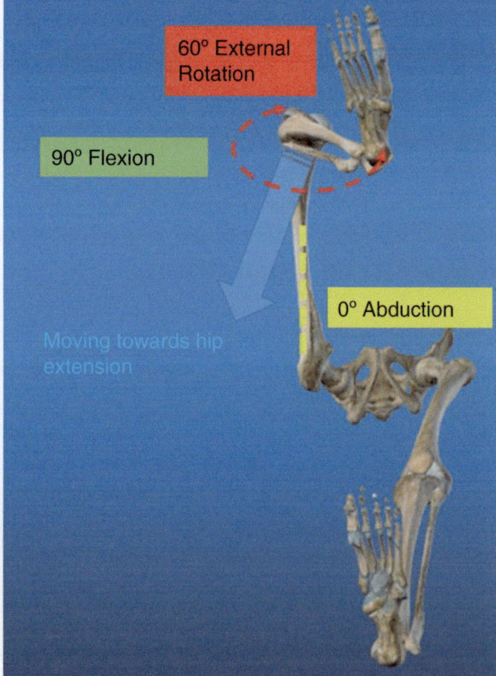

Fig. 13.3 Position 1 describes the hip in 90 of flexion, 60° of external rotation, and 30° of abduction. Position 2 varies the position of abduction to 0°. Both positions were evaluated for approximation of the greater trochanter and ischium as the hip was moved into hip extension

reliability of the Patrick-FABER test to determine contact between the greater trochanter and ischium. This physical exam maneuver was found to reproduce GTII in 24/25 (96%) specimens. Given these data, it is possible that pathologic contact between the greater trochanter and ischium may exist in certain hip positions. It is therefore plausible that repeated compression of the sciatic nerve in this space could lead to posterior hip pain in a previously undescribed clinical manner.

Causes/Risk Factors

While future studies are necessary to validate GTII as a condition responsible for extra-articular hip pain, theoretically individuals may impinge during activities where the hip moves into extension from flexion while abducted and externally rotated (Table 13.1). Other potential causes of GTII may be related to structural deformities of the hip and pelvis, space occupying lesions, or iatrogenic structural changes (Table 13.2). Coxa vara, femoral version, and over medialization of a prosthetic joint have been associated with extra-articular impingement and theoretically may be risk factors for GTII due to the close approximation of the greater trochanter and the ischium during functional movement. Legg-Calve-Perthes disease (coxa plana) may also be implicated in GTII. Alterations in femoral head and neck morphology resulting from Perthes include flat-

Table 13.1 Activities/functional positions

Ballet: Plié in the second position
Sitting crossed-legged
Baseball catchers
Yoga positions

Table 13.2 Anatomic factors

Structural deformities	Coxa vara
	Femoral version
Space occupying	Hamstring tendinopathy
	Ischial avulsion fractures
Iatrogenic	Over medialization of a prosthetic joint

tening of the femoral head and a short varus femoral neck [2]. Both of these bring the greater trochanter into closer approximation to the ilium and ischium and may lead to posterior impingement. Hamstring tendinopathy or avulsion fractures at the ischium have been implicated in narrowing the ischiofemoral space. Theoretically, these may contribute to GTII, impinging the sciatic nerve and/or quadratus femoris muscle.

Clinical Diagnosis/Imaging

GTII is currently a theoretical concept; therefore no validated clinical tests exist. Kivlan's current cadaveric study aimed to describe the relative hip position between the greater trochanter and the ischium, differentiating GTII from IFI. While this has not been studied on patients, the findings suggest a model of pathomechanics for identifying GTII. Based upon these findings, utilization of the FABER test (Fig. 13.4) could possibly be used clinically by reproducing pain in the presence of GTII; however this has yet to be validated [4].

Diagnostic injections are commonly used to confirm or rule out sources of musculoskeletal pain. A positive diagnostic injection may be beneficial in diagnostic workup for GTII. Due to the quadratus femoris space being a shared location between IFI and GTII, a positive injection would need to be accompanied by other positive diagnostic tests to differentiate between these two conditions. Magnetic resonance imaging (MRI) may have a role in diagnosing GTII by identifying edema in the quadratus femoris muscle and/or signal irregularity involving the sciatic nerve; however, these findings are also common in IFI [5, 6]. Following the current concepts in IFI, conservative measures are indicated when the IFS is within normal values. There is no currently described minimal space measure for GTII. Due to the position of the hip during GTII, static imaging is unlikely to identify this condition. Functional imaging would need to be investigated as a preferred diagnostic modality [7].

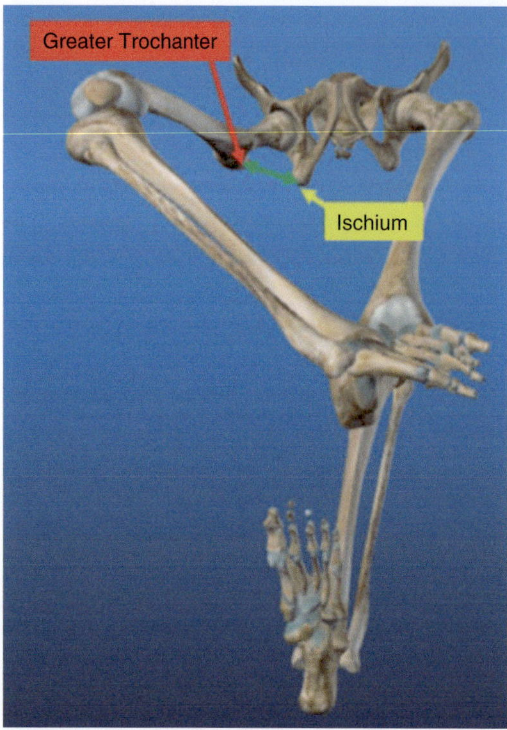

Fig. 13.4 FABER position

Intervention/Treatment

Currently, no study exists describing conservative or surgical treatment options for GTII. However, treatment concepts can be gleaned from those previously described for GTPI and IFI [8–10]. Surgical options to address anatomic factors may include relative femoral neck lengthening, ischioplasty, proximal hamstring debridement and repair, or rotational osteotomy. Relative femoral neck lengthening has been described as a treatment option for GTPI, and this may be extrapolated to GTII [2]. Moving the greater trochanter distally relative to the femoral neck increases the distance between the greater trochanter and the pelvis/ischium and could potentially decrease impingement in this site. Nonsurgical options would focus on activity modification, the correction of faulty movement patterns, and addressing nerve mobility and protection.

Conclusion

An understanding of the various causes of extra-spinal sciatic nerve compression continues to evolve. GTII is currently a theoretical concept supported by a cadaveric study that awaits confirmation as a true clinical entity. This chapter is primarily intended to create awareness of yet another potential cause of extra-spinal sciatica and ideally improve diagnostic accuracy.

References

1. Cheatham S. Extra-articular hip impingement: a narrative review of the literature. J Can Chiropr Assoc. 2016;60:47–56.
2. de Sa D. Extra-articular hip impingement: a systematic review examining operative treatment of psoas, subspine, ischiofemoral, and greater trochanteric/pelvic impingement. Arthroscopy. 2014;30(8):1026–41.
3. Kivlan BR, Martin RRL, Martin HD. Defining the greater trochanter-ischial space: a potential source of extra-articular impingement in the posterior hip region. J Hip Preserv Surg. 2016;3(4):1–6.
4. Martin HD, Palmer IJ. History and physical examination of the hip: the basics. Curr Rev Musculoskelet Med. 2013;6(3):219–25.
5. Bucknor MD, Steinbach LS, Saloner D, Chin CT. Magnetic resonance neurography evaluation of chronic extraspinal sciatica after remote proximal hamstring injury: a preliminary retrospective analysis. J Neurosurg. 2014;121:408–14.
6. Ricciardi BF, Fabricant PD, Fields KG, Poultsides L, Zaltz I, Sink EL. What are the demographic and radiographic characteristics of patients with symptomatic extraarticular femoral impingement. Clin Orthop Relat Res. 2015;473:1299–308.
7. Filler AG, Haynes J, Jordan SE, Prager J, Villablanca JP, Farahani K, McBride DQ, Tsuruda JS, Morisoli B, Batzdorf U, Johnson JP. Sciatica of nondisc origin and piriformis syndrome: diagnosis by magnetic resonance neurography and interventional magnetic resonance imaging with outcome study of resulting treatment. J Neurosurg Spine. 2005;2:99–115.
8. Bardakos NV. Hip impingement: beyond FAI. J Hip Preserv Surg. 2015;2(3):1–188.
9. Martin HD, Reddy M, Gomez-Hoyos J. Deep gluteal syndrome. J Hip Preserv Surg. 2015;2(2):1–9.
10. Reich MS, Shannon C, Tsai E, Salata MJ. Hip arthroscopy for extra-articular hip disease. Curr Rev Musculoskelet Med. 2013;6:250–7.

Ischiogluteal Bursitis 14

William Henry Márquez-Arabia,
Lorena Bejarano-Pineda,
Francisco Javier Monsalve,
and Luis Pérez-Carro

Introduction

There are more than 140 bursae described in the human body. Lately, however, they have been neglected by medical research, as the attention of physicians has been focused primarily on tendons, muscles, bones, and joints [1]. The mucosae bursae are responsible for maintaining the smoothness and frictionless movement of the body.

In 1932, Frazer et al. described a surgical resection of the ischial bursa in a patient of 50 years of age who was a sea captain and complaint of swelling in the right buttock for the last 20 years. Initially, the patient was diagnosed with a lipoma, but "the mass" was filled with fluid and weighed 2 pounds [2]. In 1974, a review of the literature of ischiogluteal bursitis was done by Swartout and Compere [3] finding only three cases about the entity. Afterward, Swartout himself developed the same condition, and he made a detailed description of the clinical presentation of this pathology.

Inflammation of the ischiogluteal bursa is an uncommon disorder that has been described in patients whose occupations require positions that cause persistent pressure in a specific region. Ischiogluteal bursitis has been called "weaver's or lighterman's bottom" [1, 4], as it can occur when spending long periods of time in a sitting position or being in jobs that involve vibration such as weaving, tractor-driving, or road equipment machines, where the ischiogluteal bursa can become inflamed [3, 5]. The ischiogluteal bursa is located between the ischial tuberosity and the gluteus maximus muscle. Specifically on the ischial area, the pain from inflammation has often been attributed to sciatic nerve disorders, ischial bone problems, or hamstring tendonitis.

Ischiogluteal bursa can be traumatized in a fall on backsides (buttocks) or by an acute or chronic shearing force in different activities or sports, resulting in chronic and sometimes disabling discomfort that can prevent athletes from participating in sports. Participants in sports that involve a sitting position such as canoeing, horseback riding, and wheelchair racing for paraplegic patients increase the risk of developing an ischiogluteal bursitis. Further, ischial tuberosity bears the

W. H. Márquez-Arabia, MD (✉)
Clínica Las Americas, Orthopedic Surgery, Medellin, Antioquia, Colombia

Sports Medicine Program, School of Medicine, Medellin, Antioquia, Colombia

L. Bejarano-Pineda, MD
Duke University Health System, Department of Orthopaedic Surgery, Durham, NC, USA

F. J. Monsalve, MD
Orthopedic Department, Medellin, Antioquia, Colombia

L. Pérez-Carro, MD, PhD
Clínica Mompia, Orthopedic Surgery Department, Santa Cruz de Bezana, Cantabria, Spain

© Springer International Publishing AG, part of Springer Nature 2019
H. D. Martin, J. Gómez-Hoyos (eds.), *Posterior Hip Disorders*,
https://doi.org/10.1007/978-3-319-78040-5_14

weight of the body in the supine position creating pressure points that may lead to ischiogluteal bursitis in debilitated patients, and particularly in those with paraplegia or with malignancy [6]. The symptoms are buttock pain or radiating pain running down the posterior thigh. The correct diagnosis can be overlooked since these clinical signs are often mistaken as being a proximal hamstring tendonitis or referred pain due to pathology of the spine or sciatic nerve [7].

Anatomy

Two types of bursae are described in the human body: constant and adventitial. Constant bursae are formed during normal embryonic development and are sac-like structures lined with endothelial cells. They are generally located between the tendon and bone or skin and serve to facilitate a gliding motion at points of high friction. Some of them may even communicate with a nearby joint. Adventitial bursae develop later in life through a process of myxomatous degeneration of fibrous tissue, in response to stress at the site of friction between adjacent structures. Endothelial lining is not present in those bursae, and such bursa will therefore not contain synovial fluid. The ischiogluteal bursa is an adventitial bursa type [8, 9]. Inflammatory bursitis often arises from repetitive subacute injury to the bursa. This repetitive injury results in local vasodilatation and increased vascular permeability, with the extravasation of serum proteins and extracellular fluid into the bursa.

The ischiogluteal bursa is an inconstant anatomical finding located deep to the gluteus maximus muscle over the ischial tuberosity. During standing, the tuberosity of the ischium is covered by the gluteus maximus muscle, but upon sitting the muscle slides up so that there is only fibrous tissue and the ischiogluteal bursa (when it is present) between the bone and the skin [3]. The sciatic and posterior femoral cutaneous nerve pass laterally to the hamstring near the ischial tuberosity, and they ride on the back of the quadratus femoris muscle. At this point, the sciatic nerve can be compressed or fixed by fibrovascular

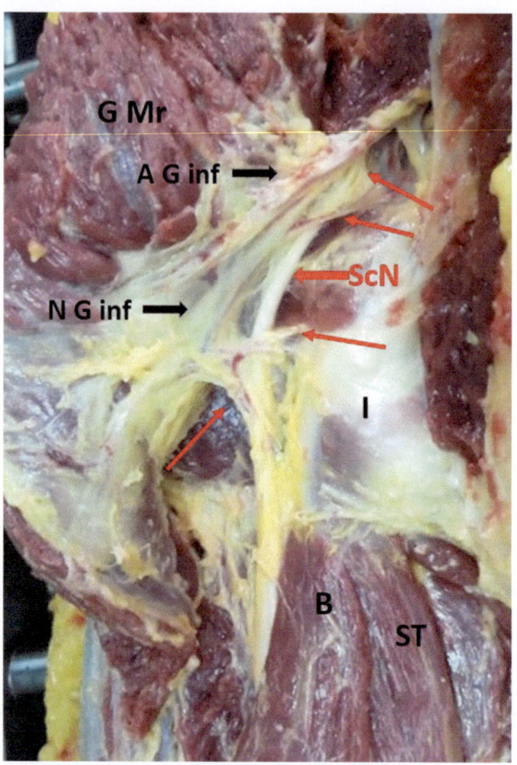

Fig. 14.1 A posterior view of the left hip of a cadaveric specimen. The gluteus maximus muscle reflected proximally. The sciatic nerve and the fibrovascular bands (red arrows) may diminish the sliding of the nerve. The inferior gluteal artery and nerve that inervate the gluteus maximus muscle (A G inf and N G inf, respectively). In the most distal area are the ischion and the hamstring proximal insertion (femoris biceps and semitendinosus muscles)

bands (Fig. 14.1) [10, 11] or can undergo compression and irritation by hamstring tendon alterations or the ischiogluteal bursa.

The hamstrings comprise the semitendinosus, the long head of biceps femoris, and semimembranosus tendons; they originate from the ischial tuberosity with the exception of the short head of the biceps femoris and insert distally below the knee on the proximal tibia. The proximal hamstring complex has a strong bony attachment on the ischial tuberosity (Fig. 14.2). The semitendinosus and the long head of biceps femoris tendons originate as a common proximal tendon from the medial portion of the tuberosity of the ischium. The oval footprint in the ischial tuberosity measures 2.7 ± 0.5 cm from

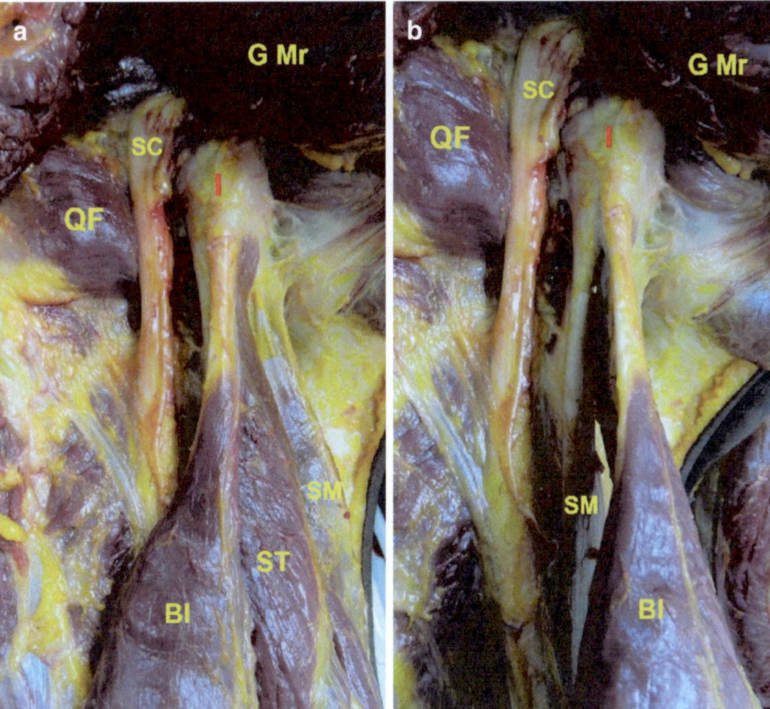

Fig. 14.2 A posterior view of the left hip of a cadaveric specimen. (**a**) The gluteus maximus muscle reflected proximally (G Mr). The sciatic nerve riding over the posterior region of quadratus femoris muscle (QF), the hamstring proximal insertion (BI, femoris biceps; ST, semitendinosus; SM, semimembranosus). (**b**) Semimembranosus muscle origin on the ischion is the most lateral and closer to the sciatic nerve

proximal to distal and 1.8 ± 0.2 cm from medial to lateral. The anatomic origin of semimembranosus tendon is more lateral in a crescent shape and measures 3.1 ± 0.3 cm from proximal to distal and 1.1 ± 0.5 cm from medial to lateral [10, 12, 13].

Etiology

Ischiogluteal bursitis often arises from repetitive subacute friction. However, other common causes are trauma (hemorrhagic bursitis), inflammatory diseases (e.g., rheumatoid arthritis, spondyloarthropathies, systemic lupus erythematosus, or Reiter's syndrome), infection (e.g., tuberculosis), and crystal deposition.

A considerable number of riders experience some degree of saddle soreness, especially in recreational activities. Tourists also describe similar symptoms at the beginning of riding on a long-distance trip. These patients usually progress to a painful ischiogluteal bursitis; however, sometimes the bursitis could be prevented with a change to a proper fitting saddle [14].

Crystal deposition as a cause of bursitis can be further categorized by the type of crystals identified in the synovial fluid with polarizing light microscopy. These crystals can be composed of monosodium urate (gout disease), calcium pyrophosphate dihydrate (pseudogout disease), or calcium hydroxyapatite [9]. Inflammatory bursitis also occurs in conjunction with systemic diseases such as syphilis, hypothyroidism, and systemic scleroderma.

Ischiogluteal bursitis has been described in patients with cachexia, severe weight loss, and cancer. It is assumed that reduction of subcutaneous fat in the buttock region results in repetitive trauma of the bursa which initiates the process of inflammation [15].

Clinical Presentation

Patients with ischiogluteal bursitis complain of pain at the lower gluteal area or inferior buttock and more specifically of localized pain over the ischial tuberosity. The pain may have a sudden onset, as a sharp or shooting sensation, and be unrelenting at night, making it difficult to find a comfortable position [3, 10]. Although the ischiogluteal bursitis is more common in patients with activities in a seated position for long periods of time, it is also present in people who are not required to constantly sit. The pain is severe in a sitting position or lying on one's back or standing and is exacerbated by standing on tip toes or bending forward [15]. Patients with ischiogluteal bursitis usually walk and stand with the trunk tilted toward the affected side; the step length is shortened, and back hyperextension is almost impossible. The pain may irradiate to the thigh or lower leg. For relief, patients often sit with the affected buttock elevated to avoid pressure on it [3]. Muscle atrophy is rare except in patients with terminal illness.

During the physical examination of a patient with ischiogluteal bursitis, an antalgic gait with elevation of the buttock to relieve pressure on the affected side is found. Pain is experienced on palpation over ischial tuberosity, which may be exacerbated by passive flexion and resisted extension of the ipsilateral hip. The pain can be reproduced by raising the leg in a straight position and be referred to the course of hamstring tendons. The Patrick test can be also positive [3, 15, 16]. In some patients, a soft tissue constituting of a painful mass might be palpated over the ischial tuberosity and be associated with inflammatory changes as increased skin temperature and redness in the buttock [17].

A rectal examination should also be carry out. In some cases, there will be a tender area of bulging inflamed tissue on the lateral wall of the affected side. Pressure on this area is severely painful.

Rubayi et al. described an infection of the ischial bursa in a patient with systemic lupus erythematosus and with a large ischial bursa infected with tuberculosis that compromised the ischium [6].

Differential Diagnosis

The evaluation of a posterior hip pain can be difficult because different pathologies can coexist and the proximity of the anatomic structures in the zone. Ischiogluteal bursitis may resemble any pathology originated in the ischium, hamstring tendons, sciatic nerve, or radicular alteration.

Posterior hip pain in elderly patients may be related to a variety of pathologies such as osteoarthritis, avascular necrosis of the femoral head, occult fracture, vascular insufficiency of gluteus maximus or medius, metastasis, and soft tissue diseases [5, 18].

The piriformis syndrome causes symptoms in a more proximal area around the hip than the ischiogluteal bursitis. Muscle stretching and palpation is also painful and may be confusing since both pathologies can produce neurologic symptoms by the irritation or compression of the sciatic nerve. A point tenderness in the ischial tuberosity helps to differentiate ischiogluteal bursitis from piriformis syndrome.

The presence of a herniated nucleus pulposus or sciatic nerve irritation may be confused with ischiogluteal bursitis. However, patients with bursitis accommodate and move by seeking the most comfortable position and are thus differentiated from patients with neuropathic pain who avoid movements. Another clue of the proper diagnosis is pain associated with hip motion.

The clinical presentation of hamstring tendon pathology is in the same anatomic area as that of ischiogluteal bursitis, but the former is generally related to sudden or repetitive stretching during sports activities, while the onset of ischiogluteal bursitis is insidious, or the patient does not remember the initiation moment.

Lumbosacral and sacroiliac alterations may also produce referred pain to the gluteal and ischiogluteal area, although those patients prefer to stand still to avoid the reproduction of pain, whereas patients with ischiogluteal bursitis will experience an increase in the intensity of pain. The palpation of a point of tenderness also helps to differentiate the source of pain.

A differential diagnosis must include a ganglion cyst, tumors in the sciatic nerve, and benign and malignant neoplasms with cystic changes in the buttock, since these pathologies can produce similar symptomatology and radiologic findings. Biopsy or surgical excision is sometimes necessary to histologically differentiate bursitis from myxoid tumors including neurofibroma, schwannoma, and myxoma [16, 19].

Finally, another structure susceptible of inflammation is the gluteal bursa which lies between the gluteus maximus and medius muscles as well as between these muscles and the underlying bone. The respective pain is localized at the upper outer quadrant of the buttock and is reproduced with resisted abduction and extension of the lower extremity [20].

Diagnosis

Plain radiograph does not provide helpful information for the diagnosis of ischiogluteal bursitis unless soft-tissue swelling or calcification in the region of the ischial tuberosity is present [21, 22]. A bone erosion in infection as tuberculous bursitis could also be evident in plain films [23].

Under normal conditions, the bursa cannot be delineated with ultrasound [24]. The diagnosis of ischiogluteal bursitis is not difficult with the use of computed tomography (CT), or magnetic resonance imaging (MRI), due to its typical location and the fluid content. Ultrasonographically, bursitis presents as a distended bursal space filled with fluid and presents soft tissue components of the wall with or without internal septa and mural nodules. Further, the bursa is compressible on ultrasound, which helps in differentiating bursitis from a solid neoplasm. The bursa may have hyperechoic or heterogeneous content that can represent crystal deposits [9, 24].

A computed tomography scan may show a soft tissue lesion with a thin wall and a central area of low attenuation adjacent to the ischial tuberosity [19].

Magnetic resonance imaging findings in ischiogluteal bursitis show low or intermediate signal intensity on T1-weighted images and markedly high signal intensity on T2-weighted images, compared to the adjacent muscle (Figs. 14.3 and 14.4) Post-contrast T1-weighted images show peripheral enhancement of the lesion. The typical features on MRI are mural nodules of the bursa which are enhanced after the intravenous administration of contrast materials,

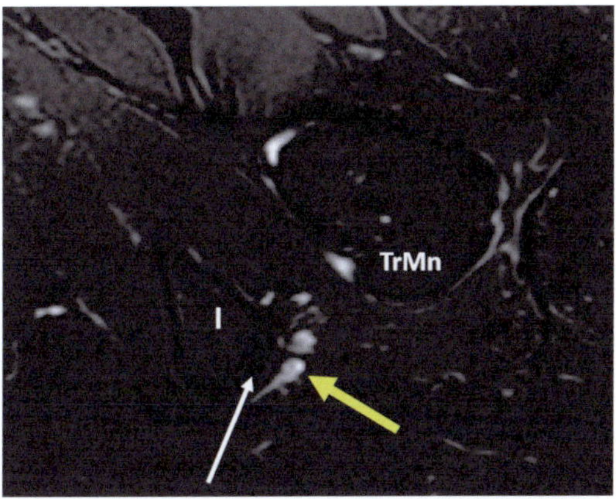

Fig. 14.3 Axial short-tau-inversion recovery (STIR) image shows hiperintensity in the ischiogluteal bursa (yellow arrow) deep to the gluteus maximus muscle. The proximal insertion of the hamstring (white arrow) on the ischion (I) and the trochanter minor (TrMn) is also identified

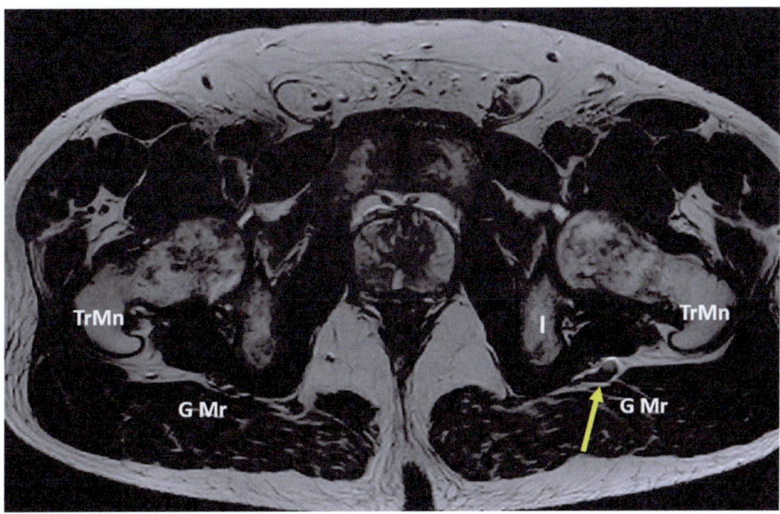

Fig. 14.4 Axial proton density (PD) image shows the ischiogluteal bursa (yellow arrow) located anterior to the gluteus maximus muscle in a left hip. (I) ischion, (TrMn) trochanter minor

and these lesions are located between the ischial tuberosity and the gluteus maximus muscle [16, 19]. The internal signal intensity of ischiogluteal bursitis is usually brighter as compared to other bursitis observed with high signal intensity on the T1-weighted image. This is probably due to an internal hemorrhage caused by the shearing force applied to the ischial tuberosity when aggravated by frequent irritation [5].

Nguyen et al. described a case with incidental detection of a large and asymptomatic ischiogluteal bursitis during F-18 FDG PET/CT (18-fluorodeoxyglucose and CT positron-emitting radioisotopes) staging for head and neck cancer [25].

Treatment

The treatment of the pain associated with ischiogluteal bursitis should be multimodal, including a combination of nonsteroidal anti-inflammatory drugs (NSAIDs), local application of heat and cold, and physical therapy. Although most of the patients benefit from this protocol, those with refractory pain can be treated with an injection of steroid and local anesthetic into the ischial bursa once concomitant infection has been ruled out. Any repetitive activity that may exacerbate the symptoms should be avoided, and the patient must use a padded cushion to sit on. To inject the ischiogluteal bursa, the patient is preferred placed in a lateral position (but prone position is used for some clinicians), with the affected side upward and the affected leg flexed at the knee. The ischial tuberosity can be identified by palpation using a sterile-gloved finger, but it is preferable to perform the procedure guided by fluoroscopy or ultrasound. Before needle placement, the patient is advised to immediately notify if he or she feels paresthesia into the lower extremity, as this symptom indicates that the needle caused impingement of the sciatic nerve. The needle is then carefully advanced through the skin, subcutaneous tissues, muscle, and tendon until it impinges on the bone of the ischial tuberosity. After careful aspiration, and if no paresthesia is present, the contents of the syringe are then gently injected into the bursa [20, 26]. After the injection, the patient must use physical modalities including local heat and gentle stretching exercises. With this treatment, most of the patients experience improvement of the symptoms. In recalcitrant cases, it is necessary to do the surgical excision of the bursa and, in such cases, the patient and the surgeon must have a careful postoperative management to avoid anal contamination. The surgical excision can be done with open surgery and in some cases with endoscopic surgery (Fig. 14.5).

The infection of the ischial bursa is uncommon; Chafetz et al. described a case in a patient with systemic lupus erythematosus and a large ischial bursa secondarily infected with tuberculosis that involved the ischium [6, 23]. In such cases, surgical drainage in the gluteal crease is required. It is also important to rule out bone ischium infection with a bone biopsy. Antibiotic treatment should be based on the identification of pathogens from cultures at the time of drainage and biopsy.

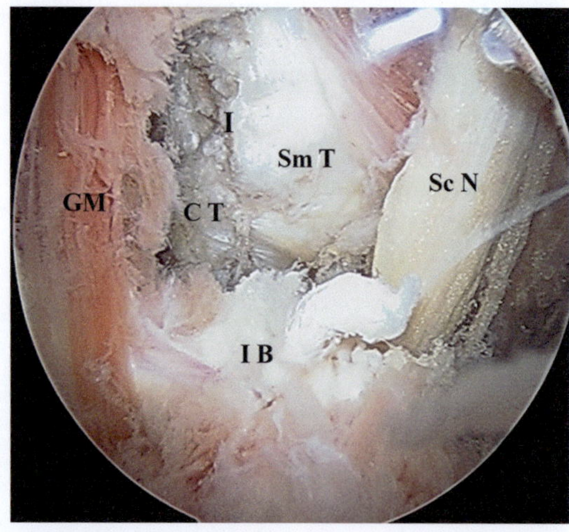

Fig. 14.5 Arthroscopic view. The proximal insertion of semimembranosus (Sm T) and the conjoint tendon (CT: femoris biceps and semitendinosus muscles) on the ischial tuberosity (I). On the left side the gluteus maximus muscle (G Mr) and on the right side the sciatic nerve (Sc N). At the bottom of the image, it is the ischiogluteal bursa (IB) deep to the gluteus maximus muscle and close to the sciatic nerve

Conclusion

Ischiogluteal bursitis is among the possible causes of posterior hip pain that are encountered in the clinical practice of an orthopedic surgeons. It may coexist with anserine tendinitis and lumbosacral and sacroiliac joint pain as well. Furthermore, it is of importance to differentiate ischiogluteal bursitis from a neoplasm around the ischium. Most of the patients benefit from conservative treatment, but surgical resection is indicated in patients with refractory pain after failed injection.

References

1. Bywaters EG. The bursae of the body. Ann Rheum Dis. 1965;24:215–8.
2. Fraser I, Belf MC. A very large bursa. Lancet. 1932;219(5658):290–1.
3. Swartout R, Compere EL. Ischiogluteal bursitis. The pain in the arse. JAMA. 1974;227(5):551–2.
4. Letter: Weaver's bottom. JAMA. 1974;228(5):565–6.
5. Cho KH, Lee SM, Lee YH, Suh KJ, Kim SM, Shin MJ, et al. Non-infectious ischiogluteal bursitis: MRI findings. Korean J Radiol. 2004;5(4):280–6.
6. Rubayi S, Montgomerie JZ. Septic ischial bursitis in patients with spinal cord injury. Paraplegia. 1992;30(3):200–3.
7. Schon L, Zuckerman JD. Hip pain in the elderly: evaluation and diagnosis. Geriatrics. 1988;43(1):48–62.
8. Butcher JD, Salzman KL, Lillegard WA. Lower extremity bursitis. Am Fam Physician. 1996;53(7):2317–24.
9. Van Mieghem IM, Boets A, Sciot R, Van Breuseghem I. Ischiogluteal bursitis: an uncommon type of bursitis. Skelet Radiol. 2004;33(7):413–6.
10. Puranen J, Orava S. The hamstring syndrome. A new diagnosis of gluteal sciatic pain. Am J Sports Med. 1988;16(5):517–21.
11. Hernando MF, Cerezal L, Perez-Carro L, Abascal F, Canga A. Deep gluteal syndrome: anatomy, imaging, and management of sciatic nerve entrapments in the subgluteal space. Skelet Radiol. 2015;44(7):919–34.
12. Cohen S, Bradley J. Acute proximal hamstring rupture. J Am Acad Orthop Surg. 2007;15(6):350–5.
13. Miller SL, Gill J, Webb GR. The proximal origin of the hamstrings and surrounding anatomy encountered during repair. A cadaveric study. J Bone Joint Surg Am. 2007;89(1):44–8.
14. Cohen GC. Cycling injuries. Can Fam Physician. 1993;39:628–32.
15. Mills GM, Baethge BA. Ischiogluteal bursitis in cancer patients: an infrequently recognized cause of pain. Am J Clin Oncol. 1993;16(3):229–31.
16. Hitora T, Kawaguchi Y, Mori M, Imaizumi Y, Akisue T, Sasaki K, et al. Ischiogluteal bursitis: a report of three cases with MR findings. Rheumatol Int. 2009;29(4):455–8.
17. Kim SM, Shin MJ, Kim KS, Ahn JM, Cho KH, Chang JS, et al. Imaging features of ischial bursitis with an emphasis on ultrasonography. Skelet Radiol. 2002;31(11):631–6.
18. Garcia-Porrua C, Gonzalez-Gay MA, Corredoira J, Vazquez-Caruncho M. Hip pain. Ann Rheum Dis. 1999;58(3):148–9.
19. Akisue T, Yamamoto T, Marui T, Hitora T, Nagira K, Mihune Y, et al. Ischiogluteal bursitis: multi-modality imaging findings. Clin Orthop Relat Res. 2003;406:214–7.
20. SD W. Pain management. 2nd ed. Amsterdam: Elsevier; 2011. 1408 p.
21. Schuh A, Narayan CT, Schuh R, Hönle W. Calcifying bursitis ischioglutealis: a case report. J Orthop Case Rep. 2011;1(1):16–8.
22. Clanton TO, Coupe KJ. Hamstring strains in athletes: diagnosis and treatment. J Am Acad Orthop Surg. 1998;6(4):237–48.
23. Chafetz N, Genant HK, Hoaglund FT. Ischiogluteal tuberculous bursitis with progressive bony destruction. J Can Assoc Radiol. 1982;33(2):119–20.
24. Cho KH, Park BH, Yeon KM. Ultrasound of the adult hip. Semin Ultrasound CT MR. 2000;21(3):214–30.
25. Nguyen BD, Roarke MC. F-18 FDG PET/CT incidental finding of large ischiogluteal bursitis. Clin Nucl Med. 2007;32(7):535–7.
26. Yasar E, Singh J, Hill J, Akuthota V. Image-guided injections of the hip. J Novel Physiother Phys Rehabil. 2014;1(2):039–48.

Posterior Femoroacetabular Impingement

15

Justin J. Mitchell, Karen K. Briggs, and Marc J. Philippon

Introduction

The hip is responsible for a significant amount of weight bearing during athletic and daily activities. Because of the contained and congruent ball and socket anatomy of the hip, any disruptions to the normal bony or soft tissue morphology can alter the normal biomechanics and distribution of force, leading to soft tissue damage in the form of capsulolabral or cartilaginous injury [1, 2]. Of these alterations in anatomy, impingement syndromes are the most common clinical presentation and can be generally categorized by either intra-articular or extra-articular impingement. Intra-articular femoroacetabular impingement (FAI) has been recognized as a cause of hip pain, chondrolabral damage, and osteoarthritis of the hip [3–5]. This results from abnormal anatomy at the femoral head-neck junction leading to decreased femoral head-neck offset (cam) or overcoverage of the acetabular rim (pincer).

However, a combined pathology from both the femoral and acetabular side is the most common pattern found in patients with symptomatic intra-articular FAI [3, 6].

In contrast, extra-articular impingement is characterized by anatomic abnormalities, or collision of structures, located outside of the hip capsule. Recent literature demonstrates increasing evidence for the presence of an extra-articular impingement condition known as ischiofemoral impingement. This is caused by abnormal contact between the lesser trochanter of the femur and the ischium and often leads to vague posterior hip or buttock pain [7, 8]. While this is a lesser-known etiology, it may contribute to posterior pain during impingement syndromes.

Understanding that the etiology and causes of posterior impingement continue to evolve, this chapter will discuss both intra-articular and extra-articular findings in posterior impingement of the hip.

Etiology and Pathomechanics Posterior Impingement

The etiology of FAI is most often unknown, except in cases of trauma in the setting of a previously asymptomatic hip. Despite this, there have been several hypotheses as to the inciting or primary cause for FAI including residual childhood diseases such as subclinical slipped capital

J. J. Mitchell, MD · M. J. Philippon, MD (✉)
The Steadman Clinic/Steadman Philippon
Research Institute, Vail, CO, USA
e-mail: drphilippon@sprivail.org

K. K. Briggs, MPH
Center for Outcomes-Based Orthopaedic Research
(COOR), Steadman Philippon Research Institute,
Vail, CO, USA

© Springer International Publishing AG, part of Springer Nature 2019
H. D. Martin, J. Gómez-Hoyos (eds.), *Posterior Hip Disorders*,
https://doi.org/10.1007/978-3-319-78040-5_15

femoral epiphyses (SCFE), Legg-Calve-Perthes disease, or even malunion of a previous femoral neck fracture, specifically when the head heals in abnormal rotatory or varus/valgus positions [9–11]. Acetabular morphologic changes that may predispose patients to pincer impingement include coxa profunda, protrusio acetabuli, or abnormal version of the acetabulum [12].

Femoral-Sided (CAM) Lesions

FAI can be caused by an abnormally shaped femoral head, specifically one which has lost its sphericity [13]. This abnormal femoral anatomy can be seen radiographically by a decreased femoral head-neck offset as well as an increase in the alpha angle (greater than 55°, as seen on the cross-table lateral radiograph), leading to a CAM lesion. When occurring in isolation, CAM lesions are most commonly found located on the anterosuperior aspect of the femoral head-neck junction in males during their late teens or early twenties [4, 14]. This bony protrusion causes abnormal contact with an otherwise normal acetabular rim when the hip is flexed and internally rotated. With deeper angles of hip flexion, the irregularly shaped femoral head loses its normal congruency and is forced into contact with the labrum and acetabulum. This motion creates sheer forces across the chondrolabral junction as the CAM lesion moves centrally, leading to tearing or avulsion of the labrum from the acetabular rim before contacting and damaging the acetabular cartilage centrally.

This anatomic variance typically affects the anterosuperior area of the labrum and cartilage within the acetabulum [3]. However, with a posteriorly based CAM lesion, the same type of impingement lesion can be seen with hip flexion or extension and external rotation, shifting the conflict to the posterior or posterosuperior labrum and acetabulum leading to posterior FAI (PFAI). This PFAI may cause further findings other than damage to the posterior acetabular cartilage and labrum. It has been postulated that as the femur impinges on the posterior acetabulum, the CAM lesion may act as a fulcrum [15], which can lead to an anterior subluxation of the femoral head, potentially resulting in anterior chondrolabral lesions. This finding matches both the clinical experience of hip arthroscopists and prior studies demonstrating patients presenting with PFAI, but also a positive anterior FAI test and chondrolabral lesions seen intraoperatively in the anterior acetabular area.

Siebenrock et al. [15] have also described PFAI in association with femoral antetorsion and valgus neck-shaft angles. Their work focused on the finding that patients with this anatomic combination present with lack of external rotation and posterior hip pain that is aggravated with hip extension and external rotation, suggesting PFAI. Their study evaluated range of motion (ROM), the location of anterior and posterior bony collision zones with impingement anatomy, and the prevalence of extra-articular impingement based on CT scan reconstructions of 13 valgus hips with increased antetorsion, 22 hips with FAI, and 27 normal hips. They found that hips with coxa valga and antetorsion showed decreased extension, external rotation, and adduction, whereas internal rotation in 90° of flexion was increased. Impingement was noted to be posteroinferior on the acetabular side; and overall impingement was found more frequently posterior or extra-articular. They concluded that valgus hips with increased antetorsion predispose to PFAI and posterior extra-articular FAI and further noted that concomitant hip dysplasia together with coxa valga and increased antetorsion could even aggravate dynamic anterior instability and lead to additional anterior impingement in deep flexion caused by the valgus neck and the decreased lateral offset. The suggestion that femoral anatomy contributes to PFAI is reinforced by the previous observations of Tonnis and Heinecke [16], who demonstrated that overcorrection of a retroverted femoral neck through osteotomy (thus creating iatrogenic antetorsion) leads to restrictions in external rotation. They further found that this overcorrection led to painful ROM, especially in flexion and external rotation.

Acetabular-Sided (Pincer) Lesions

Differing from the cam lesion, isolated pincer impingement is a result of excessive coverage of the acetabulum over a normally shaped femoral head. In contrast to isolated cam impingement, isolated symptomatic pincer impingement is most commonly seen in middle-aged females [4, 17]. This extension of the acetabular rim is often found anterosuperiorly and leads to deepening of the hip socket, which in turn creates contact of the acetabular rim against the femoral neck during flexion and internal rotation in the typical setting. However, this overcoverage can also occur posteriorly, leading similarly to posterior impingement in hip extension, abduction, or with flexion and external rotation.

In these settings, the anterior or posterior acetabular labrum collides with the femoral neck, causing more direct trauma to the labrum than is typically seen in cam lesions. The increased force and direct trauma results in increased labral degeneration and interstitial tearing [3, 18]. Because the labrum is a global extension of the acetabular rim, pincer lesions lead to a circumferential pattern of labral damage. As trauma to the labrum continues, and the injured labrum continues to experience degeneration, it is possible for chondrosis to the adjacent cartilage as well as reactive ossification to occur within the labrum. Both of these secondary reactions lead to further relative increases in overcoverage, perpetuating the impingement with at risk hip positions [19].

The acetabular cartilage is also affected in the setting of isolated pincer lesions; however, the chondral damage is typically less dramatic and limited to a narrow circumferential strip just interior to the chondrolabral junction [3]. In the setting of anterior overcoverage, the femoral neck contacts the anterosuperior acetabulum during hip flexion, forcing the femoral head posteriorly. This results in increased pressure between the posteromedial aspect of the femoral head and the posteroinferior aspect of the acetabulum. This, in turn, causes subtle posterior subluxation of the femoral head, creating PFAI symptomatology and contrecoup cartilaginous lesion on either the head itself or the posteroinferior acetabulum.

While not well described, excessive acetabular anteversion could also lead to relative posterior overcoverage and lead to PFAI symptomatology. Previous literature has demonstrated this phenomenon in patients following hip resurfacing [20, 21]. These studies showed that excessively anteverted acetabular cups or anteriorized heads effectively decreased posterior offset and placed patients at increased risk for radiographic (posterior erosion of the femoral neck just distal to the implant) and clinical evidence of PFAI. In the native hip, however, acetabular version can be difficult to appreciate, as acetabular position can be relative to pelvic tilt [22]. Acetabular anteversion decreases with anterior tilting of the pelvis, and consequently specific positions can change the orientation of the pelvis through functional ranges of motion. It has also been demonstrated that patients with increased acetabular anteversion compensate by increasing anterior pelvic tilt. These changes in pelvic position and acetabular anteversion may alter biomechanics of the hip and lead to reactive changes such as gluteal tendinopathy [23]. While further studies are required to fully elucidate the interplay in these anatomic variations, it does seem reasonable that this could lead to posterior pain and symptoms consistent with PFAI.

Combined CAM and Pincer Lesions

Mixed or combined FAI is the most common form of impingement encountered. This pattern of impingement leads to findings consistent with both femoral and acetabular pathologies aforementioned. However, it is not uncommon that intra-articular findings noted on arthroscopy will be either cam or pincer dominant. Beck et al. showed that in mixed type impingement with repeated abutment between the femoral neck and the acetabular rim can cause degeneration of the labrum similar to that seen in pincer impingement or that the labrum may be bruised and flattened or separated similar to cam impingement [3]. In severe cases of mixed impingement, intrasubstance ganglion formation or severe chondrolabral degeneration can also be seen.

Posterior Extra-articular FAI and Ischiofemoral Impingement

Extra-articular impingement of the hip is a rare cause of hip pain and may present similarly to intra-articular FAI. Because of this, the diagnosis can be challenging even for an experienced hip surgeon, and it has not been well characterized.

Extra-articular FAI results from abnormal contact between the greater trochanter, lesser trochanter, or extracapsular femoral neck against the ilium, ischium, anterior inferior iliac spine (AIIS), or acetabular rim [7, 24–30]. This abnormal contact can be caused by direct compression of the soft tissue structures around the hip (such as the capsule, surrounding musculature like the iliopsoas, or neurovascular structures) or by creating increased stress across the femoroacetabular articulation leading to impingement-induced instability [24]. Similar to intra-articular causes previously noted, these pathologies can lead to cartilage injury or labral tears but may additionally cause damage to the capsule or extracapsular musculature. Capsular laxity has been a predisposing cause for extra-articular impingement by allowing for increased hip range of motion, in turn enabling bony impingement that is anatomically difficult to achieve with normal soft tissue restraints. This laxity and extra-articular impingement could then create a potential fulcrum that further attenuates the capsule and leads to a cascade of increased capsular laxity, microinstability, and pain [8].

It is felt that these entities are related to extreme ranges of motion such as can be seen in gymnastics or dance but could also be associated with activities of daily living that require significant extension or external rotation motions. Ricciardi et al. characterized three main categories of extra-articular impingement. Type I is impingement of the greater trochanter of the femur against the anterior acetabular rim or AIIS, Type II is posterolateral impingement of the greater trochanter or femoral neck against the ischium, and Type III consisted of a complex pattern leading to both anterior and posterior impingement [24]. Overall, patients who presented and were surgically treated for extra-articular impingement were younger, more frequently female, and were more likely to have undergone a prior surgery on the ipsilateral hip compared to a matched intra-articular-only FAI cohort. Those presenting with a component of posterior extra-articular impingement were noted to have positive posterior impingement testing 75% of the time and had significantly greater

internal rotation at 90° of flexion (40° versus 15°) and femoral anteversion (21° versus 8°). They were also noted to have a lower degree of external rotation at 90° of hip flexion (40° versus 60°) and in full extension (40–48° versus 70°).

Ischiofemoral impingement (IFI) is a specific modality of posterior FAI. Beckman et al. have described IFI as a compression of the quadratus femoris between the ischium and the lesser tuberosity, leading to vague posterior hip pain or groin pain [8]. This vague pain is not uncommon, as other structures such as the psoas insertion on the lesser trochanter, the ischial origin of the hamstring tendons, or the associated bursae may also be affected in IFI [7].

This pathology is more commonly seen in women with more prominent lesser tuberosities and ischial tuberosities, and it has been demonstrated that patients with confirmed diagnoses of FAI have a smaller ischiofemoral distance and a smaller quadratus femoris space when compared to their asymptomatic counterparts. This loss in space can either be congenital or acquired, and Yoong et al. reported patients with posterior pathology such as multiple hereditary exostoses, malunited proximal femur fractures, prior proximal femoral osteotomies, or protrusion acetabula (causing medicalization of the lesser trochanter) could display similar symptoms of IFI because of bony impingement posteriorly [31].

Clinical Presentation

A thorough history is important in examining any patient with posterior hip pain. The examining physician must learn as much as possible about the quality and location of the pain, as well as the inciting motions or activities and the characteristics of the pain. As stated previously, the etiology behind the development of PFAI is often unclear, and thus a detailed history regarding trauma to the joint, athletic activities, and childhood conditions should be obtained, to possibly identify a primary cause. The clinical presentation of PFAI is often insidious, with patients initially complaining of anterior or posterior hip or groin pain, especially after prolonged sitting, walking, or following athletic activities [7, 8]. Because of the nonspecific nature of this pain, which could be present over the groin, greater trochanter, or buttocks, a high index of clinical suspicion is often required to make a diagnosis of PFAI in order to avoid missing the diagnosis or subjecting the patient to advanced imaging or invasive testing.

While the diagnosis can be nebulous, patients with PFAI will typically present with posterior hip or buttock pain that begins without an inciting event. Patients will often describe pain in position of hip flexion, abduction, and external rotation—which brings the posterior labrum, acetabulum, or pelvic structures in contact with the femoral head-neck junction or lesser trochanter. During this posterior pain, patients may also describe sciatica-type symptoms related to pinching of the sciatic nerve directly posterior to the quadratus femoris muscle [7, 8, 32].

Physical Examination

The majority of patients (50–65%) with femoroacetabular impingement have insidious onset of symptoms [6], however, immediate pain following a twisting or impact injury to the hip. Some patients also report acute symptoms without a traumatic event. The most common complaint for patients with all types of impingement is pain in the groin (approximately 80% of patients presenting with this pathology). In the setting of posterior impingement, patients will often demonstrate pain the lateral hip, buttock, posterior thigh, and lumbar spine. This pain may radiate distally in some patients, and mechanical symptoms and feeling of instability are also reported. These symptoms usually worsen with increasing activity, recurrent daily activity, or sports [6, 33].

Patient-reported history combined with a thorough physical examination of both hips can often provide the correct diagnosis. A typical stepwise approach to the hip examination is taken, and this includes visual inspection, palpation, and testing for range of motion, stability, and strength in all planes. Examining simple tasks such as standing up from a chair, moving on and off the examina-

tion table, and transferring from sitting to lying down (and vice versa) can also provide important clues as to the etiology of the pain and the functional limitations of the patient. Each examination should also include an evaluation of gait patterns, as patients may demonstrate an antalgic gait or Trendelenburg gait or sign [32].

Palpation should begin proximally, and the height of the iliac crests should be assessed for symmetry; the SI joints and lumbar spine and paraspinal musculature palpated for pain, and the muscle groups of the hip flexors and short external rotators should be carefully examined. When palpating each muscle group, the physician should specifically examine the bursae around the hip and muscular structures. When inflamed the greater trochanteric bursa and the ischial bursa can cause symptoms posterior hip pain [32].

Range of motion testing should then be performed on both the symptomatic hip and the contralateral asymptomatic hip. To avoid beginning the examination by focusing on the painful, symptomatic hip, it is helpful to begin with the contralateral hip to help put the patient at ease and diminish guarding or tension in the muscles during the remainder of the examination. Passive and active hip flexion (normal is approximately 120°), extension (normal is approximately 30°), internal rotation (normal is approximately 35°), external rotation (normal is approximately 45°), adduction (normal is approximately 20°), and abduction (normal is approximately 45°) should be measured with a goniometer and compared from side to side [34]. Strength throughout these ranges of motion should also be assessed and can be performed against resistance to evaluate for pain or weakness.

Posterior impingement can be difficult to diagnose based on a single specific test; however, physicians have utilized a combination of examination maneuvers to help correctly identify patients with this problem. The Thomas test is utilized to evaluate for the presence of a hip flexion contracture. Flexion contractures can place stress on the posterior structures and, as such, can lead to symptoms of posterior pain. With the patient positioned in the supine position, the patient is asked to flex the asymptomatic hip and grab the knee with both hands, such that it is tucked tight to the chest. The symptomatic hip is allowed to freely extend, and the patient should attempt to place the leg flat on the examination table. The test is positive for a hip flexion contracture if the symptomatic leg is unable to completely extend [32]. The posterior impingement test can also be performed in combination with the Thomas test. With the patient in the Thomas test position, place the affected limb in extension, lateral rotation, and slight abduction. The examiner then applies a posterior pressure to force the patient into extension. The test works by compressing the posterior labrum between the posterior femoral head-neck junction and the posterior rim of the acetabulum. While the test is for PFAI, posterior pain can be elicited from the labral impingement, or anterior hip pain as the femoral head abuts the capsule is considered a positive test for posterior impingement of the labrum.

The flexion/abduction/external rotation (FABER) test is also a useful test for diagnosis of PFAI. While the patient is lying supine, the affected leg is brought to the figure-four position of flexion, abduction, and external rotation, so that the ankle is placed proximal to the contralateral knee. Gentle downward force is applied to the knee of the affected extremity, while the contralateral side of the pelvis is stabilized. A positive test is demonstrated by an increased distance between the lateral aspect of the knee and the examination table, compared to the contralateral side. The logroll test and flexion, adduction, and internal rotation (FADIR) test are typically used to evaluate for anterior FAI; however, they should be used in the setting of posterior pain rule out other potential etiologies of hip pain.

Two tests were recently validated by Gómez-Hoyos et al. for diagnosing ischiofemoral impingement [35]. The long-stride walking test is expected to provoke impingement between the LT and ischium in terminal hip extension when the patient walks. The findings of this test are considered positive if the posterior pain is reproducible lateral to the ischium during extension with long strides, whereas pain is alleviated when walking with short strides. The ischiofemoral impingement test is performed with the patient in a lateral position. The examiner passively takes the patient's hip into extension. This test is intended to provoke impingement in extension with a neutral or adducted hip (re-creating the posterior pain lateral to the ischium) and relieves the impingement pain in extension with an abducted hip.

The sciatic nerve can become irritated in cases of IFI as previously mentioned, and as such, thorough neurologic evaluation with provocative lumbar testing is warranted to rule out lumbar spinal pathology when IFI is suspected [8].

Radiographic Examination

Plain radiography can often be normal in cases of PFAI; however, abnormal morphology of the proximal femur and the acetabulum can sometimes be seen on plain radiographs. In our practice, we use an AP pelvis, a cross-table lateral, and a false profile as the X-ray work-up [36]; however many other views have been described and can also be used in order to better evaluate the bony morphology [37]. AP pelvis radiograph is generally utilized to demonstrate pincer-type deformity, but some features of cam impingement can be shown such as pistol-grip deformity, head-tilt deformity, a lateral bump, and a herniation pit [38]. It is also important to measure the minimum joint space in AP radiograph, since patients with a joint space of less than 2 mm are more likely to have lower postoperative modified Harris Hip Score and are 39 times more likely to progress to a total hip replacement with surgical management of their pathology [39].

Since the nonspherical part of the femoral head is usually located at the anterosuperior or posterolateral portion of the head-neck junction, this deformity can typically be readily demonstrated in a lateral view of the femur. The femoral head-neck offset can be assessed by measuring the alpha angle as described by Notzli et al. [13].

In the original description, the alpha angle was measured in magnetic resonance (MR) scans, but several recent studies utilized plain radiographs to determine the alpha angle [36, 40–42], and angles measuring more than 50–55° are suggestive of abnormal femoral head-neck offset. When using plain radiographs, a Dunn view and the cross-table lateral seem to be the best radiographic views for alpha angle evaluation [43]. Subtle findings of sclerosis or cystic changes within the LT or ischium may also be seen because of the conflict between these structures. Plain radiographs may also reveal decreased femoral offset, or evidence of post-traumatic or congenital bony prominences, as seen with previous ischial avulsion injury or MHE. Coxa valga with an increased femoral neck angle is associated with PFAI and IFI and can also be seen with plain radiographic evaluation [16, 32].

Magnetic resonance imaging (MRI) provides details of soft tissue disorders related to PFAI. This imaging modality also reveals other causes of hip pain, which can be found concomitant with PFAI such as trochanteric bursitis, ischial bursitis, or tears to the short external rotators or abductors of the hip. Further, bony structures can be fully evaluated for viability, and the femoral can be examined for pathology such as avascular necrosis. It is essential to have a study dedicated to the hip, because a single hip MRI has a better resolution and detail when compared with a pelvic MRI which captures a broader field [44]. In PFAI, the MRI imaging will often show a posterior labral tear with bony edema within the posterior femoral head-neck junction with an associated collision lesion on the posterior acetabulum (Fig. 15.1). There may also be chondromalacia of the anterior or anterosuperior acetabular surface from a countercoup effect of the femoral head being levered anteriorly as the posterior impingement occurs. In cases of IFI, the MRI often shows increased signal and fatty atrophy in the quadratus femoris without definitive tearing of muscle. All of these MRI findings should be correlated clinically as many patients can have these imaging findings without demonstrating symptoms [8, 45].

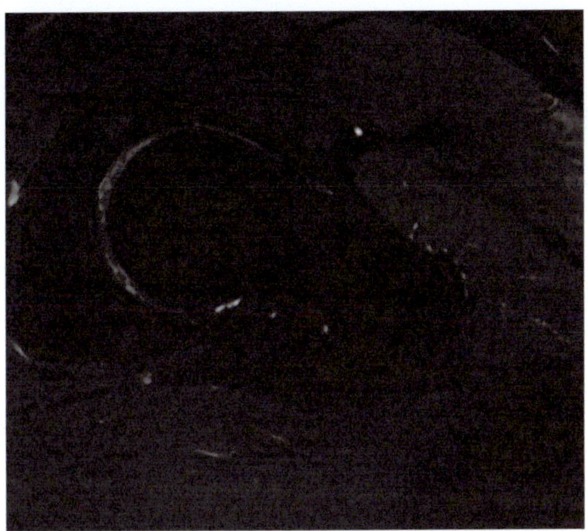

Fig. 15.1 MRI (3T) of the left hip of a 23-year-old male hockey player, demonstrating a posterior labral tear

Three-dimensional reconstructed CT scans can be used in addition to MRI to help better delineate bony pathology or abnormal anatomy. Ultrasound examination may also play a role in diagnosing the dynamic component of PFAI and IFI as static evaluations on MRI and CT scans are therefore highly dependent on the position of the limb, which may not be standardized between patients, and could miss patients who are having dynamic impingement [46].

Treatment Options for PFAI

Nonsurgical Treatment

The mainstay of initial treatment for patients with PFAI is with nonsurgical modalities including rest, ice, anti-inflammatory medications, activity modification, periarticular muscle strengthening, core stabilizing, physiotherapy, and corticosteroid or viscosupplement injections. An intra-articular injection using local anesthetic combined with corticosteroid under CT or ultrasound guidance can be both diagnostic and therapeutic. For lesions suspected to be occurring outside of the capsule (such as in IFI), a corticosteroid injection into the quadratus muscle can have similar benefits.

Surgical Treatment

Femoral and Acetabular Osteoplasty with Labral Repair

Arthroscopic treatment of PFAI aims to improve the clearance for hip motion and diminish abutment between the proximal femur and acetabular rim or extracapsular structures. A normal femoral head-neck offset is created by femoral osteoplasty while normal labral seal is maintained. This can be performed either in supine or lateral position depending on surgeon preference. In our practice, we utilize the modified supine position (the affected leg is placed in a position of 10° flexion, 15° internal rotation, 10° lateral tilt an neutral abduction) with two arthroscopic portals (anterolateral and mid-anterior portals).

After the patient is properly positioned and traction is applied, the anterolateral portal is established at 1 cm proximal and 1 cm anterior to the tip of the greater trochanter. Then, the mid-anterior portal is made 6–7 cm from the anterolateral portal at 45–60° angle with respect to the longitudinal line passing through the anterolateral portal. This location is the middle between the longitudinal lines passing through the anterior superior iliac spine and the anterolateral portal. The mid-anterior portal has a greater distance from the lateral femoral cutaneous nerve compared to the anterior portal [47]. An interportal capsulotomy connecting both portals is performed using an arthroscopic blade to allow better mobility of arthroscopic instruments. The central compartment now can be inspected to identify and treat all concomitant pathologies such as labral tears, chondral lesions, ligamentum teres tears, and a pincer lesion of the acetabular rim (Fig. 15.2).

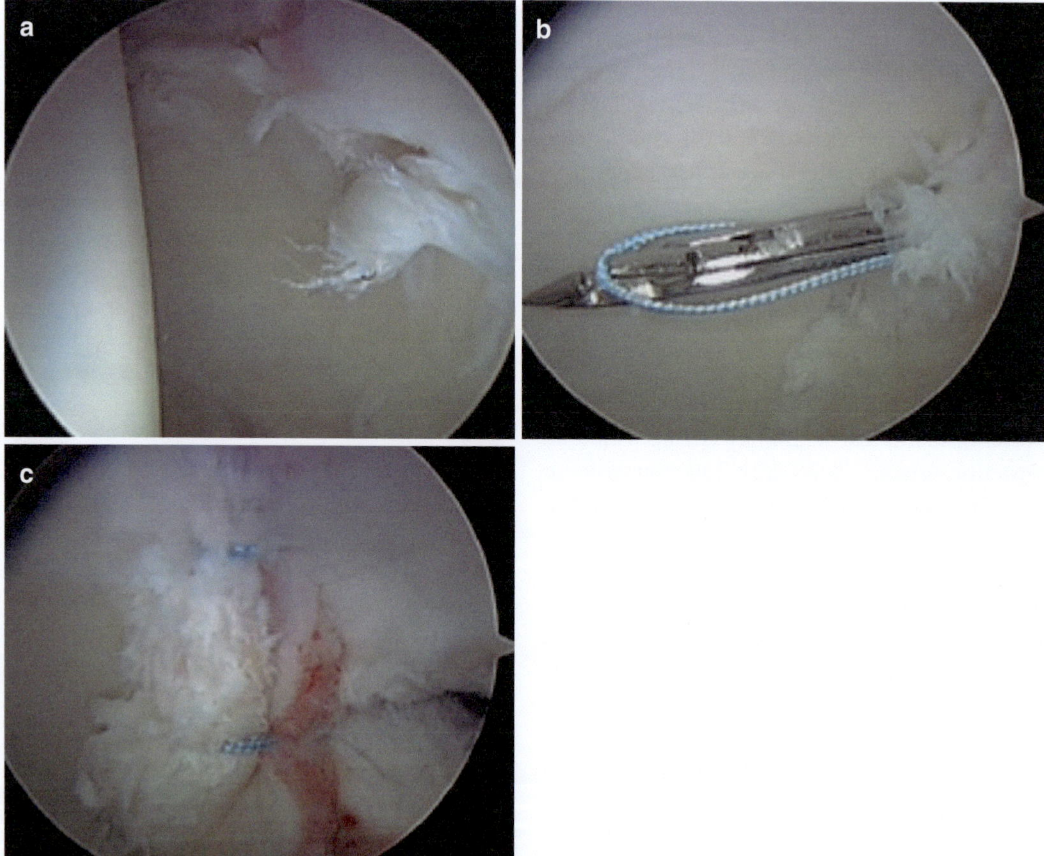

Fig. 15.2 (**a**) Arthroscopic view through the mid-anterior portal showing extensive fraying and tearing of the posterior labrum. (**b** and **c**) Suture passed under the labrum and then the labrum is reattached to acetabular rim

For femoral osteoplasty, traction is then released and the peripheral compartment is approached. The cam lesion can be usually identified as a "bump" on the femoral head-neck junction with changes in color (gray or purple typically) and texture (fibrillation, fissuring, flaps) of the cartilage over this area. While the hip is placed in 45° of flexion, femoral osteoplasty can be performed proximally at 1 cm from the peripheral edge of the labrum with the burr introduced through the anterolateral portal. The resection should taper distally along the femoral neck for 1.5–2 cm. The medial synovial fold and the lateral epiphyseal vessels should be observed and protected during the procedure, and these can be utilized as the inferior and superior boundaries of osteoplasty.

Positioning of the hip is important for accessing to different parts of the femoral head-neck junction in the peripheral compartment. The anteroinferior part of the femoral neck can be better visualized by increasing the amount of flexion of the hip. Moving the hip to a lesser degree of flexion and changing the arthroscope to the anterolateral portal facilitate burring at the superolateral part of the femoral neck. The arthroscope can be used as a capsular retractor by a levering maneuver during the procedure.

During femoral osteoplasty, the cam lesion should be adequately removed, while a smooth and concave head-neck transition is created. Overresection can increase the risk of femoral neck fracture and also has a negative effect on the labral seal. A herniation pit, which can be found in some patients, should be evacuated and usually become a shallow defect after finishing the femoral osteoplasty. For a large herniation pit, the senior author (MJP) prefers to fill the bony void with a bone graft substitute plug. Periodic examination by moving the hip in all impinging motions is crucial to ensure that adequate bony resection is achieved while good labral seal is well maintained. Capsular closure is performed using an absorbable suture. Platelet-rich plasma is injected for homeostasis purpose.

Lesser Trochanteric Osteoplasty

Lesser trochanteric (LT) osteoplasty is also a lesser-utilized treatment option for those who have failed conservative measures for IFI. This technique may be performed through an open approach or arthroscopically [27, 48]. The arthroscopic surgical technique can be performed via an anterior or posterior approach to the LT with advantages and disadvantages associated with both techniques. An anterior approach removes the risk of working near medial femoral circumflex artery and sciatic nerve but requires gaining access to the LT through a psoas tenotomy for visualization. In contrast, a posterior approach places the arthroscopic instruments near the medial femoral circumflex artery and sciatic nerve [8, 48].

Postoperative Rehabilitation

Postoperative protocol after hip arthroscopic treatment of PFAI involves restriction of weight bearing, rotation, and motion [49]. Patients are kept at 20 lb. of flat-foot weight bearing for 2–3 weeks to protect the femoral neck after osteoplasty. Four hours of continuous passive motion (CPM) machine is used for 2 weeks combined with use of a stationary bike at zero resistance for 20 min. A modified hip brace and an antirotational bolster are utilized for 2–3 weeks to limit hip external rotation and extension. This will protect the early phase of capsular healing.

Physiotherapy should start with restoration of passive motion, followed by active motion, and then strength. Passive circumduction movements are recommended to prevent adhesion. Active flexion of the hip should be gradually progressed to avoid flexor tendonitis.

Complications

Complications related to femoral osteoplasty have been reported and should be prevented, such as residual cam lesion, overresection of the femoral neck, femoral neck fracture, avascular necrosis of the femoral head, and capsular adhesion.

A residual cam lesion is one of common causes of revision surgery after arthroscopic FAI treatment [50]. This can be prevented by carefully identifying the cam deformity and performing periodic dynamic examination during femoral osteoplasty. On the other hand, overresection of the femoral neck can increase the risk of femoral neck fracture and has an adverse effect on the labral seal. Aggressive osteoplasty should be avoided. A smooth contour of the bony resection can be achieved by switching the arthroscopic portals to appreciate the three-dimensional geometry of the femoral neck.

Femoral neck fractures have been reported as complications of arthroscopic femoral osteoplasty [51] and combined arthroscopical and limited anterior approach. Mardones et al. performed a cadaveric study showing that resections up to 30% of the anterolateral head-neck junction of a morphologically normal femur did not alter significantly the load-bearing capacity of the proximal femur bone and advised that 30% should be the greatest resection performed [52]. Nonetheless, this amount of resection is seldom necessary. Weight-bearing restriction after femoral osteoplasty is emphasized to prevent this complication, and the duration should be prolonged for patients with lower bone quality.

Avascular necrosis of the femoral head is a rare complication. Both the medial synovial fold and the lateral epiphyseal vessels should be well visualized and protected during osteoplasty. Capsular adhesion is another common cause for revision surgery [50]. Progressive range of motion exercise, both passive and active motions, is utilized to prevent this problem.

Summary

Posterior femoroacetabular impingement is an abnormal conflict of the acetabular rim and the femoral head-neck junction or with the proximal femur and extracapsular structures. This condition causes pain and can lead to labral and cartilage damage and leads to early osteoarthritis of the hip. After clinical evaluation and radiographic examination, hip arthroscopy is one of the treatment options for PFAI, although surgical management is the first-line management for these patients. During hip arthroscopy, the bony abnormalities can be corrected. Femoral osteoplasty is performed to restore normal femoral head-neck offset, while the amount of bony resection is monitored by periodic examination. Postoperatively patients are kept partial weight-bearing and rehabilitation focus on range of motion. Complications related to this procedure are not common.

Financial Disclosures Board member/owner/officer/committee appointments: HIPCO, MJP Innovations, LLC, Arthrosurface, Vail Health Services, Vail Valley Surgery Center (MJP). Royalties: Smith & Nephew, Arthrocare, DonJoy, Bledsoe, Linvatec, Elsevier, Slack, Inc. (MJP). Paid consultant or employee: Smith & Nephew (MJP). Research or institutional support from companies or suppliers: Smith & Nephew, Ossur, Arthrex, Siemens, Vail Valley Medical Center, National Institute of Health, National Institute of Aging, National Institute of Arthritis and Musculoskeletal and Skin Disease (MJP/SPRI).

References

1. Crawford K, Philippon MJ, Sekiya JK, et al. Microfracture of the hip in athletes. Clin Sports Med. 2006;25:327–33.
2. Philippon MJ, Goljan P, Briggs KK. FAI: from diagnosis to treatment. Tech Orthop. 2015;27(3):167–71.
3. Beck M, Kalhor M, Leunig M, et al. Hip morphology influences the pattern of damage to the acetabular cartilage: femoroacetabular impingement as a cause of early osteoarthritis of the hip. J Bone Joint Surg Br. 2005;87:1012–8.
4. Ganz R, Parvizi J, Beck M, et al. Femoroacetabular impingement: a cause for osteoarthritis of the hip. Clin Orthop Relat Res. 2003;417:112–20.
5. Ganz R, Leunig M, Leunig-Ganz K, et al. The etiology of osteoarthritis of the hip: an integrated mechanical concept. Clin Orthop Relat Res. 2008;466:264–72.
6. Philippon MJ, Maxwell RB, Johnston TL, et al. Clinical presentation of femoroacetabular impingement. Knee Surg Sports Traumatol. 2007;15:1041–7.
7. Stafford GH, Villar RN. Ischiofemoral impingement. J Bone Joint Surg Br. 2011;93:1300.
8. Beckmann JT, Safran MR, Abrams GD. Extra-articular impingement: ischiofemoral impingement and trochanteric-pelvic. Oper Tech Sports Med. 2015;23:184.
9. Leunig M, Casillas MM, Hamlet M, et al. Slipped capital femoral epiphysis: early mechanical damage to the acetabular cartilage by a prominent femoral metaphysis. Acta Orthop Scand. 2000;71:370–5.

10. Leunig M, Beaule PE, Ganz R. The concept of femoroacetabular impingement: current status and future perspectives. Clin Orthop Relat Res. 2009;467:616–22.

11. Eijer H, Myers SR, Ganz R. Anterior femoroacetabular impingement after femoral neck fractures. J Orthop Trauma. 2001;15:475–81.

12. Philippon MJ, Stubbs AJ, Schenker ML, Maxwell RB, Ganz R, Leunig M. Arthroscopic management of femoroacetabular impingement: osteoplasty technique and literature review. Am J Sports Med. 2007;35(9):1571–80.

13. Notzli HP, Wyss TF, Stoecklin CH, et al. The contour of the femoral head-neck junction as a predictor for the risk of anterior impingement. J Bone Joint Surg Br. 2002;84:556–60.

14. Vaughn ZD, Safran MR. Arthroscopic femoral osteoplasty/chielectomy for cam-type femoroacetabular impingement in the athlete. Sports Med Arthrosc Rev. 2010;18:90–9.

15. Siebenrock KA, Steppacher SD, Haefeli PC, Schwab JM, Tannast M. Valgus hip with high antetorsion causes pain through posterior extraarticular FAI. Clin Orthop Relat Res. 2013;471(12):3774–80.

16. Tonnis D, Heinecke A. Acetabular and femoral anteversion: relationship with osteoarthritis of the hip. J Bone Joint Surg Am. 1999;81:1747–70.

17. Larson CM. Arthroscopic management of pincer-type impingement. Sports Med Arthrosc Rev. 2010;18:100–7.

18. Seldes RM, Tan V, Hunt J, et al. Anatomy, histologic features, and vascularity of the adult acetabular labrum. Clin Orthop Relat Res. 2001;382:232–40.

19. Morris WZ, Chen JY, Cooperman DR, Liu RW. Characterization of ossification of the posterior rim of acetabulum in the developing hip and its impact on the assessment of femoroacetabular impingement. J Bone Joints Surg Am. 2015;97(3):e11.

20. Ball ST, Schmalzried TP. Posterior femoroacetabular impingement (PFAI) – after hip resurfacing arthroplasty. Bull NYU Hosp Jt Dis. 2009;67:173.

21. Yoo MC, Cho YJ, Chun YS, Rhyu KH. Impingement between the acetabular cup and the femoral neck after hip resurfacing arthroplasty. J Bone Joint Surg. 2011;93:99–106.

22. Zahn RK, Grotjohann S, Ramm H, et al. Pelvic tilt compensates for increased acetabular anteversion. Int Orthop. 2015;40(8):1571–5.

23. Moulton KM, Aly A, Rajasekaran S, Shepel M, Obaid H. Acetabular anteversion is associated with gluteal tendinopathy at MRI. Skelet Radiol. 2015;44:47–54.

24. Ricciardi BF, Fabricant PD, Fields KG, et al. What are the demographic and radiographic characteristics of patients with symptomatic extraarticular femoroacetabular impingement? Clin Orthop Relat Res. 2015;476(4):1299–308.

25. Ali AM, Teh J, Whitwell D, Ostlere S. Ischiofemoral impingement: a retrospective analysis of cases in a specialist orthopaedic centre over a four-year period. Hip Int. 2013;23:263–8.

26. Ali AM, Whitwell D, Ostlere SJ. Case report: imaging and surgical treatment of a snapping hip due to ischiofemoral impingement. Skelet Radiol. 2011;40:653–6.

27. Hetsroni I, Larson CM, Dela Torre K, et al. Anterior inferior iliac spine deformity as an extra-articular source for hip impingement: a series of 10 patients treated with arthroscopic decompression. Arthroscopy. 2012;28:1644–53.

28. Johnson KA. Impingement of the lesser trochanter on the ischial ramus after total hip arthroplasty. Report of three cases. J Bone Joint Surg Am. 1977;59:268–9.

29. Tosun O, Algin O, Yalcin N, et al. Ischiofemoral impingement: evaluation with new MRI parameters and assessment of their reliability. Skelet Radiol. 2012;41:575–87.

30. Viala P, Vanel D, Larbi A, et al. Bilateral ischiofemoral impingement in a patient with hereditary multiple exostoses. Skelet Radiol. 2012;41:1637–40.

31. Yoong P, Mansour R, Teh JL. Multiple hereditary exostoses and ischiofemoral impingement: a case-control study. Skelet Radiol. 2014;43(9):1225–30.

32. Frank RM, Slabaugh MA, Grumet RC, et al. Posterior hip pain in an athletic population: differential diagnosis and treatment options. Sports Health. 2010;2(3):237–46.

33. Philippon MJ, Schenker ML. Arthroscopy for the treatment of femoroacetabular impingement in the athlete. Clin Sports Med. 2006;25:299–308.

34. Margo K, Drezner J, Motzkin D. Evaluation and management of hip pain: an algorithmic approach. J Fam Pract. 2003;52(8):607–17.

35. Gómez-Hoyos J, Martin RL, Schröder R, Palmer IJ, Martin HD. Accuracy of 2 clinical tests for ischiofemoral impingement in patients with posterior hip pain and endoscopically confirmed diagnosis. Arthroscopy. 2016;32(7):1279–84.

36. Johnston TL, Schenker ML, Briggs KK, et al. Relationship between offset angle alpha and hip chondral injury in femoroacetabular impingement. Arthroscopy. 2008;24:669–75.

37. Clohisy J, Carlisle J, Beaule P, et al. A systematic approach to the plain radiographic evaluation of the young adult hip. J Bone Joint Surg Am. 2008;90:47–66.

38. Leunig M, Beck M, Kalhor M, et al. Fibrocystic changes at anterosuperior femoral neck: prevalence in hips with femoroacetabular impingement. Radiology. 2005;236:237–346.

39. Philippon MJ, Briggs KK, Yen YM, et al. Outcomes following hip arthroscopy for femoroacetabular impingement with associated chondrolabral dysfunction: minimum two-year follow-up. J Bone Joint Surg Br. 2009;91:16–23.

40. Ochoa LM, Dawson L, Patzkowski JC, et al. Radiographic prevalence of femoroacetabular impingement in a young population with hip complaints is high. Clin Orthop Relat Res. 2010;468(10):2710–4.

41. Neumann M, Cui Q, Siebenrock KA, et al. Impingement-free hip motion: the 'normal' angle alpha after osteochondroplasty. Clin Orthop Relat Res. 2009;467:699–703.

42. Allen D, Beaulé PE, Ramadan O, et al. Prevalence of associated deformities and hip pain in patients with cam-type femoroacetabular impingement. J Bone Joint Surg Br. 2009;91:589–94.

43. Meyer DC, Beck M, Ellis T, et al. Comparison of six radiographic projections to assess femoral head/neck asphericity. Clin Orthop Relat Res. 2006;445:181–5.

44. Czerny C, Hofmann S, Neuhold A, et al. Lesions of the acetabular labrum: accuracy of MR imaging and MR arthrography in detection and staging. Radiology. 1996;200:225–30.

45. Singer AD, Subhawong TK, Jose J, et al. Ischiofemoral impingement syndrome: a meta-analysis. Skelet Radiol. 2015;44:831–7.

46. Finnoff JT, Bond JR, Collins MS, et al. Variability of the ischiofemoral space relative to femur position: an ultrasound study. PM&R. 2015;7(9):930–7.

47. Robertson WJ, Kelly BT. The safe zone for hip arthroscopy: a cadaveric assessment of central, peripheral, and lateral compartment portal placement. Arthroscopy. 2008;24:1019–26.

48. Safran M, Ryu J. Ischiofemoral impingement of the hip: a novel approach to treatment. Knee Surg Sports Traumatol Arthrosc. 2014;22:781–5.

49. Philippon MJ, Christensen JC, Wahoff MS. Rehabilitation after arthroscopic repair of intra-articular disorders of the hip in a professional football athlete. J Sport Rehabil. 2009;18:118–34.

50. Philippon MJ, Schenker ML, Briggs KK, et al. Revision hip arthroscopy. Am J Sports Med. 2007;35:1918–21.

51. Sampson TG. Complications of hip arthroscopy. Tech Orthop. 2005;20:63–6.

52. Mardones RM, Gonzalez C, Chen Q, et al. Surgical treatment of femoroacetabular impingement: evaluation of the effect of the size of the resection. J Bone Joint Surg Am. 2005;87:273–9.

Sacroiliac Joint Pain

16

William Henry Márquez-Arabia,
Francisco Javier Monsalve, Juan Gómez-Hoyos,
and Hal D. Martin

Introduction

The posterior hip pain can originate from many sites and anatomical structures, and it may result from a wide variety of extrapelvic or intrapelvic pathologies. There are more than ten causes of pain at this point starting with the lumbar spine and sacroiliac joint (SIJ) descending through the gluteal area with their muscles, nerves, bursas, and tendons.

W. H. Márquez-Arabia, MD (✉)
Clínica Las Americas, Orthopedic Surgery, Medellin, Antioquia, Colombia

Sports Medicine Program, School of Medicine, Medellin, Antioquia, Colombia

F. J. Monsalve, MD
Orthopedic Department, Medellin, Antioquia, Colombia

J. Gómez-Hoyos, MD
International Consultant, Hip Preservation Center / Baylor Scott and White Research Institute, Baylor University Medical Center, Dallas, TX, USA

Department of Orthopaedic Surgery - Health Provider, Clínica Las Américas / Clínica del Campestre, Medellin, Antioquia, Colombia

Professor - School of Medicine - Sports Medicine Program, Universidad de Antioquia, Medellín, Antioquia, Colombia

H. D. Martin, DO
Medical and Research Director, Hip Preservation Center, Baylor University Medical Center, Dallas, TX, USA

Sacroiliac joint dysfunction is believed to be an important source of low back and posterior pelvic pain [1], and it is defined as "a SIJ that is chronically painful, essentially stable, and has become disabling to the patient" [1, 2]; this alteration can be caused for different pathologies each of which will be discussed in this chapter. The SIJ has been implicated as the primary pain source in 10–25% of the patients with low back pain [3, 4]; however, the diagnosis and treatment of SIJ pathology has been poorly defined in the literature; otherwise, the diagnosis is often complicated by concomitant discogenic pain or facet joint arthritis since these structures may refer pain to the SIJ or SIJ dysfunction may develop as a result of adaptive changes [1]. In patients with pain after a lumbar fusion was found that 40–43% had symptoms arising from the SIJ [5, 6].

It is very important to understand the anatomy, biomechanics, innervation, and pathophysiology of the sacroiliac joint to help differentiate the sacroiliac joint pain from muscular, discogenic, or degenerative lumbar spine symptoms.

Anatomy

The SIJ is a C-shaped joint, and it is an irregularly shaped diarthrodial joint with cartilage surfaces. It contains synovial fluid and is itself contained in a fibrous capsule. The joint is stabilized by a thick posterior ligamentous complex that limits motion

© Springer International Publishing AG, part of Springer Nature 2019
H. D. Martin, J. Gómez-Hoyos (eds.), *Posterior Hip Disorders*,
https://doi.org/10.1007/978-3-319-78040-5_16

[7]. The pelvis is formed by the two iliac bones and the sacrum; the sacrum is wedged between the ilia, and it is composed of five fused vertebrae and forms the posterior pelvic column. the anterior sacral side of the joint is lined by thick hyaline cartilage, whereas the posterior iliac side of the joint is lined by fibrocartilage. SIJ is the largest axial joint in the human body, with a surface area of approximately 17.5 cm². SIJ is considered to be a synovial joint even though 75% of its superior joint surface is not synovial. The cartilage erodes over the years, and partial fibrous ankylosis and para-articular synostosis are common in

individuals aged more than 50 years [1, 8] (Figs. 16.1, 16.2, 16.3, and 16.4).

The anterior capsule is thin, and its overlying ventral sacroiliac ligament crosses the SIJ ventrally and caudally at the level of S1–S3 (Fig. 16.5). SIJ inserts on the periosteum close to the margins of the auricular surfaces of the sacrum and ilium, and it blends in to the iliolumbar ligament [8, 9]. In the posterior aspect should be mentioned the sacrotuberous and the sacrospinous ligament. The sacrotuberous ligament (STL) has its origin at the posterior superior iliac spine (PSIS), dorsal ligaments, sacral tubercles, sacrum, and superior coccyx. It has a spiral orientation and runs to insert on the ischial tuberosity and, in some, the tendon of the long head of the biceps femoris; the medial fibers originate from the cephalad aspect of sacrum and lateral fibers originate from the caudal aspect of the sacrum. The fascia from the dorsal aspect of the piriformis and the gluteus maximus have attachment to the STL [9].

Anterior to the sacrotuberous ligament is the sacrospinous ligament (SSL). STL extends from the lateral aspect of the apex of the sacrum and coccyx to the ischial spine. It is the division between the greater and lesser sciatic notches [10]. The pudendal nerve passes anterior to the STL and posterior to the sacrospinus ligament,

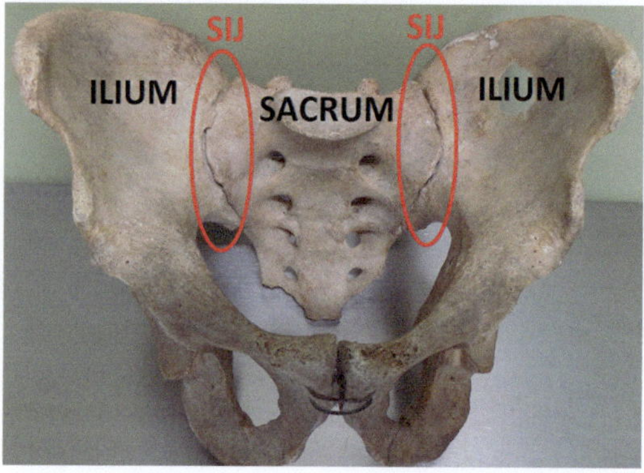

Fig. 16.1 Anatomy of the sacroiliac joint. Anteroposterior view of the pelvis showing the right and left ilium and the sacrum; both sacroiliac joint (SIJ) are highlighted

Fig. 16.2 Posterior view of the articulations and associated ligaments of the sacroiliac joint and surrounding structures: *I* Ilium, *PSIS* posterior superior iliac spine, *SIN* sacral neural foramina from S1 to S4; sacral hiatus

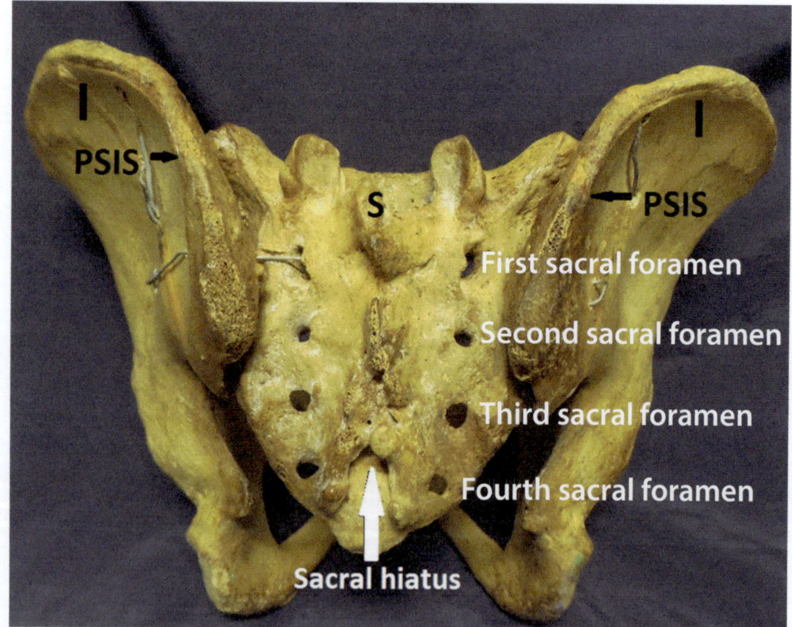

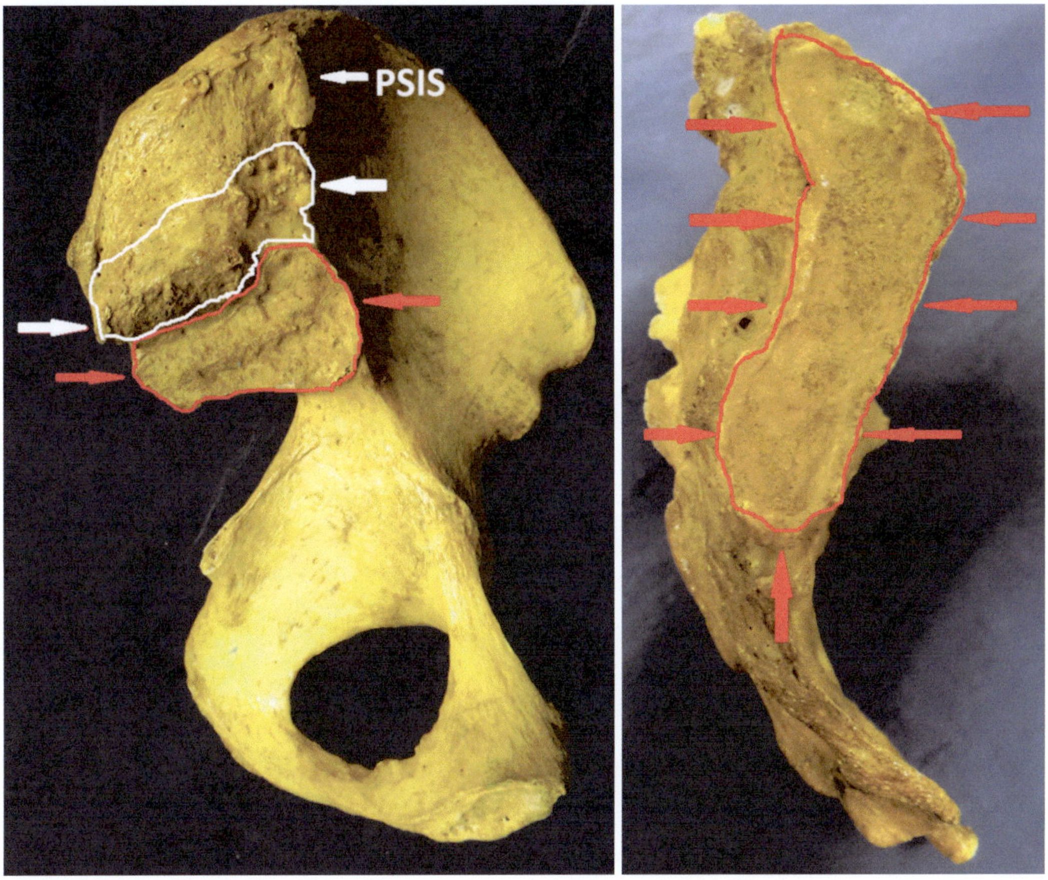

Fig. 16.3 Lateral view of ilium (left) and sacrum (right) showing the articular portion and delimiting the ventral (cartilage articular portion, red color) and dorsal (fibrous portion, white color) portions of ilium and the articular sacral aspect

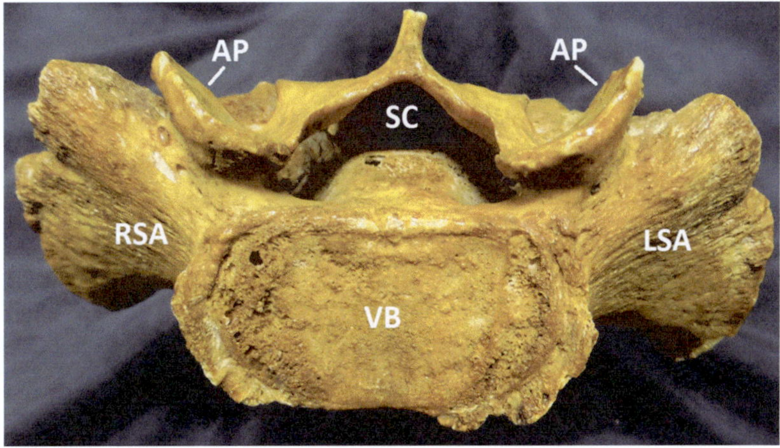

Fig. 16.4 Top view of the sacrum: *VB* vertebral body, *RSA* right sacral ala, *LSA* left sacral ala, *AP* articular portion, *SC* spinal canal

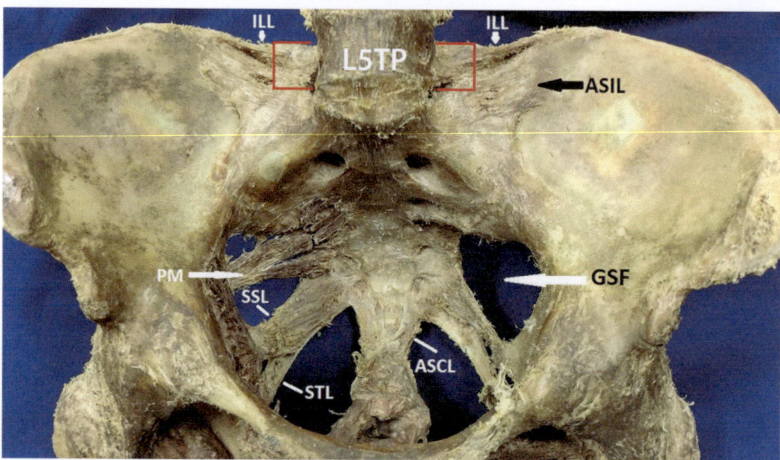

Fig. 16.5 Anterior view of the articulations and associated ligaments of the sacroiliac joint and surrounding structures: *ILL* iliolumbar ligament, *ASIL* anterior sacroiliac ligament, *GSF* greater sciatic foramen, *ASCL* anterior sacrococcygeal ligaments, *STL* sacrotuberous ligament, *SSL* sacrospinous ligament, *PM* piriformis muscle, *L5TP*, *L5* transverse process. An impingement between L5TP and the iliacus could lead to supra SIJ pain

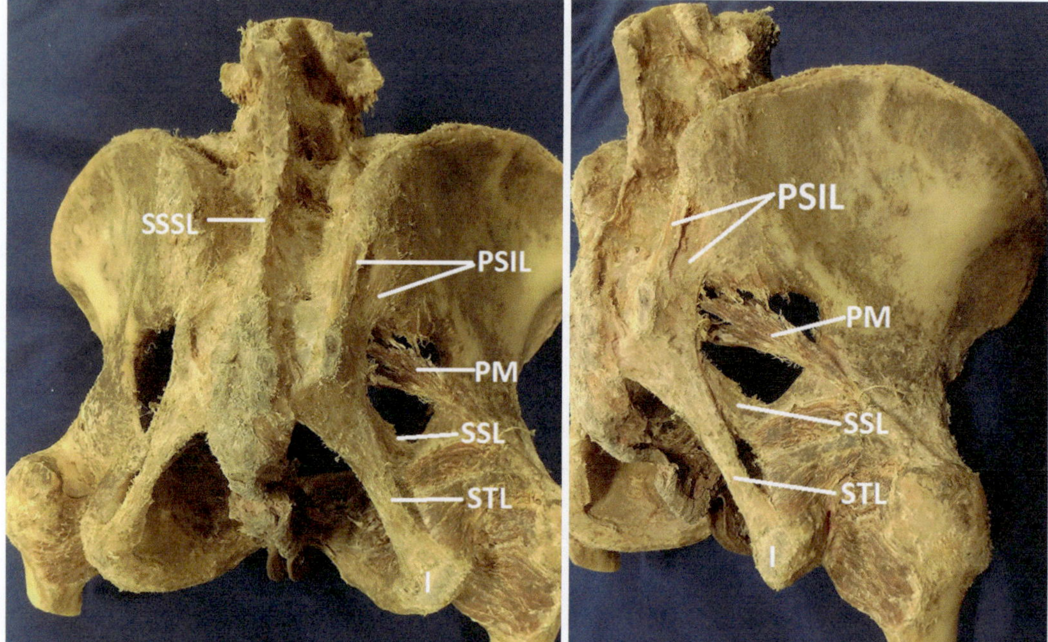

Fig. 16.6 Posterior view of the articulations and associated ligaments of the sacroiliac joint and surrounding structures: *PSIL* posterior sacroiliac ligaments, *PM* piriformis muscle, *STL* sacrotuberous ligament, *SSL* sacrospinous ligament, *SSSL* superior sacrospinous ligament

and then it runs on the back of the obturator internus muscle (Figs. 16.6 and 16.7).

The dorsal sacroiliac ligaments are composed of the long and short ligaments, and these run from the PSIS to the S3–S5 sacral tubercles. The chan lateral aspect is continuous with the gluteus maximus aponeurosis, while the medial aspect is continuous with the posterior layer of the thoracolumbar fascia. The lateral branches of the dorsal sacral rami (medial cluneal nerves) penetrate the dorsal ligaments [11]. The interosseous ligament is located

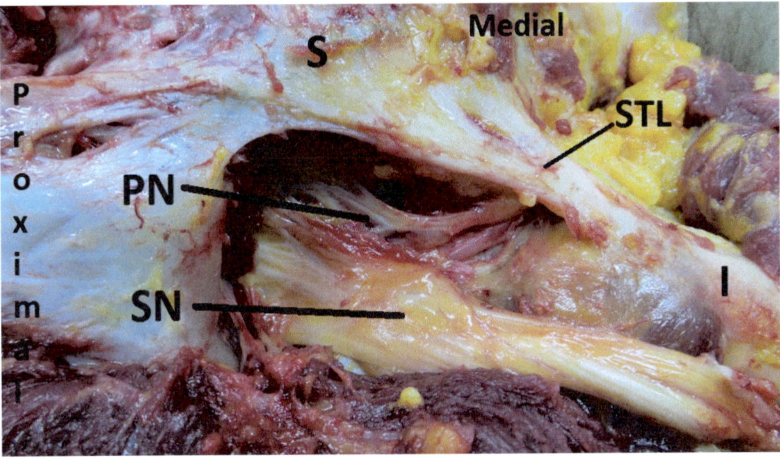

Fig. 16.7 Posterior view in cadaveric dissection showing the sacrotuberous ligament running from the sacrum (S) to ischial tuberosity (I) and its relationship with the pudendal nerve (PN) and sciatic nerve (SN)

within the most cephalad aspect between the sacrum and ilium.

Proximal to the SIJ is the iliolumbar ligament; this ligament is composed of a dorsal band, ventral band, and sacroiliac part. The dorsal band originates at the tip of the L5 transverse process and inserts onto the ventral and cephalad aspect of the iliac tuberosity and crest, and the ventral band originates at the anteroinferior aspect of the L5 transverse process, and it inserts on the anterosuperior aspect of the iliac tuberosity [12] (Fig. 16.5).

The SIJ is under the influence of muscular forces of the gluteus maximus and medius, erector spinae, latissimus dorsi, biceps femoris, psoas, piriformis, and oblique and transversus abdominis muscles as well as by the thoracodorsal fascia [8].

The L5 ventral ramus and the lumbosacral trunk course anterior to the proximal portion of the SIJ, and the S1 ventral ramus courses over the inferior anterior aspect of the SIJ [8]. The lateral branch nerves of the rami of S1, S2, S3, and S4 exit the foramen lateral to the foraminal midline [13]. These branches take various paths and enter the dorsal ligaments and interosseous ligament on the way to different areas including the SIJ.

The SIJ is innervated anteriorly by the L5–S2 ventral rami and the sacral plexus and posteriorly by lateral branches from the S1–S4 dorsal rami [14]. The receptors identified within mentioned ligaments include mechanoreceptors, proprioceptive organs, and free-nerve endings.

Biomechanics

The SIJ motion includes a combination of rotation and translation in the sagittal, coronal, and axial planes. Movement of the sacrum in the sagittal plane can be described as sacral flexion or extension. The SIJ forms a base for the spinal axis and transmits and dissipates upper trunk loads. Lumbar spine, hip, and pubic symphysis motion and myofascial imbalances may affect sacroiliac joint motion [8]. Studies conducted on cadavers with radiographic analysis systems and contrast administration report that the mobility of the SIJ varies from 1° to 4° of rotation and 1–2 mm of translation. Another study performed in healthy males measure of posterior superior iliac displacement and greater trochanter (femur) displacement during hip flexion movement in an orthostatic position resulted in a mean displacement between the reference points of 7.7 mm on the right side and 8.5 mm on the left side [15]. Sacroiliac joint motion progressively decreases in men aged between 40 and 50 years and in women aged more than 50 years.

In vitro cadaver study shows that overall motion in the SIJ is minimal and increases only slightly with transection of key posterior ligament structures [16].

A study was conducted to clarify the mobility and kinematic characteristics of the SI joint in patients with degenerative lumbar spine disorders (DLSDs) in comparison with healthy volunteers by using in vivo 3D motion analysis with voxel-based registration, and the findings reported that trunk flexion-extension in patients with DLSD, including adult spine deformity, SI joint motion is significantly increased, with increased individual difference, than in healthy volunteers. In particular, women in DLSD group had significantly more motion than did men in the group [17].

A cross-sectional study reported that patients with low back pain but without evidence of sacroiliac joint dysfunction had significantly greater external hip rotation than internal rotation bilaterally, whereas those with evidence of sacroiliac joint dysfunction had significantly more external hip rotation than internal rotation unilaterally, specifically on the side where the ilium rotates posteriorly on the sacrum [18]. This study brings to mind the importance of femoral version on proximal load strain transmission in hip flexion and extension.

A leg length discrepancy can alter biomechanics and lead to asymmetric forces through the SIJ. Utilizing two biomechanical parameters, the overall load at the contact area and the load distribution (stress) over the contact area for evaluating the effects of leg length discrepancy (LLD), a study concluded that LLD could significantly increase the load and stress at the SIJ. The peak load also increased notably as discrepancy increased. LLD increases the joint load on both short- and long-leg sides; however, this increase was greater on the longer side. As little as 1 cm of LLD can increase the load across SIJ to almost five times that of intact (shorter side) [19]. See Chap. 18.

Etiology

Sacroiliac pain can originate from structures of the sacroiliac complex or distally at the hip joint. The sacroiliac pain may result from a change in the joint's mechanics. Causes of pain generation include ligamentous or capsular tension, compression or shear forces, motion alteration, abnormal joint mechanics, and myofascial or kinetic chain imbalances resulting in inflammation and pain [8].

Certain events relate with pain originating from the SIJ such as a childbirth a significant fall directly on the buttock, during a collision in an automobile when the patient brakes with a straight leg upon impact, transferring the stress directly to the ipsilateral SIJ, leg length discrepancy, a history of inflammatory arthritis with associated spondyloarthropathies like ankylosing spondylitis, scoliosis, bone graft harvest ipsilateral side, and previous lumbosacral fusion [20].

Intra-articular sources of sacroiliac joint pain include osteoarthritis and infection. Joint infections usually occur from hematogenous spread. Infection may cause distention of the anterior joint capsule and irritate the lumbosacral nerve roots. Extra-articular pain may be caused by ligamentous, tendinous, fascial, and other soft tissue injuries that may occur posterior to the dorsal aspect of the SIJ [8, 20].

Metabolic processes may lead to early degeneration, inflammation, and pain. Other SIJ disorders include calcium pyrophosphate crystal deposition disease, gout, ochronosis, hyperparathyroidism, renal osteodystrophy, and acromegaly. Primary sacroiliac tumors are rare [8].

Clinical Presentation

Confirming the diagnosis of SIJ dysfunction can be confusing since no highly specific clinical examination techniques confirming this alteration are available. The pain originated from the SIJ may be described as aggravated by transitional activities such as climbing stairs, getting up from a chair, or getting out of a car. Activities requiring asymmetrical loading through the lower extremity or pelvis as in some sports such as skating, gymnastics, golfing, and step aerobics may provoke pain in the SIJ [21]. The diagnosis of the SI joint as a pain generator is based on physical examination of the SIJ and confirmatory diagnostic injection [22]. Three symptoms have been described to clarify if the pain comes from a dysfunctional SIJ: sitting is difficult, pain occurs when rolling over during sleep, and sharp pain that can cause the patient to stumble [20].

Dreyfuss et al. noted that pain referral above the L5 level was not found in patients with pain originating from the SIJ and suggested this finding as a possible discriminating feature [8]. In a study by Fortin et al., the SIJ of asymptomatic volunteers were subjected to stress by fluoroscopy-guided joint injections; these authors established that a sensory examination immediately after sacroiliac injection revealed an area of buttock hyperesthesia extending approximately 10 cm caudally and 3 cm laterally from the posterior superior iliac spine [23]. Pain arising from the SIJ may radiate into various anatomic regions includ-

ing the buttocks, the groin, and the entire lower limb [1] (Fig. 16.8).

To identify a painful sacroiliac joint, no specific physical examination tests have been validated. Physical examination should include a thorough neurologic examination and hip evaluation. The patient should point to the area of maximal pain, and its location should be noted. Tenderness along the sacroiliac joint line and in the sacral sulcus should be evaluated. A false-positive straight leg raise test may occur when the affected leg is elevated, and this pain is caused by sacroiliac joint motion during elevation.

The pain provocation tests most commonly relied on for diagnosing the SIJ as a pain generator include the following [24]:

- Flexion abduction external rotation (FABER or Patrick): with the patient in supine position, examiner passively positions the patient's hip in flexion, abduction, and external rotation. The examiner then gently applies an extension force to the hip by pressing down on the knee while stabilizing the contralateral pelvis. The long lever arm provided by the femur applies tensile force on the anterior aspect of the SIJ (Fig. 16.9).
- Thigh thrust (posterior shear): with patient in supine position and hips and knees flexed, examiner grasps the patient's thigh by locking patient's thigh and leg between examiner's arm and forearm. Examiner then performs upward motion followed by downward

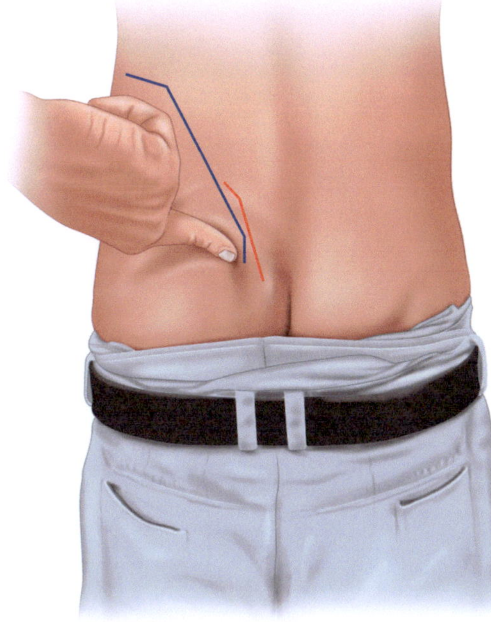

Fig. 16.8 A patient points the area of pain just medial and inferior to the posterior superior iliac spine. *Blue line* gluteus maximus origin. *Red line* sacroiliac joint pain location

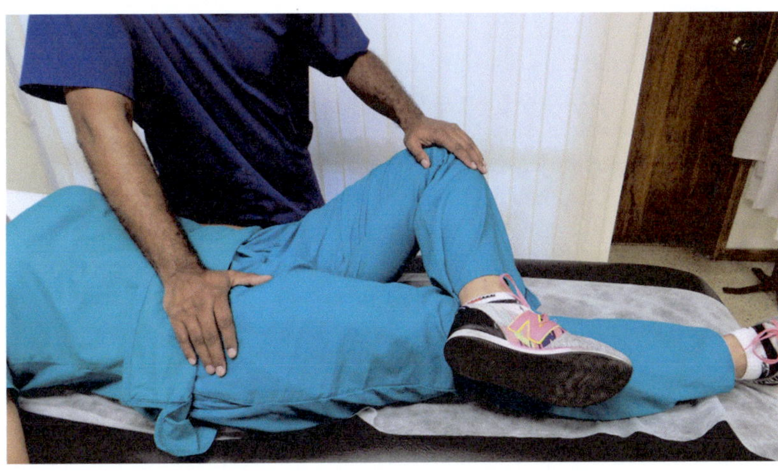

Fig. 16.9 Patrick test with the patient in supine position

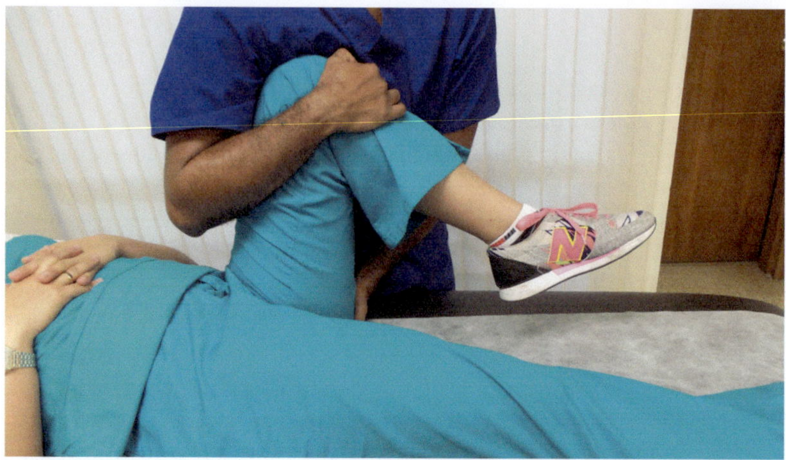

Fig. 16.10 Thigh thrust SIJ provocation test

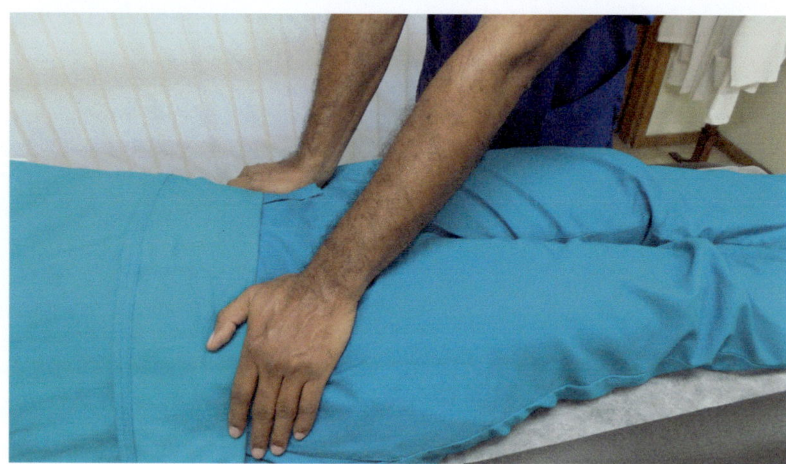

Fig. 16.11 Distraction provocation SIJ test

motion, thereby applying anteroposterior shear stress on the SIJ (Fig. 16.10).

- Iliac distraction test (pelvic gapping): with the patient in supine position, examiner faces toward patient's head and places his hands on patient's bilateral anterior superior iliac spines (ASIS). He then applies posteriorly and laterally directed force simultaneously on both ASIS. This applies tensile forces on the anterior aspect of the joint (Fig. 16.11).
- Iliac compression test (pelvic compression): with the patient in lateral decubitus, examiner places his hand over the iliac crest and applies downward (medial) pressure. This applies compression force across the SIJ (Fig. 16.12).
- Gaenslen's test: this test may be done either in the supine or lateral decubitus position. One

hip is flexed to the abdomen, and the other leg is allowed to dangle off the edge of the table. Examiner applies added downward (extension) pressure on the dangling leg. A modified version of the test is done with the patient in lateral decubitus position. The dependent knee is held up by the patient toward the chest, while examiner passively extends the other hip. This test applies torsional stress on the SIJs (Fig. 16.13).

- Sacral thrust: with the patient in prone position, examiner places his hand over the sacrum and then applies pressure directed proximal and anterior. This applies anteroposterior shear stress on the SIJ (Fig. 16.14).

If three of these are positive, then the pretest probability that a diagnostic injection will be posi-

Fig. 16.12 Compression provocation SIJ test

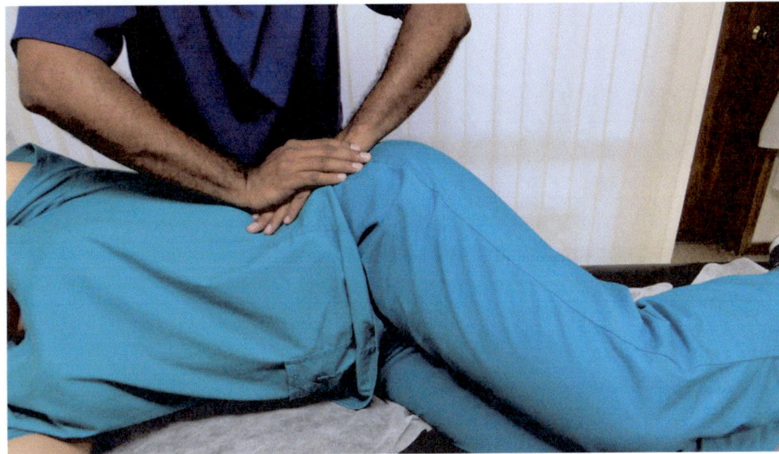

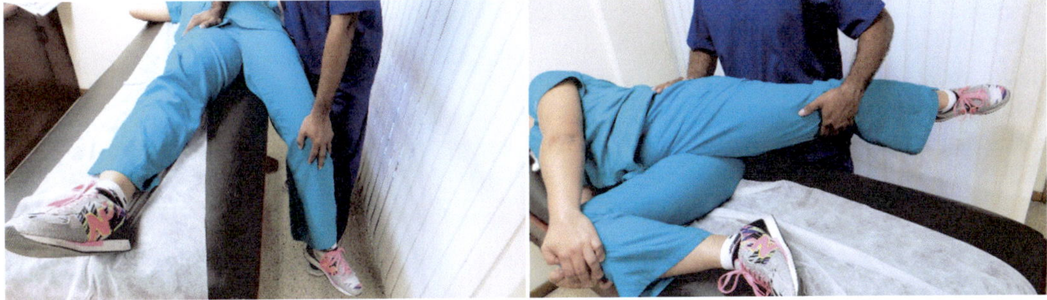

Fig. 16.13 Gaenslen's provocation SIJ test (left) and modified Gaenslen's test (right)

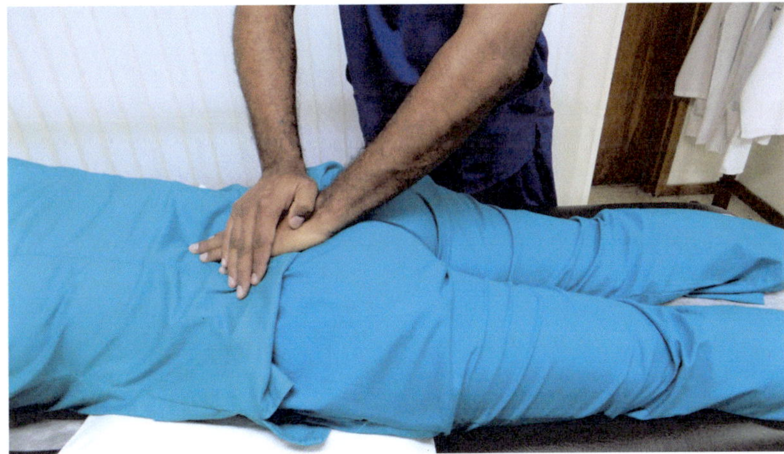

Fig. 16.14 Sacral thrust provocation SIJ test

tive is approximately 85%. Additional helpful physical examination findings are the finger test in which the patient points to the posterior superior iliac spine (PSIS) at the place where it hurts, tenderness to palpation over the PSIS, an ipsilateral positive Trendelenburg test, and pain over the PSIS with resisted supine active straight leg raise test [25]. However, motion and position tests have been repeatedly demonstrated to lack reliability and validity in the diagnosis of pain coming from the SI joint and are, thus, of no benefit in the diagnosis of SI joint pain [26–28]. It is important to distinguish a pain generated from the gluteus maximus origin from a pain originated from the SIJ.

Laboratory Test

Sacroiliitis can originate from inflammatory disease (e.g., seronegative spondyloarthopathies such as ankylosing spondylitis, psoriatic arthritis, etc.). Laboratory studies for inflammatory and rheumatologic markers (e.g., erythrocyte sedimentation rate, C-reactive protein, antinuclear antibodies, human leukocyte antigen B27, rheumatoid factor) are appropriate when an inflammatory or infectious disorder is suspected in a young patient, but, in general, these tests do not frequently add specific diagnostic value. For older patients the laboratory test must rule out malignant disease in those cases that have not improved with initial care and may have symptoms warranting further investigation [24].

Imaging Studies

The radiological evaluation of the SIJ remains challenging. No studies have clearly documented radiographic abnormalities in SIJ dysfunction. Imaging studies for the evaluation for SIJ pathology have generated a great controversy among clinicians because it is unclear whether normal and abnormal radiographic studies can help differentiate symptomatic from asymptomatic patients, except in cases of a clear evidence of seronegative spondyloarthropathy, arthritis, infection, or tumor [24].

The imaging studies must start with plain radiographs. A true anteroposterior (AP) of the sacrum and a lateral of the pelvis are the best views for imaging the SIJ. In all cases an AP of the pelvis that includes the hips is mandatory to rule out hip osteoarthritis and AP and lateral of the lumbar spine to evaluate pathologies in this segment. Computed tomography (CT), magnetic resonance imaging, and bone scan are done to

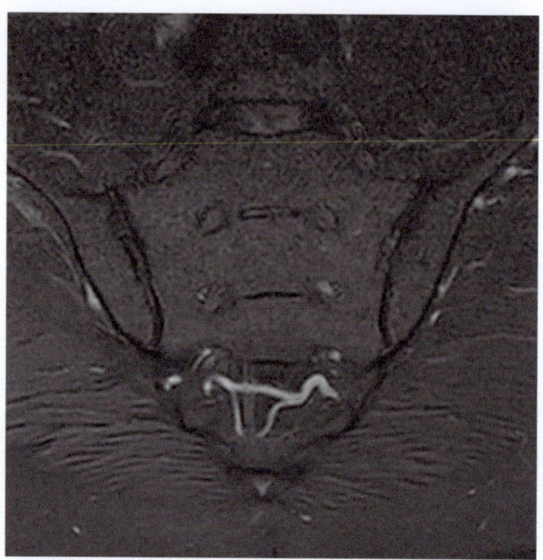

Fig. 16.15 Normal SIJ image in T2 MRI with preserved joint space and without osseous edema

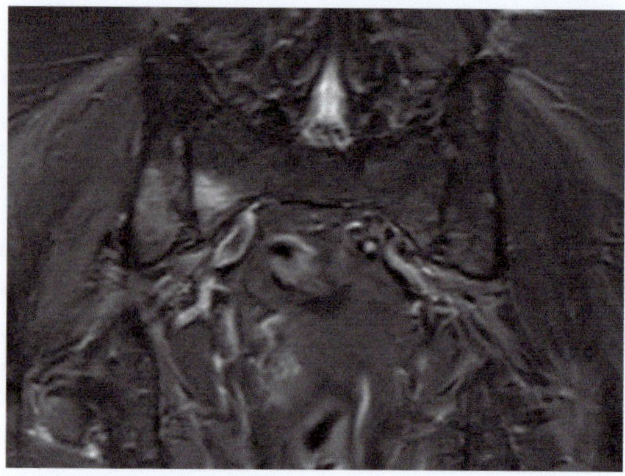

Fig. 16.16 T2 MRI coronal view showing subchondral edema of ilium and sacrum in right SIJ in a patient with noninfectious sacroiliitis

exclude other causes of pain rather than diagnose SIJ pain [8]. CT of the SIJ has poor sensitivity and specificity compared with diagnostic sacroiliac joint injections [29]. MRI is excellent to identify soft tissue disorders such as tumors, and it can help to detect early inflammatory changes in spondyloarthropathies or infection (Figs. 16.15, 16.16, and 16.17). Bone scan findings are non specific but can help identify stress fracture, inflammatory process, and tumor pathologies.

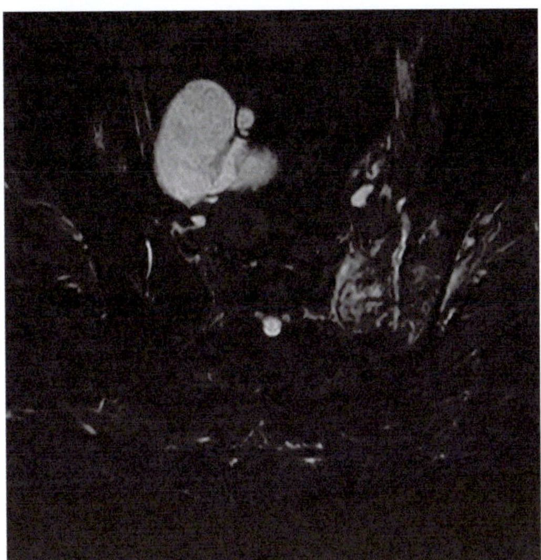

Fig. 16.17 T2 MRI coronal view showing intense subchondral edema (hypersignal) and soft tissue edema in a patient with left infectious sacroiliitis

Diagnostic Injections

Fluoroscopically guided or CT-guided, contrast-enhanced injections are the method for diagnosing or excluding the SIJ as a source of pain because of limitations of the history, physical examination, and imaging modalities. The piriformis lies immediatly anterior to the SIJ which can contribute to DGS. Pain relief obtained with SI joint injection currently is considered the "gold standard" for diagnosis of SI joint pain [24]. SIJ pain may be misinterpreted as facetogenic pain and vice versa. The therapeutic injection under fluoroscopy, combined with physical exam maneuvers, may help to obtain an accurate diagnosis by helping to rule out alternative diagnoses such as facetogenic pain, iliolumbar syndrome, and superior cluneal nerve entrapment [30]. Reported studies have used ≥75% pain relief as diagnostic of sacroiliac joint-mediated pain and ≤50% relief as not diagnostic, with 51–74% relief considered equivocal [8]. The rate of intra-articular injection seen with this clinically guided technique (no image guidance) is low; it suggests restraint in its use for injection therapy. Some image guidance (e.g., fluoroscopy, CT) is necessary to reliably inject the SIJ [31].

Treatment

The SIJ pain should undergo initial nonoperative treatment, except in cases of acute trauma resulting in gross pelvic instability. Treatment considerations include SIJ-focused physical therapy employing manual techniques, restoring balance in joint kinematics and function, establishing lumbopelvic lower extremity muscular length and strength balance, and correcting lumbopelvic-hip mechanics, core stabilization, pain modalities, therapeutic injections, anti-inflammatory medication, weight reduction, counseling, and chronic pain behavior treatment. Only if the patient has exhausted all nonoperative treatment modalities should one consider surgical treatment [8, 24]. Since the load transmission of the forces occurring at the hip are influential in SIJ pathology, it is critical that the hip biomechanics and patomechanics are properly evaluated and understood as a potential load transfer to the SIJ. Addressing joint pathology through operative and nonoperative modalities may greatly influence secondary SIJ pain.

Manual therapy can reduce pain in some cases, and an exercise program is initiated to promote restoration of soft tissue flexibility, strength, and balance, but no one of those techniques (osteopathic, chiropractic, or manual physical therapy) has shown to be superior to another. If an SIJ appears to require recurrent joint mobilization, a significant muscle imbalance may still exist [8, 21]. No manual therapy studies exist for patients with established rather than presumed sacroiliac joint pain. The physiologic basis for improvement after mobilization and/or manipulation of the sacroiliac joint is unknown. In a radiographic stereophotogrammetric analysis study of osseous positions before and after joint manipulation in ten patients with presumed sacroiliac joint pain, no positional change of the sacrum or ilium was seen, suggesting that no measurable mechanical change occurs with manipulation [32].

If pain decreases after medication and relative rest, the process of rehabilitation begins to achieve a balance between agonist and antagonist lower extremity muscle length and strength. Show improvement of a direct and indirect force transmission across the ilium and sacrum. Muscular strengthening and stretching is performed while maintaining a neutral spine position. Anatomic leg length discrepancies should be determined as early in treatment as possible so that the appropriate modifications can be accomplished with orthoses and shoe modifications [21]. Three planar alignment assessment is critical to outcome.

If after a course of therapy and nonsteroidal anti-inflammatory drugs, a patient's SIJ symptoms have not adequately resolved, the next step in the treatment process is generally injections into the joint including a mixture of anesthetic agents such as lidocaine for rapid pain reduction and bupivacaine for prolonged anesthetic response with steroids. The injection should be performed using fluoroscopic imaging [7].

A systematic review about fluoroscopically guided diagnostic and therapeutic intra-articular sacroiliac joint injections reported that patients who undergo SIJ injections with local anesthetic and steroid should have a biphasic response: immediate and delayed. When local anesthetic alone is injected, 87/246 (35%) patients had at least 75% relief; when local anesthetic and steroid were injected, 339/685 (49%) patients had at least 75% relief. The overall quality of evidence for therapeutic SIJ injections is moderate [33].

Prolotherapy (also known as proliferative therapy) involves the injection of otherwise non-pharmacological and nonactive irritant solutions such as dextrose and platelet-rich plasma into the body, usually around tendons or ligaments, in an attempt to stimulate the synthesis of an increased volume of normal collagen material in ligament, tendon, or fascia to restore function of the tissue at a specific site and relieve musculoskeletal pain; however safety and clinical outcomes have been reported, no prospective, controlled studies exist to date on the specific use of prolotherapy and SIJ dysfunction [34].

If SIJ pain persists despite the described treatments, a radiofrequency denervation can be con-

sidered. The nerves that mediate a patient's symptoms might be coagulated by radiofrequency lesioning in an effort to provide lasting relief of pain. Radiofrequency neurotomy of the L5 dorsal ramus, its branches to the sacroiliac joint, and the lateral branches of the S1–S3 dorsal rami may be performed for chronic SIJ pain. A retrospective study was performed selecting patients who underwent sensory stimulation-guided sacral lateral branch radiofrequency neurotomy; success was defined as greater than 60% consistent subjective relief and greater than a 50% consistent decrease in visual pain score, maintained for at least 6 months after the procedure, and in 14 patients the authors found 64% of patients had >50% reduction of pain [35].

In patients whose symptoms are refractory to conservative management and with SIJ pain proven by controlled diagnostic anesthetic blocks and without any pain sources in the lumbar spine, the surgical intervention could be recommended. Most of the studies involve surgical fusion of the SIJ (with two basic approaches: dorsal or lateral transarticular) and include relatively small cohorts of patients, and no comparison studies of successful fusion rates or clinical outcomes exist for the various arthrodesis techniques. Reports of small, retrospective series reveal generally positive results; however, in all of them the pain relief is rarely complete, and postoperative recovery can be protracted [36–39]. A systematic review of the literature about surgical and clinical efficacy of sacroiliac joint fusion reported rates of excellent satisfaction, determined by pain reduction, function, and quality of life in a mean of 54% in open surgical cases and a mean of 84% in patients underwent minimally invasive surgery for SIJ fusion, but the authors concluded that with the difficulty in accurate diagnosis and evidence for the efficacy of SIJ fusion itself lacking, serious consideration of the cause of pain and alternative treatments should be given before performing the operation [40]. In summary, whereas surgery appears to be clearly indicated for fracture or dislocation, its applicability to degenerative disease is less clear [34]. Assuming hip anatomy and biomechanics have been evaluated and corrected, the hip-pelvic-spine biomechanics must be understood in SIJ dysfunction. Three planar understanding of the hip-pelvic-spine biomechanics is required for successful treatment of the SIJ dysfunction.

References

1. Zelle BA, Gruen GS, Brown S, George S. Sacroiliac joint dysfunction: evaluation and management. Clin J Pain. 2005;21:446–55.
2. Dreyfuss P, Michaelsen M, Pauza K, McLarty J. The value of medical history and physical examination in diagnosing sacroiliac joint pain. Spine. 1996;21:2594–602.
3. Bernard TN, Kirkaldy-Willis WH. Recognizing specific characteristics of nonspecific low back pain. Clin Orthop. 1987;217:266–80.
4. Fortin JD, Aprill CN, Ponthieux B, et al. Sacroiliac joint: pain referral maps upon applying a new injection/arthrography technique. Part II: clinical evaluation. Spine. 1994;19:1483–9.
5. Liliang PC, Lu K, Liang CL, et al. Sacroiliac joint pain after lumbar and lumbosacral fusion: findings using dual sacroiliac joint blocks. Pain Med. 2011;12:565–70.
6. De Palma MJ, Ketchum JM, Saullo TR. Etiology of chronic low back pain in patients having undergone lumbar fusion. Pain Med. 2011;12:732–9.
7. Rashbaum RF, Ohnmeiss DD, Lindley EM, Kitchel SH, Patel VV. Sacroiliac joint pain and its treatment. Clin Spine Surg. 2016;29:42–8.
8. Dreyfuss P, Dreyer S, Cole A, Mayo K. Sacroiliac joint pain. J Am Acad Orthop Surg. 2004;12:255–65.
9. Rahl M. Anatomy and biomechanics. In: Dall BE, Eden SV, Rahl MD, editors. Surgery for the painful, dysfunctional sacroiliac joint. A clinical guide. New York: Springer; 2015. p. 15–35.
10. Lanzieri CG, Hilal SK. Computed tomography of the sacral plexus and sciatic nerve in the greater sciatic foramen. AJR Am J Roentgenol. 1984;143:165–8.
11. McGrath C, Nicholson H, Hurst P. The long posterior sacroiliac ligament: a histological study of morphological relations in the posterior sacroiliac region. Joint Bone Spine. 2009;76(1):57–62.
12. Pool-Goudzwaard AL, Kleinrensink GJ, Entius C, Snijders CJ, Stoeckart R. The sacroiliac part of the iliolumbar ligament. J Anat. 2001;199:457–63.
13. Yin W, Willard F, Carreiro J, et al. Sensory stimulation guided sacroiliac joint radiofrequency neurotomy: technique based on neuroanatomy of the dorsal sacral plexus. Spine (Phila Pa 1976). 2003;28:2419–25.
14. Barker PJ, Hapuarachchi KS, Ross JA, Sambaiew E, Ranger TA, Briggs CA. Anatomy and biomechanics of gluteus maximus and the thoracolumbar fascia at the sacroiliac joint. Clin Anat. 2014;27(2):234–40.
15. Rebello da Veiga T, Da Silva A, Gomes da Silva R, Machado Carvalho S, Orsini M, Sila J. Intraobserver reliability in three-dimensional kinematic analysis of sacroiliac joint mobility. J Phys Ther Sci. 2015;27:1001–4.
16. Vrahas M, Hern TC, Diangelo D, Kellam J, Tile M. Ligamentous contributions to pelvic stability. Orthopedics. 1995;18(3):271–4.
17. Nagamoto Y, Iwasaki M, Sakaura H, Sugiura T, Fujimori T, Matsuo Y, Kashii M, Murase T, Yoshikawa H, Sugamoto K. Sacroiliac joint motion in patients with degenerative lumbar spine disorders. J Neurosurg Spine. 2015;23(2):209–16.
18. Cibulka MT, Sinacore DR, Cromer GS, Delitto A. Unilateral hip rotation range of motion asymmetry in patients with sacroiliac joint regional pain. Spine. 1998;23(9):1009–15.
19. Kiapour A, Abdelgawad AA, Goel VK, Souccar A, Terai T, Ebraheim NA. Relationship between limb length discrepancy and load distribution across the sacroiliac joint – a finite element study. J Orthop Res. 2012;30(10):1577–80.
20. Dall B, Eden S, Rahl M, Graham Smith A. Algorithm for the diagnosis and treatment of the dysfunctional sacroiliac joint. In: Dall BE, Eden SV, Rahl MD, editors. Surgery for the painful, dysfunctional sacroiliac joint. A clinical guide. New York: Springer; 2015. p. 57–67.
21. Prather H. Sacroiliac joint pain: practical management. Clin J Sport Med. 2003;13(4):252–5.
22. Laslett M, Aprill CN, McDonald B, et al. Diagnosis of sacroiliac joint pain: validity of individual provocation tests and composites of tests. Man Ther. 2005;10(3):207–18.
23. Fortin JD, Dwyer AP, West S, Pier J. Sacroiliac joint: pain referral maps upon applying a new injection/arthrography technique. Part I: asymptomatic volunteers. Spine (Phila Pa 1976). 1994;19(13):1475–82.
24. Sembrano JN, Reiley MA, Polly DW, et al. Diagnosis and treatment of sacroiliac joint pain. Curr Orthop Pract. 2011;22(4):344–50.
25. Polly D. The sacroiliac joint. Neurosurg Clin N Am. 2017;28:301–12.
26. Freburger JK, Riddle DL. Measurement of sacroiliac joint dysfunction: a multicenter intertester reliability study. Phys Ther. 1999;79:1134–41.
27. Van der Wurff P. Clinical diagnostic tests for the sacroiliac joint: motion and palpation tests. Aust J Physiother. 2006;52:308.
28. Riddle DL, Freburger JK. Evaluation of the presence of sacroiliac joint region dysfunction using a combination of tests: a multicenter intertester reliability study. Phys Ther. 2002;82:772–81.
29. Elgafy H, Semaan HB, Ebraheim N, Coombs R. Computed tomography findings in patients with sacroiliac pain. Clin Orthop. 2001;382:112–8.

30. Eskander J, Ripoll J, Calixto F, Beakley B, Baker J, Healy P, Gunduz O, Shi L, Clodfelter J, Liu J, Kaye A, Sharma S. Value of examination under fluoroscopy for the assessment of sacroiliac joint dysfunction. Pain Physician. 2015;18:E781–6.

31. Rosenberg JM, Quint DJ, de Rosayro AM. Computerized tomographic localization of clinically-guided sacroiliac joint injections. Clin J Pain. 2000;16:18–21.

32. Tullberg T, Blomberg S, Branth B, Johnsson R. Manipulation does not alter the position of the sacroiliac joint: a roentgen stereophotogrammetric analysis. Spine. 1998;23:1124–8.

33. Kennedy D, Engel A, Kreiner S, Nampiaparampil D, Duszynski B, MacVicar J. Fluoroscopically guided diagnostic and therapeutic intra-articular sacroiliac joint injections: a systematic review. Pain Med. 2015;16:1500–18.

34. Cohen S, Chen Y, Neufeld N. Sacroiliac joint pain: a comprehensive review of epidemiology, diagnosis and treatment. Expert Rev Neurother. 2013;13(1):99–116.

35. Yin W, Willard F, Carreiro J, Dreyfuss P. Sensory stimulation-guided sacroiliac joint radiofrequency neurotomy: technique based on neuroanatomy of the dorsal sacral plexus. Spine. 2003;28:2419–25.

36. Belanger T, Dall B. Sacroiliac arthrodesis using a posterior midline fascial splitting approach and pedicle screw instrumentation: a new technique. J Spinal Disord. 2001;14:118–24.

37. Lippitt A. Recurrent subluxation of the sacroiliac joint: diagnosis and treatment. Bull Hosp Jt Dis. 1995;54:94–102.

38. Rand J. Anterior sacro-iliac arthrodesis for posttraumatic sacro-iliac arthritis: a case report. J Bone Joint Surg. 1985;67(A):157–9.

39. Waisbrod H, Krainick J, Gerbershagen H. Sacroiliac joint arthrodesis for chronic lower back pain. Arch Orthop Trauma Surg. 1987;106:238–40.

40. Zaidi H, Montoure A, Dickman C. Surgical and clinical efficacy of sacroiliac joint fusion: a systematic review of the literature. J Neurosurg Spine. 2015;23(1):59–66.

Spine and Pelvic Pathology Presenting with Posterior Hip Pain

Joshua S. Bowler, David Vier, Frank Feigenbaum, Manu Gupta, and Andrew E. Park

Introduction

Many pathologic conditions of the spine and pelvis have posterior gluteal or "hip" pain as a presenting symptom. It is critical that a thorough history is taken as well as a detailed physical examination of the patient. From this information, pertinent imaging studies may be ordered to better direct the physician toward an accurate diagnosis for the patient's symptoms. Because pain in this region can be from many different pathologic processes, it is very important that the

J. S. Bowler, MD · D. Vier, MD
Baylor University Medical Center,
Department of Orthopedic Surgery,
Dallas, TX, USA
e-mail: josuha.bowler@bswhealth.org

F. Feigenbaum, MD, FAANS, FACS
Feigenbaum Neurosurgery, Dallas, TX, USA

M. Gupta, MD
Division of Neuroradiology, Baylor University
Medical Center—Dallas, Department of Radiology,
Dallas, TX, USA
e-mail: mgupta@americanrad.com

A. E. Park, MD (✉)
Orthopaedic Surgery, Texas A&M Health Science
Center, Dallas, TX, USA

Baylor University Medical Center, Dallas, TX, USA

Department of Orthopaedic Surgery, Methodist
Hospital for Surgery, Addison, TX, USA
e-mail: a.park@texasspineconsultants.com

evaluating physician considers and evaluates the patient in a systematic fashion to properly work up the patient.

The intersection of several body systems in the posterior pelvic region mandates careful attention to the presenting complaint, the aggravating and alleviating factors. *Musculoskeletal conditions* such as sacroiliac disease, ischiofemoral impingement, facet degeneration, and hamstring injuries can usually be differentiated based on history, radiographic evaluation, and physical examination. *Neurologic conditions* such as piriformis syndrome, spinal stenosis, HNP, and Tarlov and meningeal cysts require MRI (+/− nerve conduction testing) in addition to the aforementioned diagnostics. *Vascular claudication* may be differentiated from neurogenic claudication by key components of the history, assessment of risk factors, and peripheral vascular examination. Ultrasound blood flow studies, CT angiography, and magnetic resonance angiography studies will ultimately be needed for a definitive diagnosis in such cases.

The confusion that is often caused by posterior gluteal pain and its association with various medical conditions is one that has been present as long as we have been treating disorders of the lower back, pelvis, and hip joint. A growing understanding of physiologic sagittal balance and pelvic parameters (pelvic incidence, pelvic tilt) is increasingly bringing attention on how the lower

© Springer International Publishing AG, part of Springer Nature 2019
H. D. Martin, J. Gómez-Hoyos (eds.), *Posterior Hip Disorders*,
https://doi.org/10.1007/978-3-319-78040-5_17

lumbar region and the hip joint are so intimately related. As the total lumbar lordosis is decreased (by degenerative changes of the discs or secondary to surgical fusion), the pelvis tends to assume a retroverted posture as a compensatory mechanism. This then reduces the hip's extension in a normal gait cycle, thus accentuating conditions such as ischiofemoral impingement. The radiographic parameters which may best highlight this condition relate to the patient's sacral slope, pelvic tilt, and pelvic incidence.

It is not uncommon for inexperienced practitioners to comment that they have never seen a symptomatic sacroiliac joint problem, piriformis syndrome, or Tarlov cyst (to name just a few). However, to the expert examiner in each of these fields, the diagnosis can be made and treatment rendered to resolve the patient's complaint in most instances. If the possibility of a rare or unusual condition afflicting a patient is never considered, an accurate diagnosis and appropriate treatment will certainly evade the physician.

The vast majority of the patients who present with posterior hip pain can be accurately diagnosed into one of the more common diagnoses. Among the spinal conditions to consider, spinal stenosis, lumbar disc herniation, degenerative disc disease, and lumbar facet degeneration represent the vast majority of these cases. When there is difficulty in establishing the diagnosis, it is incumbent on the physician to broaden the scope of conditions being considered and to recognize the considerable variability in presentation among the conditions on the differential diagnosis list.

In order to make an accurate diagnosis, it is often necessary to perform electrodiagnostic (EMG/NCV) studies and/or diagnostic injections to more definitively establish a diagnosis. The use of these sophisticated techniques may be the only way to differentiate some of these conditions from one another. In the following sections, the process of working up and treating the following conditions will be reviewed: peripheral vascular disease, lumbar spinal stenosis, herniated nucleus pulposus, facet degeneration/synovial cyst, degenerative disc disease, sacroiliac joint disease, piriformis syndrome, hamstring injuries, and Tarlov and meningeal cysts.

Herniated Nucleus Pulposus

Background

Lumbar disc herniation is a common cause of low back pain that can manifest as posterior hip pain. Typically, strain leads to a tear of the outer annulus fibrosus. This is usually associated with significant lower back pain. Either simultaneously or more commonly after the onset of the lower back symptoms, disc material (nucleus pulposus) from the central portion of the disc space may protrude through the opening in the annulus resulting in compression of the local neurologic structures. It is not uncommon for the pain in the lower lumbar region to resolve by the time the radicular complaints become more predominant.

Depending on the level of the disc herniation, it can cause compression of the conus medullaris in the upper lumbar levels or spinal nerve roots in the mid to lower lumbar levels. The disc can protrude and create compression at that disc level or extrude through the annulus and migrate superiorly or inferiorly. An understanding of the anatomy of the traversing and exiting nerve roots at each level is crucial in understanding the symptomatology.

A *foraminal* or *extraforaminal* herniation will compress the exiting nerve root, so at L3/4 foraminal herniation would cause compression of the L3 nerve root (Fig. 17.1a, b). The more common subarticular or lateral recess herniation typically causes compression of the *traversing nerve root*, or the nerve root below the corresponding disc level. So at L5/S1 a posterolateral disc herniation would compress the S1 nerve root on the affected side (Fig. 17.2a, b). Central disc herniations are uncommon causes of neurologic compression. Typically they are more associated with axial lower back pain than radicular symptoms. Rarely, a very large central disc herniation may cause compression of the entire cauda equina and cause cauda equina syndrome—a surgical emergency. The most common levels to exhibit symptomatic disc herniations with associated radiculopathy are at the L4/L5 and L5/S1 levels; however they can

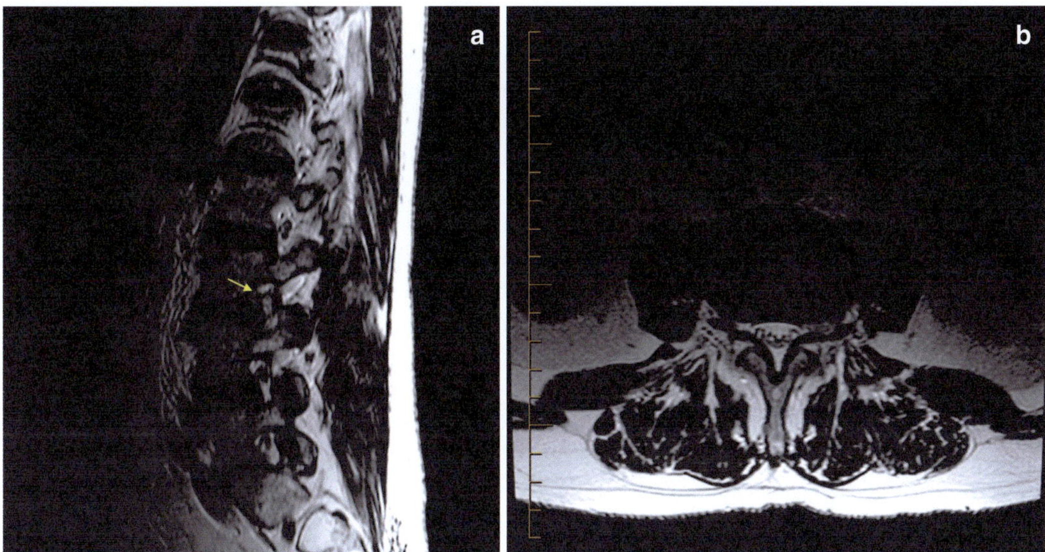

Fig. 17.1 Foraminal disc herniation. (**a**) A patient with left hip pain demonstrating a left foraminal extrusion at L3/L4 compressing the exiting L3 nerve root with severe left foraminal stenosis. (**b**) Axial image at L3/L4 demonstrating the foraminal location of the left disc herniation—compressing the left L3 nerve root

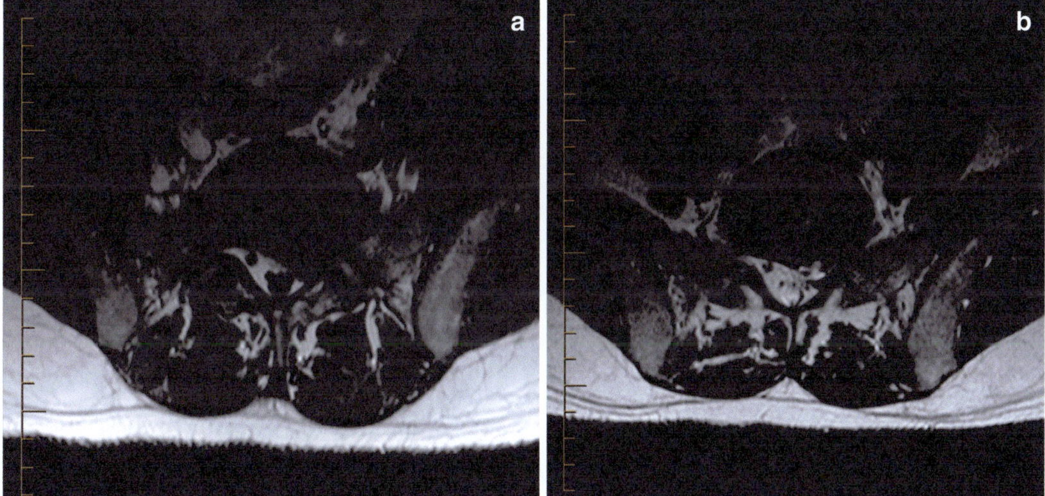

Fig. 17.2 Disc herniation with left hip pain. Images show a L5/S1 left subarticular extrusion compressing the left S1 nerve root. (**a**) Demonstrates the disc extrusion within the left subarticular recess at L5/S1 extending inferiorly to the left S1 lateral recess with compression and posterior displacement of the left S1 nerve root. (**b**) Axial T2 images demonstrating the same with profound T2 hyperintensity of the extrusion (high-intensity zone). Note how the extrusion on T2 images can blend in with the epidural fat and how much easier on T1-weighted images in this case the extrusion is seen

occur at any level in the spine from C2 to the sacrum. Subarticular disc herniations are the most common location for neurologic compression to occur.

History

Patients with a symptomatic herniated lumbar disc will often describe pain after an activity that required a higher level of physical exertion. However, a patient may experience symptoms without a definite preceding event. The presenting symptoms can vary from low back pain to buttock or leg pain that is often exacerbated by sitting or leaning forward and relieved by standing or back extension. Other symptoms include lower extremity weakness, numbness, or paresthesias. Rarely, cauda equina syndrome can manifest secondary to a herniated disc and includes lower extremity weakness, saddle anesthesia, and/or bowel/bladder incontinence. Most patients with herniated discs will have improvement of symptoms over time as the herniated disc has the capacity to spontaneously resorb. Typically, the larger and more acute the herniation is, the more likely it is to resorb. However, these are also the disc herniations most likely to cause acute radiculopathy. Other conditions with a similar presentation are spinal stenosis or synovial facet cysts which often require MRI to differentiate from HNP. All of these conditions tend to produce compression of the traversing nerve root.

Physical Exam Findings

A detailed physical examination is essential to accurately diagnose a HNP as the source of the patient's symptoms. It is very common to identify asymptomatic disc herniations on MRI or CT myelogram. Therefore, a thorough neurological examination is important in order to corroborate the level and side of nerve root compression with the identified pathology on the imaging studies. With a herniated disc, motor exam may yield weakness in a specific muscle group corresponding to compression of a specific level such as weakness of the tibialis anterior with dorsiflexion of the ankle indicating problems with the L5 nerve. Upper motor neuron signs such as hyperreflexia or clonus indicate compression at the level of the spinal cord rather than at the root level. Sensory examination in a dermatomal pattern is very helpful to further delineate the involved nerve root.

Although the classic finding of sciatica with pain radiating all the way down a particular dermatome with associated weakness of the corresponding motor unit is often seen with disc herniations, the clinical presentation can be quite varied. Often times there will be occasional sciatica pain with intervening periods of more "centralized" pain in the lower back and gluteal region. Therefore, posterior hip or gluteal pain may be the chief presenting complaint for many of these patients.

Imaging

The easiest and least expensive imaging modality to evaluate back pain is a plain X-ray. The X-ray might reveal loss of disc height in a patient with a degenerative or herniated disc. Standing radiographs will also help to identify subtle instability on flexion/extension or the presence or absence of spinal deformities such as spondylolisthesis, kyphosis, or scoliosis.

The preferred imaging modality for identification of lumbar disc herniations is an MRI. Intravenous contrast with gadolinium is often helpful in situations where prior surgery has been performed to differentiate epidural scar tissue from recurrent disc herniations. In the lumbar spine, having a combination of T1 and T2 axial and sagittal images is necessary. STIR images acquired routinely at most facilities are also very useful and should be acquired on a routine basis. This sequence maybe the only sequence to demonstrate signs of peridiscal inflammation or osseous edema. An MRI will show the location and size of the herniated disc, as well as identify other possible causes for pain/radiculopathy such as spinal stenosis or facet degeneration/cyst. However, many asymptomatic patients will have abnormal findings on the MRI as well, so treatment decisions on imaging alone is fraught with error. Any disc herniation's significance must be corroborated with the clinical exam findings. The use of contrast is also helpful when infection or tumor is suspected.

Diagnostic Tests

Imaging studies such as MRI or CT are the primary diagnostic modality for lumbar disc herniations. CT myelogram is useful in those patients not able to obtain MRI. In general there is little added information with myelography in patients who can obtain a high-quality MRI and non-contrast CT. Also unlike the cervical spine where the neural compression is most commonly osseous, in the lumbar spine that is not the case, hence making CT myelography far less necessary in the lumbar spine. EMG is often useful in evaluating which nerve root level is affected especially in a patient with a contraindication to MRI such as a pacemaker. Steroid injections can aid the diagnosis of the specific pain generator by relief with injection of a specific nerve root.

Treatment

Initial treatment is typically conservative management with the use of NSAIDs, physical therapy, muscle relaxants, or a short course of oral steroids as the symptoms from most herniated discs will resolve with a combination of conservative treatments. If a patient fails these conservative treatments, consideration for an epidural steroid injection or surgical treatment may be warranted. Surgical treatment is reserved for patients recalcitrant to conservative management, and surgery has shown improvement in pain and function compared to nonoperative treatment. The operative treatment typically performed is a microdiscectomy which includes a laminotomy with discectomy.

SI Joint Problems

The sacroiliac joint is a source of mechanical back pain that has potential to be missed by practitioners. SI joint pain is typically a chronic pain in the lower back or gluteal region of the pelvis. Problems with the SI joint can arise from a trauma or pregnancy or may also be seen in syndromes such as infection, ankylosing spondylitis, or Reiter's syndrome. It is believed that long spinal fusions to the sacrum may also result in sacroiliac pain. The imaging findings in such cases may be quite variable.

History

Patients with the SI joint as a pain generator typically present with chronic, low back pain without radiculopathy that often has an inciting event such as a fall on the buttocks or motor vehicle collision. A thorough history is important to help aid in the diagnosis of associated syndromes. Ankylosing spondylitis is an autoimmune condition with positive HLA-B27 and may have uveitis associated with the SI joint pain. Also, Reiter's syndrome is a triad of oligoarticular arthritis, conjunctivitis, and urethritis. Other conditions with similar presenting symptoms are facet disease, piriformis syndrome, and degenerative disc disease.

Physical Exam

The physical exam findings in SI joint problems will be pain with typically three or more provocative maneuvers. Many maneuvers exist and include palpating the SI joint and also the FABER test by flexing, abducting, and externally rotating the leg which should recreate the pain. Another maneuver is Gaenslen's test done by stressing both SI joints at once by having the patient lie flat on the examination table, flexing one knee to the chest and extending the other leg while it hangs off the table.

Imaging

An X-ray may show some nonspecific changes such as sclerosis, erosions, osteophytes, or ankylosis of the SI joint. Because of MRI's sensitivity

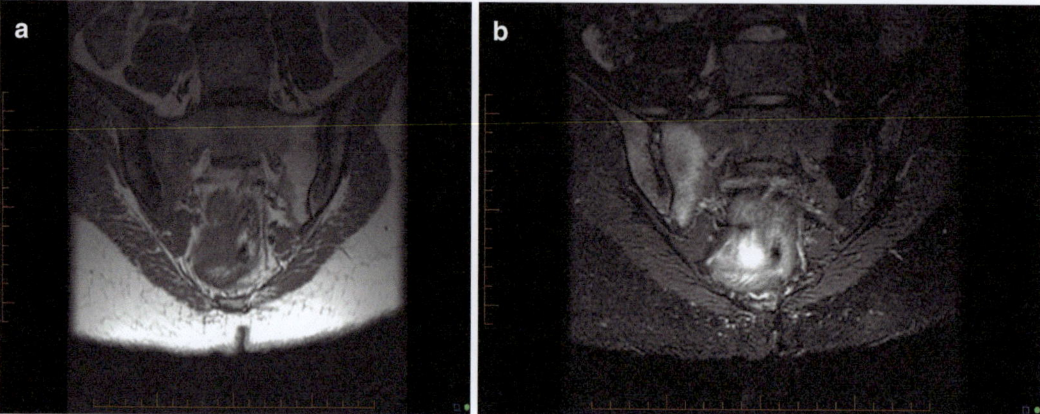

Fig. 17.3 (**a**) T1 coronal image showing areas of diminished signal within the sacrum and iliac bone along the right sacroiliac joint. T1 hyperintensity of the left sacrum likely is secondary to postinflammatory fatty infiltration. (**b**) STIR coronal image showing the increased signal on the right about the sacroiliac joint typical of sacroiliitis

to bone marrow edema and inflammatory changes, MRI with gadolinium is the preferred method of imaging. MRI will show edema, as well as synovial/joint space enhancement and fluid earlier than other methods. CT is useful when looking for abnormalities seen later in the course of the disease, such as sclerosis and ankylosis or when evaluating for subtle erosions (Fig. 17.3a, b).

Diagnostic Tests

SI joint injections with fluoroscopic guidance can not only be therapeutic but also diagnostic in cases of SI joint pain. Relief of pain after steroid or local anesthetics into the joint may be helpful in confirming the SI joint as the primary pathologic process. Lab tests can also help with diagnosis such as ESR, CRP, WBC for sacroiliitis, HLA-B27 for ankylosing spondylitis, and RF for the spondyloarthropathies. Patients with ankylosing spondylitis may ultimately autofuse this joint, and surgical treatment is not typically indicated.

Treatment

Conservative treatment is the first step such as NSAIDs and physical therapy. Continued pain may be improved with corticosteroid injections into the SI joint. The spondyloarthropathies may also require TNF inhibitors. For infection, IV antibiotics are warranted with a transition to oral antibiotics once symptoms improve.

Pharmacologic treatment for the various spondyloarthropathies is beyond the scope of treatment covered in this segment. Many new medications which modulate the immune response are being used in this capacity. Rheumatologic evaluation should be advised in such cases to direct treatment. If surgery is needed for anyone on these immune-modulating medications, careful attention must be given to stopping and restarting these medications in a timely fashion before and after surgery to minimize the risk of postsurgical infection.

Facet Disease/Synovial Facet Cyst

Facet disease is another generator of low back pain. Facet arthritis is a very common cause of low back pain as the cartilage within the joints may degenerate (Fig. 17.4a, b) Also, facet cysts filled with synovial fluid from the facet joint can form and cause some compression of the traversing neurologic structures.

Lumbar instability on flexion and extension is commonly identified among patients with a synovial cyst. Standing X-rays and flexion/extension

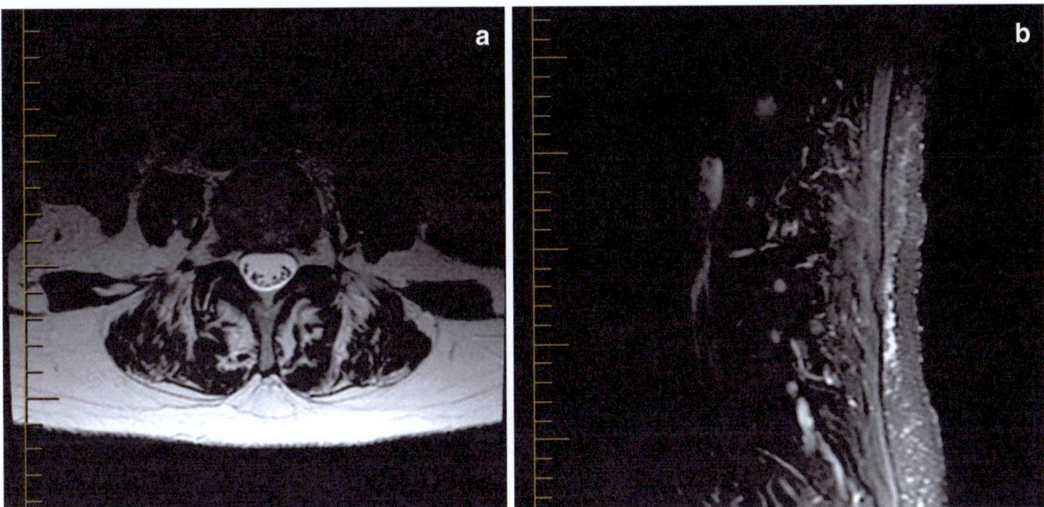

Fig. 17.4 Facet degeneration. (**a**) T2 axial image showing right facet effusion with some facet hypertrophic changes. (**b**) Sagittal STIR showing facet effusion with mild subjacent osseous edema

views should routinely be performed as it may have implications on the ultimate treatment.

History

Patients with facet arthritis will most likely have some component of low back pain and will typically present in the fifth or sixth decade of life or later. The pain typically has a mechanical component: worse with more vigorous activity and alleviated by rest. Synovial cysts occur in a broader age range and can have both axial lower back pain and radicular pain as presenting complaints. Facet cysts may wax and wane with respect to their size based on the level of the patient's activity. Thus the symptoms associated with synovial cysts may be better or worse at times as the cyst changes in size/shape.

Physical Exam

Neurologic exam may reveal tenderness to palpation of the low back near the specific arthritic facet joints. Facet syndrome typically exhibits pain with extension of the lumbar spine as the spine preferentially loads the posterior elements in extension. Pain may also be seen with lateral bending toward the affected facet joint for the same reason.

Careful neurologic examination should be performed to identify the precise nerve root which is compressed.

Imaging/Diagnostic Tests

X-rays can aid in the diagnosis of facet arthritis with the facet joints appearing sclerotic and hypertrophied on both PA and lateral radiographs. MRI is the most useful imaging study of the facet joints. Differentiating disc herniation from facet synovial cyst can only be accurately accomplished with MRI (Fig. 17.3). Also correctly identifying facet synovitis by visualizing facet joint edema, synovial fluid/thickening, and perifacet inflammation is frequently only conspicuous on MRI rather than CT or X-ray (Fig. 17.4a, b). MRI with contrast, in this scenario, can improve the sensitivity to facet joint inflammation demonstrating enhancement within and around the facet joint.

Treatment

Conservative management is the mainstay of treatment for both facet degeneration and synovial cysts. Arthritis may be improved with

NSAIDs and physical therapy and possibly ultimately with corticosteroid injections. Patients who experience substantial pain relief with corticosteroid facet injections may find better and longer-lasting relief with radiofrequency ablation of the nerve which innervates the facet joint complex.

Facet cysts may resolve over time, but if they do not regress with time and continue to cause symptoms, then surgical excision may be warranted to remove the cyst. A synovial cyst without associated spondylolisthesis may be treated with just a laminotomy to gain access to the cyst and cyst removal. Larger cysts and cysts found in conjunction with spondylolisthesis may require more expansile decompression and fusion to prevent postsurgical instability or cyst recurrence (Fig. 17.5a, b).

Hamstring Injury with Avulsion

Hamstring injuries when associated with avulsion can cause posterior hip pain. Most hamstring injuries occur at the myotendinous junction; however, the hamstring can avulse the ischial tuberosity. The hamstring includes the semitendinosus and semimembranosus and biceps femoris muscles.

History

The patient may give a history of participating in physical activity such as sprinting or water skiing during the time of injury. They may describe feelings of a "pop" during exercise with bruising and swelling afterward. Tears can be acute or chronic.

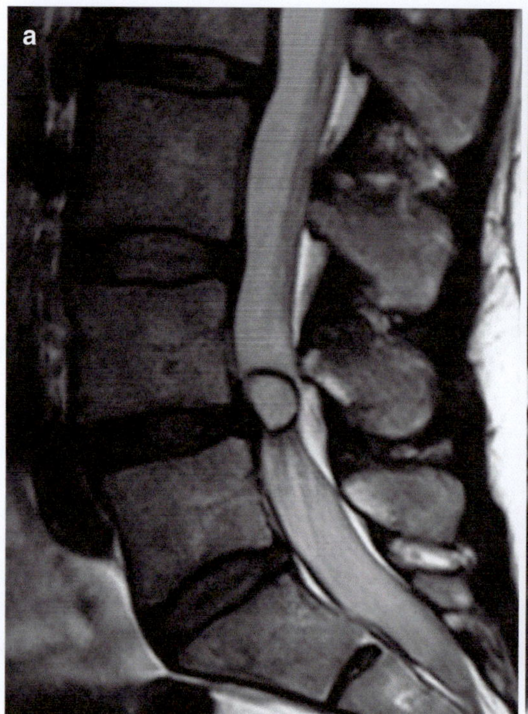
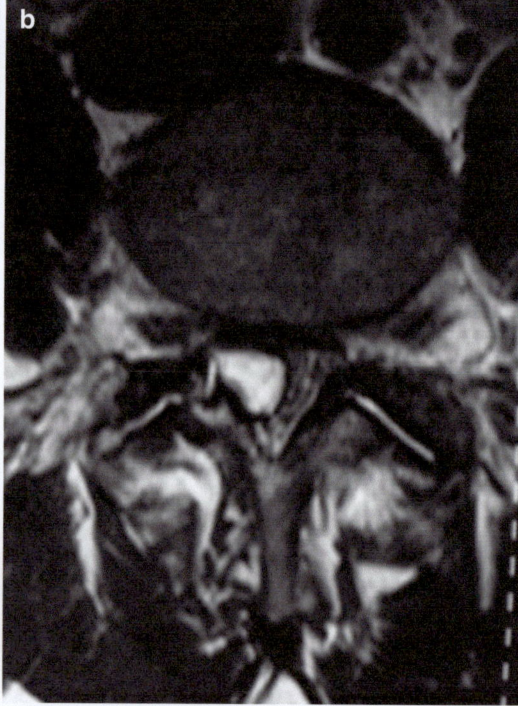

Fig. 17.5 Synovial cyst causing spinal stenosis. (**a**) Sagittal T2 image showing the synovial cyst at the L4/L5 disc level. (**b**) Axial T2 MRI image at L4/L5 disc level. Right-sided synovial cyst from the right L4/L5 facet joint. This is typically found in the setting of subtle spondylolisthesis such as in this case

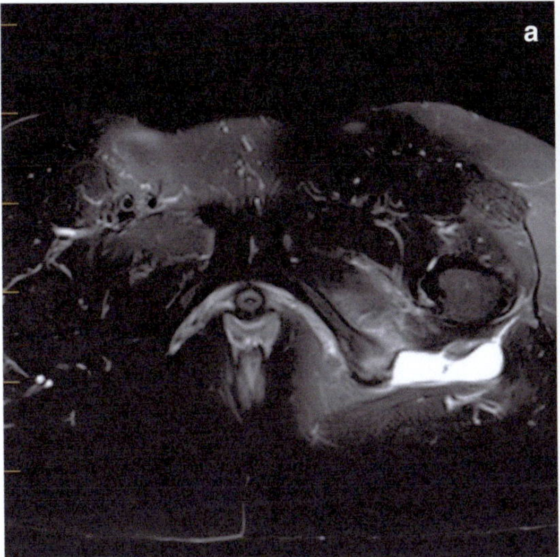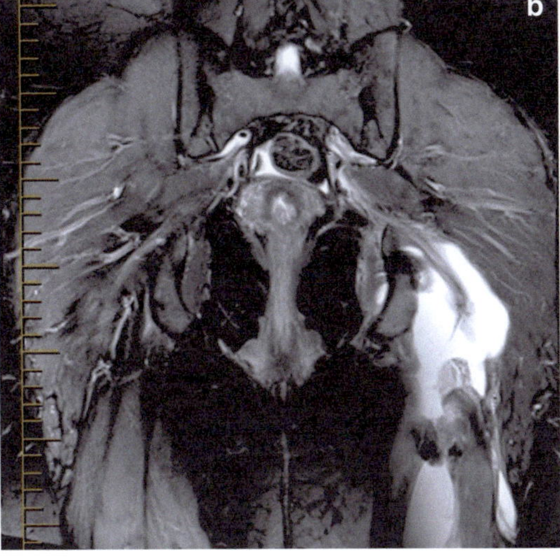

Fig. 17.6 Hamstring avulsion injury. (**a**) Axial STIR image showing absent left hamstring tendon at the level of the ischial tuberosity with edema and hemorrhage within the subjacent soft tissues. Edema is also seen in the left ischial tuberosity. (**b**) Coronal STIR image showing the complete avulsion on the left with distal retraction of the tendon (arrow) and extensive surrounding hematoma

Physical Exam

Upon physical exam, there may be extensive ecchymosis and edema as well as a palpable mass in the posterior thigh. Often times the patient will have difficulty walking or running immediately after the injury.

Imaging

Plain X-rays of the pelvis may show an avulsion at the ischial tuberosity with avulsed bone fragment. However this is less common in adults as opposed to adolescents where the apophysis will avulse due to lack of complete ossification. MRI is the exam of choice. Not only will it show the avulsed tendon but it will better show the degree of tendon retraction (Fig. 17.6).

Treatment

A hamstring injury with rupture at the myotendinous juncture warrants limited weight-bearing status for a few weeks with stretching and strengthening to follow. An avulsion injury may warrant operative repair of the hamstring tendon to the ischial tuberosity with suture anchors. The decision to operate depends on patient demands and extent of injury and disability.

Lumbar Spinal Stenosis

Background

Spinal stenosis of the lumbar spine is typically a multifactorial condition that results in narrowing of the entire spinal canal. Impingement of the spinal canal is typically caused by a combination of facet hypertrophy, disc bulge, and thickening of the ligamentum flavum. It is a common cause of posterior hip pain. The incidence of spinal stenosis increases significantly after age 60. Spinal stenosis is nearly always present in the face of a degenerative spondylolisthesis. When a spondylolisthesis is present, the stenosis will usually affect the subarticular recess preferentially.

Many authors support a multifactorial etiology in the progression of lumbar stenosis. Disc degeneration alters mechanics and loading of facet joints. The stress on the facet joint leads to hypertrophy of the facets, joint capsule, and ligamentum flavum, all of which result in decreased space in the spinal canal. Placing the lumbar spine in extension causes the ligamentum flavum to buckle and further decrease the spinal canal diameter. Thus, patients have increased symptoms when in extension.

History

Patients with lumbar spinal stenosis often complain of lower back pain, buttock and leg pain, pseudoclaudication, standing discomfort, numbness, and lower extremity weakness. These symptoms are usually exacerbated with walking, standing, descending hills, and going down stairs. Their pain will start proximally and proceed distally. Patients usually report relief of symptoms with changes in position (sitting down, leaning forward). Patients' buttock and leg pain is usually unilateral neurogenic pain that can radiate down the leg. Pain is not commonly located in the groin, as is common with hip pathology. Other symptoms can include bladder disturbances and cauda equina syndrome.

Neurogenic claudication can be distinguished from vascular claudication in that it is typically worse with extension of the back and relieved with flexion of the back, whereas vascular claudication is exacerbated by activity not position. See the section on vascular claudication for further distinguishing features.

Physical Exam

Patients with lumbar stenosis will tend to have a normal physical exam. They will usually exhibit focal tenderness to palpation in the lumbar spine that correlates with the location of impingement. Patients may also exhibit lower extremity weakness that follows a segmental pattern in accor-

dance with which nerve root is being impinged. Patients generally will *NOT* have tenderness to palpation in the buttock or groin. Symptoms will not be reproduced with passive hip ROM. If vascular claudication is suspected, ABIs are appropriate.

Similar Presenting Conditions

As highlighted in the background section, lumbar stenosis may be caused by a wide variety of conditions. The symptoms that are common to these conditions can also be present in other conditions such as vascular claudication, hip osteoarthritis, avascular necrosis of the femoral head, piriformis syndrome, trochanteric bursitis, Tarlov cysts, facet cysts, sacroiliac joint disease, and peripheral neuropathy.

Imaging

Proper imaging is critical to the diagnosis of lumbar spinal stenosis. Imaging studies should include AP, lateral and oblique radiographs, flexion-extension radiographs, MRI, and/or CT myelogram. It is very important to obtain standing lumbar radiographs. On the standing X-rays the following issues should be specifically reviewed: standing posture, presence or absence of spondylolisthesis, or instability on flexion and extension. It is not unusual that MRI or CT will miss a subtle spondylolisthesis due to the recumbent position that the images are obtained. Oblique radiographs may be helpful to identify pars lesions or spondylolysis. From cross-sectional images, MRI is again the diagnosis of choice. The stenosis will be visible, but the dominant cause of the stenosis (disc, facet, ligamentum flavum, epidural lipomatosis) and where the stenosis is located will be visible (Fig. 17.7). CT myelography is beneficial in those patients in whom MRI cannot be obtained, but myelography is not a simple or straightforward procedure in patients with severe spinal stenosis.

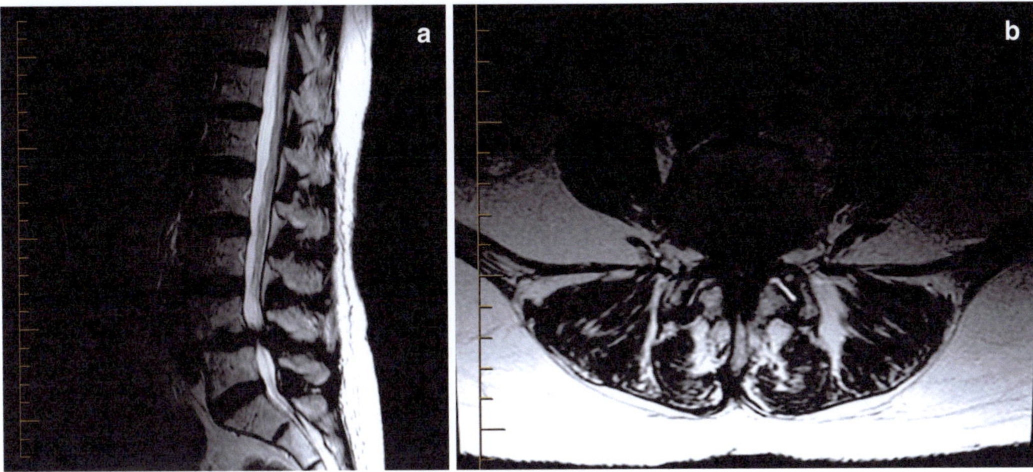

Fig. 17.7 Spinal stenosis. (**a** and **b**) Sagittal and axial T2 images showing spondylolisthesis and severe spinal and subarticular stenosis at L4/L5 from a combination of spondylolisthesis, disc bulge, facet degeneration, and ligamentum flavum buckling

Special Diagnostic Testing

EMG is a useful tool to differentiate lumbar spinal stenosis from peripheral neuropathy or piriformis syndrome. Ankle-brachial index should be part of the assessment if vascular claudication in suspected.

Treatment

Nonsurgical interventions for lumbar spinal stenosis have marginal long-term efficacy. They include drug therapy, physical therapy, and epidural steroid injections. Drug therapy should consist of acetaminophen and NSAIDs initially. Narcotics and muscle relaxants should be used sparingly and only on a short-term basis. Physical therapy should focus on core strengthening, lumbar stabilization, flexibility, and aerobic conditioning. Epidural steroid injections can provide pain relief for patients on a short-term basis, but they have not been shown to change the natural progression of disease or decrease the need for future surgical intervention.

Patients whose symptoms are recalcitrant to nonsurgical treatment regimens are candidates for surgical intervention. The mainstay of surgical intervention for lumbar spinal stenosis is direct nerve root decompression via laminectomy or laminotomy. Spinal fusion surgery is generally not indicated for patient with spinal stenosis without instability or other spinal deformities (i.e., scoliosis). Indirect nerve root decompression via distraction of the disc space or other interspinous process device (Coflex, X-stop) may be reasonable in some selected cases. However, the results of the SPORT (Spine Patient Outcomes Research Trial) study demonstrate the very good and reproducible outcomes that may be achieved via lumbar laminectomy.

Degenerative Disc Disease

As patients age, the composition of vertebral discs is altered. The number of viable cells decreases, as does the amount of proteoglycans within the nucleus of the disc space. The decrease in proteoglycans leads to a loss of hydration within the disc. The resultant structural changes include an expansion of the inner layers of the annulus and decreased disc height and ultimately lead to altered biomechanics (as previously discussed in the lumbar spinal stenosis section). These degenerative changes are termed degenerative disc disease (DDD). DDD causes an increase in mechanical load and stress on the ligaments and facet joints around the degenerative disc. This leads to abnormal motion and hypertrophy of the affected facets.

Common comorbidities associated with DDD include diabetes mellitus, vascular insufficiency, and smoking; however no causal link has been established.

History

The primary manifestation of DDD is back pain without radiculopathy. Patients will complain of midline pain in the lumbar spine that can usually be well-localized. This pain may be exacerbated by axial loading, sitting, and bending. It is also important to differentiate whether the pain is acute or chronic.

Acute low back pain is described as lower back pain of less than 3 months duration that is functionally limiting. It is not usually accompanied by neurologic symptoms, is usually self-limiting, and typically resolves within a short time frame. EMG and other nerve conduction studies generally are not warranted.

While most causes of acute low back pain resolve over time, some acute pathology requires immediate attention. These include metastatic disease, infection, vertebral fracture, cauda equina syndrome, and herniated nucleus pulposus. As such, it is imperative that a thorough history includes questions of cancer history, unexplained weight loss, fever, recent sickness or infection, changes in mental status, recent trauma or fall, urinary retention, saddle anesthesia, numbness, tingling, and neurologic deficit. Positive findings to any of these lines of question should alert the provider to investigate further.

Evaluation of chronic low back pain can be multifaceted and nuanced. In general, pain should be localized to a specific region of the spine, and the patient should be asked to distinguish the nature of the pain. As with acute low back pain, chronic low back pain must be evaluated for pathology that requires immediate attention, such as fracture, neoplasm, or infection. It is also criti-

cal to screen for underlying psychiatric disease, secondary gain, and inconsistencies in history and exam findings.

Physical Exam

On physical exam, patients with DDD will demonstrate midline TTP over specific areas of the lower back that correspond to the levels where DDD changes are occurring. It is important to differentiate this mechanical pain from myofascial pain. They may also have a decreased or painful range of motion. Tension signs such as straight leg testing and bowstring testing will usually be normal.

Similar Presenting Conditions

As discussed in the history section, metastatic disease, infection, vertebral fracture, cauda equina syndrome, and herniated nucleus pulposus can all mimic some of the symptoms of DDD. In addition, there are many abdominal conditions that can present with low back pain as a primary symptom. These include abdominal aortic aneurysm, renal colic, pelvic inflammatory disease, UTI, and retrocecal appendicitis.

Imaging

Radiographs may show disc height loss or may be normal. If DDD is suspected, MR is again the imaging study of choice. Characteristic findings of DDD on MRI would include disc height loss and a low signal (black disc) on T2-weighted image without significant herniation or stenosis. As progressive pathologic disc degeneration ensues, osteophyte formation, intradiscal/nuclear gas, annular tears/high-intensity zones, and Modic changes in the subjacent vertebral bodies can be seen though not necessarily in that order. At this point the findings are starting to move beyond the realm of normal (aging related) degeneration and toward pathologic degeneration (internal disc disruption).

Special Diagnostic Testing

Provocative discography has been used as a means of confirming DDD as the source of low back pain. A positive test shows concordant pain response, shows abnormal disc morphology on fluoroscopy, and has negative lumbar spine control levels. While diagnostically accurate, discography is somewhat controversial. Possible injury to the disc at control levels and the subjective nature of how the results are interpreted by the examiner have been some of the shortcomings of this technique.

Treatment

Nonoperative management includes rest, activity modification, taking of NSAIDs and muscle relaxants, bracing, and physical therapy focusing on stretching, strengthening, and weight control. Other interventions that have shown benefit include behavioral modification, smoking cessation, and activity modification.

Immediate surgical intervention is necessary for cases of neoplasia, infection, fracture, HNP, or in patients who develop neurological deficits including those with cauda equina syndrome. In such cases, surgical intervention should be tailored to treat the specific cause and will not be covered in detail in this section.

Surgical management of confirmed DDD should only be pursued if the patient has had persistent symptoms that do not resolve with a 6-month regimen of nonoperative treatment as previously described. Options for surgical intervention include lumbar discectomy and fusion, transforaminal interbody fusion or lumbar total disc replacement.

Piriformis Syndrome

Background

Compression of the sciatic nerve after it leaves the pelvis can cause posterior hip and leg pain known as piriformis syndrome. This entrapment can occur anterior to the piriformis and posterior to the gemelli and obturator internus at the level of the ischial tuberosity.

History

Patients with piriformis syndrome will complain of posterior gluteal pain that migrates down the back of the leg that is often described as burning or aching in nature. See Chap. 8.

Physical Exam

Patients with piriformis syndrome can demonstrate tenderness to palpation lateral to the ischial tuberosity and/or weakness or diminished sensation in the lower leg. The definitive test for piriformis syndrome is conducted by passively placing stress on the piriformis and short external rotators. This is known as the FAIR Test due to the proper positioning (flexion, adduction, internal rotation). The FAIR Test is positive when placing the patient in this position and leads to a reproduction of symptoms.

Imaging

In patients with piriformis syndrome, radiographs are usually negative. Initially MRI of the pelvis was thought to also bear little additional information but has now proven to be a useful test. Findings frequently seen include piriformis enlargement (of multiple causes), muscle inflammation and scaring, and congenital muscular variants of size and attachment (Fig. 17.8).

Lumbar MRI is helpful in ruling out spinal causes of nerve compression that could mimic a lower entrapment neuropathy.

Special Diagnostic Testing

Electrodiagnostic studies such as EMG and nerve conduction studies are useful in the diagnosis of piriformis syndrome and may demonstrate

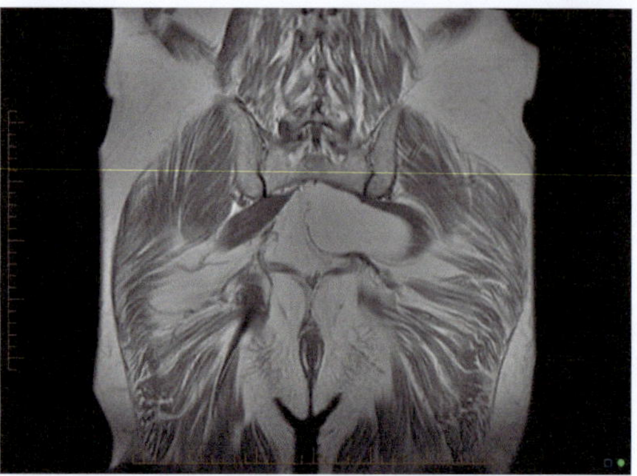

Fig. 17.8 Piriformis syndrome. T1 coronal image showing a left piriformis lipoma (arrow) in someone presenting with left piriformis syndrome. Normal right piriformis on the right (arrow)

functional impairment of sciatic nerve. However, negative results do not exclude piriformis syndrome as the diagnosis.

Treatment

Nonoperative management includes rest, taking of NSAIDs and muscle relaxants, physical therapy focusing on stretching the piriformis muscles and short external rotators, and corticosteroid injections directed near the piriformis muscle.

Surgical management is indicated only in refractory cases without response to conservative treatment and consists of piriformis muscle release or external sciatic neurolysis.

Peripheral Vascular Disease

Background

Arterial insufficiency is due to narrowing of the arteries in the lower extremities. Atherosclerosis leads to a narrowing of the arterial blood supply, such that when a patient has an increased oxygen demand (during exercise or walking for example) the diminished blood supply is not able to keep up with oxygen demand from the muscle tissue, resulting in intense pain and cramping of the legs. The popliteal artery is the most common location

of arterial insufficiency because it is the smallest diameter artery that is still a common location for atherosclerotic buildup. Incidence of arterial insufficiency increases with age. Most patients will be over 50 at first onset of symptoms. Hypertension, diabetes, smoking, and obesity are strongly correlated with arterial insufficiency. See Chap. 19.

History

The hallmark presenting symptom of arterial insufficiency is "vascular claudication." Claudication is defined as cramping activity-related leg pain. It has insidious onset over many years and leads to decreased activity levels. Patients relate that they are no longer able to walk for as long as they used to due to cramping pain in their feet, calves, and thighs. Patients report relief of symptoms with rest. Patients can also present with numbness and tingling in their feet. Symptoms can be unilateral or bilateral. In earlier stages, the symptoms are unaffected by changes in position. However, as disease advances, even standing can cause symptoms.

Physical Exam

Patients with arterial insufficiency can present with diminished or absent distal pulses, cold extremities, cyanosis, or atrophy in the affected limb. Atrophic changes can include loss of hair, atrophied muscles, and shiny skin. ABIs will be diminished in the affected limb.

Similar Presenting Conditions

It is important to distinguish between *neurogenic claudication* and vascular insufficiency as the source of pain in patients who present with claudication as their chief complaint. In general, vascular claudication is worsened with activity, while neurogenic claudication is worsened with position. Thus, a patient who relates relief of symptoms with decreased activity and notices no difference with postural changes is more likely to have vascular insufficiency. Conversely, extension of the lumbar spine closes down the area available for the spinal cord and increases neurogenic claudication. Thus, it is worsened by standing, walking upright, and walking downhill, but activity that places the back in flexion, such as walking downhill, riding a bicycle, or leaning over while pushing a shopping cart, will improve symptoms. Another determining factor in differentiation is the peripheral exam. Vascular claudication is more likely to present with abnormal pulses, skin changes, cyanosis, and cold extremities.

Imaging

Doppler ultrasound is the gold standard for initial noninvasive evaluation and readily identifies stenosis and occlusion of the vasculature. CT angiography and MR angiography are now routinely used for characterization of the location and degree of stenosis. Direct catheter angiography and arteriography can be useful for patients requiring more detailed surgical evaluation.

Treatment

Nonoperative management includes lifestyle modification and control of chronic medication conditions such as hypercholesterolemia, hypertension, and diabetes mellitus.

Operative management includes angioplasty, stenting, and arterial bypass grafting. Amputation often becomes necessary as a salvaging procedure in patients with uncontrolled diabetes.

Other Musculoskeletal Conditions/ Considerations

This chapter will not specifically address other conditions such as complications secondary to total hip arthroplasty or hip resurfacing. Ischiofemoral impingement and other intra-articular conditions of the hip joint are discussed elsewhere and are beyond the scope of this chapter.

Tarlov Cysts

Background

Tarlov (perineurial) cysts are one of the several distinct types of spinal meningeal cyst commonly found in the lumbosacral region (Fig. 17.9). They share the potential to cause symptomatic spinal nerve root compression and bone remodeling presenting as sacral or posterior hip pain. Unfortunately, knowledge concerning these cysts has historically been limited, and past teachings have been to avoid them at all costs. This most likely stems from their reputation for poor surgical outcomes and a high rate of complications, particularly cerebrospinal fluid (CSF) leakage. Though not a prerequisite for causing symptoms, Tarlov cysts can sometimes be radiologically impressive in size and extent (Fig. 17.10). These factors, along with the complexity of the presenting symptoms, can combine to pose a daunting treatment quandary, even for the most seasoned spine surgeon or pain management practitioner alike.

Unfortunately, when the diagnosis of a symptomatic Tarlov cyst is missed and standard evaluations for hip and SI joint pathology are unsurprisingly normal, patients are often relegated to endless pain clinic and physical therapy or simply told that there is nothing wrong and that their problem is psychological. Still worse, patients can be misdiagnosed with other orthopedic, spinal, gynecological, urological, or gastroenterological disorders and subjected to an endless array of unneeded interventions. Topping this list are misguided SI joint fusion, an assortment of spinal surgeries, hysterectomy (often while still of childbearing age), exploratory laparotomy, and bladder procedures (Fig. 17.11).

This section is therefore intended to give the reader an understanding of sacral Tarlov cysts and their presentation so that misdiagnosis can be prevented and patients can receive appropriate care.

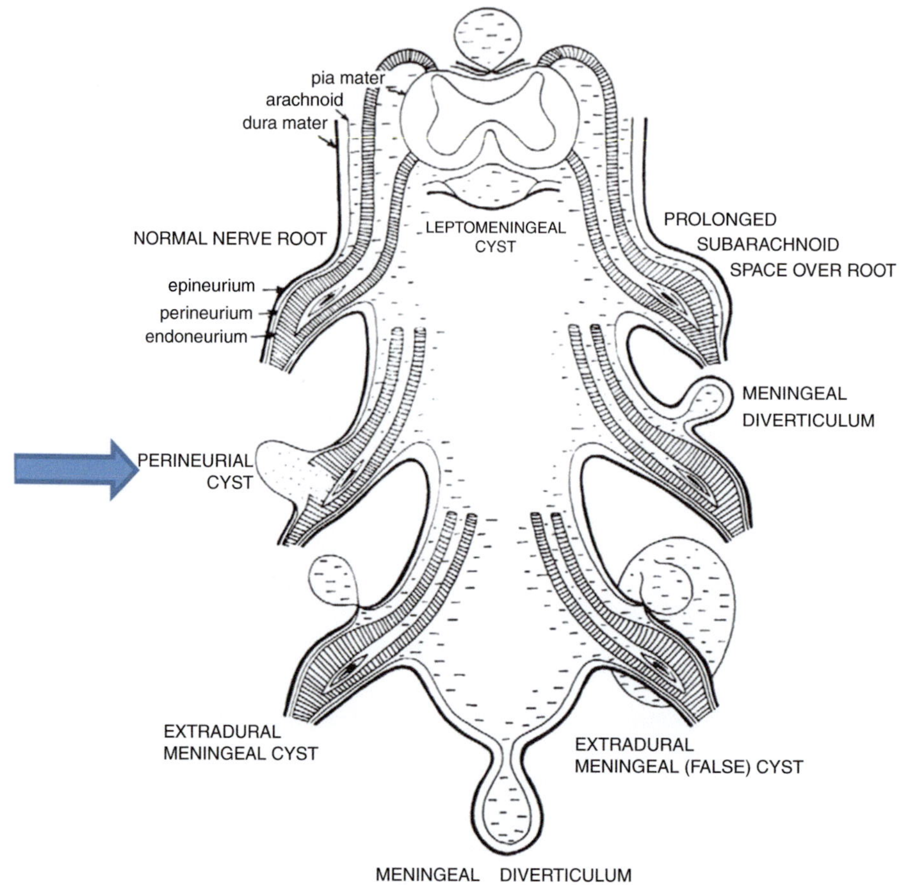

Fig. 17.9 Image from the original publication by IM Tarlov describing different types of meningeal cysts in the sacrum arising from the spinal sac, including perineurial cysts (arrow), which were later named after him

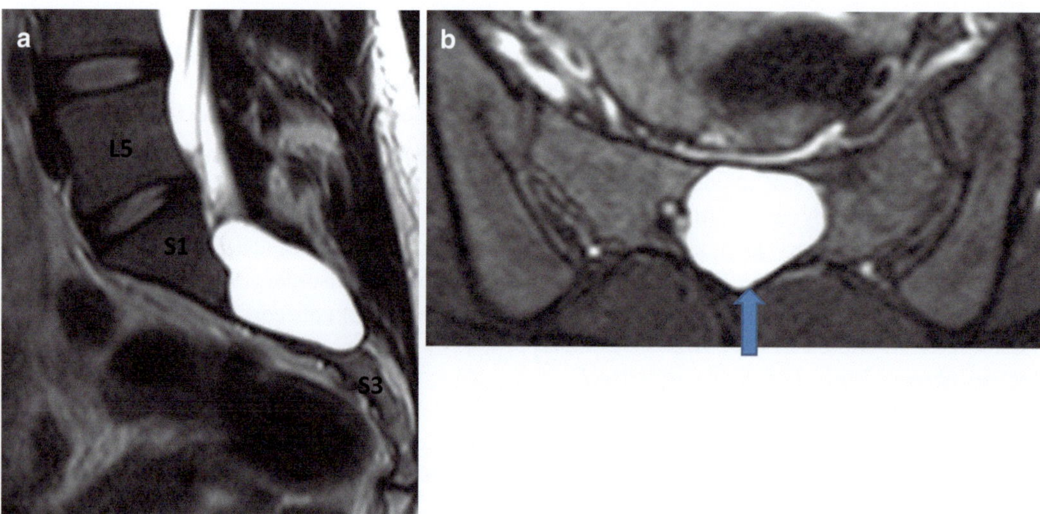

Fig. 17.10 A large sacral Tarlov cyst is seen on sagittal (**a**) and axial (**b**) T2-weighted MRI. The cyst fills the entire spinal canal from S1 to S3, compressing the nerve roots of the sacral cauda equina. The bone remodeling caused by the cyst is extensive, with the S2 vertebra almost no longer visible on the sagittal image. In fact, the cyst appears to have penetrated completely through the back of the sacral lamina dorsally on the axial view

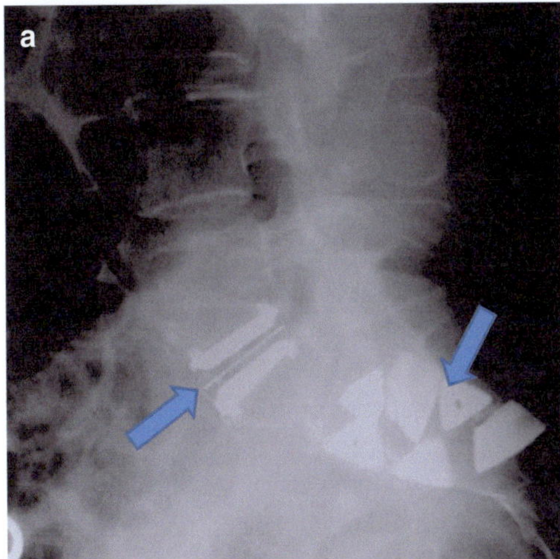

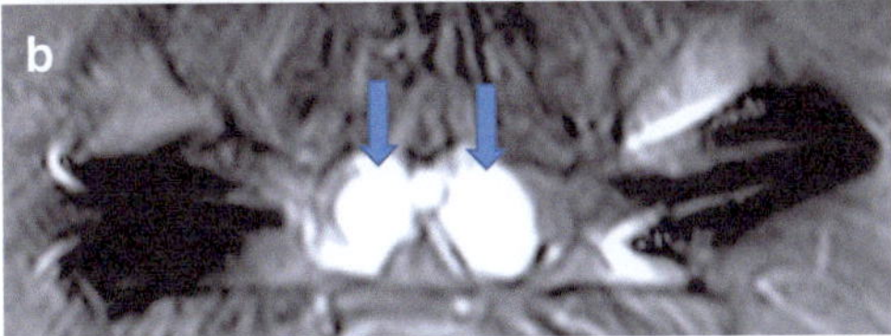

Fig. 17.11 The diagnosis of symptomatic Tarlov cysts was missed in this patient with posterior hip and sacral symptoms. Instead, she underwent artificial disc placement at L5/S1 (left arrow) and bilateral sacroiliac joint fusion procedures (right arrow), whose hardware can be seen on lateral X-ray of the pelvis (**a**). Despite the flanking presence of metal artifact from the patient's sacroiliac fusion procedures, an axial MRI of the sacrum (**b**) reveals two large Tarlov cysts filling the spinal canal (arrows), which turned out to be the true source of her symptoms

Pathophysiology

As defined by IM Tarlov himself, a Tarlov (perineurial) cyst is a dilation of a spinal nerve root arising proximal to the dorsal nerve root ganglion (Fig. 17.9). Although the term was originally intended to describe perineurial cysts alone, in current practice it is often misapplied to other types of spinal meningeal cysts due to their similar radiographic appearance.

The exact mechanism leading to Tarlov cyst formation has not yet been elucidated. By some mechanism, spinal fluid enters and accumulates within a nerve root, either as a result of being trapped there or due to laxity in the dura of the nerve root sleeve. Fluid accumulation in the nerve root then causes it to balloon, sometimes to the point of producing symptoms by compressing adjacent structures. Although they can form at any spinal level, symptomatic Tarlov cysts are most commonly found affecting the sacral nerve roots. They most often involve the portion of the nerve root in the spinal canal but can also develop anywhere along the course of a spinal nerve, including in the neural foramen and the retroperitoneal pelvis (Fig. 17.12).

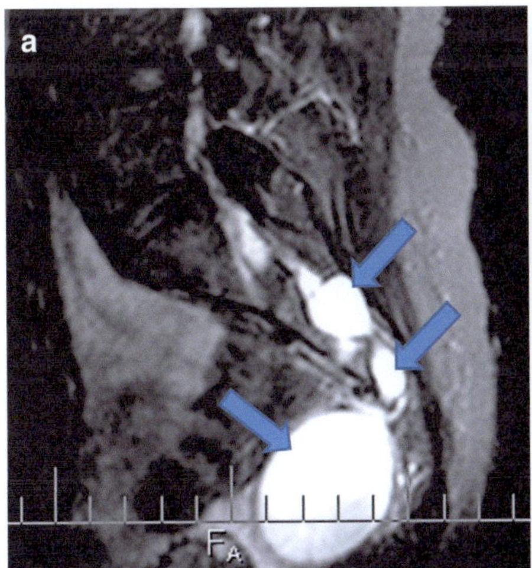

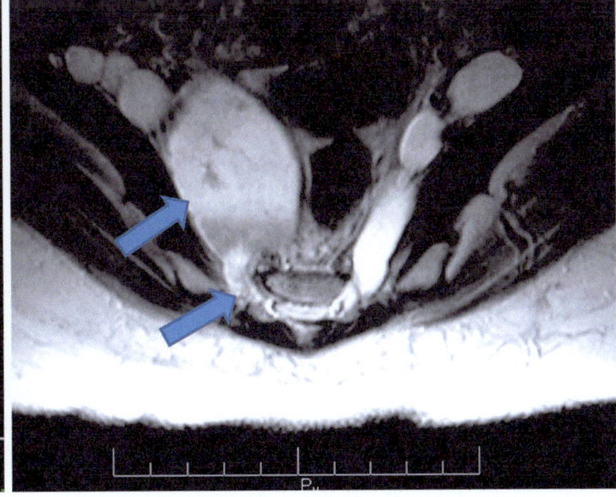

Fig. 17.12 A Tarlov cyst can develop along any portion of a spinal nerve root throughout its course, as seen in this patient with multiple cysts. On sagittal MRI (**a**), Tarlov cysts are seen in the spinal canal (upper arrow), in the foramina exiting the sacrum (middle arrow), and in the retroperitoneal pelvis (lower arrow). On axial MRI (**b**), both the intraforaminal (lower arrow) and retroperitoneal (upper arrow) portion of the same S3 nerve root have become cystic. The contralateral S3 nerve root is also cystic in appearance

Symptoms

Tarlov cysts can cause symptoms by producing mechanical compression of adjacent spinal nerve roots in the spinal canal. In the sacrum, this can result in a corresponding pattern of sacral radiculopathy symptoms (Table 17.1). The variety of symptoms displayed and their laterality depend on the location of the cyst/cysts and the extent to which they are compressing adjacent nerves. Compression of the S1 and S2 nerve roots typically produces sacral pain radiating to the buttock, posterior hip, and down to the back of the leg to the bottom or lateral aspect of the foot. Numbness in a similar distribution and weakness in plantar flexion and the intrinsic muscles of the foot are also often present.

Sacral and posterior hip pain almost always limits the ability to sit, with patients constantly squirming in their chair and avoiding seated activities. Interestingly, patients often adopt curious seated postures, constantly leaning far to one side in order to decrease direct pressure on the sacrum or hip. They also tend to carry special cushions with them to sit on for similar reasons despite the awkward nature of carrying a cushion or pillow in public.

Compression of S2, S3, or S4 can produce perineal pain and numbness. Neurogenic bladder symptoms are not uncommon, with the patient experiencing urinary urgency and frequency, as well as urinary retention requiring the patient to perform Valsalva or press on their abdomen (Crede maneuver) in order to empty their bladder completely. They can also have neurogenic bowel symptoms, with constipation requiring extensive laxative use or manual assistance to have a bowel movement. Some also describe the loss of sensation to know when to empty their bladder or bowel. Patients frequently describe dyspareunia, or painful intercourse, due to their perineal pain or sexual dysfunction due to the loss of perineal sensation.

The presence of sacral or posterior hip pain in combination with the above sacral radiculopathy symptoms should prompt an evaluation for Tarlov cyst or other pathology affecting the sacral nerve roots.

Imaging

MRI is currently the best modality for diagnosing spinal meningeal cysts, such as Tarlov cysts. The water content in the cerebrospinal fluid makes them stand out, particularly on T2-weighted imaging. Since Tarlov cysts arise from spinal nerve roots, they tend to be found laterally in the spinal canal, as opposed to centrally, which is more typical of other cyst types. Since each Tarlov cyst is a nerve root, it contains neural elements, and a careful search can sometimes reveal the fascicle bundle within a Tarlov cyst, particularly on axial images (Fig. 17.13).

Table 17.1 Common symptoms due to sacral Tarlov cysts

Sacral pain radiating to the hip, buttock, and down the back of the leg to the bottom of the foot
Numbness or tingling in a similar distribution
Weakness in plantar flexion and the intrinsic muscles of the foot
Perineal pain and numbness
Neurogenic bladder symptoms
Urinary urgency, frequency, and retention with the need to perform Valsalva or the Crede maneuver in order to empty completely
Neurogenic bowel symptoms
Constipation requiring the extensive use of laxatives or manual facilitation
Dyspareunia (painful intercourse)
Sexual dysfunction
Inability to tolerate sitting

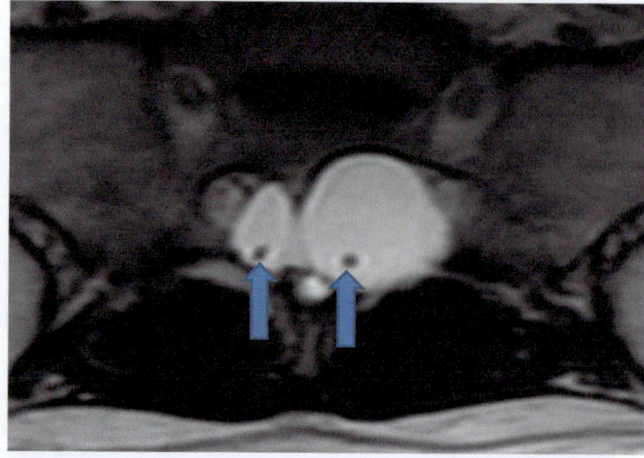

Fig. 17.13 Two Tarlov cysts are seen side by side filling the spinal canal in the sacrum on axial MRI. The spinal fluid filling the cysts appears bright. Each cyst is a spinal nerve root containing a nerve fascicle bundle that is clearly seen (arrows)

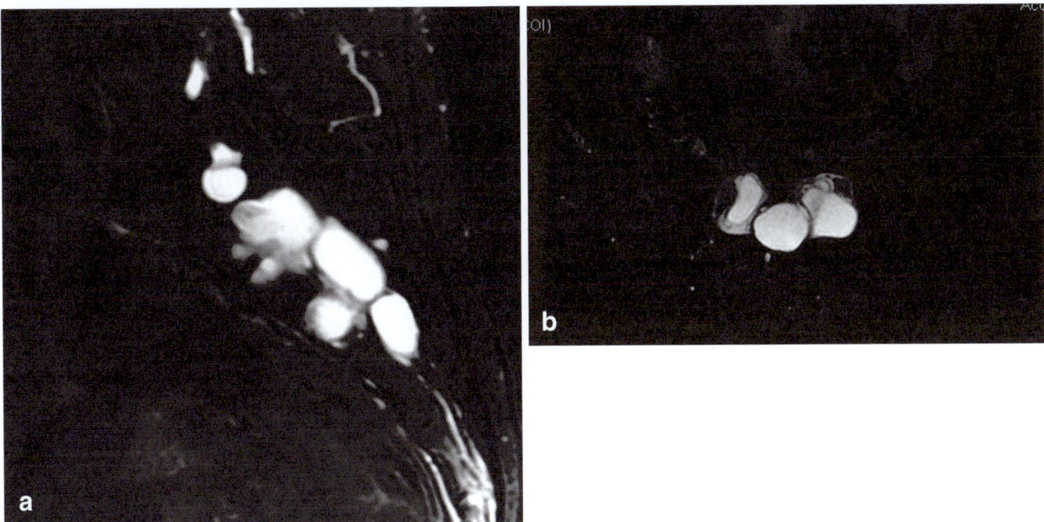

Fig. 17.14 This symptomatic patient had multiple Tarlov cysts in the spinal canal, as seen on sagittal (**a**) and axial (**b**) pelvic MRI. Interestingly, she was also known to have a connective tissue disorder, suggesting a causal relationship

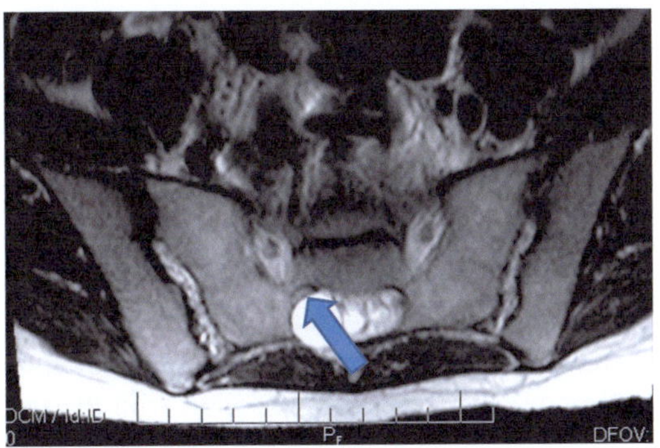

Fig. 17.15 In this patient with right S2 distribution symptoms, axial sacral MRI reveals a compressed right S2 nerve root (arrow tip) by a Tarlov cyst affecting the right S3 nerve root (obscured by arrow)

Tarlov cysts can be single, or multiple can be present in the same patient (Fig. 17.14). The likelihood of causing symptoms increases with the number of cysts, as their cumulative effect is to occupy a greater volume of the spinal canal typically reserved for the spinal nerve roots alone. In other words, multiple small cysts in the same area of the spinal canal have the same compressive effect as one large cyst of the same overall volume.

MRI also allows optimal visualization of the surrounding neural structures, such as adjacent spinal nerve roots under compression (Fig. 17.15). These relationships are critical for diagnosis, particularly when the laterality and distribution of a patient's symptoms can be correlated with a specific nerve root that is observed on MRI to be blatantly compressed by a Tarlov cyst. These relationships are also obviously important for surgical planning purposes. The addition of contrast to an MRI is useful for identifying other potential pathologies affecting the sacral nerve roots, such as tumors, including spinal schwannomas, neurofibromas, and meningiomas.

Although patients with larger cysts tend to have better surgical outcomes, it is not necessary for a cyst to be "big" to cause symptoms. Instead, it is more important to know its location and which nerves it is compressing. If the radiographic appearance of a Tarlov cyst can be correlated with the laterality and distribution of symptoms, then the cyst is suspect, regardless of its size.

Although one's attention when reviewing a lumbar MRI is easily distracted by a radiographically impressive sacral cyst, it is critical to review the entire imaging study for other potential sources of sacral and hip symptoms. A search for alternate pathology that might explain symptoms should also be made higher up in the lumbar spine, toward the sacroiliac joints, and in the pelvis, particularly as it relates to the lumbosacral plexus. Further clues can sometimes be found suggesting the presence of sacral nerve root dysfunction. For example, an abnormally distended bladder may reflect neurogenic urinary retention caused by a Tarlov cyst compressing the sacral nerve roots (Fig. 17.16).

CT scanning is of limited value in diagnosing Tarlov cysts since neural structures are not visualized. In certain instances it can be useful for delineating the extent of bone remodeling/erosion caused by a cyst or for identifying painful sacral insufficiency fractures (Fig. 17.17). CT myelography is a lesser alternative to MRI but may be necessary when patients harbor non-MRI-compatible hardware. However, the appearance of spinal meningeal cysts is variable and unreliable on CT myelography when compared to MRI. This is particularly true when the penetration of spinal fluid into a cyst is very slow and the dye does not have time to enter and fill the cyst. For this reason, additional cysts can sometimes be identified when delayed CT myelography images are obtained. Regardless, the absence of a spinal meningeal cyst cannot reliably be determined with CT myelography.

In antiquated theories, CT myelography was thought to be useful for distinguishing Tarlov cysts from other types of spinal meningeal cysts based on how fast they filled. However, these theories are illogical and have fallen by the wayside, primarily since the extent to which spinal meningeal cysts communicate with the spinal sac is not cyst specific. In other words, the size of the opening between the spinal sac and a meningeal cyst is not constant based on the cyst type.

Some spine surgeons erroneously use CT myelography to decide which Tarlov cysts to treat surgically, thinking that if the cyst is not seen on a CT myelogram, then the risk of postoperative cerebrospinal fluid leakage is eliminated. This assumption is essentially a gamble, because it can be safely said that, with rare exception, all Tarlov cysts are in communication with the spinal sac and have the potential to leak spinal fluid following surgery, regardless of how fast they filled with dye on a preoperative CT myelogram.

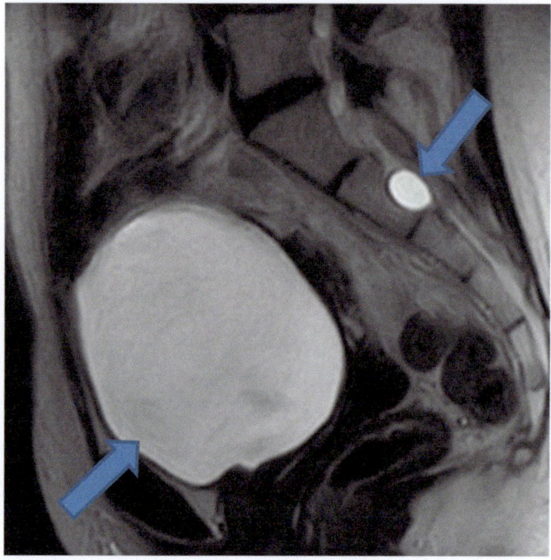

Fig. 17.16 Evidence of urinary retention caused by a Tarlov cyst (right arrow) compressing the sacral nerve roots is seen in the form of a severely distended bladder (left arrow)

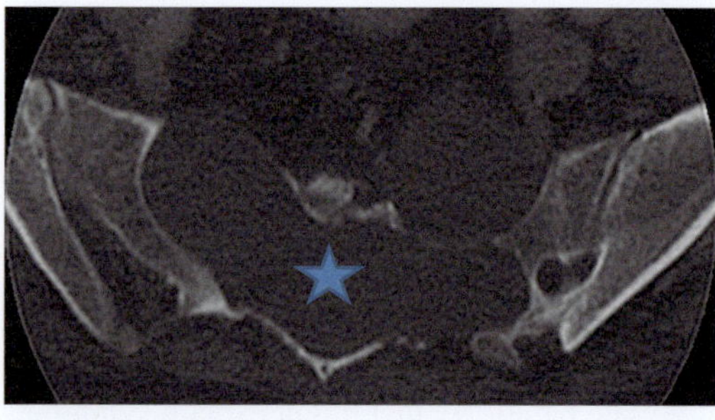

Fig. 17.17 The extent to which Tarlov cysts can produce sacral osseous destruction is evident on this axial CT of the sacrum where spinal canal (star) and foramina are dramatically enlarged and there is extensive bone loss. The patient presented after a fall with pelvic-spinal dislocation due to sacral insufficiency fractures

Electrodiagnostics

The use of EMG and nerve conduction studies in the evaluation of sacral Tarlov cysts is usually of little benefit since they routinely do not assess nerve function below the level of S1. Dysfunction of the S2–S4 nerve roots, which are the most likely to be impacted by symptomatic sacral Tarlov cysts, is therefore missed. For this reason it is not unusual to encounter patients with blatant sacral nerve root dysfunction and a completely normal electrodiagnostic study. Some centers perform EMG studies which do evaluate the lower sacral nerve roots, but patient discomfort is significant since it requires placement of multiple needles in the perineum.

Treatment

In cases where a Tarlov cyst is the suspected etiology, the presence of neurological deficit or progressively worsening symptoms should prompt referral to a clinician experienced in their diagnosis and treatment. An attempt at conservative management can be made in patients without neurological deficit provided a careful evaluation for lumbosacral spinal nerve dysfunction has been made. Conservative management efforts typically involve physical therapy and pain management focused on lumbar spine, hip, and SI joint but are usually ineffective or make symptoms worse. In some centers pelvic floor therapy is an option for perineal and pelvic symptoms, although data on its effectiveness is sparse.

For the most part, needle procedures near a spinal meningeal cyst should be limited to selective nerve blocking in experienced hands for the purposes of diagnosis. For example, if a patient with left S2 distribution symptoms has a Tarlov cyst compressing the left S2 nerve root, then a diagnostic left S2 nerve root block followed by temporary symptomatic relief can help confirm the diagnosis.

Practitioners should resist the urge to order percutaneous drainage procedures. Tarlov cysts are in direct communication with the spinal fluid of the spinal sac. Drainage alone is therefore pointless, since the cyst simply refills again, with the patient having been exposed to risks such as cerebrospinal fluid infection, hemorrhage, or nerve injury. Some centers inject materials into Tarlov cysts, such as fibrin glue, simplistically thinking that it will somehow prevent further entry of spinal fluid into the cyst. However, this technique has multiple shortcomings, with prior publications describing postinjection meningitis and adhesive arachnoiditis, since any substance introduced into a Tarlov cyst is also introduced into the CSF of the central nervous system. Additionally, fibrin glue injection complicates subsequent definitive surgical treatment by mak-

ing nerve fascicles within a Tarlov cyst more difficult to identify intraoperatively and protect.

Tarlov cysts cannot simply be resected since each cyst is a spinal nerve root. This is particularly true in the sacrum; nerve root sectioning can result in unacceptable deficits, such as the loss of bowel and bladder function. Alternate surgical approaches, such as performing a laminectomy to "give the nerves space" without treating the Tarlov cyst/s, have been tried and failed, as might be expected.

Attempting Tarlov cyst surgery without specific experience in their treatment often leads to a long, punishing misadventure, even among those with extensive skills in other areas of spine surgery. To complicate matters further, Tarlov cysts often appear similar to other types of spinal meningeal cysts on preoperative imaging, and the cyst type is sometimes not definitely known until it is evaluated intraoperatively. There is significant variability in the surgical strategy required to treat different types of meningeal cysts and the ability recognize and treat each cyst type is needed. Therefore, reliance on intraoperative improvisation is ill-advised, and a strong argument can be made that surgery for these complex cysts is best accomplished by those with specific experience in their treatment.

Bibliography

1. Devin CJ, McCullough KA, Morris BJ, Yates AJ, Kang JD. Hip-spine syndrome. J Am Acad Orthop Surg. 2012;20:434–42.
2. Savage JW, Patel AA. Fixed sagittal plane imbalance. Global Spine J. 2014;4:287–96.
3. Jauregui JJ, Banerjee S, Issa K, Cherian JJ, Mont MA. Does co-existing lumbar spinal canal stenosis impair functional outcomes and activity levels after primary total hip arthroplasty? J Arthorplasty. 2015;30:1569–73.
4. Lazennec J, Brusson A, Rousseau M. Hip-spine relations and sagittal balance clinical consequences. Eur Spine J. 2011;20(suppl 5):S686–98.
5. Fogel GR, Esses SI. Hip spine syndrome: management of coexisting radiculopathy and arthritis of the lower extremity. Spine J. 2003;3:238–41.
6. Ben-Galim P, Ben-Galim T, Rand N, et al. Hip-spine syndrome: the effect of total hip replacement surgery on low back pain in severe osteoarthritis of the hip. Spine (Phila Pa 1976). 2007;32:2099–102.

7. Offierski CM, MacNab I. Hip-spine syndrome. Spine. 1983;8:316–21.

8. Fardon DF, Milette PC. Nomenclature and classification of lumbar disc pathology. Recommmendations of the combined task forces of the North American Spine Society, American Society of Spine Radiology, and American Society of Neuroradiology. Spine (Phila Pa 1976). 2001;26(5):E93–E113.

9. Jordan J, Konstantinou K, O'Dowd J. Herniated lumbar disc. BMJ Clin Evid. 2011;2011:1118.

10. Boden SD. The use of radiographic imaging studies in the evaluation of patients who have degenerative disorders of the lumbar spine. J Bone Joint Surg Am. 1996;78(1):114–24.

11. Borenstein DG, O'Mara JW Jr, et al. The value of magnetic resonance imaging of the lumbar spine to predict low-back pain in asymptomatic subjects: a seven-year follow-up study. J Bone Joint Surg Am. 2011;83-A(9):1306–11.

12. Rhee JM, Schaufele M, Abdu WA. Radiculopathy and the herniated lumbar disc. Controversies regarding pathophysiology and management. J Bone Joint Surg Am. 2006;88(9):2070–80.

13. Casey E. Natural history of radiculopathy. Phys Med Rehabil Clin N Am. 2011;22(1):105.

14. Aydin S, Abuzayed B, et al. Discal cysts of the lumbar spine: report of five cases and review of the literature. Eur Spine J. 2010;19(10):1621–6.

15. Egund N, Jurik A. Anatomy and histology of the sacroiliac joints. Semin Musculoskelet Radiol. 2014;18(03):332–40.

16. Forst S, Wheeler M. The sacroiliac joint: anatomy, physiology and clinical significance. Pain Physician. 2006;9:61–8.

17. Schaeren S, Broger I, Jeanneret B. Minimum four-year follow-up of spinal stenosis with degenerative spondylolisthesis treated with decompression and dynamic stabilization. Spine (Phila Pa 1976). 2008;33(18):E636–42. https://doi.org/10.1097/BRS.0b013e31817d2435.

18. Abdu WA, Lurie JD, Spratt KF, et al. Degenerative spondylolisthesis: does fusion method influence outcome? Four-year results of the spine patient outcomes research trial. Spine (Phila Pa 1976). 2009;34(21):2351–60. https://doi.org/10.1097/BRS.0b013e3181b8a829.

19. Fischgrund JS, Mackay M, Herkowitz HN, Brower R, Montgomery DM, Kurz LT. Volvo award winner in clinical studies. Degenerative lumbar spondylolisthesis with spinal stenosis: a prospective, randomized study comparing decompressive laminectomy and arthrodesis with and without spinal instrumentation. Spine (Phila Pa 1976). 1997;22(24):2807–12. http://www.ncbi.nlm.nih.gov/pubmed/9431616. Accessed 27 Apr 2016.

20. Weinstein JN, Lurie JD, Tosteson TD, et al. Surgical compared with nonoperative treatment for lumbar degenerative spondylolisthesis four-year results in the Spine Patient Outcomes Research Trial (SPORT) randomized and observational cohorts. J Bone Joint Surg Am. 2009;91(6):1295–304. https://doi.org/10.2106/JBJS.H.00913.

21. Tosteson ANA, Tosteson TD, Lurie JD, et al. Comparative effectiveness evidence from the spine patient outcomes research trial: surgical versus non-operative care for spinal stenosis, degenerative spondylolisthesis, and intervertebral disc herniation. Spine (Phila Pa 1976). 2011;36(24):2061–8. https://doi.org/10.1097/BRS.0b013e318235457b.

22. Martin CR, Gruszczynski AT, Braunsfurth HA, Fallatah SM, O'Neil J, Wai EK. The surgical management of degenerative lumbar spondylolisthesis: a systematic review. Spine (Phila Pa 1976). 2007;32(16):1791–8. https://doi.org/10.1097/BRS.0b013e3180bc219e.

23. Radcliff K, Hilibrand A, Lurie JD, et al. The impact of epidural steroid injections on the outcomes of patients treated for lumbar disc herniation: a subgroup analysis of the SPORT trial. J Bone Joint Surg Am. 2012;94(15):1353–8. https://doi.org/10.2106/JBJS.K.00341.

24. Radcliff KE, Rihn J, Hilibrand A, et al. Does the duration of symptoms in patients with spinal stenosis and degenerative spondylolisthesis affect outcomes?: analysis of the Spine Outcomes Research Trial. Spine (Phila Pa 1976). 2011;36(25):2197–210. https://doi.org/10.1097/BRS.0b013e3182341edf.

25. Weinstein JN, Tosteson TD, Lurie JD, et al. Surgical versus nonsurgical therapy for lumbar spinal stenosis. N Engl J Med. 2008;358(8):794–810. https://doi.org/10.1056/NEJMoa0707136.

26. Weinstein JN, Lurie JD, Tosteson TD, et al. Surgical versus nonsurgical treatment for lumbar degenerative spondylolisthesis. N Engl J Med. 2007;356(22):2257–70. https://doi.org/10.1056/NEJMoa070302.

27. Hopayian K, Song F, Riera R, Sambandan S. The clinical features of the piriformis syndrome: a systematic review. Eur Spine J. 2010;19(12):2095–109. https://doi.org/10.1007/s00586-010-1504-9.

28. Jawish RM, Assoum HA, Khamis CF. Anatomical, clinical and electrical observations in piriformis syndrome. J Orthop Surg Res. 2010;5:3. https://doi.org/10.1186/1749-799X-5-3.

29. Pokorný D, Jahoda D, Veigl D, Pinskerová V, Sosna A. Topographic variations of the relationship of the sciatic nerve and the piriformis muscle and its relevance to palsy after total hip arthroplasty. Surg Radiol Anat. 2006;28(1):88–91. https://doi.org/10.1007/s00276-005-0056-x.

30. Cass SP. Piriformis syndrome: a cause of nondiscogenic sciatica. Curr Sports Med Rep. 2015;14(1):41–4. https://doi.org/10.1249/JSR.0000000000000110.

31. Smoll NR. Variations of the piriformis and sciatic nerve with clinical consequence: a review. Clin Anat. 2010;23(1):8–17. https://doi.org/10.1002/ca.20893.

32. Feigenbaum F, Henderson F. Surgical management of meningeal cysts, including perineurial (Tarlov)

cysts and meningeal diverticula. Semin Spine Surg. 2006;18:154–60.

33. Feigenbaum F, Henderson F. Tarlov cysts. In: Benzel E, editor. Spine surgery. 3rd ed. Philadelphia: Elsevier; 2012. p. 1135–40.

34. Hayashi K, Nagano J, Hattori S. Adhesive arachnoiditis after percutaneous fibrin glue treatment of a sacral meningeal cyst: case report. J Neurosurg Spine. 2014;20(6):763–6.

35. Patel M, Louie W, Rachlin J. Percutaneous fibrin glue therapy of meningeal cysts of the sacral spine. AJR Am J Roentgenol. 1997;163:367–70.

36. Tarlov IM. Spinal perineurial and meningeal cysts. J Neurol Neurosurg Psychiatry. 1970;33:833–43.

37. Voyadzis J, Bhargava P, Henderson F. Tarlov cysts: a study of 10 cases with review of the literature. J Neurosurg Spine. 2001;95:25–32.

Vascular Causes of Posterior Hip Pain

18

Luke Spencer-Gardner

Introduction

The etiology of posterior hip pain is varied and is often assumed to arise from either musculoskeletal or neurologic origins. Vascular etiologies of posterior hip pain are less often encountered in the typical orthopedic practice; however, in the absence of musculoskeletal or neurologic causes for posterior hip pain, the diagnosis of buttock claudication of a vascular origin should be considered [1].

Claudication is defined as reproducible muscular pain or discomfort as a result of walking that is not resolved with continued walking and is relieved by rest [2]. Buttock claudication typically occurs in the setting of peripheral arterial disease, although thromboembolic, inflammatory, and iatrogenic causes have been described [3–9]. Regardless of the etiology, the hip specialist should have an understanding of the etiology and clinical presentation of this condition. This chapter will present the vascular anatomy of the pelvis and deep gluteal space, discuss the etiology of buttock claudication, outline the clinical presentation and work-up of suspected buttock claudication, and, finally, discuss the treatment options and outcomes for this condition.

L. Spencer-Gardner, MD
Baylor University Medical Center, Hip Preservation Center, Dallas, TX, USA

Vascular Anatomy of the Pelvis and Deep Gluteal Space

A detailed understanding of the vascular anatomy of the pelvis and deep gluteal space is necessary when considering the etiology and treatment of buttock claudication. The abdominal aorta divides into the common iliac arteries at the level the fourth lumbar vertebrae. Each iliac artery then divides into an internal and external iliac artery, anterior to the sacroiliac joint, at the level of the L5 and S1 vertebrae. The internal iliac artery (IIA) supplies the pelvic viscera; however, branches of the IIA supply the buttocks, medial thigh, and perineum [10]. The IIA is approximately 4 cm long and courses posteromedially into the true pelvis toward the greater sciatic notch where it divides into anterior and posterior branches. The branches of the anterior division of the IIA include the following arteries: umbilical, obturator, inferior vesicle (males), vaginal artery (females), middle rectal, internal pudendal, and inferior gluteal (Figs. 18.1 and 18.2). The branches of the posterior division of the IIA include the following arteries: superior gluteal artery (SGA), iliolumbar artery, and lateral sacral arteries [10]. The anatomic course and distribution of the internal and external IIA are included in Table 18.1. Collateral supply in the distribution of the IIA is well documented with contributions from the contralateral IIA system,

© Springer International Publishing AG, part of Springer Nature 2019
H. D. Martin, J. Gómez-Hoyos (eds.), *Posterior Hip Disorders*,
https://doi.org/10.1007/978-3-319-78040-5_18

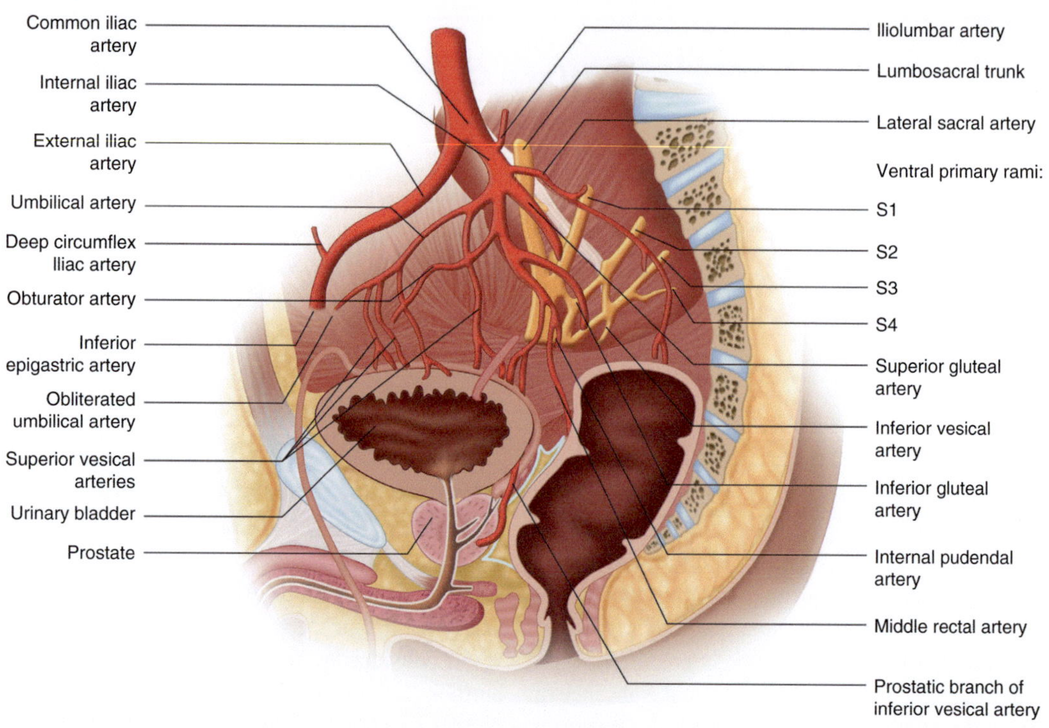

Fig. 18.1 Common iliac artery and its branches (male)

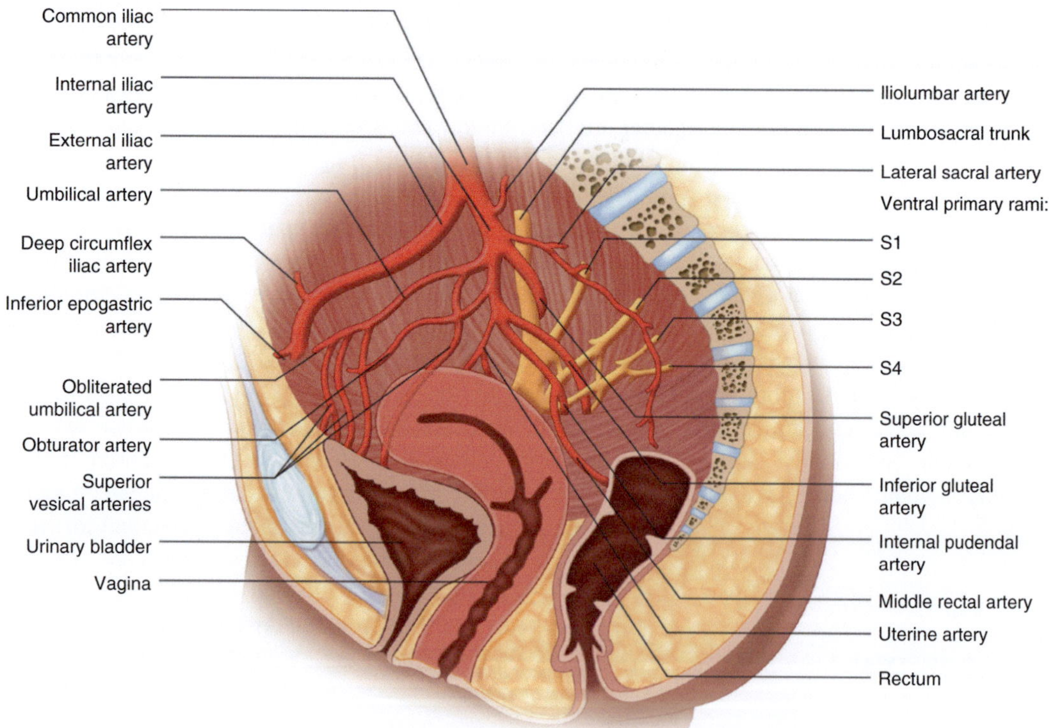

Fig. 18.2 Common iliac artery and its branches (female)

Table 18.1 Arteries of the pelvis

Artery	Origin	Course	Branches	Distribution
Internal iliac artery (IIA)	Common iliac	Courses posteromedial into the true pelvis toward the greater sciatic notch	Anterior division, posterior division	Primary blood supply to pelvic viscera, gluteal muscles, and perineum
Anterior division of IIA	IIA	Courses anteriorly in the pelvis and divides into visceral branches, obturator, and inferior gluteal arteries	Umbilical, superior vesical, obturator, inferior vesical, artery to ductus deferens, prostatic, uterine, vaginal, internal pudendal, middle rectal, inferior gluteal	Pelvic viscera, gluteal region, and adductor muscles of the thigh
Posterior division of IIA	IIA	Courses posteriorly giving rise to parietal branches	Iliolumbar, lateral sacral, superior gluteal	Pelvic wall and gluteal region

anastomoses between the inferior mesenteric and IIA systems via the rectal network, and anastomoses between ipsilateral medial and lateral femoral circumflex arteries with the IGA and SGA, respectively, reported to be protective of ischemia in cases of iatrogenically induced IIA occlusion [11–13].

Etiology

Buttock claudication results from reduced blood flow in vascular distributions of the IIA involving the pelvic viscera and the deep gluteal space musculature. When the restriction of blood flow is no longer compensated by collateral flow, activity-related pain, cramping, and fatigue of the proximal lower limb musculature of the buttock and thigh and end-organ dysfunction such as impotence may ensue. In the case of isolated IIA or SGA occlusion, circulation in the distal lower limb is not affected owing to the preservation of the blood flow in the external iliac artery and subsequently the femoral artery. The vascular insult occurs most commonly due to stenosis resulting from atherosclerosis, but thrombosis, aneurism, and systemic vasculitis have also been described as rare causes [3–8]. Iatrogenic causes have been reported due to IIA embolization to prevent endoleak at the time of endovascular aortic aneurism repair [9].

Clinical Diagnosis

A vascular etiology of buttock pain should be considered in the absence of musculoskeletal or neurologic causes and in the presence of risk factors and clinical findings typical of vascular claudication. Differentiating vascular claudication from neurogenic claudication can present a diagnostic challenge [14, 15]. Neurogenic claudication typically begins in the buttocks radiating down the affected limb distally and is exacerbated or relieved by postural changes. Symptoms are often exacerbated with standing, and relieved by forward flexion of the spine, or sitting. The clinical presentation of buttock claudication will depend on the level of vascular occlusion. Patient with buttock pain from vascular claudication may describe activity-related pain, cramping, and fatigue of the buttock and proximal lower limb musculature and end-organ dysfunction such as impotence or colonic ischemia. Aortoiliac occlusive disease, otherwise known as Leriche syndrome, results from a proximal occlusion near the aortic bifurcation. The classic triad of buttock claudication, impotence, and absent femoral pulses is the hallmark of this condition [16]. Pure buttock claudication in the setting of a more distal occlusion at the level of the IIA or SGA is more subtle as the femoral pulses may be normal due to the absence of disease in the external iliac artery and beyond [4, 6] (Batt, Berthelot). Risk factors for PAD include smoking, diabetes, older age (>40 years), hypertension, hyperlipidemia, hyperhomocysteinemia, and coronary or renal arterial disease [2]. Physical examination findings such as weak or absent distal pulses, the absence of distal hair growth, dry skin, and poorly healing wounds will again depend on the level of involvement and may be absent in the case of isolated buttock claudication. Medical history of vascular pathology and any prior treatment should be documented. Buttock claudication after endovascular aortic aneurism repair is a known complication due to the need to embolize the IIA, and therefore, any prior history of aortic aneurism repair should raise the clinical index of suspicion. If the diagnosis of PAD as the cause of buttock pain is suspected clinically, typically the ankle-brachial index (ABI) is measured; however, in the setting of isolated buttock claudication, the ABI may be normal [17]. Likewise, arterial duplex studies may not be able to adequately localize the site of the lesion given anatomic constraints, yet gluteal duplex studies have been reported as a useful tool to exclude vascular disease [18]. Noninvasive vascular studies combined with exercise testing have been used as a screening measure to identify patients with buttock claudication prior to more invasive studies. A decrease of 15 mm Hg of transcutaneous oxygen tension (tcPO2) on the buttocks during exercise testing is a sensitive and specific indicator of decreased perfusion in the IIA vascular network [19]. Although these noninvasive tests may provide additional information, buttock claudication lacks a validated diagnostic test [1]. Reproduction of the pain alleviated with short periods of test is helpful in the diagnosis.

Additional imaging modalities may be required to precisely localize the level of suspected occlusion; however, their use should be reserved for cases where all appropriate investigations have been completed to rule out other causes. Computed tomography angiography (CTA) and magnetic resonance angiography (MRA) will locate the lesion and allow for definitive diagnosis to be made; however, these tests should be reserved for patients in whom revascularization will be considered given the risks of contrast administration and the costs involved [20]. Oblique projections may

be required when evaluating the SGA as a potential site of occlusion as the external iliac artery may obscure the origin of the SGA on standard projections [21]. Prior to ordering these tests, referral to a vascular specialist for continued evaluation and treatment is recommended.

Treatment and Prognosis

Patients with lower extremity arterial disease have been found to have reduced functional capacity and lower quality of life [2, 22]. Nonoperative treatment of buttock claudication applies the principles of evidence-based interventions for PAD and includes modification of risk factors, medical treatment, and a supervised exercise program, with the goal of improved functional capacity and quality of life.

Risk factor modification includes smoking cessation, utilization of lipid-lowering medications, optimization of blood glucose control, and medical treatment of hypertension. Medical treatment combines the use of medications indicated for risk factor modification and antiplatelet agents such as aspirin and clopidogrel [2]. Medications aimed at risk factor modification and antiplatelet action have been found to have little direct effect on claudication. In contrast, cilostazol, a type 3 phosphodiesterase inhibitor, has been found to improve pain-free and maximal walking distance in several studies [23–26]. Quality of life and physical function have also been improved with the use of cilostazol in the setting of PAD [25, 26].

Exercise programs are a mainstay of nonoperative treatment for intermittent claudication in patients deemed medically fit to participate. The benefits of exercise programs are the result of improved oxygen extraction and metabolic efficiency in the effected muscle groups [2]. In the most recent Cochrane review, supervised programs completed at least twice weekly were found to be of significant benefit compared with placebo in increasing walking time and distance. Patients participating in exercise programs were also found to have improved physical and mental outcome scores when compared to controls [27].

If nonoperative interventions fail to provide adequate relief, revascularization procedures are then considered. Transluminal percutaneous angioplasty (TPA) is typically utilized in favor of open approaches, particularly in cases of more distal stenosis or occlusion. Stenotic lesions are treated via balloon catheter angioplasty, and occlusions are treated with recanalization, with stenting performed on a case by case basis.

Several case studies have been published on the endovascular treatment of buttock claudication, typically involving revascularization of the IIA or the SGA [12, 28–30].

Prince et al. reported their results of the largest series in the literature of endovascular treatment of buttock claudication due to IIA stenosis. In a retrospective review of their series of 34 patients, partial or complete relief of buttock claudication was reported in 79% of cases, at a mean follow-up of 3 months postoperatively [31]. The second largest study included 22 cases which were treated with PTA. At a mean follow-up of 14.7 months, there was 100% success of symptom alleviation with significant increases in mean walking distance from 85 m preoperatively to 225 m postoperatively ($p < 0.001$) [32]. Batt et al. presented the largest series on the outcomes of the treatment of isolated SGA stenosis. Their series included 34 patients with buttock claudication who underwent PTA of the SGA with selective stent use. At a mean follow-up of 4 years, 60% were free of recurrence. Thirteen patients had recurrence, and of those repeat angioplasty was successful in 8/13 with restenosis. Failure of repeat angioplasty was more likely in cases of reocclusion. They concluded that angioplasty was a safe and efficacious treatment option for buttock claudication due to isolated SGA lesions [21]. In his commentary on Batt et al.'s paper, de Borst agreed that the intervention was safe and effective in the short term but reservations were expressed regarding the durability of the results and the methodology of the follow-up protocol [1]. Regardless, there appears to be a growing body of evidence supporting the concept and advancing the field toward more accurate diagnosis and effective management of buttock claudication.

Iatrogenically induced buttock claudication from prophylactic occlusion of the IIA prior to Endovascular aortic repair (EVAR) for the treatment of aortic aneurism is a commonly recognized source of buttock claudication, with symptoms reported in 52% of patients postoperatively [33]. Preventative measures including proximal occlusion of the IIA, which allows the maximal perfusion from collaterals, preoperative collateral circulation evaluation, and unilateral embolization are recommended to avoid this problem [34]. The use of an iliac branch graft as a modification of the EVAR which allows perfusion of the IIA through a side branch of the graft prevented the occurrence of buttock claudication [35].

Conclusion

The etiology of posterior hip and buttock pain is varied. In the absence of identifiable neurologic or orthopedic causes, a vascular etiology should be considered. The presence of clinical risk factors and key findings on history and physical examination should lead the clinician to include buttock claudication in the differential diagnosis. Diagnostic testing including ABI, duplex ultrasonography, and tcPO2 of the buttock during exercise testing can further confirm the diagnosis of buttock claudication as a component of PAD. Nonoperative treatment options including risk factor modification, medication, and a supervised exercise program are the first line of treatment. Under the direction of a vascular specialist, further diagnostic imaging can be utilized to localize and ultimately treat the cause of buttock claudication that is refractory to nonoperative treatment.

References

1. de Borst GJ, Moll FL. Commentary: endovascular treatment for buttock claudication: the proof of the pudding is in the eating! J Endovasc Ther. 2014;21(3):407.
2. Hiatt WR. Medical treatment of peripheral arterial disease and claudication. N Engl J Med. 2001;344(21):1608.

3. Kato H, Sugimura T, Akagi T, Sato N, Hashino K, Maeno Y, Kazue T, Eto G, Yamakawa R. Long-term consequences of Kawasaki disease. A 10- to 21-year follow-up study of 594 patients. Circulation. 1996;94(6):1379.

4. Berthelot JM, Pillet JC, Mitard D, Chevalet-Muller F, Planchon B, Maugars Y. Buttock claudication disclosing a thrombosis of the superior left gluteal artery: report of a case diagnosed by a selective arteriography of the iliac artery, and cured by per-cutaneous stenting. Joint Bone Spine. 2007;74(3):289.

5. Chaer RA, Faries PL, Lin S, Dayal R, McKinsey JF, Kent KC. Successful percutaneous treatment of gluteal claudication secondary to isolated bilateral hypogastric stenoses. J Vasc Surg. 2006;43(1):165.

6. Batt M, Desjardin T, Rogopoulos A, Hassen-Khodja R, Le Bas P. Buttock claudication from isolated stenosis of the gluteal artery. J Vasc Surg. 1997;25(3):584.

7. Dix FP, Titi M, Al-Khaffaf H. The isolated internal iliac artery aneurysm – a review. Eur J Vasc Endovasc Surg. 2005;30(2):119.

8. Elsharawy MA, Cheatle TR. Buttock claudication secondary to isolated internal iliac artery stenosis. Eur J Vasc Endovasc Surg. 2000;19(1):87.

9. Choi HR, Park KH, Lee JH. Risk factor analysis for buttock claudication after internal iliac artery embolization with endovascular aortic aneurysm repair. Vasc Spec Int. 2016;32(2):44.

10. Moore KL, Dalley AF, Agur AM. Clinically oriented anatomy. Philadelphia, PA: Lippincott Williams & Wilkins; 2013.

11. Yano OJ, Morrissey N, Eisen L, Faries PL, Soundararajan K, Wan S, Teodorescu V, Kerstein M, Hollier LH, Marin ML. Intentional internal iliac artery occlusion to facilitate endovascular repair of aortoiliac aneurysms. J Vasc Surg. 2001;34(2):204.

12. Kofoed SC, Bismuth J, Just S, Baekgaard N. Angioplasty for the treatment of buttock claudication caused by internal iliac artery stenoses. Ann Vasc Surg. 2001;15(3):396.

13. Chait A, Moltz A, Nelson J. The collateral arterial circulation in the pelvis: an angiographic study. Am J Roentgenol. 1968;102(2):392.

14. Haig AJ, Park P, Henke PK, Yamakawa KS, Tomkins-Lane C, Valdivia J, Loar S. Reliability of the clinical examination in the diagnosis of neurogenic versus vascular claudication. Spine J. 2013;13(12):1826.

15. Nadeau M, Rosas-Arellano MP, Gurr KR, Bailey SI, Taylor DC, Grewal R, Lawlor DK, Bailey CS. The reliability of differentiating neurogenic claudication from vascular claudication based on symptomatic presentation. Can J Surg. 2013;56(6):372.

16. Frederick M, Newman J, Kohlwes J. Leriche syndrome. J Gen Intern Med. 2010;25(10):1102.

17. Batt M, Baque J, Bouillanne PJ, Hassen-Khodja R, Haudebourg P, Thevenin B. Percutaneous angioplasty of the superior gluteal artery for buttock claudication: a report of seven cases and literature review. J Vasc Surg. 2006;43(5):987.

18. Bruninx G, Salame H, Wery D, Delcour C. Doppler study of gluteal arteries. A useful tool for excluding gluteal arterial pathology and an important adjunct to lower limb Doppler studies. J Mal Vasc. 2002;27(1):12.

19. Abraham P, Picquet J, Vielle B, Sigaudo-Roussel D, Paisant-Thouveny F, Enon B, Saumet JL. Transcutaneous oxygen pressure measurements on the buttocks during exercise to detect proximal arterial ischemia: comparison with arteriography. Circulation. 2003;107(14):1896.

20. Conte MS, Pomposelli FB. Society for Vascular Surgery Practice guidelines for atherosclerotic occlusive disease of the lower extremities management of asymptomatic disease and claudication. Introduction. J Vasc Surg. 2015;61(3 Suppl):1S.

21. Batt M, Baque J, Ajmia F, Cavalier M. Angioplasty of the superior gluteal artery in 34 patients with buttock claudication. J Endovasc Ther. 2014;21(3):400.

22. Vogt MT, Cauley JA, Kuller LH, Nevitt MC. Functional status and mobility among elderly women with lower extremity arterial disease: the study of osteoporotic fractures. J Am Geriatr Soc. 1994;42(9):923.

23. Dawson DL, Cutler BS, Meissner MH, Strandness DE Jr. Cilostazol has beneficial effects in treatment of intermittent claudication: results from a multicenter, randomized, prospective, double-blind trial. Circulation. 1998;98(7):678.

24. Dawson DL, Cutler BS, Hiatt WR, Hobson RW 2nd, Martin JD, Bortey EB, Forbes WP, Strandness DE Jr. A comparison of cilostazol and pentoxifylline for treating intermittent claudication. Am J Med. 2000;109(7):523.

25. Money SR, Herd JA, Isaacsohn JL, Davidson M, Cutler B, Heckman J, Forbes WP. Effect of cilostazol on walking distances in patients with intermittent claudication caused by peripheral vascular disease. J Vasc Surg. 1998;27(2):267.

26. Beebe HG, Dawson DL, Cutler BS, Herd JA, Strandness DE Jr, Bortey EB, Forbes WP. A new pharmacological treatment for intermittent claudication: results of a randomized, multicenter trial. Arch Intern Med. 2041;159(17):1999.

27. Lane R, Ellis B, Watson L, Leng GC. Exercise for intermittent claudication. Cochrane Database Syst Rev. 2014;7:CD000990.

28. Senechal Q, Auguste MC, Louail B, Lagneau P, Pernes JM. Relief of buttock claudication by percutaneous recanalization of an occluded superior gluteal artery. Cardiovasc Intervent Radiol. 2000;23(3):226.

29. Morse SS, Cambria R, Strauss EB, Kim B, Sniderman KW. Transluminal angioplasty of the hypogastric artery for treatment of buttock claudication. Cardiovasc Intervent Radiol. 1986;9(3):136.

30. Cook AM, Dyet JF. Percutaneous angioplasty of the superior gluteal artery in the treatment of buttock claudication. Clin Radiol. 1990;41(1):63.

31. Prince JF, Smits ML, van Herwaarden JA, Arntz MJ, Vonken EJ, van den Bosch MA, de Borst

GJ. Endovascular treatment of internal iliac artery stenosis in patients with buttock claudication. PLoS One. 2013;8(8):e73331.

32. Donas KP, Schwindt A, Pitoulias GA, Schonefeld T, Basner C, Torsello G. Endovascular treatment of internal iliac artery obstructive disease. J Vasc Surg. 2009;49(6):1447.

33. Pavlidis D, Hormann M, Libicher M, Gawenda M, Brunkwall J. Buttock claudication after interventional occlusion of the hypogastric artery--a mid-term follow-up. Vasc Endovasc Surg. 2012;46(3):236.

34. Kritpracha B, Pigott JP, Price CI, Russell TE, Corbey MJ, Beebe HG. Distal internal iliac artery embolization: a procedure to avoid. J Vasc Surg. 2003;37(5):943.

35. Fernandez-Alonso L, Fernandez-Alonso S, Grijalba FU, Farina ES, Aguilar EM, Alegret Sole JF, Pascual MA, Centeno R. Endovascular treatment of abdominal aortic aneurysms involving iliac bifurcation: role of iliac branch graft device in prevention of buttock claudication. Ann Vasc Surg. 2013;27(7):851.

Surgical Approaches to the Posterior Hip

Bernardo Aguilera-Bohórquez
and Miguel Eduardo Sanchéz-Otamendi

Background

An extensive knowledge of the anatomy is required when performing surgical approaches to the posterior hip; this will allow for an accurate identification of the anatomical landmarks and their structural relationship with internal organs.

Traditionally, pathologies or injuries of the posterior hip had been described separately. This chapter aims to summarize all these isolated topics in one compilation.

The chapter is divided into three sections: (a) intra-articular, (b) deep gluteal space, and (c) sacrum, which allows us to describe and analyze all approaches in a detailed manner.

Superficial Anatomy of the Posterior Hip

The most important anatomical landmarks to identify are:

B. Aguilera-Bohórquez, MD (✉)
M. E. Sanchéz-Otamendi, MD
Orthopaedics and Traumatology, Centro Médico Imbanaco de Cali, Young Adult Hip Arthroscopy and Preservation Unit, Cali, Colombia
e-mail: baguilera@imbanaco.com.co

Bony Landmarks

- Posterior superior iliac crest
- Posterior superior iliac spine (PSIS)
- Posterior inferior iliac spine (PIIS)
- Greater trochanter
- Ischial tuberosity
- Sacrum
- Sacroiliac joint
- Coccyx

Muscular and Skin Landmarks

- Gluteal fold
- Intergluteal cleft (Fig. 19.1)

Deep Anatomy

The hip joint is surrounded by a great amount of muscles. Twenty-one muscles are actively involved in the function of the joint. Only nine of these muscles cover the posterior region of the hip. They are distributed in three muscular layers:

- *Superficial layer*: tensor fascia lata and gluteus maximus.
- *Medium layer*: gluteus medius and minimus, located in the lateral and superior portion of the joint.

© Springer International Publishing AG, part of Springer Nature 2019
H. D. Martin, J. Gómez-Hoyos (eds.), *Posterior Hip Disorders*,
https://doi.org/10.1007/978-3-319-78040-5_19

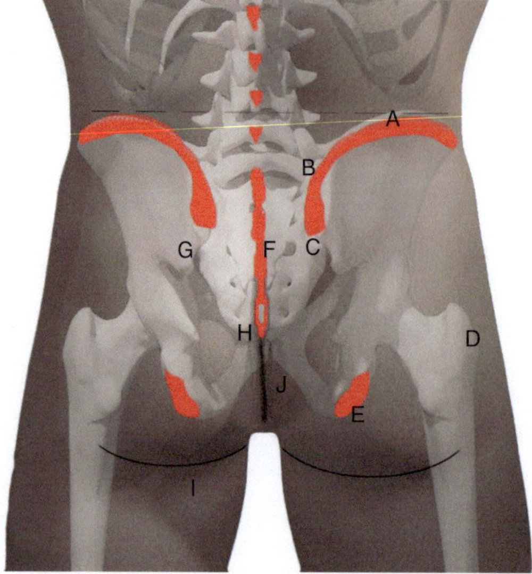

Fig. 19.1 Skin and bony landmarks (**a**) Posterior superior iliac crest, (**b**) Posterior superior iliac spine (PSIS), (**c**) Posterior inferior iliac spine (PIIS), (**d**) Greater trochanter, (**e**) Ischial tuberosity, (**f**) Sacrum, (**g**) Sacroiliac joint, (**h**) Coccyx, (**i**) Gluteal fold, (**j**) Intergluteal cleft (the bony landmarks are highlighted in red color)

- *Deep layer*: directly related to the posterior aspect of the joint. It is formed by the piriformis, gemellus superior, obturator internus and gemellus inferior (these last three muscles converging in a tendon). Additionally in this layer we find the quadratus femoris which covers the lesser trochanter and the posterior medial insertion of the iliopsoas tendon.

The piriformis muscle deserves a special mention because it is a constant reference point for neurovascular structures of the deep gluteal space, being the main internal landmark in the posterior surgical approaches.

The neurovascular structures located *above* the piriformis muscle are:

- *Superior gluteal vessels.* The superior gluteal artery emerges above the piriformis muscle and divides into two branches that are close to the posterior superior iliac spine, hence it is at high risk to be injured during procedures in this area.
- *Superior gluteal nerve.* It emerges next to the superior gluteal vessels, and then divides into several branches, passing between the gluteus

Table 19.1 Anatomic variants of the sciatic nerve in relation to the piriformis muscle (Beaton and Anson's Classification [27])

Type I	Sciatic nerve emerges undivided below the piriformis muscle
Type II	The sciatic nerve divisions pass between and below the piriformis muscle
Type III	The sciatic nerve divisions pass above and below the piriformis muscle
Type IV	Sciatic nerve emerges undivided through the piriformis muscle
Type V	The sciatic nerve divisions pass between and above the piriformis muscle
Type VI	Sciatic nerve emerges undivided above the piriformis muscle

medius and minimus and provides motor innervation to these two muscles and to the tensor fascia lata muscle.

The neurovascular structures located *below* the piriformis muscle are:

- *Sciatic nerve.* It usually runs under the piriformis muscle, emerging at its inferior border.
- *Posterior femoral cutaneous nerve.* It lies medial to the sciatic nerve behind the pelvitrochanteric muscles.
- *Inferior gluteal vessels and nerves.* They lie medial to the sciatic nerve, and travel deep to the gluteus maximus where they divide into several branches.
- *Pudendal vessels and nerves.* They travel medial to the sciatic nerve, course along the ischial spine and the sacrospinous ligament, and then loop back around to enter the perineum through the lesser sciatic foramen.

A number of anatomical variations exist around the posterior region of the hip, such as the sciatic nerve going through the piriformis muscle (Table 19.1). This variant changes the relationship among all the anatomical structures of the region, which may cause confusion to the surgeon, putting all the structures that travel underneath the piriformis muscle at a risk for injury.

Surgical Approaches

The literature has always separately described different techniques for surgical approaches to the posterior hip when referring to specific pathologies.

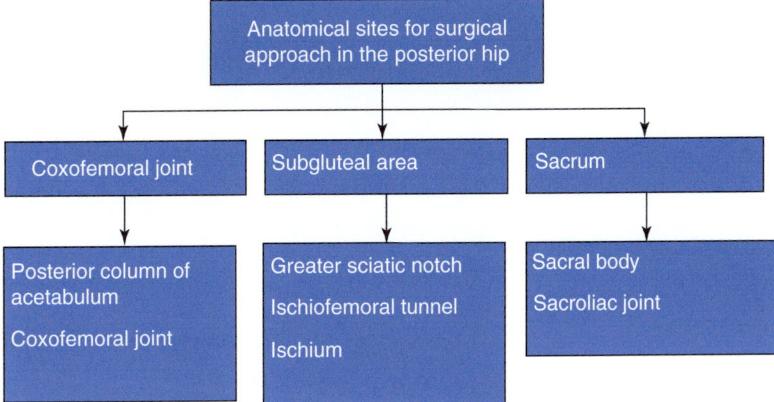

Fig. 19.2 Anatomical sites for surgical approach in the posterior hip region

This chapter will try to address all different techniques, which allows the reader to have a complete guideline on how to approach the posterior hip.

The region will be divided into three different anatomic zones and these zones will be separated into specific areas according to the pathology being treated (Fig. 19.2).

Posterior Coxofemoral Joint

Approach of the Coxofemoral Joint and Posterior Acetabulum Column [1, 2]

The posterior approaches of the hip address the intra-articular pathologies and of the posterior column of the acetabulum. All of the approaches share common characteristics, however they have variations that depend on the specific site of intervention.

Common characteristics of the posterior approaches:

- Posterior retraction of the gluteus maximus, which may change depending on the approach and the goal of the procedure.
- Release of the external rotator muscles. Preservation of the vascular structures depends on the goal of the surgery (joint preservation).
- Osteotomy of the greater trochanter preserving the insertion of the abductor muscles. This is necessary when the approach needs to be extended to intervene the superior and anterior portion of the acetabulum.

Posterior Approach: Kocher-Langenbeck's (K-L) Approach [3–6]
Indications of the Procedure

- Posterior exposure of the posterior column of the acetabulum
- Reduction of femoral head or neck fractures
- Coxofemoral luxation not reducible by external maneuvers
- Fractures of acetabulum and femoral head

Patient's position: prone or lateral decubitus. If a fracture is being treated, some authors suggest placing a supracondylar traction, keeping the knee with a minimal flexion of 45°.

Anatomical landmark: greater trochanter, posterior superior iliac spine, and the lateral face of the longitudinal axis of the femur.

Procedure
It begins with a skin incision from the greater trochanter towards the PSIS, without going further than 6 cm away from the spine in order to avoid the superior gluteal vessels. Subsequently direction is changed, and the incision is continued distally from the greater trochanter over the lateral aspect of the thigh approximately 10 cm or more if needed (Fig. 19.3)

Dissection of the subcutaneous cellular tissue to expose the fascia lata (Fig. 19.4)

- The fascia lata is cut parallel to the fibers of the gluteus maximus or aligned with the skin incision (Fig. 19.5).
- The gluteus maximus is dissected separating its fibers until exposing the greater trochanter.

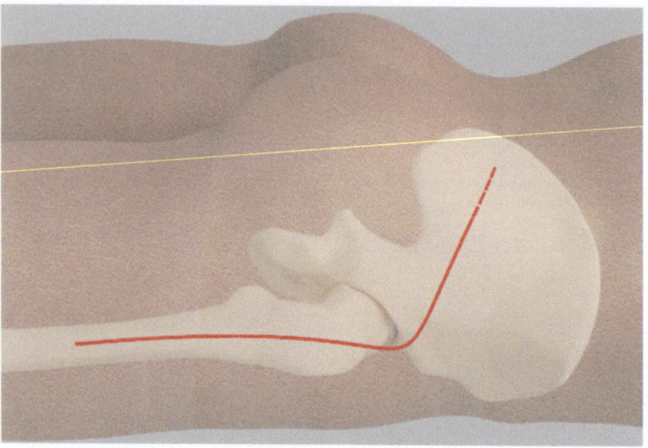

Fig. 19.3 Kocher-Langenbeck A. approach

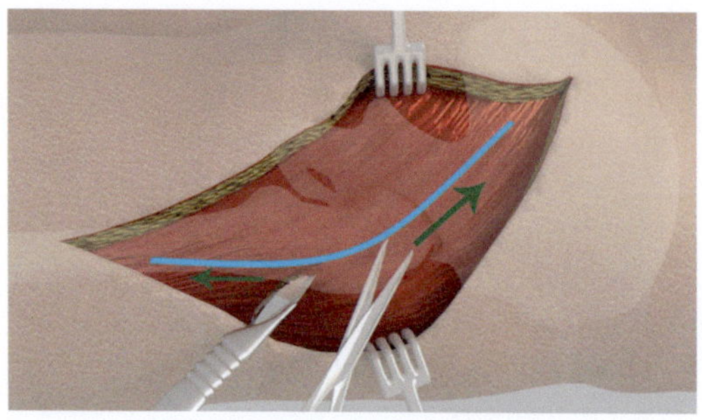

Fig. 19.4 Kocher-Langenbeck B. approach

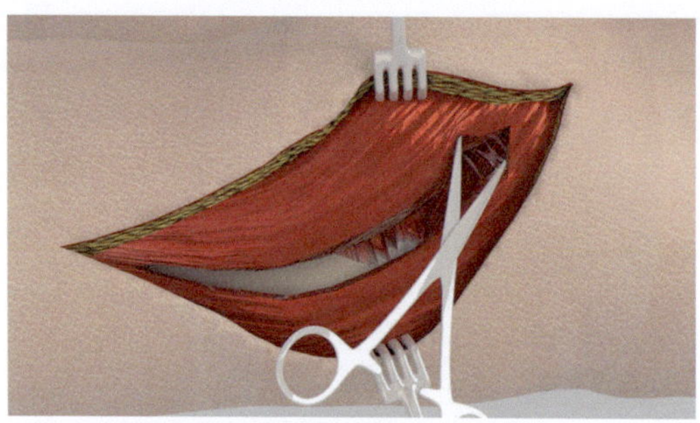

Fig. 19.5 Kocher-Langenbeck C. approach

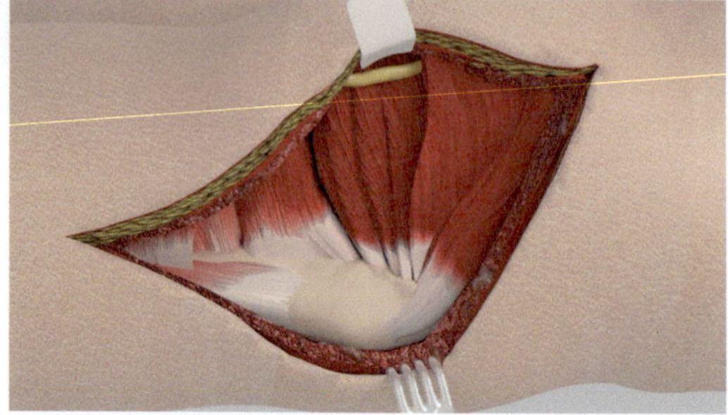

Fig. 19.6 Kocher-Langenbeck D. approach

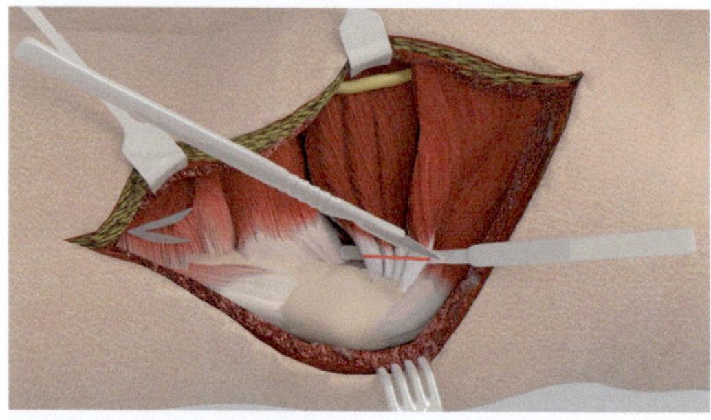

Fig. 19.7 Kocher-Langenbeck E. approach

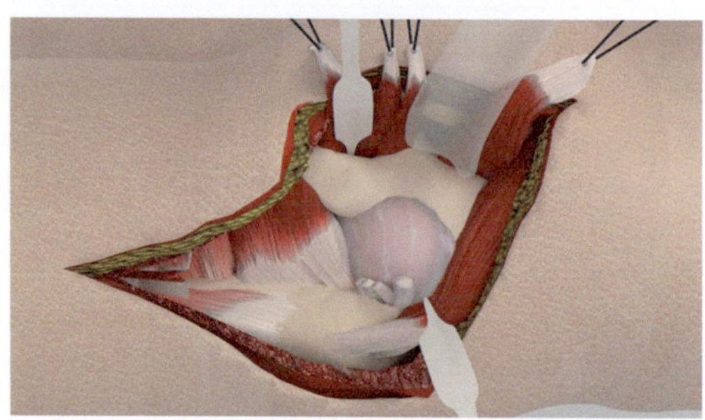

Fig. 19.8 Kocher-Langenbeck F. approach

At this point the branch of the inferior gluteal nerve in the anterior superior portion of the gluteus maximus needs to be preserved.

- Taking the greater trochanter as a reference, the quadratus femoris is localized and maintained intact, in order to preserve the ascending branch of the medial circumflex femoral artery that courses underneath it (Fig. 19.6).
- The sciatic nerve is identified.
- The tendon of the piriformis muscle is identified.
- The internal obturator and the superior and inferior gemellus are identified, leaving a remnant for reinsertion. They are lifted towards the middle, exposing the joint capsule below them and preserving the sciatic nerve that is medial to the mentioned muscles (Fig. 19.7).
- The gluteus medius and minimus are loosened subperiosteally from the ilium, and the superior gluteal nerve and vessels are identified and preserved as they exit at the greater sciatic notch.
- At this point the posterior acetabulum and the posterior column are exposed (Fig. 19.8).
- Once the joint capsule is dissected, Hohman separators are used to define the superior and

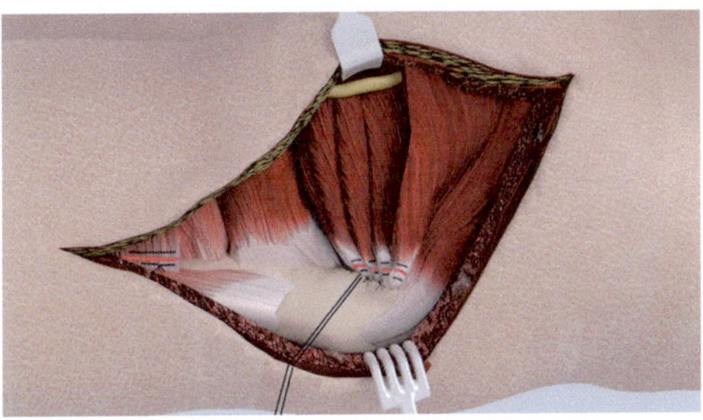

Fig. 19.9 Kocher-Langenbeck G. approach

inferior plane, and a longitudinal H or U-shaped capsulotomy is performed.

- Hohman separators are placed in the borders of the acetabulum, to obtain enough exposure to perform the procedure.
- Once the procedure is finished, a thorough washing is performed extracting the osteocartilaginous fragments, irrigation with good amount of saline is performed, and the joint capsule is sutured and the rotators are repaired (Fig. 19.9).

Exposure of the posterior surface of the acetabulum is obtained from the ischial tuberosity to the inferior portion of the iliac wing. In addition, access to the quadrilateral sheet can be obtained by palpation through the greater or lesser sciatic notch [7].

Advantages

– Direct visualization of the joint and the posterior column of the acetabulum, fractures of the femoral head with adequate resection of the osteocartilaginous fragments may be managed with this approach.
– Potentially extendible approach.

Disadvantages

– Gluteus maximus divulsion.

Common Complications

Sciatic nerve lesion by accidental section or stretching during the retraction or during coagu-

lation maneuvers to control the bleeding of the superior gluteal vessels.

Technique Variation

There is a minimally invasive variation of the Kocher-Langenbeck's approach. In this variation just the proximal portion of the traditional procedure is performed. That is to say going obliquely from the tip of the trochanter towards the PSIS, then the fibers of the gluteus maximus are separated, following the same recommendations made for the K-L approach to avoid lesions of the superior gluteal nerve. Using this approach the tuberosity may also be exposed, which would allow the placement of pins or plates for fragment fixation.

Indications

- Acetabulum fractures with compromise of the posterior portion.
- Some transverse fractures and fractures of the posterior column.
- It can be extended to perform a traditional K-L approach if necessary.

Modified Gibson's Approach

The Modified Gibson's approach is a modification of the Kocher-Langenbeck's approach when access to the iliac wing and the superior and anterior acetabulum is needed. The Modified Gibson is also useful in obese or muscular patients [5, 8].

Indications

- Same as Kocher-Langenbeck's approach

Patient's position: prone or lateral decubitus. The traction table may be used as in the Kocher-Langenbeck's approach.

Skin Demarcation

- Iliac crest
- Greater trochanter and lateral portion of the femur

Procedure

- A straight incision of approximately 20–30 cm is made. It starts in the lateral surface of the proximal femur aligned with the diaphysis passing over the tip of the greater trochanter until the level of the iliac crest (Fig. 19.10).
- Dissection of the subcutaneous tissue over the gluteus maximus to reach the fascia lata and the iliotibial band is performed. The anterior border of the gluteus maximus can be identified due to the constant presence of superior gluteal artery branches that go through the fascia, between the gluteus maximus and medius.
- The incision of the fascia must be initiated lateral to the greater trochanter and towards the iliac crest in front of the anterior border of the gluteus maximus.
- The gluteus medius muscle is separated from the fascia at this level and the gluteus maximus is retracted posteriorly. Its mobilization may be improved by performing a partial section of the femoral insertion (Fig. 19.11).
- At this point of the procedure the deepest layers are exposed and one can proceed as in the Kocher-Langenbeck's procedure (Fig. 19.12).

Advantages

- Better anterosuperior access to the coxal bone.
- Less risk of iatrogenic lesion of the gluteus maximus innervation.
- It decreases the necessity to perform an osteotomy of the trochanter, however it can be performed if necessary.
- Better cosmetic results especially in obese women.

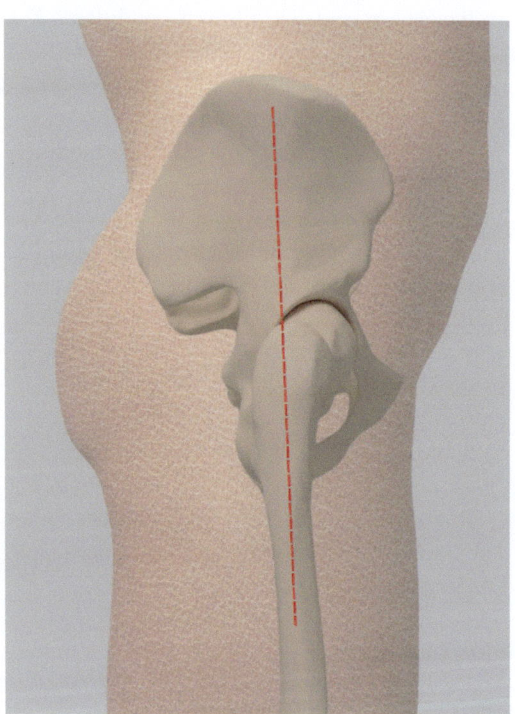

Fig. 19.10 Gibson's A. approach

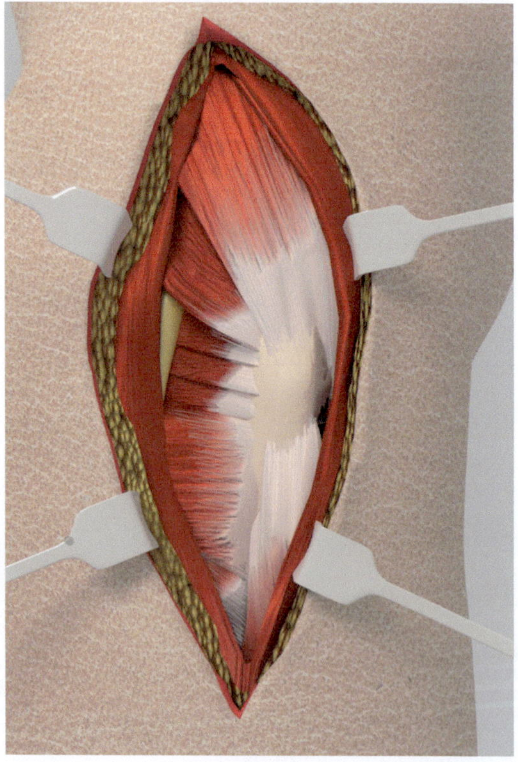

Fig. 19.11 Gibson's B. approach

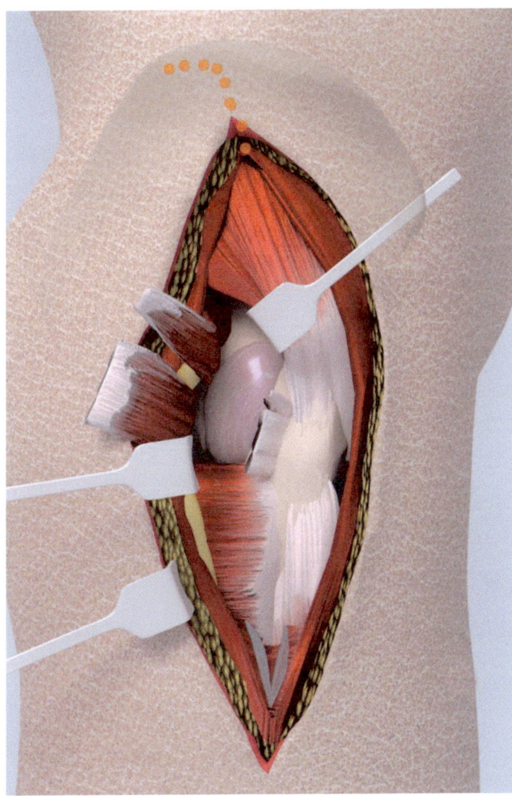

Fig. 19.12 Gibson's C. approach

Disadvantages

- It must be avoided when exposure of the greater sciatic notch is needed.

Moore's Approach

This is a modification of Harris's approach. Currently it is one of the most used approaches for hip replacement surgery because it does not involve the abductor mechanism allowing for a faster rehabilitation [5, 9, 10].

Indications

- Total hip replacement
- Total hip replacement revision where exposure of the femur is needed.
- Hemiarthroplasty
- Osteosynthesis of transverse fractures of the acetabulum or its posterior column.
- Open reduction of posterior hip luxations.

- Arthrotomy and hip drainage of infections.
- Vascular bone grafts

Patients' position: prone or lateral decubitus
Anatomical landmark and skin demarcation: greater trochanter and PSIS.

Procedure

- The incision begins 10 cm from the PSIS over a line that goes distal, lateral, and parallel to the fibers of the gluteus maximus to avoid the superior gluteal vessels. The line extends to the posterior border of the greater trochanter. At this point it changes direction and travels distally and parallel to the femoral axis with a total length of 7–12 cm (Fig. 19.13).
- The fascia lata is incised and the gluteus maximus is dissected to expose the external rotators. The gluteus maximus is separated posteriorly with a Chanley's separator (Fig. 19.14).
- The sciatic nerve must be visualized and protected, located in the posterior portion of the approach, immediately above the medial portion of the external rotators (Fig. 19.15).

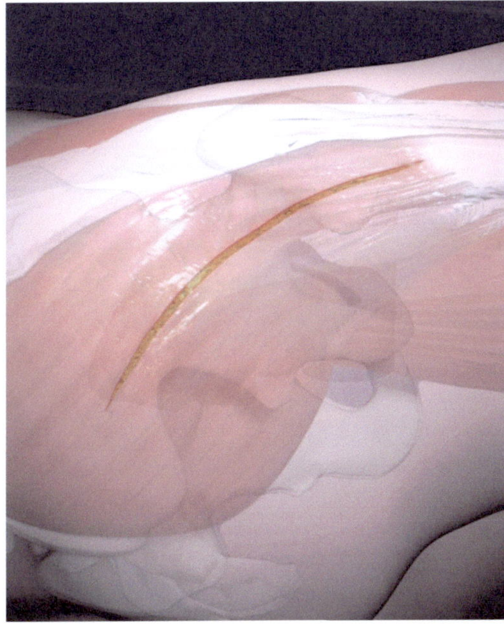

Fig. 19.13 Moore's A. approach

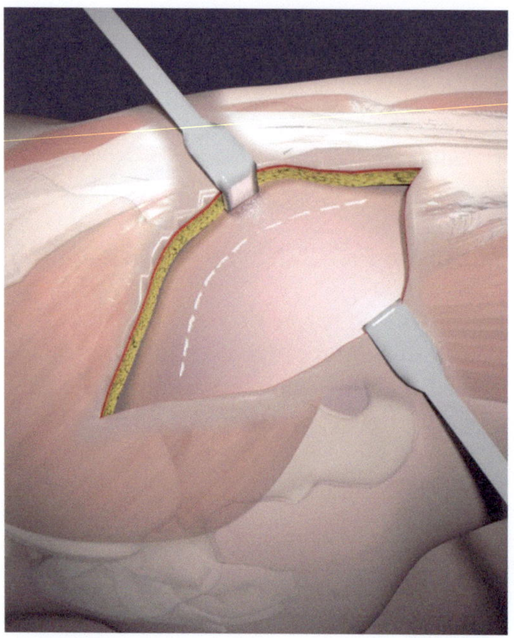

Fig. 19.14 Moore's B. approach

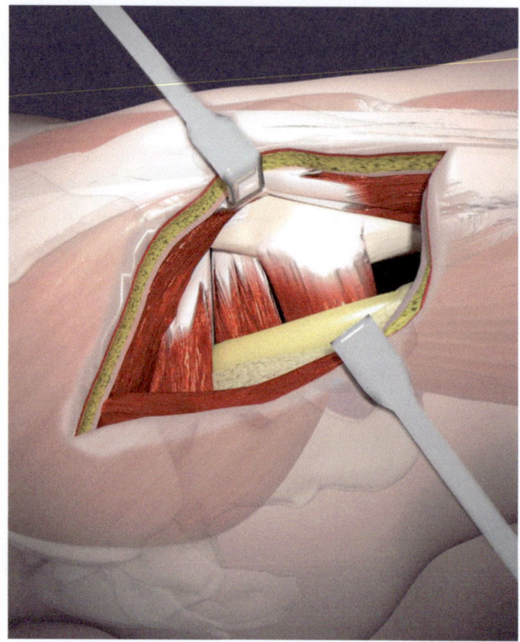

Fig. 19.16 Moore's D. approach

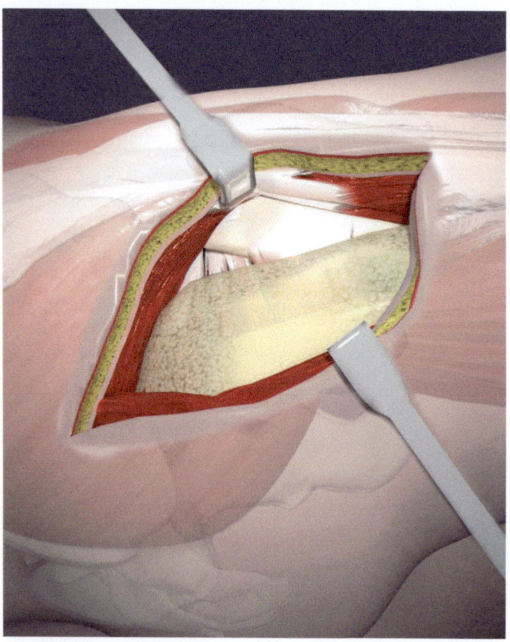

Fig. 19.15 Moore's C. approach

- The piriformis muscle and the short rotators (both gemellus and internal obturator) are sectioned near to their insertion at the greater trochanter and tagged for identification and reinsertion if needed (Fig. 19.16).

- Once the rotator muscles are medially placed, the posterior face of the joint capsule becomes exposed. The rotator muscles and the joint capsule are frequently cut together, however they can be cut separately and repaired when the procedure is finished (Fig. 19.17).
- H or U-shaped capsulotomy is performed and the femoral head is luxated by flexion and internal rotation of the hip (Fig. 19.18).
- At this point, an osteotomy of the femoral head may be performed which allows for exposure of the acetabulum by careful placement of the separators on its borders.

Advantages

- Reproducible
- It allows the surgical assistants an adequate visualization of the field
- Excellent exposure of the joint
- Extensible

Disadvantages

- Instability of the posterior hip
- Bleeding of the medial circumflex femoral artery

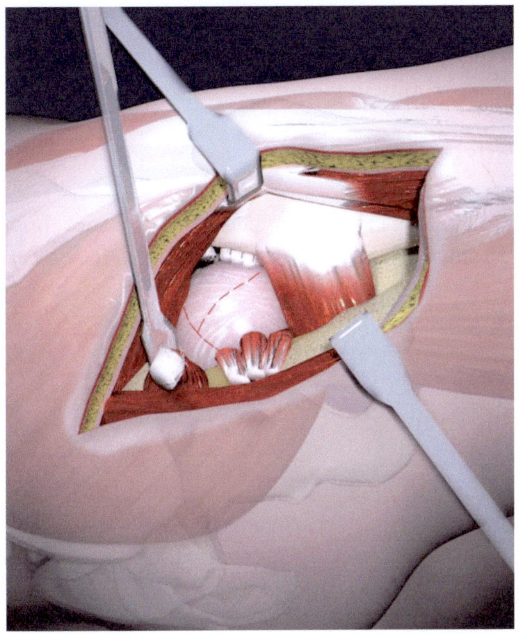

Fig. 19.17 Moore's E. approach

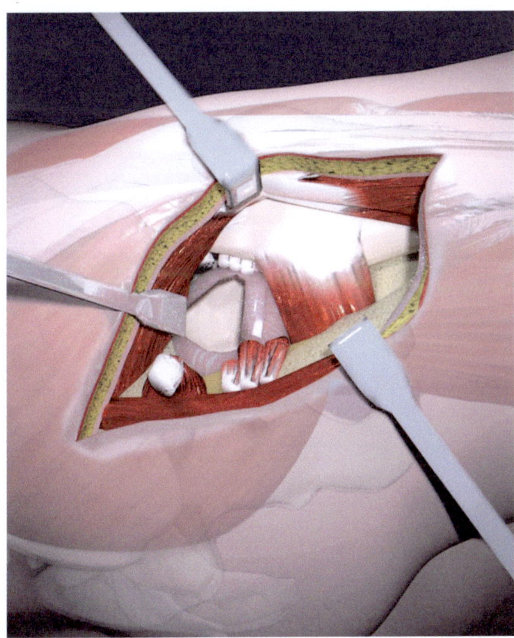

Fig. 19.18 Moore's F. approach

Complications

– Injury of the gluteus medius
– Injury of the sciatic nerve

This approach may be extended, however it is limited proximally by the inferior gluteal nerve which is located about 5 cm from the tip of the greater trochanter. Distally, once the muscle layers are lifted including detaching the gluteus maximus, a greater exposure of the femur is obtained [11].

Deep Gluteal Space and Ischiofemoral Space

Open Approach for Hamstring Muscles Repair

Indications: Rupture of the origin or proximal portion of the hamstring muscles.

Absolute indication: Rupture of the hamstring muscles with retraction greater than 3 cm.

Patient's position: Prone position with 30–40° knee flexion, a pillow can be placed at the ankles to obtain an adequate flexion.

Anatomical Landmarks

– Ischium
– Inferior gluteal fold

Open Technique
• The incision is performed at the gluteal fold. Depending on the type of lesion it can be done either horizontally or longitudinally (Fig. 19.19a).
• If there is retraction of the proximal hamstring origin, the incision must be longitudinal to allow exploration distal to the gluteal region, and horizontal if there is no retraction.
• Dissection of the subcutaneous tissue, identification of the inferior border of the gluteus maximus (Fig. 19.19b).
• A large incision is made in the aponeurotic fascia at the inferior border of the gluteus maximus, which allows for proximal retraction, taking caution when placing the separators (Fig. 19.19c).
• The ischium is identified and the proximal hamstring attachment in the lateral and posterior face of the ischial tuberosity is immediately visualized (Fig. 19.19d).

- Before starting any repair maneuver, it is essential to identify and protect the sciatic nerve and the posterior femoral cutaneous nerve, which is located just lateral to the muscle insertion.
- Peritendinous tissue at the hamstring origin is cut open in order to evaluate the damage.
- In the ruptures without retraction, an osseous scarification is performed to prepare the reinsertion site.
- It is important to highlight that the origin of the hamstring muscles is not at the ischial tuberosity but it is 2 cm lateral and proximal to it.
- Muscle reinsertion is performed with suture anchors or osseous tunnels.

- Hermetic closure of the wound must be done to decrease the risk of infection due to the proximity to the perianal region.

Advantages

- It can be extended to perform a posterior thigh approach and any distally retracted lesion can be located and repaired.
- It allows exploration of the sciatic nerve until the popliteal fossa.

Disadvantages

- Risk of infection due to closeness to the perianal region.

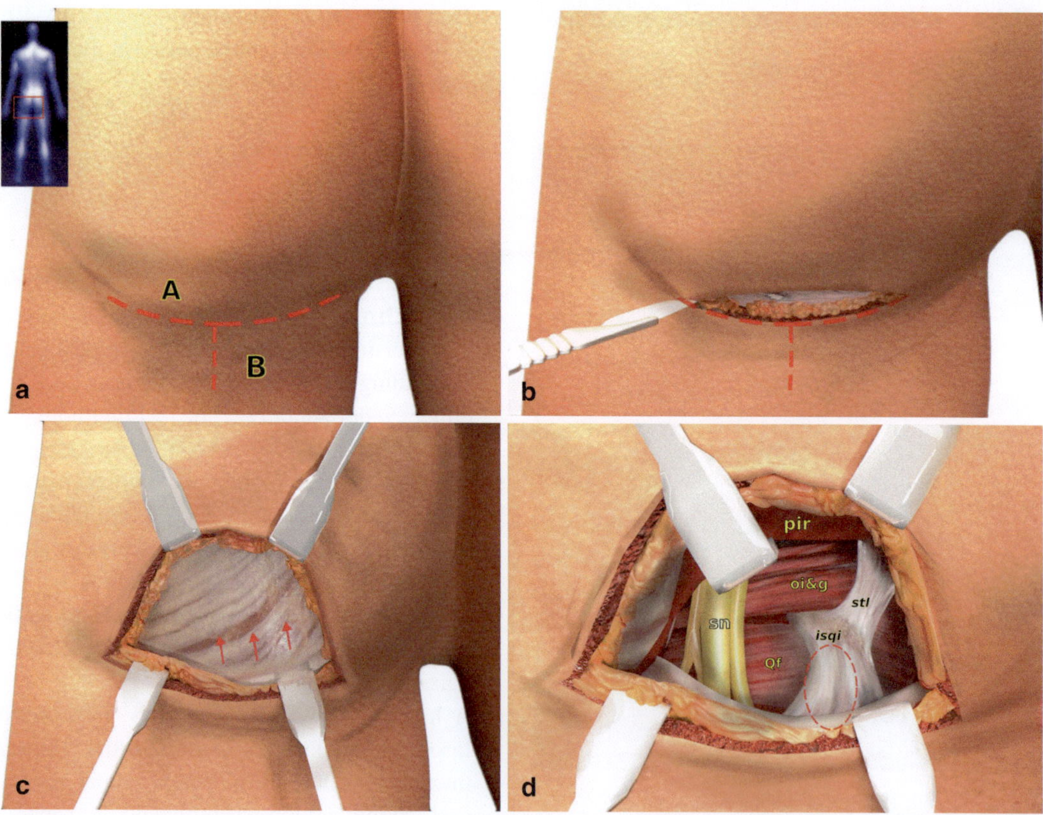

Fig. 19.19 (**a**) Open approach. Ischium and hamstring canal. (**b**) Open approach. Ischium and hamstring canal. Red dash line: inferior border of gluteus maximus. (**c**) Open approach. Ischium and hamstring canal. Red dash line: inferior border of gluteus maximus, Red arrows: proximal retraction of gluteus maximus after the incision of aponeurotic fascia. (**d**) Open approach. Ischium and hamstring canal. *Stl* sacrotuberous ligament, Dashed line: conjoined tendon origin (semitendinosus and biceps femoris) and semimembranosus origin (more lateral), *pir* m. piriformis, *qf* m. quadratus femoris, *Sn* sciatic nerve, *oi&g* obturator internus and superior and inferior gemellus muscles

– Risk of injury of the inferior gluteal nerve and/or vessels.
– Difficulty to sit down.

Complications

– Infection
– Lesion of the inferior gluteal artery or nerve

Open Technique: Endoscopic Assisted Minimally Invasive Procedure [12]

Indications: Rupture of proximal hamstring attachment with retractions lesser than 3 cm.

Patient's position: Prone position in translucent surgical table with 30–40 knee flexion

Anatomical Landmark and Skin Demarcation

Palpation of ischium and inferior gluteal fold
Fluoroscopic location of the ischiofemoral space
  and ischial tuberosity

Technique

1. Transverse incision (of about 8 cm) from superior lateral to inferior medial between the ischiofemoral space and the ischium (Fig. 19.20a).
2. Dissection of subcutaneous tissue to expose the fascia of gluteus maximus.

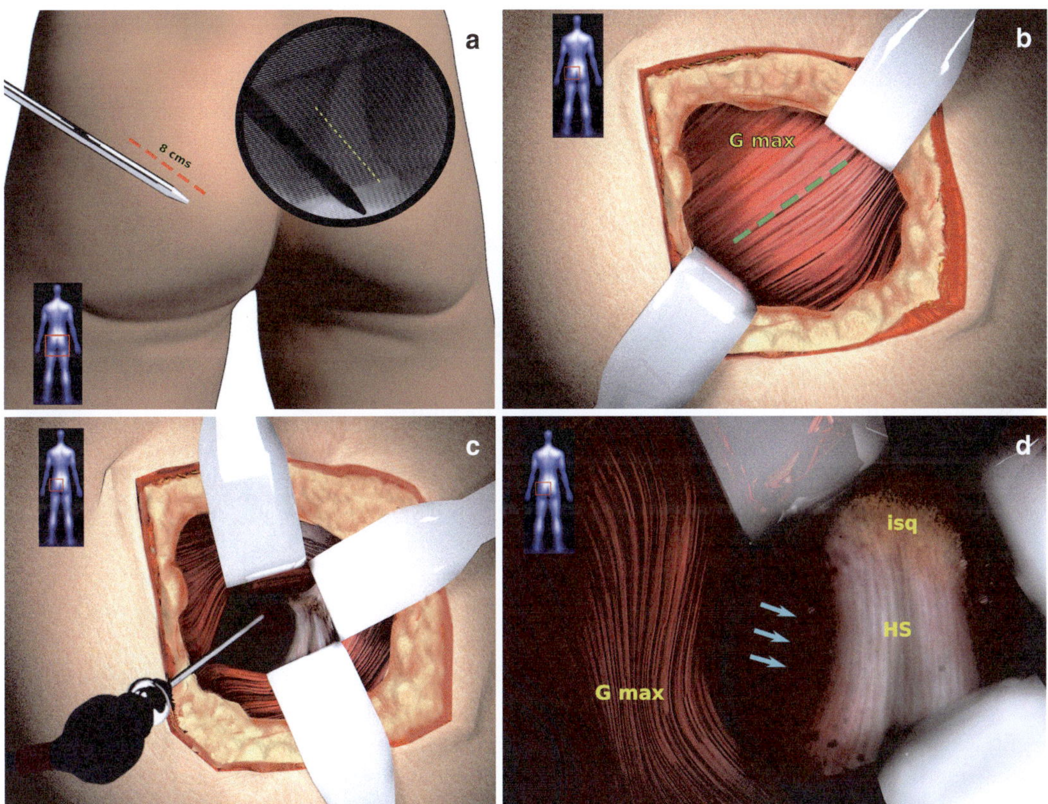

Fig. 19.20 (a) Endoscopic assisted minimally invasive procedure ischium and hamstring canal. The ischium and the lesser trochanter are targeted with fluoroscopy. The orientation of the 8 cm incision (Red dashed line) is superolateral to inferomedial on the ischiofemoral space. (b) Endoscopic assisted minimally invasive procedure ischium and hamstring canal. *Gmax* gluteus maximus, Green dashed line: dissection is made through the gluteus maximus following the muscle fibers until the external border of the ischium. (c) Endoscopic assisted minimally invasive procedure ischium and hamstring canal. The endoscope is introduced. (d) Endoscopic assisted minimally invasive procedure ischium and hamstring canal. *G max* gluteus maximus, *isq* ischium, *Hs* Hamstring tendons, Blue arrows: lateral border of ischium

3. A longitudinal dissection is made through the gluteus maximus at the junction between the proximal two thirds and the distal third following the muscle fibers until the external border of the ischium (Fig. 19.20b).
4. The space is maintained with deep angle separators.
5. The endoscope (30° or 70°) is introduced and the lesion is identified (Fig. 19.20c).
6. The necessary procedures are performed by a combination of an open and an endoscopic technique (Fig. 19.20d).
7. Debridement and exposure of the osseous bed, repair is performed with suture anchors as in the open technique.

Advantages

- It is technically less challenging than full-endoscopic technique.
- More detailed visualization of the lesion with the endoscope.
- It allows an adequate attack angle for placing suture anchors.
- There is less risk of infection when compared to the open technique (risk can be compared with the infection risk of the full-endoscopic technique).
- It allows visualization and preservation of the sciatic nerve during the procedure.
- There is no risk of fluid extravasation.

Disadvantages

- It is not adequate for major lesions and/or with retraction.

Complications

- Vascular lesions
- Infection

Recommendations

- The incision must be angled and guided by fluoroscopy

- Sciatic nerve exploration must be done at the beginning of the procedure as well as neurological intraoperatory monitoring to decrease the risk of nerve injury.
- Hermetic wound closure to decrease the risk of infection due to the proximity of the perianal region.

Endoscopic Technique
Indications

- Repair of acute or chronic lesions of the proximal hamstring origin with little retraction (less than 3 cm).
- Bursectomy of the ischial tuberosity.
- Entrapment of the sciatic nerve in the ischiofemoral tunnel.

Arthroscopic Technique 1 [13]
Patient's position: prone position in translucent surgical table with 30–40 knee flexion.

Anatomical Landmarks and Skin Demarcation

Ischial tuberosity
Gluteal fold

Procedure

- Two portals are established: first the lateral portal, place 2–3 cm lateral to the ischial tuberosity (Fig. 19.21a).
- Blunt dissection is performed with a switching stick through the gluteus maximus and a submuscular plane is obtained.
- The switching stick is directed towards the ischium and the space immediately medial and lateral to it is developed.
- The medial portal 2–3 cm medial to the ischial tuberosity is established (Fig. 19.21b).
- Divulsion of the medial and distal ischial space is performed, always in the medial and central zone of the ischium to avoid sciatic nerve lesion.

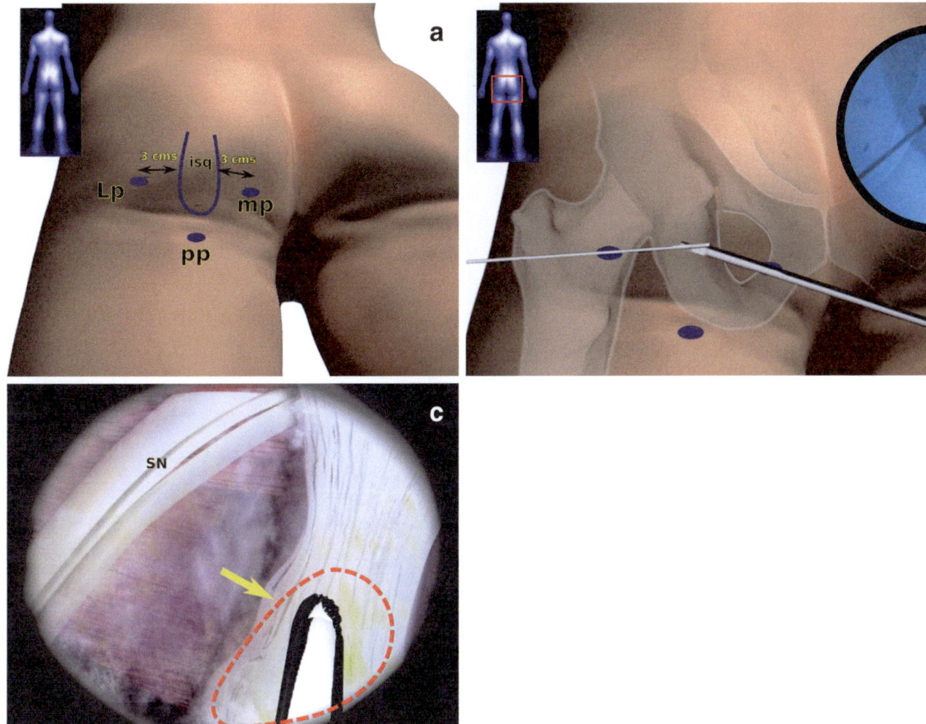

Fig. 19.21 (**a**) Ischium and ischiofemoral tunnel arthroscopic approach. *Lp* lateral portal, *mp* medial portal, *pp* distal portal. (**b**) Ischium and ischiofemoral tunnel arthroscopic approach. Lateral and medial portal established with fluoroscopic confirmation, *mp* medial portal, *pp* distal portal. (**c**) Ischium and ischiofemoral tunnel arthroscopic approach. *SN* sciatic nerve, dashed red line: Hamstring tendons at ischium, Yellow arrow: lateral side of ischium

- Once the medial and lateral borders of the ischium are identified, the lateral face is exposed and both the sciatic nerve and the posterior femoral cutaneous nerve are explored using blunt dissection (Fig. 19.21c).
- Finally, a distal portal located 4 cm from the ischial tuberosity is created. This portal will be used as an accessory portal.
- Be aware that the hamstring origin has an oval shaped footprint that is lateral and proximal with common attachment of the semitendinosus muscle and the long head of the biceps femoris, and a separate semilunar shaped footprint that is medial and distal for the semimembranosus muscle.
- Once all the portals are established, the management of the pathologies can proceed.

Advantages

- Chronic and acute lesions with little retraction (less than 3 cm) can be managed with this procedure.

Recommendations

- The portals must be equidistant from one another and in relation with the ischial tuberosity.
- The distance between the ischium and the portals can vary depending on the muscle mass and the size of the gluteal region.
- It is important to keep the minimal irrigation pressure necessary to allow an adequate visualization and to avoid extravasation.

Arthroscopic Technique 2 [14, 15]

Patient's position: Prone position in translucent surgical table, with knee flexion of 20–30°.

Anatomical Landmark and Skin Demarcation

- Ischial tuberosity
- Gluteal fold

Procedure

- Two portals at the level of the gluteal fold are established.
- A posterior portal located right on the ischial tuberosity and a second posterior lateral portal.
- The submuscular plane is developed with a blunt switching stick and the ischial tuberosity is identified and delimited.
- The posterior medial portal can be created always under direct visualization and fluoroscopic control.

Advantages

- Since the portals are at the level of the gluteal fold, this procedure can be switched to the open technique.
- Several additional portals can be used, especially for anchoring device placement, always under fluoroscopic visualization using spinal needle.

General Advantages of Endoscopic Technique

- Minimal alteration of the anatomy
- It allows an adequate evaluation due to the superior visualization
- Less risk of bleeding

General Disadvantages of Endoscopic Technique

- Potential risk of neurological lesion especially when creating the first portal (which is done blindly)
- It requires high technical skills.
- Longer surgical time, especially during the learning curve.

General Complications of Endoscopic Technique

- Lesions of the sciatic nerve, posterior femoral cutaneous nerve, and inferior gluteal nerve.
- Vascular lesions
- Extravasation of irrigation fluids to the pelvis.

Approach of Ischiofemoral Space [16]

Open Approach of Ischiofemoral Space

Patient's position: semiprone position.

Anatomical landmark and skin demarcation: The place for the incision is drawn at the gluteal fold with the patient in a standing position to obtain better cosmetic results.

Procedure

- Incision is made at the gluteal fold to reach the gluteus maximus, dissecting the subcutaneous tissue to reach the fascia at the inferior border of the gluteus maximus.
- Dissection of the inferior border of the gluteus maximus, deep enough to palpate the ischial tuberosity.
- Dissection is performed laterally to the tuberosity and ischium to expose the sciatic nerve, carefully retracting the gluteus maximus. Be aware that this maneuver may injure the inferior gluteal neurovascular bundle.
- The posterior femoral cutaneous nerve must be identified. It may be located medial or superficial to the sciatic nerve.
- Once all the nerves are identified and preserved, one can proceed to the identification of the hamstring tendons and the ischiofemoral space.
- Inflammatory tissue or bursitis is removed.
- The lateral border of the hamstring muscles and the medial border of the sciatic nerve are identified and neurolysis of the sciatic nerve is performed if necessary. Normal mobility of the sciatic nerve must be maintained.
- If the ischiofemoral space needs to be extended, the quadratus femoris is identified to palpate the lesser trochanter, and through a central opening the resection of the lesser trochanter is performed.

- It is necessary to be aware of the presence of the first perforating artery in the inferior portion of the quadratus femoris and a branch of the medial circumflex femoral artery in the superior border.
- Evaluation of the characteristics of the tendons looking for obvious tendinopathies is performed and these areas are removed.
- The surgical wound is closed in layers with absorbable sutures.

Endoscopic Approach of the Ischiofemoral Space [17]

Indications

- Entrapment of the sciatic nerve in the ischiofemoral tunnel
- Ischiofemoral impingement

Patient's Position

- Patient is on a fracture table in supine position or in a lateral position. Initially the leg is on neutral rotation and afterwards in maximal internal rotation with 20° of abduction.

Procedure

- The peritrochanteric space is entered by two proximal and distal portals that are established approximately 5 cm apart, parallel to the posterior border of the femur, and centered at the level of the lesser trochanter (Fig. 19.22a–d).
- 30° and 70° arthroscopes are used for visualization of the peritrochanteric space and ischiofemoral decompression.

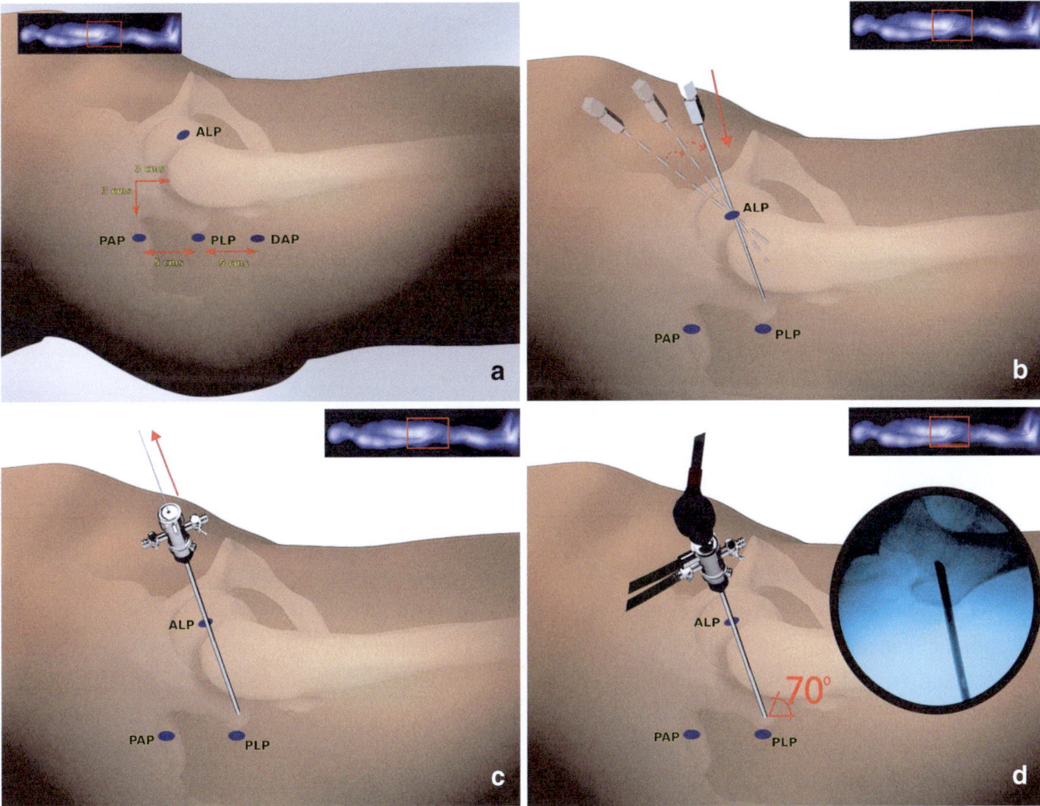

Fig. 19.22 (**a**) Endoscopic portals—ischiofemoral space. *Alp* anterolateral portal, *PAP* proximal accessory portal, *PLP* posterolateral portal, *DAP* distal accessory portal. (**b**) Endoscopic ischiofemoral space. Approach of the peritrochanteric space until reaching the posterior border of the greater trochanter. (**c**) Endoscopic ischiofemoral space. (**d**) Endoscopic ischiofemoral space. Use of fluoroscopy to locate the arthroscope. (**e**) Endoscopic ischiofemoral space. Identification of the sciatic nerve and quadratus femoris muscle. (**f**) Endoscopic ischiofemoral space. The quadratus femoris is identified and an opening is made on its medial third to avoid injury of the medial circumflex femoral vessels. (**g**) Endoscopic ischiofemoral space. The quadratus femoris window and exposition of the lesser trochanter and insertion of iliopsoas

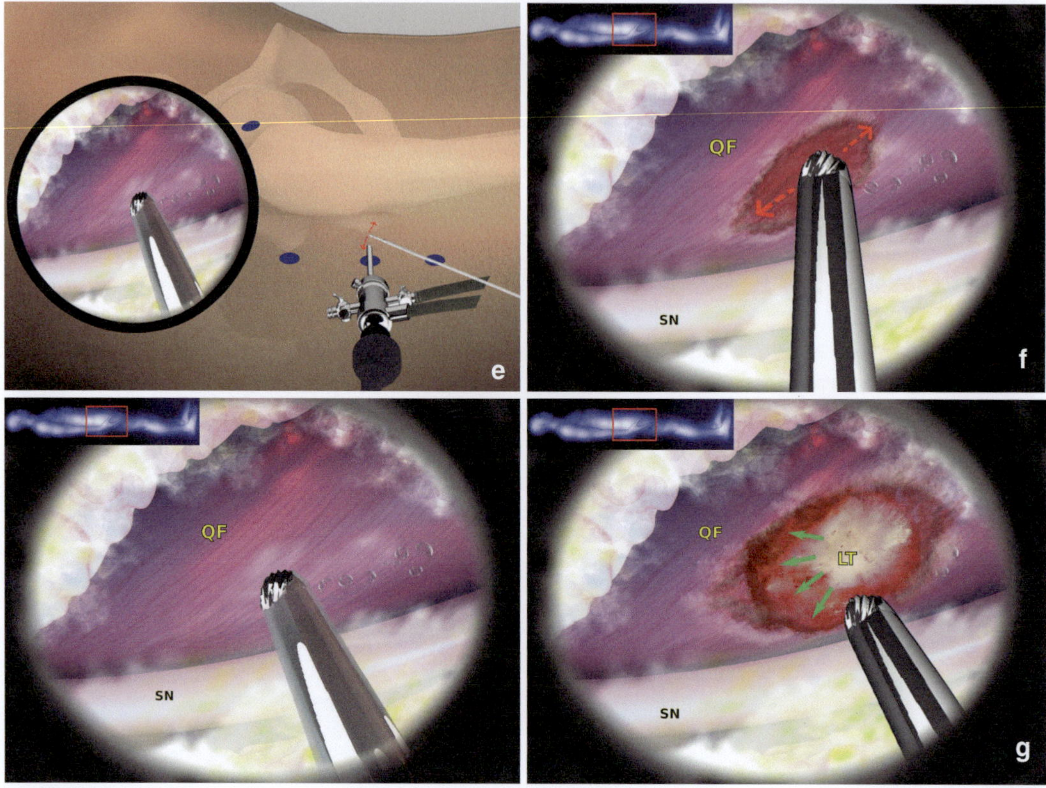

(continued)

- Once the peritrochanteric space posterior to the proximal femur has been entered, the gluteal sling? Seven and the sciatic nerve (located posterior and lateral to the femur) are identified (Fig. 19.22e).
- A blunt switching stick can be used to gently dissect and palpate the tissues to improve visualization.
- The quadratus femoris is identified and an opening is made on its medial third. Care must be taken to protect and avoid injury of the medial circumflex femoral vessels, which run along the superior border of the quadratus femoris and bifurcate at the level of the tendon (Fig. 19.22f).
- Fluoroscopy may be used to confirm the location relative to the lesser trochanter.
- Next, the leg is internally rotated about 20–40° to bring the lesser trochanter into the field of view.
- The camera is usually kept in the proximal portal and the instruments in the distal portal, which protects the irrigation through the circumflex vessels (Fig. 19.22g).
- The sciatic nerve is posterior to where the surgeon is working and can be protected by keeping the instruments in front of it (in front of the sciatic nerve itself).
- The resection of the posterior aspect of the lesser trochanter is done by progressive and

careful abrasion. The posterior femoral cortex will define the level of resection.
- Fluoroscopy is used to guide the resection.
- This particular subperiosteal approach maintains the insertion of the iliopsoas tendon on the anterior portion of the lesser trochanter and the femur.

Advantages

- Preservation of the insertion of the iliopsoas tendon on the anterior portion of the lesser trochanter.
- It allows concomitant treatment of other hip pathologies.
- It gives a fixed and reproducible reference point for the level of the osteotomy of the lesser trochanter.

General Disadvantages of Endoscopic Techniques

- Risk of sciatic nerve damage.
- Risk of injury to circumflex vessels.
- Risk of performing excessive osteotomy of the sub trochanteric femur.

Approaches for Posterior Hip Nerve Injuries

Open Approach for Posterior Thigh and Hip Nerve Injuries

The sciatic nerve can be exposed as it leaves through the greater sciatic notch towards the posterior region of the thigh [18].

Indications

- Extrapelvic entrapment of the sciatic nerve, posterior femoral cutaneous and pudendal nerve.
- Tumors of soft and vascular tissues located in the subgluteal space.

Patient's position: Prone position in translucent table.

Anatomical Landmarks and Skin Demarcation

- Posterior superior iliac spine
- Greater trochanter
- Gluteal fold

Procedure

- The incision begins at the PSIS and it is directed diagonally and distally in line with the fibers of the gluteus maximus towards the greater trochanter of the femur.
- Approximately 2.5 cm medial to the greater trochanter, the incision is curved towards the middle line, passing just distal to the gluteal fold and until its middle point.
- The incision can be extended to the posterior aspect of the thigh about 10 cm proximal to the skin fold of the popliteal fossa (Fig. 19.23).
- The posterior femoral cutaneous nerve is identified and protected at the level of the inferior border of the gluteus maximus.
- The incision goes deep through the gluteal fascia, and the fibers of the gluteus maximus are separated.
- The fascia of the thigh is incised longitudinally in relation to the gluteal fold, and the distal attachment of the gluteus maximus is separated from the iliotibial band (Fig. 19.24).
- The gluteus maximus and its neurovascular bundle are retracted medially to expose both the sciatic nerve and the piriformis muscle. The piriformis is tenotomized (Fig. 19.25).
- When the nerve injury is more distal to the ischium, the skin incision must be extended

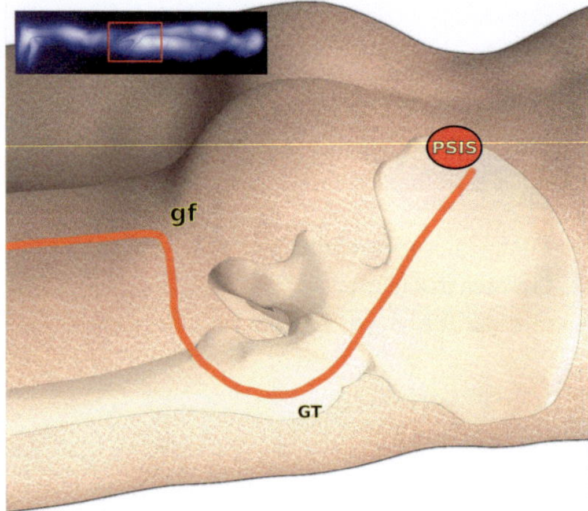

Fig. 19.23 Open approach of the sciatic nerve A. *PSIS* posterior superior iliac spine, *GT* greater trochanter, *Gf* gluteal fold

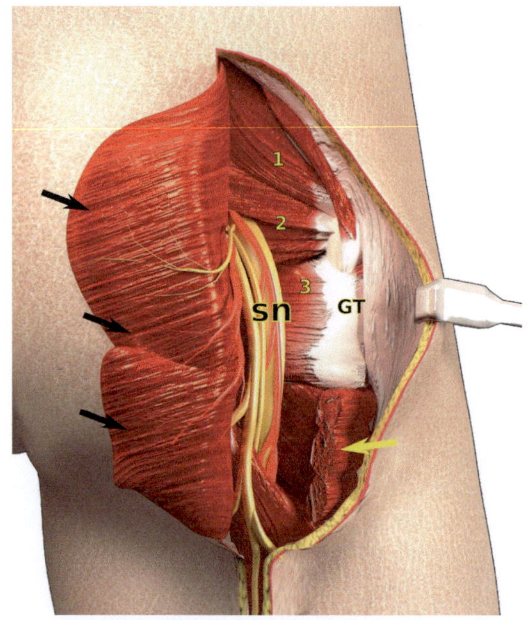

Fig. 19.25 Open approach of the sciatic nerve C. Black Arrows: The gluteus maximus and its neurovascular bundle are retracted medially, Yellow Arrow: distal attachment of the gluteus maximus separated, *Sn* sciatic nerve, 1: pir: m. piriformis, 2: obturator internus and superior and inferior gemellus muscles, 3: m. quadratus femoris

Advantages

- Wide exposure of the nerve from the greater sciatic notch to the posterior region of the thigh.
- Preservation of vascular planes.

Disadvantages

- The extensive detachment of the gluteus maximus is a time-consuming procedure and often requires the use of hip immobilizers.
- If the gluteal vessels are injured, they can retract up to the pelvis. In this case, a laparotomy may be needed to control the bleeding.

Transgluteal Approach for Posterior Thigh and Hip Nerve Injuries

All the posterior surgical approaches are essentially transgluteal techniques. The two most used techniques to treat sciatic nerve injuries in the subgluteal space are the Kocher-Langenbeck's approach and Moore's approach. They allow a quick exposure of the zone with shorter post-operative recovery.

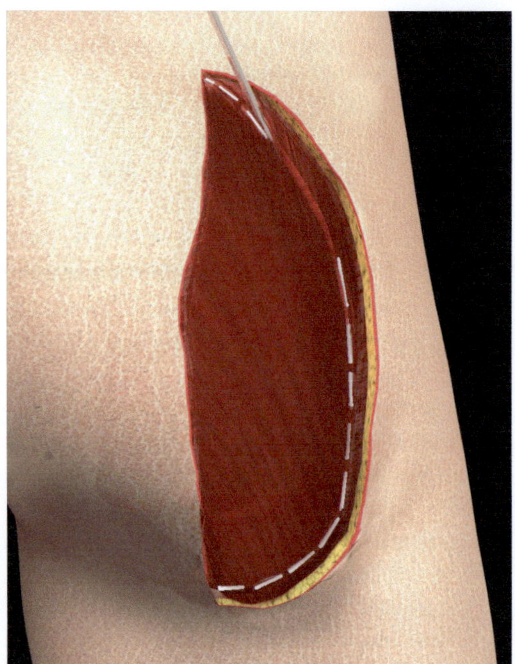

Fig. 19.24 Open approach of the sciatic nerve B. White dashed line: The incision goes deep through the gluteal fascia, and the fibers of the gluteus maximus are separated

from the middle of the gluteal fold to the posterior aspect of the thigh. Caution must be taken to protect the posterior femoral cutaneous nerve that is right under the deep fascia.

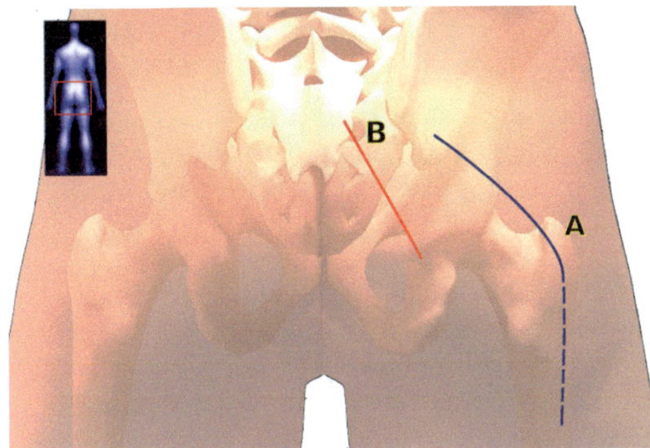

Fig. 19.26 Transgluteal approach of the sciatic nerve (blue line). A: transgluteal approach to sciatic nerve and piriformis, B: transgluteal approach to pudendal nerve

The divulsion of the gluteus maximus allows adequate exposure of the posterior femoral cutaneous nerve and the sciatic nerve as it passes through the greater sciatic notch. However the exposure of distal neurovascular structures is limited, and caution must be taken to avoid injury of superior and inferior gluteal nerves and vessels during the separation of the fibers of the gluteus maximus (Fig. 19.26).

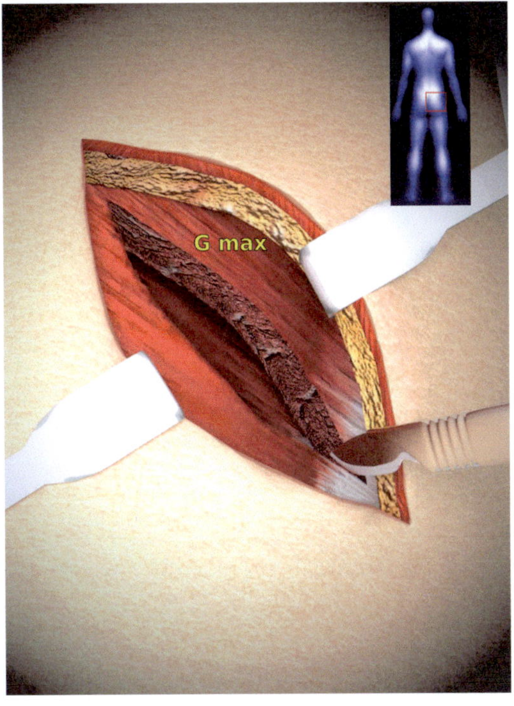

Fig. 19.27 Open transgluteal approach of the sciatic nerve A. *G max* gluteus maximus

Open Transgluteal Approach of the Sciatic Nerve [19, 20]

Indications

- Neurolysis of the sciatic nerve
- Tenotomy of the piriformis muscle

Patient's position: Lateral decubitus

Anatomical Landmarks and Skin Demarcation

Greater trochanter

Procedure

- The incision begins at the level of the posterolateral border of the tip of the greater trochanter and it is directed posteriorly following the fibers of the gluteus maximus.
- Dissection and separation of the fascia and fibers of the gluteus maximus (Fig. 19.27).

- The piriformis tendon is identified and tagged. The tendon is sectioned at the insertion on the greater trochanter and proximal dissection is performed until it goes through the greater sciatic notch (Fig. 19.28).
- Identification and neurolysis of the sciatic nerve by blunt dissection starting at the greater sciatic notch.
- Washing and hemostasis
- Layered closure

Endoscopic Approach of the Sciatic Nerve in the Subgluteal Space [21]
Indications

- Entrapment injuries of the sciatic nerve from its exit through the greater sciatic notch until the level of the quadratus femoris.

Patient's Position

- Supine position in a traction table, standard preparation for hip arthroscopy, no traction.

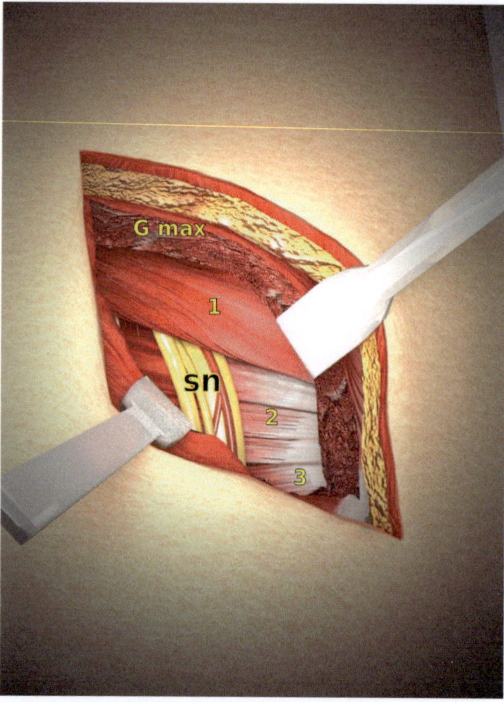

Fig. 19.28 Transgluteal approach of the sciatic nerve B. *Gmax* gluteus maximus dissected, *Sn* sciatic nerve, 1: pir: m. piriformis, 2: obturator internus and superior and inferior gemellus muscles, 3: m. quadratus femoris

Anatomical Landmarks and Skin Demarcation

- Greater trochanter
- Gluteal fold

Procedure

- Two standard hip arthroscopic portals (anterolateral and posterolateral) are established in the peritrochanteric space using 70° lenses (Fig. 19.29a).
- Another accessory portal is created 3 cm proximal and 3 cm posterior to the tip of the greater trochanter. This allows for a better visualization.
- The femoral insertion of the gluteus maximus and the quadratus femoris are identified and decompression of the sciatic nerve is performed, from distal to proximal (Fig. 19.29b).
- The mobility of the sciatic nerve is evaluated with internal and external rotation while the hip is flexed and internal and external rotation while the hip is extended.
- Once the cause of the nerve entrapment is identified, one can proceed to perform the release by blunt dissection (Fig. 19.29c).

Advantages

- It allows to address concomitant hip pathology
- Patient will be more comfortable while sitting or lying down.
- Better cosmetic results

Approaches for Pudendal Nerve Injuries

Transperineal Approach [22, 23]
This is the first approach described for this type of injury.

Indications: Distal entrapment of the nerve (after Alcock's canal).

Patient's position: Prone position, lithotomy position. Under general or raquideal anesthesia.

Procedure

- Vertical incision of the skin between the anus and the ischial tuberosity.
- Opening of the ischiorectal fossa with scissors.
- The inferior rectal nerve is identified and traced (using a finger)? back to the Alcock's canal.
- Opening of the Alcock's canal (this technique does not open the "clamp" between the sacro-spinal and sacro-tuberous ligaments)
- Hemostasis control.
- Skin closure with nylon sutures that allow drainage through them.

Disadvantages

- It requires deep dissection of the ischiorectal fat which is highly vascularized.
- It is difficult to reach the junction of the sacro-tuberous and sacrospinous ligaments (impingement zone) which may compromise the release of the critical compression area.

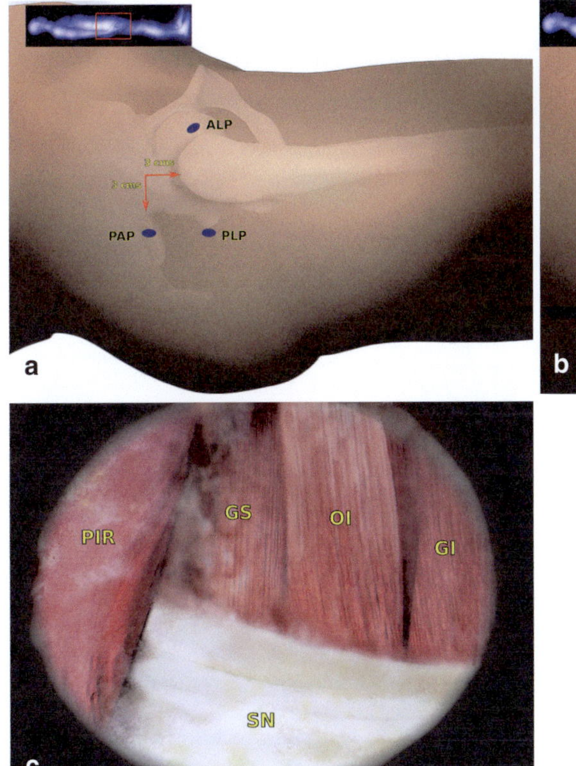

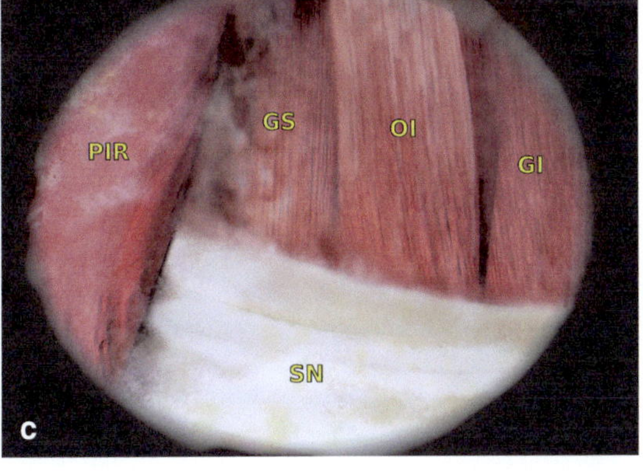

Fig. 19.29 (**a**) Endoscopic port of the subgluteal space. *ALP* anterolateral portal, *PAP* proximal accessory portal, *PLP* posterolateral portal. (**b**) Endoscopic Approach of subgluteal space. After approaching the posterior part of the peritrochanteric space, the sciatic nerve and the qua-dratus femoris are identified to direct proximally towards the sciatic emergency. (**c**) Endoscopic approach of subgluteal space. *Sn* sciatic nerve, *pir* m. piriformis, *OI* obturator internus, *GS* superior Gemellus muscles, *GI* inferior Gemellus muscles

- Risk of infection due to the location.
- Pain over the perianal scar when sitting down.

Transgluteal Approach of the Pudendal Nerve [24]

Professor Robert in France first described it, and it is probably the most used method for surgical decompression of the pudendal nerve.

Indications: extra and intrapelvic entrapment of the pudendal nerve

Patient's position: prone or genupectoral position.

Procedure

- Gluteal oblique incision (in line with the gluteus maximus fibers) of about 7 cm, it must be centered in the transverse line of the superior portion of the coccyx (Fig. 19.30).

- Dissection and deinsertion of the gluteus maximus from the sacrotuberous ligament (Figs. 19.31 and 19.32)
- Transverse section of the sacrotuberous ligament at the level of the ischiatic spine.
- Visualization of the pudendal neurovascular bundle and its release from the dorsal aspect of the sacrospinous ligament.
- Medial retraction of the ischiorectal fat using a separator and exposure of the pudendal canal.
- Digital release of the nerve.
- If the obturator fascia is thickened or the falciform process is compromised, the release is done by an incision.
- The sacrospinous ligament is sectioned and the nerve can be transposed in front of the ischiatic spine.

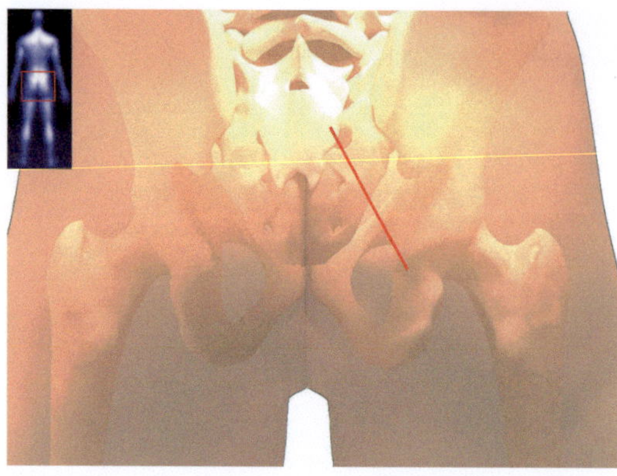

Fig. 19.30 Transgluteal approach of the pudendal nerve A

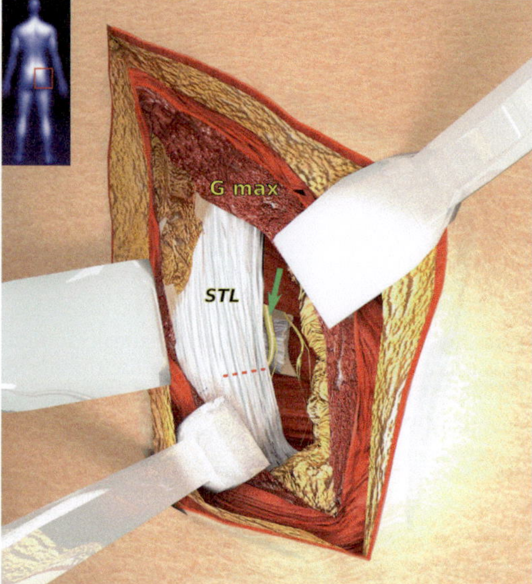

Fig. 19.31 Transgluteal approach of the pudendal nerve B. Green arrow: pudendal nerve, *Gmax* gluteus maximus, *Stl* sacrotuberous ligament, Red dashed line: incision of sacrotuberous ligament

- The diameter, shape, and aspect of the nerve and the presence of fibrosis and dilations of the satellital veins must be evaluated.
- Layered closure is performed

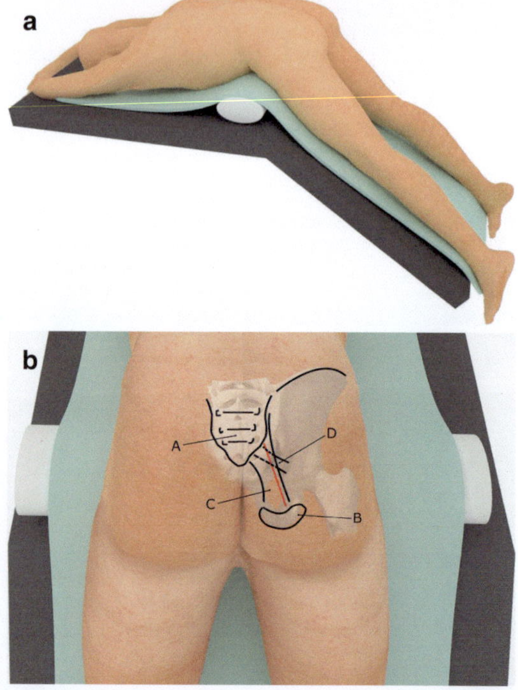

Fig. 19.32 Transgluteal approach to expose the pudendal nerve. (**a**) Patient's setup in a prone position with hip flexion. (**b**) Posterior hip anatomy landmarks are the sacrum (A), ischial tuberosity (B), sacrotuberous ligament (C), sacrospinous ligament (D)

The sacrifice of the two ligaments does not have adverse effects in the sacroiliac joint. Some surgeons use a modified version of the transgluteal approach and avoid cutting the ligaments, however this leads to a poor visual field. Some authors describe reconstruction of the ligaments with Achilles' tendon allograft.

Advantages

- There is better visualization of the nerve during the procedure.
- Less risk of bleeding.
- Less risk of infection.

Coccyx and Sacroiliac Joint

Approach of the Sacroiliac Joint [7]

Indications

- Luxations or fractures of the sacroiliac joint
- Sacroiliac joint arthrosis

Patient's position: prone position

Anatomical Landmark and Skin Demarcation

Posterior iliac crest
Posterior superior iliac spine
Middle sacrum line (over the dorsal spines) (Fig. 19.33)

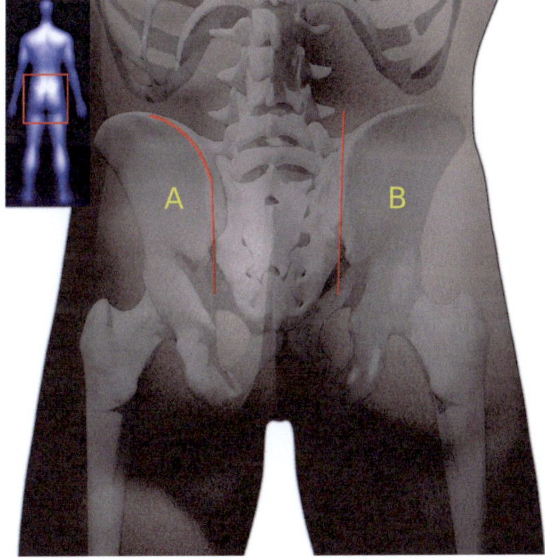

Fig. 19.33 Approach of the sacroiliac joint. Anatomical landmarks. B: The skin incision is vertical of about 12–15 cm long and located 2 cm lateral to the PSIS. A: If the extension towards the posterior superior iliac crest is necessary, the incision will be curved, going laterally along the iliac crest

Modified Surgical Technique: Procedure

- The skin incision is vertical of about 12–15 cm long and located 2 cm lateral to the PSIS. If the extension towards the posterior superior iliac crest is necessary, the incision will be curved, going laterally along the iliac crest. The incision must allow for exposure of the greater sciatic notch and the inferior part of the sacroiliac joint. It also must allow enough medial subfascial dissection to release the attachment of the gluteus maximus from the sacrum.
- The incision must be deep enough to reach the fascia of the gluteus maximus and allow the creation of a full thickness fasciocutaneous flap (different from the traditional description that creates a subcutaneous flap just superficial to the fascia of the gluteus maximus with subsequent dead space formation)
- The medial subfascial dissection is meticulously performed and the muscular portion of the gluteus maximus is carefully released from the fascia.
- The fascia of the gluteus maximus has septal extensions that invaginate in the muscle approximately every 10 mm. Special care must be taken to maintain the correct plane without injuring the fascia and minimizing the muscular damage. Maintaining an intact fascia is necessary for anatomic closure. The medial dissection is complete when the origin of the gluteus maximus in the sacrum is identified.
- Once the origin of the gluteus maximus is identified, the muscle is released from the aponeuroses of the thoracolumbar fascia, the iliac crest, the PSIS, and the multifidus fascia. Next, the gluteus maximus is released from the sacral crest to allow a better exposure. An adequate portion of the tendon must be preserved to facilitate an anatomical repair.
- If the pattern of the fracture requires an exposure closer to the greater sciatic notch, caution must be taken to avoid injury of the superior

gluteal vessels and nerves that emerge above the piriformis muscle in this area.

- It is possible to visualize the anterior aspect of the sacroiliac joint and palpate the ventral sacral foramina, to evaluate the reduction by dissection of the attachment of the piriformis muscle from the anterior portion of the sacrum with a curved periosteal elevator.
- If it is necessary for fracture fixation, the erector spinae muscle and the multifidus muscle can be lifted and medially dissected from the dorsal surface of the sacrum to gain complete exposure. If this procedure is performed, caution must be taken to preserve the fasciculations of the multifidus muscle to the PSIS and the posterior sacroiliac ligaments.
- Debridement of the nonviable muscle and careful washing of the zone must be performed, a drain in the abductor muscles with opening to the skin lateral to the surgical wound is placed, and then one can proceed with closure.
- The distal origin of the gluteus muscle is attached first to the remnant periosteum over the dorsomedial and medial surface of the sacrum, and in the proximal region to the multifidus fascia using an absorbable suture. The proximal attachment of the gluteus maximus is then sutured to the thoracolumbar fascia.
- Several reinforcement sutures must be used to avoid the avulsion of the gluteus maximus origin and if possible to secure the medial extension of the gluteus maximus fascia that is part of the subfascial flap, minimizing the potential dead space.
- A second drain is left superficial to the gluteus maximus and under the fascia. The gluteus maximus fascia is repaired with an absorbable suture. Finally a conventional closure of the subcutaneous space, subdermal, and subcuticular layer is performed.

Advantages

- Anatomical landmarks of easy recognition.
- En-bloc and lateral subperiosteal displacement of the gluteus maximus avoiding injury of the superior gluteal nerve.
- Adequate exposure of the sacroiliac joint by osteotomy.

Disadvantages

- Location of the wound, which may interfere with supine position for resting.
- Dead space due to the flap.
- Risk of injury of superior gluteal vessels and nerve
- Closeness to perianal region.

Complications

- Injury of superior gluteal vessels and nerve if the approach goes past the posterior iliac crest.
- Infection.

Approach of Both Sacroiliac Joints or Sacrum (Mears and Rubash's Modification) [5]

Indications

- Unstable luxations of both sacroiliac joints
- Vertical comminuted fractures of the sacrum as part of a pelvic ring disruption

Patient's position: Prone position

Anatomical Landmarks and Skin Demarcation

Posterior iliac crest
Posterior superior Iliac Spine
Midline of the sacrum (above the dorsal spines)

Procedure

- A transverse straight incision 1 cm lower to the posterior superior iliac spine and through the middle portion of the sacrum is performed (Fig. 19.34).
- If the sciatic nerve needs to be explored either on one or both sides, the end of the incision may be distally curved in order to allow exposure of the sciatic nerves from the sacrum to the greater sciatic notch.

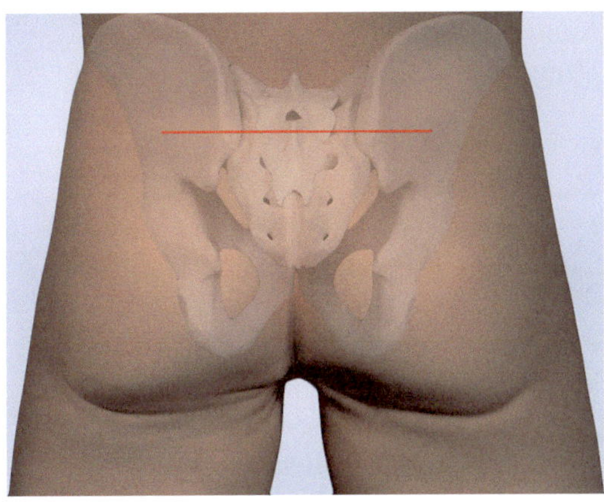

Fig. 19.34 Approach of both sacroiliac joints

- Incision through the deep fascia to expose the superior aspect of the origins of both gluteus maximus in the posterior iliac spines.
- The paravertebral muscles are lifted and a medial to lateral osteotomy of the posterior superior iliac spines is performed. Care must be taken to avoid injury of the origin of the gluteus maximus muscle.
- The tips of the spinous processes of the sacrum are osteotomized as necessary.
- If the sacroiliac joints need to be exposed, it is necessary to either split the gluteus maximus muscle or to make an incision on its origin at the posterior superior iliac spine and go laterally, in order to expose the posterior portion of the iliac bone and to perform a larger osteotomy of the posterior ilium.

Advantages

- Exposure of both joints and the body of the sacrum
- Visualization of the ligaments and the sacral foramina.

Disadvantages

- Location of the wound (near to the anus).

- Location of the wound may interfere with supine position for resting.
- Risk of dead space formation
- Risk of injury of superior gluteal vessels and nerves.
- Instability due to resection of the posterior sacroiliac ligaments.

Complications

Infections
Flap necrosis
Hematomas

Arthroscopic Approach of the Sacroiliac Joint (As an Aid for Joint Arthrodesis) [25]

Indications

- Type C pelvic fractures (Tile classification) documented with CT scan and characterized by luxation of the sacroiliac joint combined with diastasis of the pubic symphysis or fracture of the obturator foramen.

Patient's Position

- Prone position on a radiolucent surgical table without traction with a 30° flexion of the hip by using cushioned sacks under the pelvis.

Anatomical Landmarks and Skin Demarcation

Procedure

- The initial portal is directed to the joint space and is placed 2.5 cm from the midline. The direction of this portal is established by palpating the posterior iliac crest and then inclining in a 60° angle in the sagittal plane.
- Once at the sagittal plane, the cephalocaudal location varies according to the area to be

explored. The location of the instrument must be confirmed with fluoroscopy.

- Once the joint is exposed, another rigid cannula is inserted to establish the working portal. These portals are interchangeable in order to improve access to the joint.
- An incision is then made in the center of the lumbosacral joint to allow the insertion of the screw into L5, S1, and S2 pedicles.
- The subcutaneous space is dissected until reaching the fascia of the posterior iliac crest, where the erector spine muscle partially rises, allowing the extension of the access to the sacroiliac joint.

Advantages

It is minimally invasive in a potentially contaminated place.

It allows the debridement of the anterior aspect of the sacroiliac joint.

It allows the introduction of bone grafts under direct visualization.

Disadvantages

It is a technically difficult procedure

It is not highly reproducible

Lack of information about results

Complications

Instruments damage

Approach to the Coccyx and the Sacrococcygeal Joint [11, 26]

Indications

- Partial or total resection of the coccyx

Patient's Position

- Prone position (Kraske's position) with the buttocks separated and tightly fixed by using adhesives in order to facilitate the exposure of the coccyx.

Anatomical Landmarks and Skin Demarcation

- The incision must be longitudinal beginning at the level of the sacrococcygeal junction to the tip of the coccyx, with a distal margin of no less than 4 cm from the anus.

Procedure: Surgical Technique (Gardner's Modification)

- The incision of approximately 6–7.5 cm long is made in the midline over the intergluteal fold, ending at 4 cm from the anus.
- The incision is deepened with electrocautery to the level where the posterior aspect of the coccyx is exposed.
- The zone of instability is identified by palpation and direct visualization, and is carefully demarcated with the electric scalpel, always maintaining the cut close to the bone until exposing the lateral borders of the coccyx. Caution must be taken in order to achieve adequate hemostasis of the coccygeal vessels that run on each side of the coccyx.
- Then one can proceed to expose the anterior aspect of the coccyx, which is very close to the rectum, because of this a meticulous dissection is mandatory. Starting at the level of the sacrococcygeal junction disk or the abnormally mobile segment, advance slowly to the tip of the coccyx. At this point many surgeons prefer to perform a dissection that leaves an anterior subperiosteal plane, leaving intact the ligamentous and muscular insertions in front of it, which has shown to significantly decrease the risk of post-surgical infections.
- The residual portion of the coccyx, and even the most proximal portion of the sacrum from the sacrococcygeal junction, may be removed by using a gouge.
- It is recommended to make the final closure in three layers, a negative pressure drain can be used and it must be removed after 24 or 48 h.
- Placement of the final dressing is important, as it must isolate the surgical wound from the anal margin.

Advantages

It allows management of chronic pain due to sacrococcygeal alterations.

Disadvantages

- Location of the incision
- Risk of bleeding, highly vascularized area
- Risk of sensitivity alterations
- High risk of contamination

Complications

- Injury of the rectum
- Intraoperative bleeding
- Wound infection.

Comments of the Author

The posterior space is small, but it contains many neurological and vascular structures, which requires a perfect anatomical knowledge of the area.

Pathologies or injuries of the posterior hip have previously been described separately, this chapter aimed to compile all these isolated topics.

The chapter was divided into three subareas: (a) articular, (b) subgluteal space, and (c) sacrum, which allowed for describing and analyzing with more details on every approach. We hope this gives to the reader a specific guideline to this area.

References

1. Farrell C, et al. Motor nerve palsy following primary total hip arthroplasty. J Bone Joint Surg. 2005;87-A(12):2619–25.
2. Carr J, Leach P. Small-incision surgical exposure for select fractures of the acetabulum: the gluteus maximus-splitting approach. J Orthop Trauma. 2006;20(8):573–5.
3. Matta J. Operative indications and choice of surgical approach for fractures of the acetabulum. Tech Orthop. 1986;1:13–21.
4. Rommens P. Abordaje de Kocher-Langenbeck para el tratamiento de las fracturas acetabulares. Tec Quir Ortop Traumatol. 2004;13(3):120–31.
5. Crenshaw A. General principles. Chapter 1 Surgical techniques and approaches. In: Canale ST, Beaty JH, editors. Campbell's operative orthopaedics. 11th ed. Philadelphia: Mosby; 2007. p. 90–1.
6. Matta J. Operative indications and choice of surgical approach for fractures of the acetabulum. Tech Orthop. 1986;13–21.
7. Fowler TT, et al. The posterior approach to pelvic ring injuries: a technique for minimizing soft tissue complications. Injury. 2013;44:1780–6.
8. Moed BR. The modified Gibson approach to the acetabulum. Oper Orthop Traumatol. 2014;26(6):591–602. https://doi.org/10.1007/s00064-011-0111-1.
9. Chechik O, et al. Surgical approach and prosthesis fixation in hip arthroplasty world wide. Arch Orthop Trauma Surg. 2013;133:1595–600. https://doi.org/10.1007/s00402-013-1828-0.
10. White R, Archibeck M. Abordaje posterolateral. In: Barrack & Rosenberg editores. Master en Cirugía Ortopédica: Cadera. 2nd ed. Madrid: España Marban Libros; 2009. p. 29–41.
11. Gardner RC. An improved technic of coccygectomy. Clin Orthop Relat Res. 1972;85:143–5.
12. Gómez-Hoyos J, et al. Dry endoscopic-assisted mini-open approach with neuromonitoring for chronic hamstring avulsions and ischial tunnel syndrome. Arthrosc Tech. 2015;4(3):e193–9.
13. Dierckman B, Guanche C. Endoscopic proximal hamstring repair and ischial bursectomy. Arthrosc Tech. 2012;1(2):e201–7.
14. Domb B, et al. Endoscopic repair of proximal hamstring avulsion. Arthrosc Tech. 2013;2(1):e35–9.
15. Jackson T, et al. Endoscopic transtendinous repair for partial-thickness proximal hamstring tendon tears. Arthrosc Tech. 2014;3(1):e127–30.
16. Young Ian J, et al. Surgical release for proximal hamstring syndrome. Am J Sports Med. 2008;36(12):2372–8.
17. Howse E, et al. Ischiofemoral space decompression through posterolateral approach: cutting block technique. Arthrosc Tech. 2014;3(6):e661–5.
18. Jobe Mark T, Martinez Santos F. Peripheral nerve injuries: sciatic nerve. Volume IV, Part XVI, Chapter 59. In: Canale ST, Beaty JH, editors. Campbell's operative orthopaedics. 11th ed. Philadelphia: Mosby; 2007. p. 3691–2.
19. Benson ER, Schutzer SF. Posttraumatic piriformis syndrome: diagnosis and results of operative treatment. J Bone Joint Surg Am. 1999;81:941–9.
20. Patil PG, Friedman AH. Surgical exposure of the sciatic nerve in the gluteal region: anatomic and historical comparison of two approaches. Oper Neurosurg. 2005;56(1):165–71. https://doi.org/10.1227/01.NEU.0000144169.84261.9D.
21. Martin HD, et al. The endoscopic treatment of sciatic nerve entrapment/deep gluteal syndrome. Arthroscopy. 2011;27(2):172–81.
22. Shafik A. Pudendal canal syndrome. Description of a new syndrome and its treatment: report of 7 cases. Coloproctology. 1991;13:102–10.
23. Shafik A, et al. Surgical anatomy of the pudendal nerve and its clinical implications. Clin Anat. 1995;8:110–5.
24. Robert R, et al. Decompression and transposition of the pudendal nerve in pudendal neuralgia: a

randomized controlled trial and long-term evaluation. Eur Urol. 2005;47:403–40.

25. Ould-Slimane M, et al. Sacro-iliac joint arthroscopy for arthrodesis after traumatic dislocation. Cadaver and clinical feasibility study. Orthop Traumatol Surg Res. 2014;100:159–63.

26. Nathan T, Fisher BE, Robert CS. Coccydynia. A review of pathoanatomy, aetiology, treatment and outcome. J Bone Joint Surg. 2010;92-b(12):1622–7.

27. Beaton LE, Anson BJ. The relation of the sciatic nerve and its subdivisions to the piriformis muscle. Anat Rec.1937;70:1–5.

Physical Therapy and Rehabilitation in Posterior Hip Pathology

RobRoy L. Martin, Ryan P. McGovern,
Ricardo Gonçalves Schröder,
and Benjamin R. Kivlan

Rehabilitation for those with posterior hip pain begins with a standard comprehensive physical examination that not only determines a diagnosis but also classifies individuals into treatment categories and identifies impairments that need to be addressed with physical therapy intervention. The identified impairments can be prioritized and treated within the context of the particular diagnosis. As the examination relates to identifying impairments in individuals with posterior hip pain, particular attention needs to be paid to strength, flexibility, range of motion, and neuromuscular control. An assessment of biomechanical abnormalities should also be included in the examination, with a focus on identifying leg length discrepancy, dynamic valgus of the knee joint during loading, and excessive pronation. In those with posterior hip pain, interventions should be directed at a prioritized problem list that considers static and dynamic alignment abnormalities. A physical therapy-based evaluation algorithm and classification system are available to manage individuals with posterior hip pain [1, 2]. This algorithm- and classification-based treatment system includes considerations for the lumbosacral spine and intra-articular and extra-articular sources of hip posterior pain.

Lumbosacral Spine

Pain radiating from the lumbosacral spine needs to be considered when individuals present with posterior hip pain. Gait and postural deviations that result from hip impairments can negatively affect lumbosacral spine alignment and function. A physical therapy assessment of the lumbosacral spine includes an evaluation of pelvic landmark symmetry, lumbar spine range of motion, sacroiliac joint special tests, lumbosacral segmental mobility, and response to sustained and repeated lumbar movements. When the lumbosacral spine is found to contribute to an individual's symptoms, physical therapy intervention can be directed according to manipulation/mobilization, stabilization, and specific movement direction

R. L. Martin, PhD, PT, CSCS (✉)
Department of Physical Therapy, Rangos School
of Health Sciences, Duquesne University,
Pittsburgh, PA, USA

Centers for Sports Medicine, University of Pittsburgh,
Pittsburgh, PA, USA
e-mail: martinr280@duq.edu

R. P. McGovern, MS, ATC
Rangos School of Health Sciences, Rehabilitation
Sciences, Duquesne University, Pittsburgh, PA, USA
e-mail: mcgover1@duq.edu

R. G. Schröder, PT
Hip Preservation Center, Baylor University Medical
Center, Dallas, TX, USA

B. R. Kivlan, PhD, PT, OCS, SCS
Department of Physical Therapy, Rangos School
of Health Sciences, Duquesne University,
Pittsburgh, PA, USA
e-mail: kivlanb@duq.edu

© Springer International Publishing AG, part of Springer Nature 2019
H. D. Martin, J. Gómez-Hoyos (eds.), *Posterior Hip Disorders*,
https://doi.org/10.1007/978-3-319-78040-5_20

preference (flexion, extension, or lateral shift) treatment categories [3, 4].

The mobilization category describes treating individuals who have a decreased lumbosacral segmental mobility and/or positive tests for sacroiliac joint dysfunction [3, 4]. The mobilization treatment technique involves positioning the patient, with respect to the lumbar spine, in side bending toward and rotation away from the painful side. A force directed anterior to posterior is applied to the anterior superior iliac spine on the symptomatic side in a Grade 5 thrusting maneuver (Fig. 20.1). Individuals who fall into this category are also given lumbopelvic range of motion and strengthening exercises. The stabilization category describes treating individuals who are thought to have hypermobility/instability of the lumbosacral spine [3, 4]. Therefore, individuals in the stabilization category have increase segmental lumbar mobility, generally appear to be very flexible, and present with weakness in the muscles that support the spine. Strengthening and stabilization exercise for muscles that support the lumbopelvic spine are emphasized for individuals who fall into this category. The spe-

cific movement direction preference category describes individuals who report an improvement in symptoms with repeated and/or sustained lumbar flexion, extension, or side bending [3, 4]. The movements that produced a favorable response are incorporated into a comprehensive exercise program for individuals in this category.

Conditions in the hip and lumbosacral spine commonly coexist because of the interaction between the hip and lumbosacral complex. Following intervention directed at the lumbosacral spine and the results of reassessment of previously positive signs and symptoms, the evaluation may need to continue to assess intra- and extra-articular hip structures as a contributor to the individual's posterior hip pain.

Intra- vs. Extra-Articular Hip Pain

Once the lumbosacral spine is evaluated, the clinician must determine if there is an intra-articular and/or extra-articular source of symptoms. The flexion-abduction-external rotation (FABER), internal range of motion with over-pressure (IROP), flexion-adduction-internal rotation (FADIR), and scour tests are recommended tests [5–10]. If the FABER, FADIR, IROP, and/or scour tests reproduce symptoms, an intra-articular source of symptoms should be considered as a source of the posterior hip pain.

Intra-Articular Hip Pain

Related to intra-articular hip pathology, posterior impingement can be a cause of posterior hip pain. In these individuals, the lateral and posterior rim tests are typically found to reproduce pain. Intervention individuals with posterior impingement address underlying arthrokinematic and range of motion restrictions with appropriate joint mobilization. An inferior joint glide, moving the femur on the acetabulum, is employed to increase hip flexion range of motion (Fig. 20.2). A distraction joint mobilizations with movement using a manual therapy belt can be done to improve pain-free range of motion, in particular internal rotation (Fig. 20.3). This mobilization

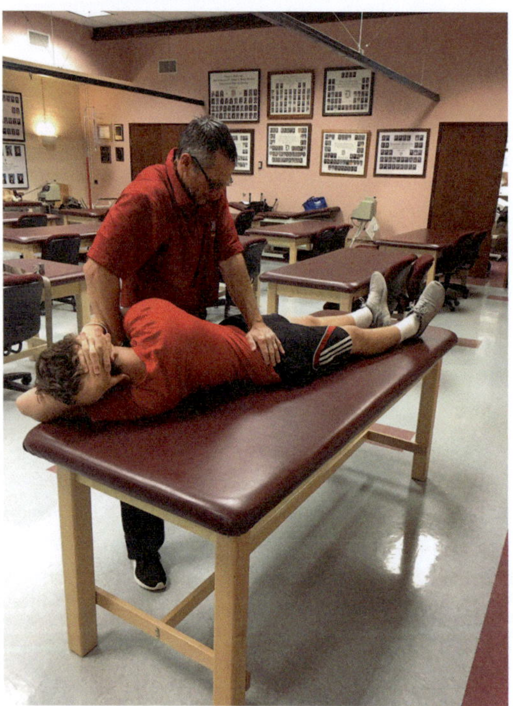

Fig. 20.1 Mobilization treatment technique

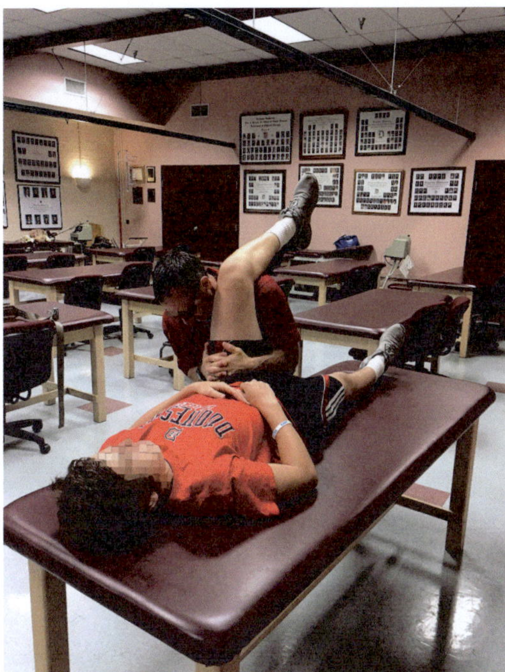

Fig. 20.2 An inferior joint glide of the hip

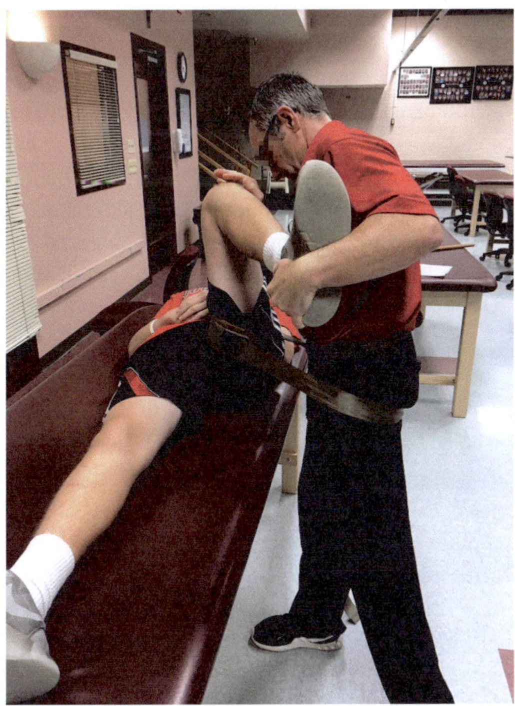

Fig. 20.3 Distraction mobilizations of the hip

with movement technique, in addition to increasing range of motion, may facilitate pain reduction by stimulating joint mechanoreceptors [11]. If the FABER, FADIR, IROP, and scour tests do not reproduce the individual's symptoms, an extra-articular source of posterior hip pain should be considered.

Extra-Articular Hip Pain

Musculotendinous pathologies, nerve entrapments, and boney impingement can act as sources of extra-articular posterior hip pain. A comprehensive and consistent physical examination needs to be performed to properly identify source(s) of extra-articular hip pain.

Musculotendinous Pathology

In those with musculotendinous sources of hip pain, provocation of symptoms should occur with palpation, passive lengthening, and/or resisted movement directed at the involved tissues. As it relates to posterior hip pain, particular attention should be given to the gluteus medius, piriformis, deep external rotators (obturator internus, quadratus femoris, inferior and superior gemellus), adductors, and hamstring muscles. The symptoms of musculotendinous pathologies can also be dynamically reproduced during gait and functional tasks. For example, gait can reproduce pain during the initial load and terminal swing phases in those with ischial tunnel syndrome and/or proximal hamstring pathologies. Also, individuals with a gluteus medius pathology may report symptoms of pain and have excessive pelvic sway during the stance phase of gait.

Intervention techniques for individuals with musculotendinous pathologies will depend on the phase of the healing that can be defined as either acute inflammatory, subacute, or chronic remodeling [12]. An acute injury can be identified in those with redness, warmth, and/or swelling. Additionally, individuals in the acute phase healing are usually not able to achieve full active movement against gravity when using the involved muscle [12]. Acute injuries are treated with modalities to promote healing, decrease pain, and reduce inflammation. Additionally, submaximal isometric exercises, passive range of motion, and lumbopelvic stabilization exercises should be included as part of the intervention plan. All of these intervention techniques should be pain-free. The ability to concentrically move through full range of motion can be used as the criteria to progress individuals to the subacute phase of healing [12]. Subacute injuries are treated with concentric exercises, including functional closed chain/weight-bearing exercises. Treatment progression includes the addition of more dynamic lumbopelvic stabilization, general stretching, and progressive balance exercises. Criteria to progress to the chronic remodeling phase of healing can include range of motion that is similar to the uninvolved side and strength that approximates 75% of uninvolved side [12]. Pain with resisted testing should be minimal for those in the chronic remodeling phase of healing. Interventions for individuals in the chronic remodeling phase should emphasize eccentric exercises and sport-specific training [12].

Manual therapy soft tissue interventions can also be employed in those with musculotendinous pathology. The goals of this intervention are to increase range of motion, reduce pain, decrease swelling, increase flexibility, and/or improve muscle performance. Manual therapy soft tissue techniques can include traditional massage, trigger point therapy, and active release. Soft tissue techniques can include the use of specialized instruments in treatment administration. These instrument-assisted soft tissue mobilization techniques attempt to induce biological changes that promote the reabsorption of scar tissue and to stimulate the regeneration of soft tissues [13, 14]. These techniques may also try to mechanically mobilize tissues that are restricting the gliding of tissue [15].

Nerve Entrapment

Posterior hip pain can also be caused by nerve entrapment in the deep gluteal space. Entrapment can be caused by the piriformis, gluteal, hamstring, and gemelli-obturator internus muscles, as well as fibrous bands in the area. Pain at the level of the external rotators and piriformis muscles can indicate sciatic nerve entrapment at that location. Pain lateral to the ischium can indicate ischiofemoral impingement involving the sciatic nerve, while pain medial to ischium is suggestive of pudendal nerve entrapment. The seated palpation test can be used to distinguish the source of entrapment based on location of tenderness [16]. This test requires the patient to sit on the examiner's hand while the examiner simultaneously palpates three locations in the gluteal area: (1) piriformis (lateral/superior) at the level of the external rotators, (2) hamstring on the ischium, and (3) obturator internus and soft tissue medial to the ischium [16].

Intervention strategies for those with nerve entrapment can include neural gliding, soft tissue mobilization, stretching and strengthening exercises, aerobic conditioning, and cognitive behavior education [17]. Neural gliding is a specific technique that attempts to improve neurodynamics by restoring movement of the nerve in relation to surrounding structures [17]. The hypothesized benefits of neural gliding techniques include facilitation of normal nerve mobility, reduction of nerve adherence, dispersion of noxious fluids, reduction of intraneural edema, increased neural vascularity, and improvement of axoplasmic flow. These techniques may also affect central mechanisms by decreasing nociceptive behavior in the spinal cord [17]. To perform the neural glide technique, an understanding of neurokinematics is required. For example, sciatic nerve glide would require combined movements of hip flexion, knee extension, and ankle dorsiflexion to "slide" the nerve (Fig. 20.4). The clinician must perform neural gliding using pain-free range of motion in a slowly controlled progressive manner in order to prevent overstretching of the nerve.

In addition to neural gliding, soft tissue mobilization and exercises may also try to mechanically mobilize nerve and surrounding tissue. Stretching, whether done independently by a patient or performed by a clinician, attempts to relieve nerve compression by lengthening shortened musculotendinous structures. One specific exercise for the sciatic nerve involves the combined movements of hip flexion, abduction, and external rotation to symptom provocation followed by movements of hip adduction, internal rotation,

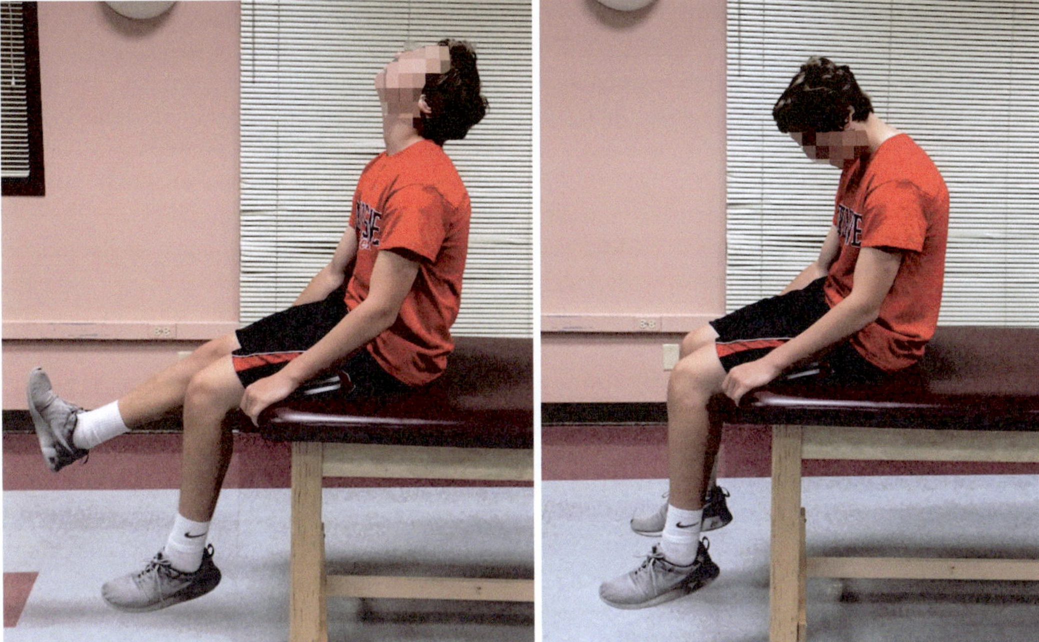

Fig. 20.4 Sciatic nerve glide

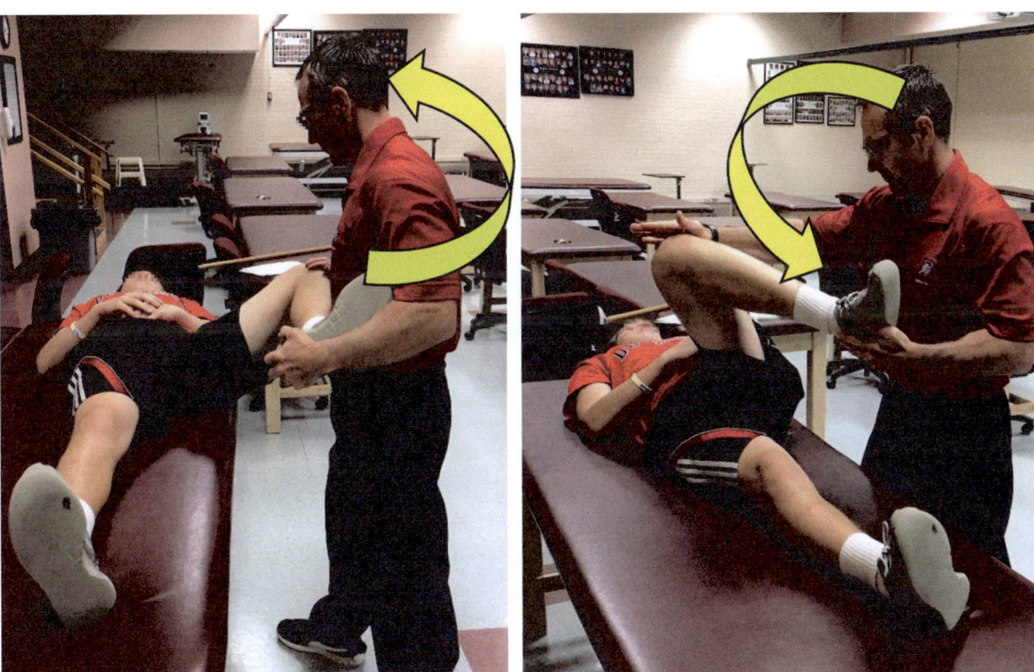

Fig. 20.5 Exercise to mobilize the sciatic nerve

and extension (Fig. 20.5). This movement combination is felt to mobilize the sciatic nerve in the deep gluteal region. Also included in the intervention plan are lumbosacral and hip strengthening exercises. The goal of these exercises is to facilitate proper load transfer and neuromuscular control between the lumbosacral spine, pelvis, and lower extremity.

Ischiofemoral Impingement

Posterior hip pain from ischiofemoral impingement (IFI) is a result of a compressive injury to the structures between the ischium and lesser trochanter. Structures that can be impinged in this space include the quadratus femoris muscle, hamstrings tendon, and sciatic nerve [18]. The long stride and IFI tests have demonstrated high diagnostic accuracy in identifying those with IFI [19]. Muscle weakness impairments in the hip region, particularly with abduction, may lead to a lack of pelvic control and dynamic hip adduction during the stance phase of gait.

Treatment of those with IFI should emphasize the stabilization and alignment of the lumbar spine, pelvis, and hip. Ischiofemoral impingement is often associated with decreased terminal hip extension. This lack of hip extension can cause increased compensatory lumbar extension and a risk of developing low back pain. The correction of an excessive pelvic adduction and lack of hip extension during ambulation must be emphasized as part of the intervention plan. Therefore, exercise directed at strengthening the gluteus medius in weight bearing should be included. Because the quadratus femoris and sciatic nerve can be involved in individuals with IFI, soft tissue mobilization and nerve gliding may also need to be included in the intervention plan.

Impairment-Based Examination

A clinical examination not only identifies a diagnosis but also serves to identify impairments that may contribute to the development of posterior hip pain. The impairments can be prioritized and treated within the context of the diagnosis. A comprehensive examination should assess the entire lower kinetic chain for strength, range of motion, flexibility, and neuromuscular deficits as well as biomechanical abnormalities. The components of the examination can be found in Fig. 20.6. As the examination relates to identifying impairments in individuals with posterior hip pain, particular attention needs to be paid to range of motion of the lumbar spine and hip; flexibility of gluteus medius, gluteus minimus, piriformis, hamstrings, iliotibial band, and iliopsoas muscles; and strength with abduction, extension, external rotation, and flexion movements. An assessment for leg length discrepancy, dynamic valgus, and excessive pronation should also be included in the examination.

Static and dynamic alignment is also important to consider in those with posterior hip pain. For example, those with hamstring injuries may have poor sagittal plane pelvic alignment. An excessive posteriorly tilted pelvis may be a result of limited hamstring flexibility. A lack of dynamic control of the lower limb during gait with excessive internal rotation and adduction of the hip is termed dynamic valgus. Eccentric overload in the piriformis and deep external rotators can occur in individuals with dynamic valgus. The inclusion of education in proper static and dynamic alignment can enhance postural control and be an important intervention strategy.

The interaction of range of motion, flexibility, strength, balance, proprioception, and neuromuscular control may be best assessed with functional performance tests. These tests, which can include balance tests, hop/jump tests, and field agility tests, can be used to assess individuals with posterior hip pain. The deep squat, single-leg balance, and the medial triple hop tests have evidence of validity in those with hip-related pathology [20]. The deep squat test assesses an individuals' ability of their lower body to a position of maximum hip and knee flexion and requires adequate strength and postural control in the lower body and trunk (Fig. 20.7). The single-leg balance test is a static measurement of postural control and balance requiring adequate gluteus medius muscle activation in order to keep the pelvis level to the ground [20]. Provocation of pain during this test may be another important factor in detecting tendinopathy of the gluteus medius and minimus [21]. The medial and lateral hop tests measure the distance of a singular hop or multiple hops in medial and lateral directions. The lateral hop test is thought to simulate forces encountered during cutting or changing of direction [20]. The medial triple hop test demonstrated evidence of validity in subjects with hip pain [22].

Name:_____________________ **Date:**_________ **Age:**______ **Sex:**_______ **Height:**________ **Weight:**_________

Date of onset: _________ **Involved limb:** R L Both   **Dominant Limb:** R L N/A

Pertinent Health Information

Chief complaint:	Occupation:
Mechanism of injury:	Fitness level/activities:
Location of pain:	Health status/co-morbidities:
Previous injury/treatment:	Systemic symptoms:

Gait

	Yes/No	Right/Left
Antalgic		
Trendelenburg		
Knee valgus		
Excessive pronation		

	+/-
Long stride test	

Pain during (circle): Initial Contact - Loading Response - Mid Stance Terminal Stance - Pre Swing - Initial Swing - Mid Swing - Terminal Swing

Standing

	Right	Left
Shoulder height		
Iliac crest height		
Leg Length		

Lumbar	ROM	+/- Pain
Flexion		
Extension		
Side bending right		
Side bending left		

Note response to sustained or repeated movement:

	+/- Right	Left
Standing flexion test		

Seated

	Right			Left		
	ROM	Strength	Pain	ROM	Strength	Pain
ER						
IR						

	R/L	+/-
Seated palpation test		
Seated piriformis test		

Supine

	Right			Left		
	ROM	Strength	Pain	ROM	Strength	Pain
Flexion						
Extension						
Abduction						
Adduction						

	+/- Right	Left
FADIR		
FABER		
IROP		
Scour test		
DEXRI		
DIRI		
Post rim test		
Thomas test		
SLR		
SI compress		
SI distraction		

Sidelying/Prone

Sidelying	Right			Left		
	ROM	Strength	Pain	ROM	Strength	Pain
Abduction						
Adduction						

	+/- Right	Left
Ober test		
Active piriformis test		
Lateral rim test		
IFI test		

Prone	ROM	Strength	Pain	ROM	Strength	Pain
Extension						
ER						
IR						

	Right	Left
Craig's test		

Functional Performance Tests

Deep squat	
Medial hop test	
Lateral hop test	
Triple hop test	
Single Leg Stance/Balance	

Spring testing

Fig. 20.6 Hip evaluation form

Impairment-Based Treatment Plan

In those with posterior hip pain, interventions should be directed at a prioritized problem list that addresses deficits in strength, range of motion, flexibility, and neuromuscular control while considering biomechanical abnormalities, static alignment, and dynamic alignment. Exercises to improve strength, range of motion, and flexibility are commonly used in a treatment plan. However, the reestablishment of neuromuscular control of the lower extremity is important

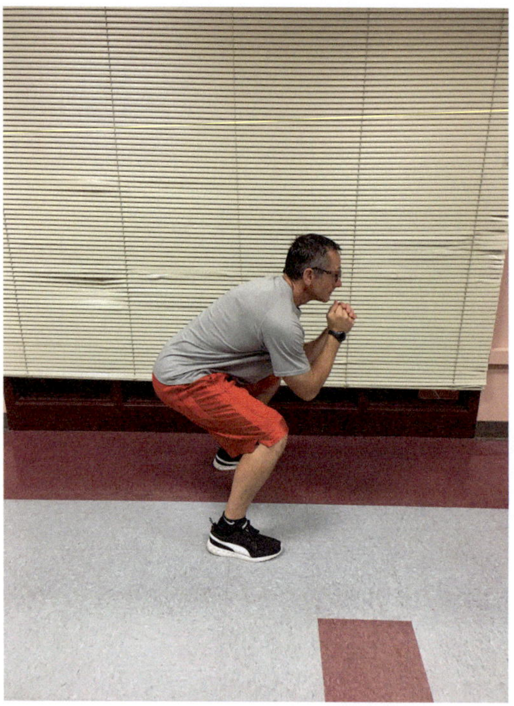

Fig. 20.7 Deep squat test

in restoring functional movement patterns. Therefore, a comprehensive treatment plans need to include interventions that address neuromuscular control.

Strength

Strengthening of musculature involved in posterior hip pain can be addressed from a muscle performance perspective with considerations for strength, power, and endurance, as well as whether the muscle is functioning in a concentric, eccentric, or isometric manner. Which perspective is emphasized with an exercise prescription will be dependent upon the fiber type of targeted muscle(s) and type of contraction that mimics the muscle activation patterns during the individual's desired functional activity. Muscle fibers may be categorized as type I, tonic, or type II, phasic fibers. Type I muscle fibers are involved in endurance activities and are trained with a low-load high-repetition training prescription. Type II muscle fibers are involved in strength and power and are best trained with a high-load

low-repetition prescription. When selecting exercises, those that produce a higher level of muscle activation as indicated by electromyography (EMG) would also seem beneficial. The gluteus medius, gluteus maximus, and erector spinae are commonly impaired in those with hip pathology, thus are the focus of exercise prescription. These muscle groups have been well studied with regard to muscle fiber type composition and EMG activity during commonly performed exercises.

The gluteus medius is one of the primary muscles impaired in those with hip pathology. The main functions of the gluteus medius are to produce hip abduction and to act as a pelvic stabilizer during activities in single-leg stance. The majority of the muscle is made up of type I fibers [23] and therefore would benefit a low-load high-repetition exercise prescription. There have been a number of studies investigating gluteus medius muscle activation during various exercises. A summary of EMG studies is provided in Table 20.1. Research has identified the highest

Table 20.1 Electromyographic maximum volitional isometric contraction (%MVIC) for gluteus maximus and gluteus medius therapeutic rehabilitation exercises

Gluteus medius		Gluteus maximus	
Exercise	%MVIC	Exercise	%MVIC
Side plank abduction with dominant leg on bottom	103 [24]	Front plank with hip extension	106 [24]
Side plank abduction with dominant leg on top	89 [24]	Lateral step up	90 [25]
Single limb squat	82 [24]	Gluteal squeeze	81 [24]
Side-lying hip abduction	81 [26]	Rotational single-leg squat	78 [27]
Clamshell (hip clam) progression 4	77 [24]	Standing hip abduction with band at ankle	73 [28]
Front plank with hip extension	75 [24]	Side plank abduction with dominant leg on top	73 [24]
Side bridge	74 [29]	Side plank abduction with dominant leg on bottom	71 [24]
Single-leg supine bridge (on stable surface)	73 [30]	Single limb squat	71 [24]

level of EMG activity occurs in the side plank exercises [24]. The single-leg squat also produced high EMG activity and would represent a functional single-leg exercise [24]. These exercises are depicted in Fig. 20.8.

The gluteus maximus is another common muscle targeted in rehabilitation process in those with hip pathology. The gluteus maximus is a large muscle that primarily acts as a hip extensor as well as hip external rotator and abductor (upper fibers). When the lower extremity is fixed, the gluteus maximus will act as a trunk extensor and contribute in producing a posterior pelvic tilt. Additionally, activation of gluteus maximus was found to increase compressive force across the sacroiliac joint [31], and therefore exercises to strengthen the gluteus maximus may be helpful in those with sacroiliac joint dysfunction. There seems to be some controversy as to the proportion of type I and II fibers that make up the gluteus maximus [23, 32]. This may mean a prescription should include both low-load high-repetition and high-load low-repetition exercises. Gluteus maximus muscle activation during various exercises has also been studied with a summary of these studies provided in Table 20.1. The front plank with hip extension was found to produce a high level of EMG activity [24]. The lateral step up was also an exercise that produced a high level of EMG activity and would represent a functional single-leg exercise [25]. These exercises are depicted in Fig. 20.8. An important consideration to note is the reinforcement to pelvic positioning during exercise. Performing posterior pelvic tilt during exercise targeting the gluteus maximus seems to produce greater muscle activation as opposed to anterior pelvic tilt position [33].

In view of posterior hip pain and proper lumbopelvic position, the erector spinae muscle group is important to be considered. The erector spinae functions to produce spine extension and rotation, as well as dynamic stability in the lumbar spine. The erector spinae displays a greater proportion of type I fibers [34–36] and therefore would benefit from low-load high-repetition exercise prescription. The four-point kneeling arm and leg lift exercise was found to be an effective exercise to activate the erector spinae muscle group [37]. The muscle group was also highly active during the good morning exercise [38]. These exercises are depicted in Fig. 20.8.

Ultimately, the results of the physical examination will identify which muscle groups are impaired and need to be the focus of strengthening intervention. The most comprehensive approach may include a combination of high-load low-repetition and low-load high-repetition exercises with concentric, eccentric, and isometric type of contractions. The most practical exercises included in the exercise prescription will be based on an analysis of the individual's desired activities and movement patterns associated with these activities. The selected exercises would then attempt to mimic the muscle performance and type of contraction associated with the activity.

Flexibility and Range of Motion

When assessing muscular imbalances, one must be aware that muscle contractures do not happen in isolation. Muscles, tendons, and ligaments must disperse an applied load across the joints to provide stabilization and movement, while the sensorimotor system provides control for the motion. Intervention strategies for patients with deficits in flexibility and range of motion can be addressed through static stretching, dynamic stretching, and contract-relax stretching.

The goal of stretching is to overcome the passive resistance of the soft tissue in order to increase available motion [39]. Static stretching (<30 s) is utilized to increase range of motion and muscle flexibility by temporarily altering the viscoelastic and mechanical muscular proprieties [40]. Static stretching is usually performed during postexercise cooldown to achieve a more permanent change in flexibility [41]. Static stretching should not precede high-speed, explosive, reactive, or strengthening activities because of the reduced reflex sensitivity, decreased maximal voluntary contraction, and potential of activation following long-duration (90 s) stretching [42, 43].

Gluteus Medius

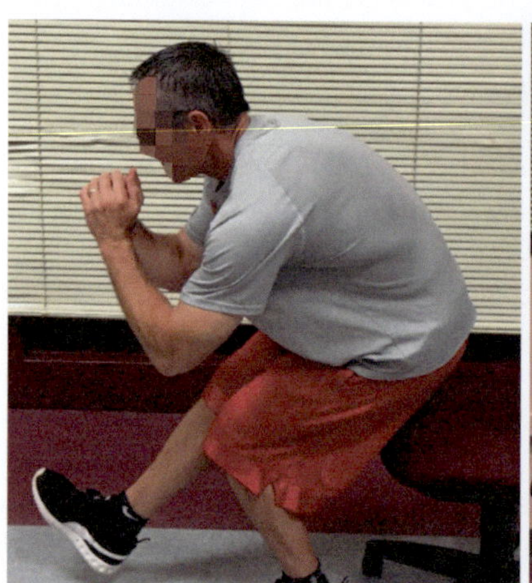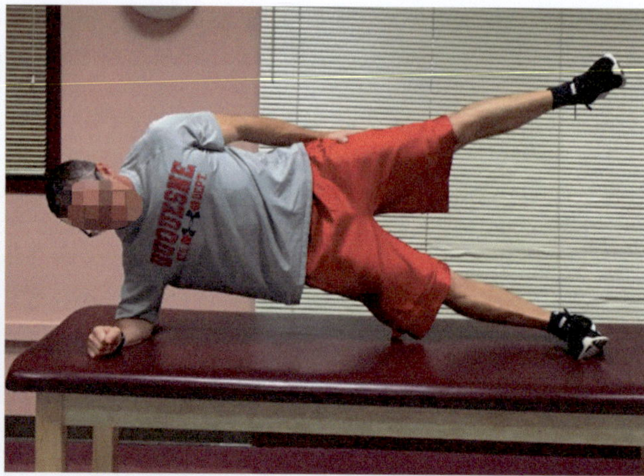

Gluteus Maximus

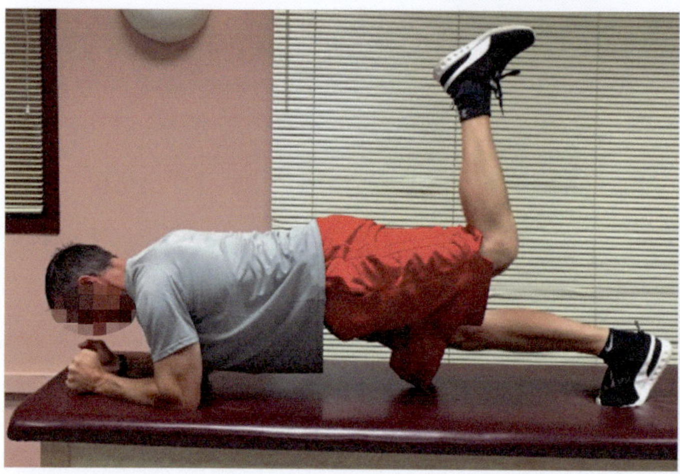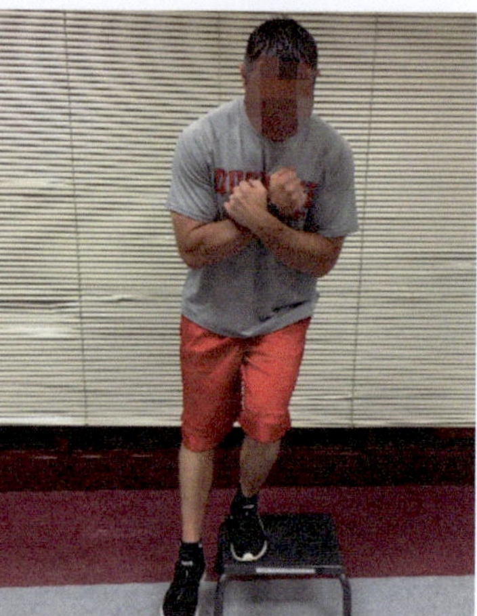

Erector Spinae

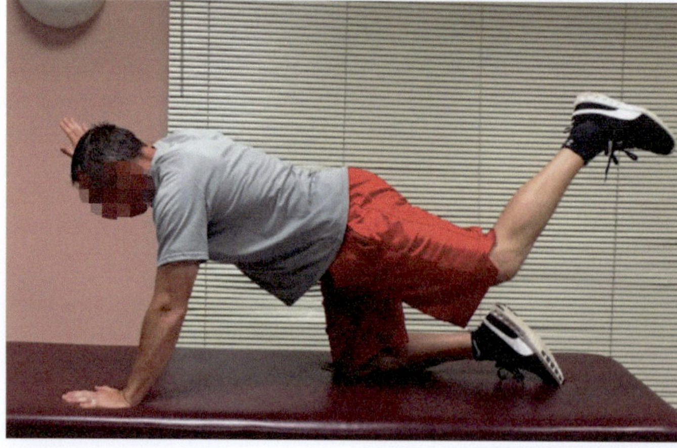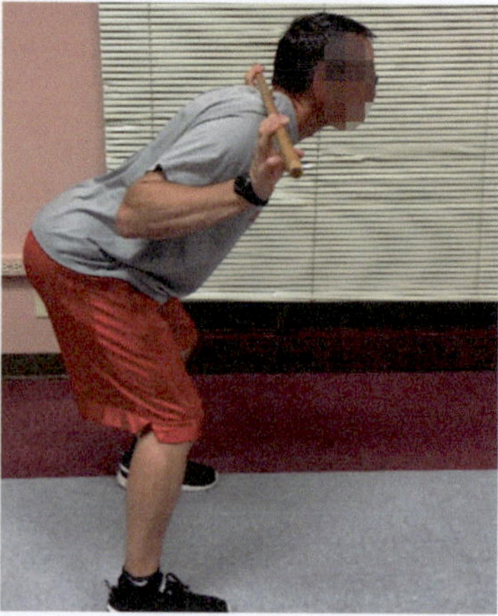

Fig. 20.8 Exercise for the gluteus medius, gluteus maximus, and erector spinae

Dynamic stretching involves active movement through and beyond available range of motion and can be applied prior to high-level performances. Dynamic stretching can improve muscular performance due to the elevation in muscle and body temperature [44], post-activation potentiation in the stretched muscle [45, 46], stimulation of the nervous system, and/or decreased inhibition of the antagonist muscles [47]. Dynamic stretching is preferable to static stretching when preparing for physical activity [41].

Proprioceptive neuromuscular facilitation (PNF) uses muscle contraction to enhance the effect of the applied stretch. Contract-relax and hold-relax PNF stretching techniques utilize an isotonic or isometric contraction, respectively, of the agonist to muscle group applied during a PNF stretching technique. Muscle contraction preceding the stretching triggers an autogenic inhibition mechanism, creating a subsequent reduction in muscle tension through stimulation of the Golgi tendon organs. This mechanism lowers resistance to stretch and can assist in improving range of motion [48–50].

In those with posterior hip pain, the hamstrings, piriformis, and deep external rotators (obturator internus, quadratus femoris, inferior and superior gemellus) are commonly targeted with stretching intervention. The cross-leg stretch is a common stretching position for piriformis and deep external rotators, which are displayed in Fig. 20.9. It should be noted that, similar to the strengthening exercise prescription, strategies to increase range of motion and flexibility should be based on impaired movements identified with the comprehensive physical examination. The best intervention program to increase flexibility and range of motion may include a combination of static, dynamic, and PNF stretching techniques.

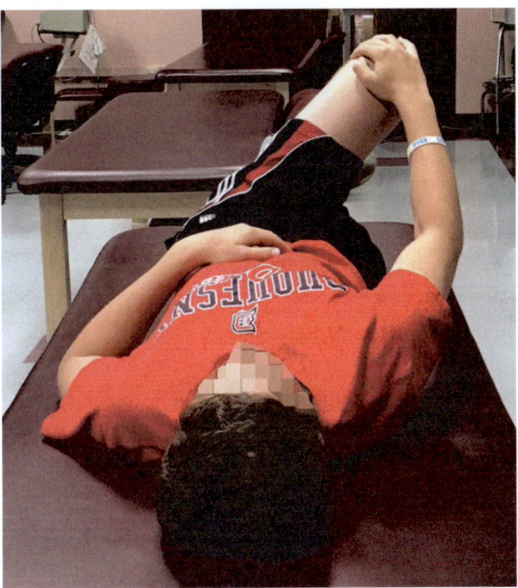

Fig. 20.9 Cross-leg stretch for piriformis and deep external rotators

customized to meet the desired functional demands of the individual. Typically, neuromuscular control exercises are initiated with static balance activities and progress to more dynamic movement patterns. Other variables such as base of support, surface, and complexity of movement pattern may be manipulated to challenge neuromuscular control of the individual. Neuromuscular control exercises may be initiated on stable surfaces and progress to unstable surfaces and/or may begin with the individual in double-limb support and progress to single-limb support. Exercises also progressed from single to multiple plane movements. Criteria for progression of the exercises include establishment of proper static alignment on stable surfaces before movement patterns on unstable surfaces are employed. Exercises are progressively added to gradually challenge the neuromuscular control of the entire lower kinetic chain.

Neuromuscular Control

Neuromuscular control may be best thought of as an intervention that incorporates motion, strength, and stability in a functional movement pattern. Therefore, the exercises included in a neuromuscular rehabilitation program are often

Biomechanical Abnormalities

Biomechanical abnormalities can be the underlying cause of strength, range of motion, flexibility, and neuromuscular deficits. Abnormal biomechanical findings may be categorized as correctable or uncorrectable deficits. Correctable deficits include leg length discrepancy, dynamic knee valgus, and excessive pronation. The deficit in leg length can be addressed through the administration of a heel lift that corrects approximately ½ of the measured deficit. Dynamic knee valgus when identified can be addressed by strengthening exercises for the hip external rotators and abductors and performing activities that promote neuromuscular control of the lower extremity. Excessive foot pronation can be assessed using the Foot Posture Index-6 [51]. When excessive pronation is identified, it may be addressed through anti-pronation taping. Positive response to these taping techniques indicates that the individual may also benefit from either over-the-counter or custom-made orthotics. Uncorrectable deficits include boney structural abnormalities, such as femoral version. For individuals with uncorrectable deficits, identified abnormalities may serve as potential prognostic indicators for outcome of conservative rehabilitation.

Conclusion

A comprehensive examination should be performed to determine a diagnosis, classify individuals into treatment categories, and identify impairments that need to be addressed with physical therapy intervention. A physical therapy-based evaluation algorithm and classification- based treatment categories include considerations for the lumbosacral spine and intra-articular and extra-articular sources of hip posterior pain. Strength, range of motion, flexibility, strength, and neuromuscular control deficits, as well as biomechanical abnormalities, should be addressed as appropriate within the context of the individual's diagnosis.

References

1. Martin RL, Enseki KR. Nonoperative management and rehabilitation of the hip. In: Sekiya JK, Safran MR, Ranawat AS, Leunig ML, editors. Techniques in hip arthroscopy and joint preservation surgery. Philadelphia: Elsevier Saunders; 2011. p. 67–73.
2. Martin RL, Kivlan BR. Classification-based treatment of hip pathology in older adults. Top Geriatr Rehabil. 2013;29(4):218–26.
3. Delitto A, Erhard RE, Bowling RW. A treatment-based classification approach to low back syndrome: identifying and staging patients for conservative treatment. Phys Ther. 1995;75(6):470–85. Discussion 85-9.
4. Fritz JM, George S. The use of a classification approach to identify subgroups of patients with acute low back pain. Interrater reliability and short-term treatment outcomes. Spine. 2000;25(1):106–14.
5. Clohisy JC, Knaus ER, Hunt DM, Lesher JM, Harris-Hayes M, Prather H. Clinical presentation of patients with symptomatic anterior hip impingement. Clin Orthop Relat Res. 2009;467(3):638–44.
6. Johnston TL, Schenker ML, Briggs KK, Philippon MJ. Relationship between offset angle alpha and hip chondral injury in femoroacetabular impingement. Arthroscopy. 2008;24(6):669–75.
7. Maslowski E, Sullivan W, Forster Harwood J, Gonzalez P, Kaufman M, Vidal A, et al. The diagnostic validity of hip provocation maneuvers to detect intra-articular hip pathology. PM & R. 2010;2(3):174–81.
8. Philippon M, Schenker M, Briggs K, Kuppersmith D. Femoroacetabular impingement in 45 professional athletes: associated pathologies and return to sport following arthroscopic decompression. Knee Surg Sports Traumatol Arthrosc. 2007;15:908–14.
9. Sutlive TG, Lopez HP, Schnitker DE, Yawn SE, Halle RJ, Mansfield LT, et al. Development of a clinical prediction rule for diagnosing hip osteoarthritis in individuals with unilateral hip pain. J Orthop Sports Phys Ther. 2008;38(9):542–50.
10. Tannast M, Kubiak-Langer M, Langlotz F, Puls M, Murphy SB, Siebenrock KA. Noninvasive three-dimensional assessment of femoroacetabular impingement. J Orthop Res. 2007;25(1):122–31.
11. Paungmali A, O'Leary S, Souvlis T, Vicenzino B. Hypoalgesic and sympathoexcitatory effects of mobilization with movement for lateral epicondylalgia. Phys Ther. 2003;83(4):374–83.
12. Tyler TF, Nicholas SJ, Campbell RJ, McHugh MP. The association of hip strength and flexibility with the incidence of adductor muscle strains in professional ice hockey players. Am J Sports Med. 2001;29(2):124–8.
13. Kivlan BR, Carcia CR, Clemente FR, Phelps AL, Martin RL. The effect of Astym(R) therapy on muscle strength: a blinded, randomized, clinically controlled trial. BMC Musculoskelet Disord. 2015;16:325.
14. McCormack JR. The management of bilateral high hamstring tendinopathy with ASTYM(R) treatment and eccentric exercise: a case report. J Man Manipulative Ther. 2012;20(3):142–6.
15. Looney B, Srokose T, Fernandez-de-las-Penas C, Cleland JA. Graston instrument soft tissue mobilization and home stretching for the management of plantar heel pain: a case series. J Manipulative Physiol Ther. 2011;34(2):138–42.

16. Martin HD, Shears SA, Johnson JC, Smathers AM, Palmer IJ. The endoscopic treatment of sciatic nerve entrapment/deep gluteal syndrome. Arthroscopy. 2011;27(2):172–81.
17. Schmid AB, Nee RJ, Coppieters MW. Reappraising entrapment neuropathies – mechanisms, diagnosis and management. Man Ther. 2013;18(6):449–57.
18. Kassarjian A, Tomas X, Cerezal L, Canga A, Llopis E. MRI of the quadratus femoris muscle: anatomic considerations and pathologic lesions. AJR Am J Roentgenol. 2011;197(1):170–4.
19. Hatem MA, Palmer IJ, Martin HD. Diagnosis and 2-year outcomes of endoscopic treatment for ischiofemoral impingement. Arthroscopy. 2015;31(2):239–46.
20. Kivlan BR, Martin RL, Christoforetti JJ. Functional testing for hip dysfunction in the performing arts. International Society of Hip Arthroscopy, Boston, MA; 2012.
21. Lequesne M, Mathieu P, Vuillemin-Bodaghi V, Bard H, Djian P. Gluteal tendinopathy in refractory greater trochanter pain syndrome: diagnostic value of two clinical tests. Arthritis Rheum. 2008;59(2):241–6.
22. Kivlan BR, Carcia CR, Clemente FR, Phelps AL, Martin RL. Reliability and validity of functional performance tests in dancers with hip dysfunction. Int J Sports Phys Ther. 2013;8(4):360–96.
23. Sirca A, Susec-Michieli M. Selective type II fibre muscular atrophy in patients with osteoarthritis of the hip. J Neurol Sci. 1980;44(2–3):149–59.
24. Boren K, Conrey C, Le Coguic J, Paprocki L, Voight M, Robinson TK. Electromyographic analysis of gluteus medius and gluteus maximus during rehabilitation exercises. Int J Sports Phys Ther. 2011;6(3):206–23.
25. Simenz CJGL, Lutsch BN, Suchomel TJ, Ebben WP. Electromyographical analysis of lower extremity muscle activation during variations of the loaded step-up exercise. J Strength Cond Res. 2012;26(12):3398–405.
26. Distefano LJ, Blackburn JT, Marshall SW, Padua DA. Gluteal muscle activation during common therapeutic exercises. J Orthop Sports Phys Ther. 2009;39(7):532–40.
27. Webster KA, Gribble PA. A comparison of electromyography of gluteus medius and maximus in subjects with and without chronic ankle instability during two functional exercises. Phys Ther Sport. 2013;14(1):17–22.
28. Brandt M, Jakobsen MD, Thorborg K, Sundstrup E, Jay K, Andersen LL. Perceived loading and muscle activity during hip strengthening exercises: comparison of elastic resistance and machine exercises. Int J Sports Phys Ther. 2013;8(6):811–9.
29. Ekstrom RA, Donatelli RA, Carp KC. Electromyographic analysis of core trunk, hip, and thigh muscles during 9 rehabilitation exercises. J Orthop Sports Phys Ther. 2007;37(12):754–62.
30. Philippon MJ, Decker MJ, Giphart JE, Torry MR, Wahoff MS, LaPrade RF. Rehabilitation exercise progression for the gluteus medius muscle with consideration for iliopsoas tendinitis: an in vivo electromyography study. Am J Sports Med. 2011;39(8):1777–85.
31. Snijders CJ, Vleeming A, Stoeckart R. Transfer of lumbosacral load to iliac bones and legs. Part 1: Biomechanics of self-bracing of the sacroiliac joints and its significance for treatment and exercise. Clin Biomech (Bristol, Avon). 1993;8(6):285–94.
32. Johnson MA, Polgar J, Weightman D, Appleton D. Data on the distribution of fibre types in thirty-six human muscles. An autopsy study. J Neurol Sci. 1973;18(1):111–29.
33. Queiroz BC, Cagliari MF, Amorim CF, Sacco IC. Muscle activation during four Pilates core stability exercises in quadruped position. Arch Phys Med Rehabil. 2010;91(1):86–92.
34. Jorgensen K, Nicholaisen T, Kato M. Muscle fiber distribution, capillary density, and enzymatic activities in the lumbar paravertebral muscles of young men. Significance for isometric endurance. Spine (Phila Pa 1976). 1993;18(11):1439–50.
35. Mannion AF, Dumas GA, Cooper RG, Espinosa FJ, Faris MW, Stevenson JM. Muscle fibre size and type distribution in thoracic and lumbar regions of erector spinae in healthy subjects without low back pain: normal values and sex differences. J Anat. 1997;190(Pt 4):505–13.
36. Sirca A, Kostevc V. The fibre type composition of thoracic and lumbar paravertebral muscles in man. J Anat. 1985;141:131–7.
37. Kim JS, Kang MH, Jang JH, Oh JS. Comparison of selective electromyographic activity of the superficial lumbar multifidus between prone trunk extension and four-point kneeling arm and leg lift exercises. J Phys Ther Sci. 2015;27(4):1037–9.
38. Vigotsky AD, Harper EN, Ryan DR, Contreras B. Effects of load on good morning kinematics and EMG activity. PeerJ. 2015;3:e708.
39. Reid DA, McNair PJ. Passive force, angle, and stiffness changes after stretching of hamstring muscles. Med Sci Sports Exerc. 2004;36(11):1944–8.
40. Taylor DC, Dalton JD Jr, Seaber AV, Garrett WE Jr. Viscoelastic properties of muscle-tendon units. The biomechanical effects of stretching. Am J Sports Med. 1990;18(3):300–9.
41. Behm DG, Chaouachi A. A review of the acute effects of static and dynamic stretching on performance. Eur J Appl Physiol. 2011;111(11):2633–51.
42. Kokkonen J, Nelson AG, Cornwell A. Acute muscle stretching inhibits maximal strength performance. Res Q Exerc Sport. 1998;69(4):411–5.
43. Young WB, Behm DG. Effects of running, static stretching and practice jumps on explosive force production and jumping performance. J Sports Med Phys Fitness. 2003;43(1):21–7.
44. Fletcher IMJB. The effect of different warm-up stretch protocols on 20 meters sprint performance in trained rugby union players. J Strength Cond Res. 2004;18(4):885–8.
45. Hough PA, Ross EZ, Howatson G. Effects of dynamic and static stretching on vertical jump performance

and electromyographic activity. J Strength Cond Res. 2009;23(2):507–12.

46. Torres EM, Kraemer WJ, Vingren JL, Volek JS, Hatfield DL, Spiering BA, et al. Effects of stretching on upper-body muscular performance. J Strength Cond Res. 2008;22(4):1279–85.

47. Jaggers JR, Swank AM, Frost KL, Lee CD. The acute effects of dynamic and ballistic stretching on vertical jump height, force, and power. J Strength Cond Res. 2008;22(6):1844–9.

48. Gribble PA, Guskiewicz KM, Prentice WE. Effects of static and hold-relax stretching on hamstrings range of motion using the flex LE1000. J Sport Rehabil. 1999;8(3):195–208.

49. Magnusson SP, Simonsen EB, Aagaard P, Dyhre-Poulsen P, McHugh MP, Kjaer M. Mechanical and physical responses to stretching with and without pre-isometric contraction in human skeletal muscle. Arch Phys Med Rehabil. 1996;77(4):373–8.

50. Moore MA, Hutton RS. Electromyographic investigation of muscle stretching techniques. Med Sci Sports Exerc. 1980;12(5):322–9.

51. Redmond AC, Crosbie J, Ouvrier RA. Development and validation of a novel rating system for scoring standing foot posture: the Foot Posture Index. Clin Biomech (Bristol, Avon). 2006;21(1):89–98.

The Pelvic Floor

21

Valerie L. Bobb, Lorien Hathaway, and Cyndi Hill

Conservative management of posterior hip syndromes requires a multidisciplinary and multimodal approach as specific pain generators can be challenging to identify. Intrapelvic physical therapy assessment and treatment is an essential component in the overall comprehensive diagnostic evaluation and successful outcome for this complex diagnosis [1]. The hip has a relationship anatomically to both intra- and extrapelvic structures, and posterior hip issues often coexist with or may even be misinterpreted as an intrapelvic issue [1, 2]. An understanding of intrapelvic anatomy from a neurological, musculoskeletal, and functional perspective is needed if one is to adequately and fully treat this population successfully [1]. The role of pelvic floor physical therapy is to examine and provide expertise with regard to the musculoskeletal system of the pelvis; thus, urological and gynecological pelvic organ issues

such as infection or visceral pain etiologies should be ruled out via the appropriate medical practitioner, especially considering that many pelvic floor disorders are accompanied by complaints such as generalized pelvic and perineal pain, lower urinary tract symptoms, defecation disorders, coccygodynia, rectal and pelvic girdle pain, dyspareunia, and sexual dysfunction [3].

Anatomy

Bones, Muscles, and Ligaments

When learning about the functional anatomy of the pelvic floor, it is imperative to understand that it is an integration of a static support via the bony structure combined with musculotendinous, fascial, neural, and visceral systems [3]. Per Wei and De Lancey [4], the term "pelvic floor" may be used to refer to all the structures of support within the pelvic cavity. Pelvic floor support is provided via the abdominal peritoneum, endopelvic fascia, deep pelvic floor muscles, perineal membrane, and the superficial pelvic floor muscles. Additionally it should be noted that visceral support is provided through the bladder, urethra, uterus, prostate, and rectum. The attachments of the pelvic floor muscles, the muscles themselves, the endopelvic fascia, and their fascial attachments combined with the static support of the bony pelvis work together to

V. L. Bobb, PT, DPT, WCS, ATC (✉)
Women's and Men's Health Pelvic Therapy,
University of Washington Medical Center,
Seattle, WA, USA
e-mail: BobbV@uw.edu

L. Hathaway, PT, DPT, WCS, BCB-PMD
Baylor Scott & White Institute for Rehabilitation
(A Division of Select Medical), Outpatient
Services – Plano Alliance, Plano, TX, USA
e-mail: lhathaway@BSWRehab.com

C. Hill, PT, DPT
Kinetic Physical Therapy, Chester Springs, PA, USA
e-mail: cyndih@kineticpta.com

© Springer International Publishing AG, part of Springer Nature 2019
H. D. Martin, J. Gómez-Hoyos (eds.), *Posterior Hip Disorders*,
https://doi.org/10.1007/978-3-319-78040-5_21

form a structural and functional support system for the pelvic contents [5].

The pelvis itself is composed of a bony ring with cartilaginous, ligamentous, and tendinous attachments, some of which originate from inside the pelvis and some from structures near or adjacent to it. The bony pelvis absorbs and transmits forces from the spine and lower limb [6]. This system of bones and ligaments provides structure to support the musculature found within the bony pelvis. Specifically, the pelvic diaphragm is formed by the levator ani muscle group and the coccygeus muscle [7]. Additionally, the obturator internus muscle performs the dual function of hip joint stabilization and formation of pelvic wall parietal fascial anatomy [8, 9].

The levator ani is made up of three primary paired muscle groups: the pubococcygeus, iliococcygeus, and puborectalis [7]. The pubococcygeus originates lateral to the pubic symphysis and on the posterior surface of the superior pubic ramus and the fascia of the obturator internus muscle. It then travels posteriorly and inserts onto the inner surface of the spine of the ischium and the coccyx. The iliococcygeus originates from the ischial spine as the combined surface of the tendinous arch of the pelvic fascia and the obturator internus fascia or arc de tendinous inserts into the anococcygeal ligament and coccyx. The puborectalis originates from the superior and inferior pubic rami. The puborectalis forms a muscular sling around the rectum as it joins the midline and posterior to the rectum. The coccygeus is a small triangular-shaped muscle which originates from the ischial spine and inserts on the lower sacrum and coccyx and is attached on its external surfaces to the sacrospinous ligament [5–7]. The perineal body or central tendon of the perineum forms a fibrous and muscular mass located between the anal and urogenital triangles and provides important support to the pelvic floor serving as an anchor for the female vagina and anal canal in both sexes [7]. The pelvic muscles, external anal sphincter, and posterior vaginal wall all attach to the perineal body. The more superficial muscles of the pelvic floor and pelvic or urogenital diaphragm, the bulbospongiosus, ischiocavernosus, deep and superficial transverse perineum, and

urethral sphincter muscles, also have attachments here. The superficial pelvic muscles or perineal diaphragms as they are commonly called assist the deeper pelvic diaphragm muscles in sphincteric and support functions. Additionally the external anal sphincter works in conjunction with the levator ani to help coordinate fecal continence and defecation [6]. The muscles of the pelvic floor, via their attachments to the perineal body, pelvic side walls, and bony pelvis, help to support the contents of the abdominopelvic cavity as well as to maintain the position of pelvic viscera. They contract reflexively during times of increased intra-abdominal pressure and assist in compression of the urethra and rectum as well as vagina in females. These muscles aid in continence via contraction and defecation and urination by way of relaxation [7] as well as contribute to sexual function [3].

Two ligamentous structures are of significant importance in the evaluation of intrapelvic structures: the sacrotuberous and sacrospinous. These two ligaments serve to connect the sacrum and ischium on either side of the pelvis [7]. The sacrotuberous ligament absorbs and distributes forces for the lower extremities through direct fascial attachments to the hamstrings – due to a shared fascial insertion – and the thoracodorsal fascia [10]. The sacrotuberous ligament is broad, flat, and fibrous and spans the space between the lateral edge of the sacrum and ischial tuberosity [7]. The sacrotuberous ligament's anterior surface partially joins with both the sacrospinous ligament and the piriformis [7]. In some individuals it has been noted that the pudendal nerve may actually be adhered to the deep surface of the sacrotuberous ligament inferior and just medial to the greater sciatic notch in the retro-sciatic region. At the ischial tuberosity, the ligament becomes a dense/fanning band known as the falciform process [11]. The sacrospinous ligament attaches medially from the lateral sacrum and coccyx to the ischial spine. The upper border of the sacrospinous ligament forms the lower border of the greater sciatic foramen, while its lower border outlines the lesser sciatic foramen. It is through this lesser foramen that the internal pudendal vessels and nerves travel to enter the pelvis [6].

Nerves

Intrapelvic neural anatomy is of importance when evaluating and treating pelvic floor as objectively defining specific peripheral nerve involvement in the pelvis can be difficult due to the relationship of pelvic floor lower motor neurons with the sacral spinal cord, autonomic nervous system, and the cortex via the corticospinal tract [6]. The diffuse, plexus-like neural and vascular supply of the autonomic nervous system is thought to be a significant contributor to intra- and extrapelvic pain issues. Neurological cross-sensitization from convergent sensory and somatic input of the pelvic region can result in the dysfunction of neural pathways and resultant central sensitization of the nervous system. This central sensitization or "pathological state characterized by generalized or side-spread hypersensitivity" [12] can cause muscle or visceral dysfunction in both intra- and extrapelvic tissues. Muscular issues include myofascial trigger points, heightened resting tone or activity, and decreased strength. Visceral issues often involve diffuse pain in the abdominal and pelvic region as well as bowel and bladder symptoms. Also of note, the rectum rests on the pelvic surface of the sacrum and coccyx, ending just superior to the pelvic floor muscles. Proximity of the sacroiliac joint and lumbosacral plexus to the sigmoid colon and rectum are possible pain generators as this plexus is just dorsal to the rectum, ventral to the sacrum and piriformis. Pressure from chronically hardened stool with constipation could contribute to neural, joint, and soft tissue irritation around the sacroiliac joint. The sacral plexus, S3–S4, may be relevant in cases of pain associated to sitting, constipation, or a history of vaginal delivery due to tissue compression, traumatic irritation, and the prolonged and repetitive stressing of tissues that often occur in such instances [2]. Compression of the L5–S2 due to endopelvic lesions might also occur at the greater sciatic notch [13, 14].

Such a complex system requires a focused urological and gynecological history to detect any suggestions of intrapelvic nerve entrapment. Reports of pain such as with menstruation, a history of endometriosis, painful intercourse, bladder or bowel issues, or a prior pelvic or abdominal surgical history can help to identify intrapelvic nerve entrapment disorders as a source of dysfunction [13, 15]. The important nerve branches associated with clinical syndromes of or near the pelvic floor are the sciatic, obturator, femoral, lateral femoral cutaneous, and pudendal [10]. However, of specific note with regard to posterior hip pain and the intrapelvis are the sciatic [16, 17] and the pudendal nerves [18].

The fourth and sometimes fifth sacral nerve roots exit the sacral foramens lateral to the sacrum. After leaving the foramens, the roots are found on the posterior surface of the pelvis limited on the lateral side by the piriformis muscle and ventrally by the cardinal ligament of the uterus. Upon crossing the cardinal ligament, these sacral nerves pass through the suprapiriformis space, cross the muscle, and travel toward the lower part of the greater sciatic notch. Here the roots join to form the sciatic nerve at the infra-piriformis [13, 14] deep gluteal space [18]. Intrapelvically, the sciatic nerve is primarily affected in locations above and below this deep gluteal space [19]. The sciatic nerve's close proximity anatomically to the gluteal and iliac vessels makes it vulnerable to compression. Varicose gluteal veins, congenital pelvic arteriovenous malformations, and aneurysms of the distal aorta as well as issues with the iliac and intrapelvic arteries have been implicated in triggering symptoms via sciatic compression [20]. Additionally, issues may occur as the sciatic nerve is compressed at the greater sciatic notch or at the sacral nerve roots due to endometriosis or damage during intrapelvic gynecological procedures [13, 14]. Symptoms of this extra-spinal, intrapelvic sciatic nerve compression include pelvic and lower extremity pain, sensory disturbances (paresthesia or dysesthesias), myotomal weakness, gait dysfunction, and reflex impairment [20].

The pudendal nerve is made up of fibers from the ventral rami of the sacral plexus. The pudendal nerve initially passes through the greater sciatic foramen over the spine of the ischium. At the area of the ischial spine, the pudendal nerve runs superficial to the sacrospinous and deep to the sacrotuberous ligaments. It then reenters through the lesser sciatic foramen along the lateral wall of the ischiorectal fossa to enter the pelvis accompanied by the internal pudendal vessels through the pudendal or Alcock's canal [11, 21]. This canal is formed by the splitting of the obturator internus fascia. This portion of the obturator internus is thickened and fibrous and is attached to the falciform process of the sacrotuberous ligament [11]. Prior to entering Alcock's canal, the pudendal nerve gives off an inferior rectal branch which enters the ischiorectal fossa. Occasionally this inferior rectal nerve will arise directly from the sacral plexus and join the pudendal nerve laterally to the beginning of Alcock's canal before separating to enter the ischiorectal fossa. Midway through Alcock's canal, the pudendal nerve then divides into both the perineal branch and the dorsal nerve of the clitoris/penis. These two branches then travel together to the canal's end. Upon exiting the canal, the perineal branch further divides into sensory branches to the perineum and motor branches to the superficial pelvic floor muscles and the external anal and urethral sphincter muscles. There are some proponents of the belief that the pudendal nerve may also supply some muscle branches to the deeper levator ani pelvic floor muscles, although evidence shows these are primarily innervated via the sacral plexus. The dorsal nerve of the clitoris/penis is a terminal branch responsible for sensation to the dorsal aspect of the penis and infra-pubic region [22].

Individuals with pudendal nerve entrapment typically present with pain, a sensation of burning or tearing, stabbing, or electrical-like sharp or shooting pain medial to the ischium. A sensation of the presence of a foreign body made worse with sitting as well as alleviation of symptoms when sitting on a toilet are also common complaints. Symptoms are often relieved with standing [23] and are usually absent on awakening [11, 24]. Pudendal nerve irritation or entrapment symptoms also often include pain and numbness in all or part of the nerve's distribution specifically the perineal or "saddle" area, low medial buttock, rectum, terminal urinary tract, and/or proximal, medial thigh [11]. Additionally, dysfunction of the rectal and urogenital systems due to pudendal nerve issues might include urinary and defecatory storage and emptying dysfunctions such as urinary and fecal incontinence, constipation, and urinary urgency, frequency, and obstructive voiding [25]. Sexual dysfunction such as female continuous arousal and dyspareunia and male erectile dysfunction and testicular pain may also be noted [24, 26, 27].

Obturator Internus

Of key importance in pelvic anatomy is the obturator internus (OI) muscle whose belly is located intrapelvically but then becomes tendinous as it exits the pelvis through the lesser sciatic foramen. The nerve to the OI arises from the sacral plexus with fibers from the L5–S2 spinal nerves [24] and runs posterior to the surface of the sacrospinous ligament before turning into the greater sciatic foramen, supplying the muscle from the pelvic surface [10]. The OI originates on the medial surface of the pubis and along the obturator foramen and membrane. The bulk of the muscle is located along the medial ischial wall [1, 10, 21, 28–33]. The muscle becomes narrow and tendinous or band like as it leaves the pelvis via the lesser sciatic foramen and curves sharply around the ischium travelling laterally, anterior to the sciatic nerve [1, 10, 29–31, 33–36]. The OI then travels posterior to the ischial tuberosity where it makes a 120° turn upward to insert along with the superior and inferior gemelli onto the medial portion of the greater trochanter [6]. Interestingly, cadaver studies have found that another of the deep hip external rotators, the inferior gemellus, originates from the lateral surface of the ischial tuberosity as well as intrapelvically with its origin found just beneath the OI and covered by the falciform process of the sacrotuberous ligament. The OI tendon inserts in the same area as that of the piriformis, and in some cadavers, a blending of the OI and piriformis tendinous insertions on the greater trochanter has been noted [37]. One study found that the OI and piriformis muscles were actually fused in 48/112 cases, thus indicating a strong relationship and interaction between the piriformis, OI, and therefore sciatic nerve [1].

Aggravation of the sciatic and posterior femoral cutaneous nerves can occur due to aggravation by the OI tendon when under abnormal tension, especially in the early stages of hip flexion [37]. Additionally sciatic neuropathy caused by excessive compressive forces of the OI on the sciatic nerve at its pelvic outlet may be present when the hip joint is internally rotated due to compression via the OI of both the arterial blood flow and sciatic nerve itself [32]. Symptomology may include palpatory pain on the lateral aspect of the ischial tuberosity and radiating posterior leg pain [11].

The fascial border of the medial aspect of the OI helps to form the Alcock's canal through which, as stated prior, the pudendal nerve travels into the pelvic cavity [33]. Abnormal tension or spasm of the OI is present in a large percentage of individuals with pudendal nerve symptomology. Deformation of the pudendal neurovascular bundle in the Alcock's canal and subsequent edema secondary to compressive forces at the ischial spine can occur due to the abnormal tensioning of the OI and its concomitant tendon [11]. Pain medial to the ischium may indicate pudendal nerve entrapment [18, 28, 38] with a common finding being sensitivity to palpation of the OI muscle via manual compression deep on the medial aspect of the ischial tuberosity. Additionally pain or sensitivity at the ischial margin near the inferior aspect of the sciatic notch and tenderness of the greater trochanteric region of the hip may be noted. Adduction of the thigh in a seated position, passive hip internal and external rotation, and resisted hip abduction of the flexed and internally rotated thigh may reproduce symptoms. Per Travell and Simons, deep tenderness in the posterior hip and upper 1/3 of the greater trochanter is likely caused by one of the hip external rotators such as the OI, and pain immediately posterior to the greater trochanter can be a result of entrapment of the nerve to the OI. Bursae of the OI may be found deep in its tendon as it winds around the sciatic notch and additionally are occasionally found between the common tendon of the OI tendon and capsule of the hip joint [1]. These bursae can be a source of posterior hip and ischial tunnel region pain when irritated or inflamed [35].

Anatomy Conclusion

Successful pelvic floor physical therapy evaluation and treatment requires knowledge of both intra- and extrapelvic anatomy and the overall relationship to structure and function. Intrapelvic issues often arise as a result of hip or bony pelvis issues, while pelvic floor dysfunction changes joint loading and often leads to a sequela of posterior hip dysfunction [10]. Intrapelvic pain and dysfunction due to inherent musculoskeletal issues may lead to the recruitment of nearby global hip muscles in order to compensate for intrinsic pelvic incoordination, overactivity, structural, or weakness issues [39–41]. Conversely, functional adaption of the pelvic floor for disorders within the pelvic-hip-spine complex may occur [39] when these structural abnormalities are present and thus contribute to the development of secondary pelvic pain due to pelvic muscle over-recruitment and activation, fatigue, or imbalance [9]. Specifically, activities in which hip rotation is required necessitate that individuals with hip instability issues excessively engage the hip rotator, adductor, and abductor musculature to maintain required stability. This need to provide stability over greater range of mobility could cause the extrapelvic hip muscles to fatigue and/or become unbalanced with regard to length, strength, and coordination components and ultimately lead to an increased resting state or overactivity of the obturator internus and pelvic floor muscles, possible nerve irritation or entrapment, and ultimately posterior and lateral hip, buttock, and intrapelvic pain [39].

Function

The pelvic floor muscles have many functions that are often broken down based on a specific specialty's perspective. However the pelvic floor is a functional unit that should not be fragmented into singular functions without a good understanding of the broad overall purpose.

Bowl shaped and in the transverse plane, the pelvic floor supports all the pelvic organs. The pelvis also contains a constant level of normal tone allowing the sphincters to remain close and not allowing urine or fecal matter to leak out [4]. As the diaphragm descends into the abdominal cavity, the pelvic floor will also descend slightly, maintain a constant intra-abdominal pressure, but maintain its tone in order to maintain the subject's continence. However, the tone will change based on dynamic movement, adjusting to an increase in intra-abdominal pressure. If a subject lifts a heavy box and requires more activation of the stabilization muscles (multifidi, TrA, gluteus maximus), the pelvic floor will react to the increase in intra-abdominal pressure and increase its tone to maintain continence and add stability to the system [42].

The OI works as a functional unit with the other lateral hip external rotators [32]. The OI has been proposed to have a primary role in hip stabilization along with the internally rotating gluteus medius and other deep hip external rotators. These muscles likely have a significant role in stabilizing the femoral head on the acetabulum as well as a role in modulating hip joint stiffness and providing subtle proprioceptive adjustments for the hip joint as well as compression of hip and acetabular surfaces. As one of the local stabilizers to the hip, the OI is well positioned anatomically, biomechanically, and physiologically to provide dynamic stabilization producing a significant force over a small muscle length. Additionally, the OI force lines work advantageously to provide compression of the femoral head in the acetabulum, and it is notable that the OI is even thought to have attachment to the capsule of the hip joint itself, further supporting a proprioceptive role. As a predominately slow-twitch fiber muscle, the OI is suited to tonic contraction and is therefore fatigue resistant [9]. Hip pathology may cause pain and movement adaptation and thus promote an increased resting state in the OI causing the muscle to "rest" or relax in a contracted position and thus become irritated and painful due to overactivity and guarding [39].

Diane Lee describes the pelvic floor as the bottom of the canister of the "core." Cadaveric studies show that, when the pelvic floor contracts as a unit, there is an increase in force closure of the SIJ and lumbar spine. More importantly it is not just the contraction but the coordination of the pelvic floor muscle with the transverse abdominis, gluteus medius, piriformis, and gluteus maximus. Activation of the pelvic floor should depend on the level of the load, mobility requirements, predictability, and real or perceived risks to the system [42]. Stiffening of all muscle groups through a static co-contraction is the simplest strategy and leaves the lowest room for error. When the task is perceived as a high load, low predictability, and the individual perceives the threat as high, the individual's CNS system will rely on this strategy. This leads to a higher compression forces, increased energy expenditure, and higher intra-abdominal pressure. In a situation perceived as low risk, high predictability, and low load, the system will rely on a dynamic strategy that allows more mobility and less compression and less excessive intra-abdominal pressure [42]. The CNS relies on accurate input from a variety of sources (mechanoreceptors, visual input) including past experience and beliefs. Individuals in pain may perceive activities as more threatening than they truly are and rely more on the co-contraction strategies leading to overloaded muscles and changes in movement and breathing patterns [42].

This system will be altered in a hip that is not functioning correctly, particularly in a patient that has a history of pelvic floor dysfunction (see "History" section). An adequate pelvic floor exam can add information to complete the picture of deep gluteal syndrome. Because the pelvic floor adds stability in both dynamic and static postures, the pelvic floor may be overworked in a lumbo-pelvic-hip complex that has compromised hip strength [42]. The pelvic floor can be overactive, compensating from a poor movement pattern and lack of coordination. Over time, the pelvic floor may become shortened, or the patient may lack the coordination to voluntarily relax the pelvic floor. This can lead to additional pelvic pain syndromes as well as stress or urgency incontinence. A thorough examination by a skilled therapist will be able to determine pelvic floor or intrapelvic involvement as well as the difference between a shortened pelvic floor or a pelvic floor lacking coordination. A shortened pelvic floor is often characterized with urgency/frequency symptoms and pain with penetration, rigidity to palpation, lack of ability to bear down during exam, and low tolerance to exam. An overactive pelvic floor that lacks coordination is also characterized by urgency/frequency and pain with penetration but also includes urinary and fecal incontinence symptoms. On examination, the pelvic floor will be tender to palpation and have poor relaxation during tasks that would require relaxation (bearing down, defection, or breathing) and non-relaxing abdominal muscles [43].

The pelvic floor muscle could have also started out weak resulting in a lack of coordination with the hip muscles and adding to a strain on the deep gluteals and nerves. This is the less likely scenario; however a proper exam will guide the therapist to proper treatment.

Examination

The pelvic floor is the largest structure in the pelvis, but it is seldom considered in the evaluation of pelvic and hip pain. This muscular group can be a significant source of pain and is easily palpated in exam. An internal pelvic floor exam should only be performed by a clinician trained in this technique.

History

It is important to get a comprehensive history prior to the physical exam. Because many of the nerves that affect the hip/pelvic region start in the abdomen (such as the genitofemoral, ilioinguinal, iliohypogastric nerves), it is important to understand all relevant history for both the abdomen and then pelvic floor. A thorough history of all abdominal surgeries should be taken (and all incisions later palpated for adhesions and reproduction of pain). For women, a gynecological history including pelvic infections, urogenital infections, and all pregnancy and birth questions should be asked. Regarding birth, questions specifically regarding type of birth, length of labor,

length of pushing, use of instrumentation, and any tearing or injury during birth are important. For men, a comprehensive urogenital history should be taken including surgeries and infections. This gives the therapist an idea of both acute and chronic injury in the abdomen and pelvic floor.

Orthopedic Screen

A thorough examination will generally include an orthopedic survey of the spine, pelvis, and hips [44]. The physical therapist seeks to quantify the degree of dysfunction and identify musculoskeletal or neuromuscular factors contributing to the patient's condition, such as pelvic obliquity, leg length discrepancy, hip mobility imbalance, sacroiliac joint subluxation, or sciatica, among others [44]. Various special tests used to rule in or rule out dysfunction that might be contributing to the patient's complaints may include, but are not limited to, the following:

- Stork test: to assess load transfer in the pelvis [45].
- Active straight leg raise: to assess load transfer [45, 46].
- SIJ compression/distraction: to assess for sacroiliac contributions to the patient's symptoms with gapping and compression of sacroiliac joint. Pain reproduction can lead to further investigation of SIJ involvement to the patient's symptoms [45, 47].
- Gaenslen's test: indicates the presence or absence of a SIJ lesion, pubic symphysis instability, or hip pathology [48].
- FAIR (flexion, adduction, internal rotation): also known as piriformis test; used to screen the piriformis muscle and to detect tightness or other discomforts of the sciatic nerve as it passes through or under the piriformis muscle [49].
- FABER (flexion, abduction, external rotation): also known as Patrick's test; indicates pathology located in the hip or sacroiliac joint or posterior pelvic girdle pain [45].

- Hip scour: tests for nonspecific joint pathology.
- 90-90 straight leg raise test: assesses hamstring tightness.

See the chapter Physical Examination.

External Pelvic Floor Examination

After physical examination tests are completed, an intravaginal or intrarectal examination will help quantify the resting tension of the pelvic floor and hip musculature and investigate possible sources of pain and dysfunction.

The pelvic floor is dome-shaped muscle complex with contraction occurring in three planes. Although there is no single standard for assessing the function of the pelvic floor, a focused approach to the physical examination, including an assessment of muscular tightness, trigger points, reproduction of symptoms, and the patient's ability to contract and relax the pelvic floor muscles (coordination), is useful through vaginal and rectal digital palpation [50].

Assessment begins with visual inspection of the vulva, perineum, and anus. The clinician inspects for any tissue changes in color, discharge, or presence of hemorrhoids. Mobility is then assessed. The patient is asked to perform a pelvic floor contraction (i.e., to contract the muscles used to stop urine or gas). When effective, contraction results in an upward lift of the perineum and anus or movement of the penis. The patient should also have complete relaxation. The patient is then asked to bear down to check for coordination and mobility of pelvic floor lengthening. Finally the patient is asked to cough. The patient should have a slight contraction or no movement of the pelvic floor. Bulging of the pelvic floor during a cough demonstrates a lack of coordination [51, 52].

External palpation of the urogenital triangle includes the ischiocavernosus, bulbospongiosus, and transverse perineal muscles and the perineal body [50]. The therapist is asking the patient for tenderness or reproduction of symptoms as well as palpating quality of muscle tissue (normal muscle tissue, increased tension, etc.). If the patient is complaining of vulvar burning, a cotton swab test should be performed to rule out vestibulodynia [53].

The anal wink test is commonly used to evaluate the function of the sacral nerve roots [54]. This test is conducted by lightly stroking the external anal sphincter with a cotton swab. An intact anal reflex (evidenced by an "anal wink") is indicative of intact nerve pathways. The absence of a reflex could indicate sacral disease or sphincter denervation [54].

Internal Pelvic Floor Examination

The internal portion of the female examination will begin by palpating the introitus for sensitivity and reproduction of symptoms and then move to the deep levator ani bilaterally, with specific attention to findings of banding, spasm, or tenderness [44]. The clinician angles posteriorly and laterally toward the thickest part of the muscle. The clinician feels for a "cliff" and then retracts slightly to approximate the sight of the deep levator ani. To further confirm accurate palpation, the clinician can ask the patient to "push your knee into my hand" to activate the OI. A contraction of the OI will help with orientation, and bringing the finger slightly more superficial will estimate the site of the deep levator ani. A contraction of the pelvic floor muscles ("squeeze and lift" "stop urine from flowing") should confirm placement. (See Fig. 21.1.)

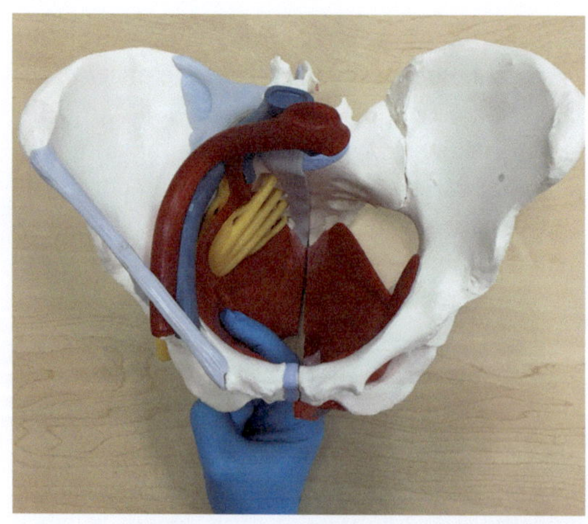

Fig. 21.1 Palpation point for muscle testing of levator ani

The initial part of the deep internal exam is for tenderness and spasm. Spasm of a portion of the levator ani may often be detected and will be a palpable band resembling a guitar string within the muscle or focal trigger points [44]. The patient will often report pain with palpation of these tight bands. Again the clinician is looking for reproduction of the patient's symptoms. Any scarring is also noted.

Asking the patient to squeeze and relax their pelvic floor muscles will allow the clinician to evaluate strength and endurance of the deep levator ani muscles. It will also give the clinician insight into coordination of the pelvic floor muscle contraction and relaxation as well as proprioception [7]. Strength, endurance, and coordination are measured as described by Laycock [55]. For patients with pain, special attention is paid to total muscle excursion and relaxation ability.

With further palpation of the internal musculature, the obturator internus (OI) can help orient the clinician to the anatomy of the pelvic floor, as the muscle belly is easy to feel when contracted. Palpating laterally, the clinician asks the patient to abduct the knee against resistance, while the hip is flexed. The iliococcygeus covers the lower two-thirds of the OI. Following OI posteriorly will lead to the ischial spine. With the finger pressed posterolaterally and superiorly to the ischial spine, the piriformis muscle can be examined. In the patient with normal pelvic musculature, palpation of the levator ani and piriformis typically elicits a sensation of pressure, whereas a patient with pelvic floor myalgia will report significant pain [44]. The discomfort experienced by these patients often reproduces their primary complaint. Another typical finding during examination is a distinct asymmetry between the right and left elements of the pelvic diaphragm. This shortening or contracture will be ipsilateral to the patient's pain [44].

Moving the examining finger anteroinferiorly from here allows palpation over the pudendal nerve in Alcock's canal, which lies interior to the arcus tendineus. Placing the leg in internal rotation stretches the pudendal nerve, allowing the examiner to check for pain [56]. The symptoms could present as sensations such as burning, tingling, and shooting pain. These sensations may expand into the groin, abdomen, legs, and buttocks. A Tinel's test should also be performed to test the sensitivity of the pudendal nerve. If the patient experiences sharp, shooting pain along the sensory nerve path of the pudendal nerve with palpation, the test is considered positive. The pudendal nerve can be palpated externally and internally at Alcock's canal, at the ischial spine, and at the dorsal branch [57, 58].

Rectal examination in both men and women is also important, not only to assess the anal sphincter but also to evaluate the coccygeus, levator ani muscles, sacrococcygeal ligaments, and attachments to the sacrum and coccyx [50]. In men, all the musculature will be palpated rectally.

Patients who continue to live with unresolved hip pain and/or dysfunction may very well be living with undiagnosed pelvic floor dysfunction. Including a thorough pelvic floor examination during evaluation of hip disorders will lend to a greater understanding of the genesis of pain and musculoskeletal dysfunction and successful treatment of the condition.

Treatment

Clinically patients with hip dysfunction typically present with an overactive pelvic floor component if his/her pelvic floor is involved. Therefore this chapter focuses on treatment for overactive or painful pelvic floor.

Respiration

Restoring posture and breathing mechanics should be the part of the initial treatment addressed in patients that have pelvic floor component of deep gluteal syndrome. Most people with chronic pain have adapted compensatory breathing patterns including shallow breathing utilizing the upper accessory muscles [59]. Restoring proper posture will help return the pelvic floor and the fascial layers to proper length. Restoring proper diaphragmatic breathing allows a small pelvic floor stretch with each breath. This will help with nerve mobility which improves blood flow and downregulates a sensitive nervous system [59], increases lymphatic flow, and restores normal piston relationship. It is important that this is practiced in proper posture in order to stretch restricted area of the muscle and to not reinforce poor habits [60]. Diaphragmatic breathing education and a daily exercise should be given within the first visits.

Manual Therapy

Manual therapy has been shown in research as an effective way to decrease restriction in fascial layers and muscle [58]. The purpose of manual therapy in this area is no different than traditional manual therapy. The goals are to improve circulation, restore proper tissue integrity, decrease ischemia in tissue and nerve, and decrease adverse neural tension of peripheral nerve branches [58, 61]. It is important to return a normalized tissue system. If connective tissue restrictions remain, it can cause further muscle tightness, trophic changes, and restriction in the neural containers causing peripheral nerve symptoms [61]. After a thorough exam, the therapist should address all restricted areas both externally and internally. Common treatments include connective tissue manipulation (skin rolling) both anteriorly and posteriorly, from the knee to the diaphragm with the therapist addressing restriction with other techniques such as myofascial release or trigger point release as warranted (Fig. 21.2). Trigger point release, myofascial

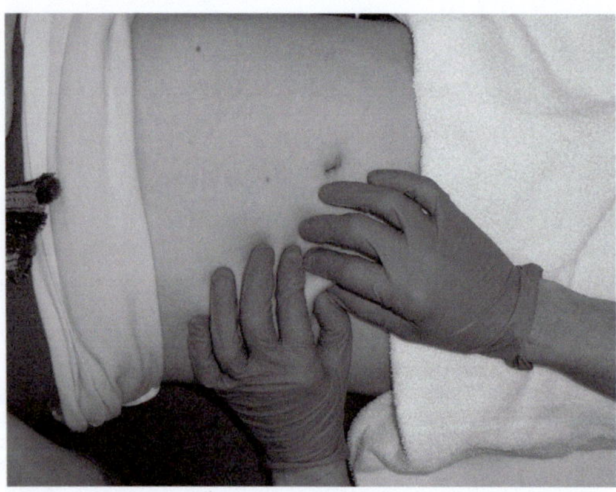

Fig. 21.2 Connective tissue manipulation

release through manual techniques with assistance, such as Graston, or without, can be performed based on the therapist's discretion. Trigger points are commonly found in the posterior hip musculature, abdominals, and the pelvic floor. Any abdominal scar restriction should be addressed as well [62]. Internally sustained pressure and/or a sweeping motion can be done to release trigger points and improve pelvic floor mobility. In females this is done intravaginally and in males intrarectally. Here the OI can be addressed if it is found to be a pain generator. However, it is important to investigate why the soft tissue restriction has developed and to not just treat the soft tissue with manual therapy. Through the examination, the physical therapist should be investigating weakness, coordination, or poor movement strategies that may be leading to soft tissue dysfunction. When appropriate, correcting these issues should be incorporated into treatment.

If there is sciatic or pudendal nerve involvement, manual nerve gliding or flossing should also be incorporated. A trained pelvic floor therapist can integrate nerve flossing into his or her manual therapy treatment. Nerve flossing is done by mobilizing the fascial tissue surrounding the area of the expected nerve path. The techniques vary from mild mobilization to more aggressive mobilization with the patient performing active movements [63]. It is important that the patient is given home nerve glides to perform in order to maintain this new mobility. While the pudendal nerve cannot be directly mobilized, it is mobilized through sciatic nerve gliding and incorporating deep breathing with stretching of the pelvic floor through a partial or full squat. The nerve glides begin with the patient in a partial squat, based on patient's tolerance with the patient holding onto a stable surface. The patient is instructed to lift up his/her chin to take the tension off if he/she is uncomfortable. The hips and feet should be wide and in slight external rotation. Slowly the patient will lower into a deeper squat, keeping the ischial tuberosities wide, based on tolerance. It is important to remember this is a gliding and sliding motion and should not be forced [64]. It is also important to note that the hip position and squat depth may have to be modified based on the patient's hip complaint.

Alternative Treatments

As an adjunct other therapies may be used. Surface EMG (SEMG) biofeedback is commonly used in the clinic. SEMG is measured with an intrarectal or intravaginal sensor and is dependent on good contact. The patient must be motivated and capable of reading the output on the machine with guidance. SEMG purely shows muscle recruitment and is not a measurement in strength. In most cases of pelvic-involved hip pain, the therapist is focusing on relaxation of the pelvic floor, or down training. The patient is commonly holding tension in the pelvic floor, has increased resting tension, or has incoordination to relax when appropriate. In some patients, SEMG can be a valuable tool to give a visual and/ or auditory output to help the patient "connect" with his/her pelvic floor. Down training's goal is to decrease the electrical output of the EMG. This is commonly done through cueing for diaphragmatic breathing, visualization of relaxing, separating ischial tuberosities, actively perineal bulging, or doing contract/relax contraction. Down training is commonly thought to be more difficult for patients to learn than up training (strengthening) [53].

If muscles are not relaxing as appropriate, the physical therapist may consult with the physician regarding injections. Trigger point injections and Botox injections are prescribed by physicians for the pelvic floor region. These interventions are not performed by a physical therapist, but a physical therapist may be the first practitioner to identify the need.

Neuromuscular Reeducation

As normal mobility of the pelvic floor is restored, it is important to incorporate neuromuscular reeducation and strengthening exercises to strengthen the normalized muscle tissue and coordinate the pelvic floor with all of its synergistic muscle groups. This should be done in conjunction with the other progressive resistive exercises for the hip described in previous chapters. It is important to focus on coordination of the pelvic floor muscles with the transverse abdominis and posterior hip muscles for postural stabilization and dynamic stabilization (Figs. 21.3, 21.4, and 21.5).

Treatment Conclusion

Finally, therapists must not forget the sensitive nervous system in their treatment if the patient has been screened for chronic pain. There are many techniques that decrease the sympathetic nervous system response in a patient with chronic pain. Many of these patients will benefit from a comprehensive approach of both tissue dysfunc-

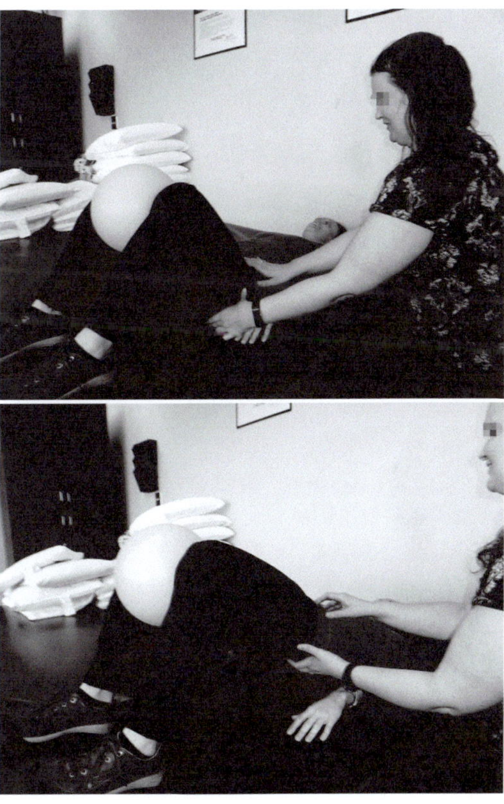

Fig. 21.3 Top: beginning level neuromuscular education. Bridge cueing for TrA and PFM contraction. Bottom: finish position

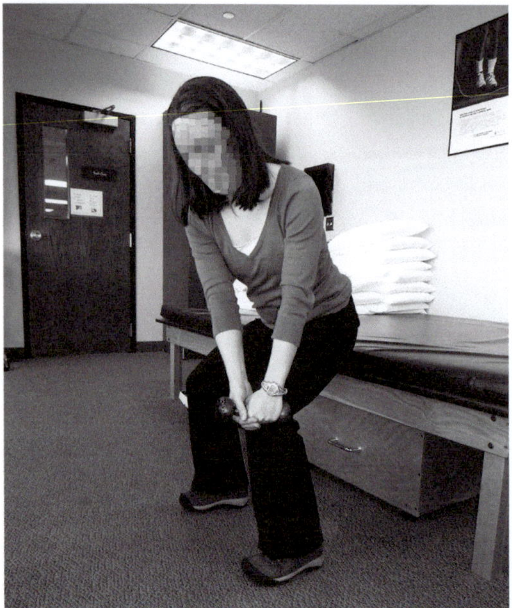

Fig. 21.4 Advanced neuromuscular education—transition to functional activity

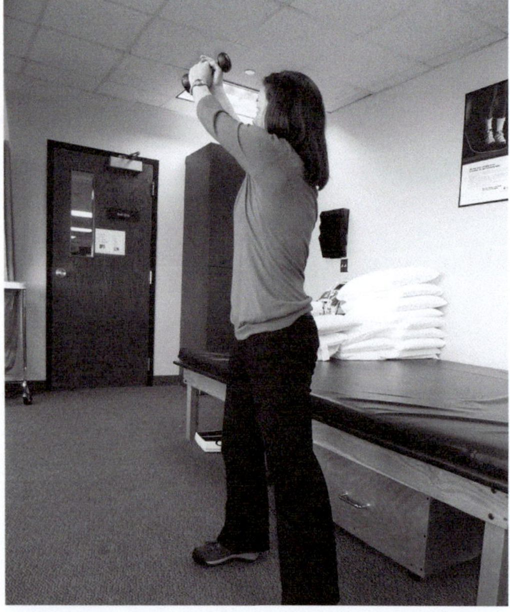

Fig. 21.5 Woodchop with PFM contraction

tion and modulation of the nervous system. Vandyken and Hilton describe a comprehensive approach to the treatment of persistent pelvic pain.

Pain education: educating the patient on the brain's role in chronic pain (neurophysiology) has been shown in RCT as effective in changing pain cognition and improving physical performance [65].

Connective tissue mobilization: mobilization is used to have direct effect on tissue dysfunction but also may directly impact the state of the autonomic nervous system.

Deep breathing: retraining lateral costal and diaphragmatic breathing.

Relaxation training: decreases anxiety and improves self-esteem.

Cardiovascular exercise: evidence suggests CV exercise lowers a person's stress response.

Guided imagery: utilizes the power of the mind to reduce anxiety.

Yoga: adopted for the patient's dysfunction, addresses body awareness and coordinates breathing and balance.

Affirmations/positive thinking: thoughts are nerve impulses that can drive pain; positive affirmation can decrease anxiety and restore patient's control.

Addressing sleep dysfunction: good sleep hygiene improves mood, quality of life, and healing.

Therapists should provide education on these pieces and/or partner/refer to experts in these fields [64].

The most important component of incorporating the pelvic floor into treatment of posterior hip pain is a therapist skilled in the treatment of pelvic floor. It is important to find one that can perform all components of the examination and manual therapy and has an advanced understanding of the pelvic floor's influence on the posterior hip and lumbar spine structures.

References

1. Cox JM, Bakkum BW. Possible generators of retrotrochanteric gluteal and thigh pain: the gemelli–obturator internus complex. J Manip Physiol Ther. 2005;28(7):534–8.
2. George SE, Clinton SC, Borello-France DF. Physical therapy management of female chronic pelvic pain: anatomic considerations. Clin Anat. 2013;26(1):77–88.

3. Doggweiler R, Stewart AF. Pelvic floor therapies in chronic pelvic pain syndrome. Curr Urol Rep. 2011;12(4):304–11.

4. Wei JT, De Lancey JO. Functional anatomy of the pelvic floor and lower urinary tract. Clin Obstet Gynecol. 2004;47(1):3–17.

5. Hartmann D, Sarton J. Chronic pelvic floor dysfunction. Best Pract Res Clin Obstet Gynaecol. 2014;28(7):977–90.

6. Prather H, Dugan S, Fitzgerald C, Hunt D. Review of anatomy, evaluation, and treatment of musculoskeletal pelvic floor pain in women. PM&R. 2009;1(4):346–58.

7. Irion J, Irion G. Women's health in physical therapy: principles and practices for rehabiliation professionals. Philadelphia, PA: Lippincott-Williams & Wilkins; 2009.

8. Neumann DA. Kinesiology of the hip: a focus on muscular actions. J Orthop Sports Phys Ther. 2010;40(2):82–94.

9. Retchford T, Crossley K, Grimaldi A, Kemp J, Cowan S. Can local muscles augment stability in the hip? A narrative literature review. J Musculoskelet Neuronal Interact. 2013;13(1):1–12.

10. Aung HH, Sakamoto H, Akita K, Sato T. Anatomical study of the obturator internus, gemelli and quadratus femoris muscles with special reference to their innervation. Anat Rec. 2001;263(1):41–52.

11. Filler AG. Diagnosis and treatment of pudendal nerve entrapment syndrome subtypes: imaging, injections, and minimal access surgery. Neurosurg Focus. 2009;26(2):E9.

12. Devor M. Pathophysiology of damaged nerves in relation to chronic pain. In: Textbook of pain. Philadelphia, PA: Elsevier; 1999. p. 129–64.

13. Possover M, Forman A. Neuropelveological assessment of neuropathic pelvic pain. Gynecol Surg. 2014;11(2):139–44.

14. Possover M, Schneider T, Henle K. Laparoscopic therapy for endometriosis and vascular entrapment of sacral plexus. Fertil Steril. 2011;95(2):756–8.

15. Lemos N, Possover M. Laparoscopic approach to intrapelvic nerve entrapments. J Hip Preserv Surg. 2015;2(2):92–8. hnv030.

16. Barton PM. Piriformis syndrome: a rational approach to management. Pain. 1991;47(3):345–52.

17. Wyant GM. Chronic pain syndromes and their treatment II. Trigger points. Can Anaesth Soc J. 1979;26(3):216–9.

18. Martin HD, Reddy M, Gómez-Hoyos J. Deep gluteal syndrome. J Hip Preserv Surg. 2015;2(2):99–107.

19. Torriani M, Souto SC, Thomas BJ, Ouellette H, Bredella MA. Ischiofemoral impingement syndrome: an entity with hip pain and abnormalities of the quadratus femoris muscle. Am J Roentgenol. 2009;193(1):186–90.

20. Ailianou A, Fitsiori A, Syrogiannopoulou A, Toso S, Viallon M, Merlini L, et al. Review of the principal extra spinal pathologies causing sciatica and new MRI approaches. Br J Radiol. 2014;85(1014):672–81.

21. Gajraj NM. Botulinum toxin a injection of the obturator internus muscle for chronic perineal pain. J Pain. 2005;6(5):333–7.

22. Schraffordt SE, Tjandra JJ, Eizenberg N, Dwyer PL. Anatomy of the pudendal nerve and its terminal branches: a cadaver study. ANZ J Surg. 2004;74(1–2):23–6.

23. Martin HD. Subgluteal space and associated disorders. In: Operative hip arthroscopy. Berlin: Springer; 2013. p. 309–29.

24. Popeney C, Ansell V, Renney K. Pudendal entrapment as an etiology of chronic perineal pain: diagnosis and treatment. Neurourol Urodyn. 2007;26(6):820–7.

25. Possover M, Forman A. Voiding dysfunction associated with pudendal nerve entrapment. Curr Bladder Dysfunct Rep. 2012;7(4):281–5.

26. Berman JR, Goldstein I. Female sexual dysfunction. Urol Clin North Am. 2001;28(2):405–16.

27. Pink L, Rancourt V, Gordon A. Persistent genital arousal in women with pelvic and genital pain. J Obstet Gynaecol Can. 2014;36(4):324–30.

28. Martin HD, Shears SA, Johnson JC, Smathers AM, Palmer IJ. The endoscopic treatment of sciatic nerve entrapment/deep gluteal syndrome. Arthroscopy. 2011;27(2):172–81.

29. Lee SC, Rha DW, Kim HJ, Yang HM, Lee SH, Koh D. Ultrasound-guided injection of the intrapelvic portion of the obturator internus in a cadaver model. Reg Anesth Pain Med. 2014;39(4):347–50.

30. Murata Y, Ogata S, Ikeda Y, Yamagata M. An unusual cause of sciatic pain as a result of the dynamic motion of the obturator internus muscle. Spine J. 2009;9(6):e16–8.

31. Shinohara H. Gemelli and obturator internus muscles: different heads of one muscle? Anat Rec. 1995;243(1):145–50.

32. Meknas K, Christensen A, Johansen O. The internal obturator muscle may cause sciatic pain. Pain. 2003;104(1–2):375–80.

33. Valovska A, Zaccagnino MP, Weaver MJ, Valovski I, Kaye AD, Urman RD. Intrapelvic obturator internus muscle injections: a novel fluoroscopic technique. Pain Physician. 2015;18:E237–43.

34. Smith J, Wisniewski SJ, Wempe MK, Landry BW, Sellon JL. Sonographically guided obturator internus injections: techniques and validation. J Ultrasound Med. 2012;31(10):1597–608.

35. Swezey RL. Obturator internus bursitis: a common factor in low back pain. Orthopedics. 1993;16(7):783–5. Discussion 785-6.

36. Dalmau-Carola J. Myofascial pain syndrome affecting the piriformis and the obturator internus muscle. Pain Pract. 2005;5(4):361–3.

37. Rohde RS, Ziran BH. Obturator internus tendinitis as a source of chronic hip pain. Orthopedics. 2003;26(4):425–6.

38. Hatem MA, Palmer IJ, Martin HD. Diagnosis and 2-year outcomes of endoscopic treatment for ischiofemoral impingement. Arthroscopy. 2015;31(2):239–46.

39. Prather H, Spitznagle TM, Dugan SA. Recognizing and treating pelvic pain and pelvic floor dysfunction. Phys Med Rehabil Clin N Am. 2007;18(3):477–96.
40. Laycock J, Jerwood D. Pelvic floor muscle assessment: the PERFECT scheme. Physiotherapy. 2001;87(12):631–42.
41. Spitznagle TM, Robinson CM. Myofascial pelvic pain. Obstet Gynecol Clin N Am. 2014;41(3):409–32.
42. Lee D. The pevlic girdle an integration of clinical experience and research. Amsterdam: Elsevier; 2011.
43. Washington University Program in Physical Therapy. Diagnosis dialog: pelvic floor conditions. 2015. https://dxdialog.wusm.wustl.edu/ Presentations%20and%20Publications/Forms/ AllItems.aspx?RootFolder=%2fPresentations%20 and%20Publications%2fSection%20on%20 Women%27s%20Health%20%2d%20Table%20 of%20Pelvic%20Floor%20Conditions&FolderCTID =&View=%7bA55622A3%2dED08%2d4684%2d8C 32%2d116BFC4546E4%7d. Accessed 28 Feb 2016.
44. Swisher E, Rich J, Weiss PM. Pelvic floor spasm the missing link in chronic pelvic pain. Contemp OB GYN. 2012;57(10):38–46. 9p.
45. Vleeming A, Albert HB, Ostgaard HC, Sturesson B, Stuge B. European guidelines for the diagnosis and treatment of pelvic girdle pain. Eur Spine J. 2008;17(6):794–819.
46. Mens JM, Vleeming A, Snijders CJ, Koes BW, Stam HJ. Reliability and validity of the active straight leg raise test in posterior pelvic pain since pregnancy. Spine (Phila Pa 1976). 2001;26(10):1167–71.
47. Laslett M, Aprill CN, McDonald B, Young SB. Diagnosis of sacroiliac joint pain: validity of individual provocation tests and composites of tests. Man Ther. 2005;10(3):207–18.
48. Dutton M. Orthopaedic examination, evaluation and intervention. 2nd ed. New York: McGraw Hill; 2008.
49. Flynn T, Cleland J, Whitman J. Users' guide to the musculoskeletal examination: fundamentals for hte evidence-based clinician. Louisville, KY: Evidence in Motion; 2008.
50. Faubion SS, Shuster LT, Bharucha AE. Recognition and management of nonrelaxing pelvic floor dysfunction. Mayo Clin Proc. 2012;87(2):187–93.
51. Bø K, Sherburn M. Evaluation of female pelvic-floor muscle function and strength. Phys Ther. 2005;85(3):269–82.
52. Messelink B, Benson T, Berghmans B, Bø K, Corcos J, Fowler C, et al. Standardization of terminology of pelvic floor muscle function and dysfunction: report from the pelvic floor clinical assessment group of the International Continence Society. Neurourol Urodyn. 2005;24(4):374–80.
53. Shelley B, Neville C, Strauhal M, Jenkyns P. Pelvic physical therapy level I. American Physical Therapy Association Section on Women's Health 2010.
54. Doughty D. Urinary & fecal incontinence: current management concepts. 3rd ed. St Louis: Elsevier; 2006.
55. Laycock J, Haslem J. Therapeutic management of incontinence and pelvic pain. 2nd ed. London: Springer; 2008.
56. FitzGerald MP, Kotarinos R. Rehabilitation of the short pelvic floor. I: background and patient evaluation. Int Urogynecol J Pelvic Floor Dysfunct. 2003;14(4):261–8.
57. Hibner M, Desai N, Robertson LJ, Nour M. Pudendal neuralgia. J Minim Invasive Gynecol. 2010;17(2):148–53.
58. Rummer E, Prendergast S. The role of physical therapy in treating myofascial pelvic pain syndrome. In: IASP SIG on pain of urogenital origin-Newsletter, vol. 1(2); 2009.
59. Busch V, Magerl W, Kern U, Haas J, Hajak G, Eichhammer P. The effect of deep and slow breathing on pain perception, autonomic activity, and mood processing-an experimental study. Pain Med. 2012;13(2):215–28. 14p.
60. Wiebe J. The pelvic floor piston:foundation for fitness; 2014. DVD.
61. Prendergast S, Rummer E. The role of physical therapy in the treatment of pudendal neuralgia. IPPS Vision. 2007;15(1):1–4.
62. Padoa A, Rosenbaum TY, editors. The overactive pelvic floor. Berlin: Springer; 2016.
63. Butler D. The sensitive nervous system. Adelaide: NOI Group; 2000.
64. Vandyken C, Hilton S. The puzzle of pelvic pain: a rehabilitation framework for balancing tissue dysfunction and central sensitization II: a review of treatment considerations. J Womens Health Phys Ther. 2012;36(1):44–54. 11p.
65. Moseley GL, Nicholas MK, Hodges PW. A randomized controlled trial of intensive neurophysiology education in chronic low back pain. Clin J Pain. 2004;20(5):324–30.

Index

© Springer International Publishing AG, part of Springer Nature 2019
H. D. Martin, J. Gómez-Hoyos (eds.), *Posterior Hip Disorders*,
https://doi.org/10.1007/978-3-319-78040-5